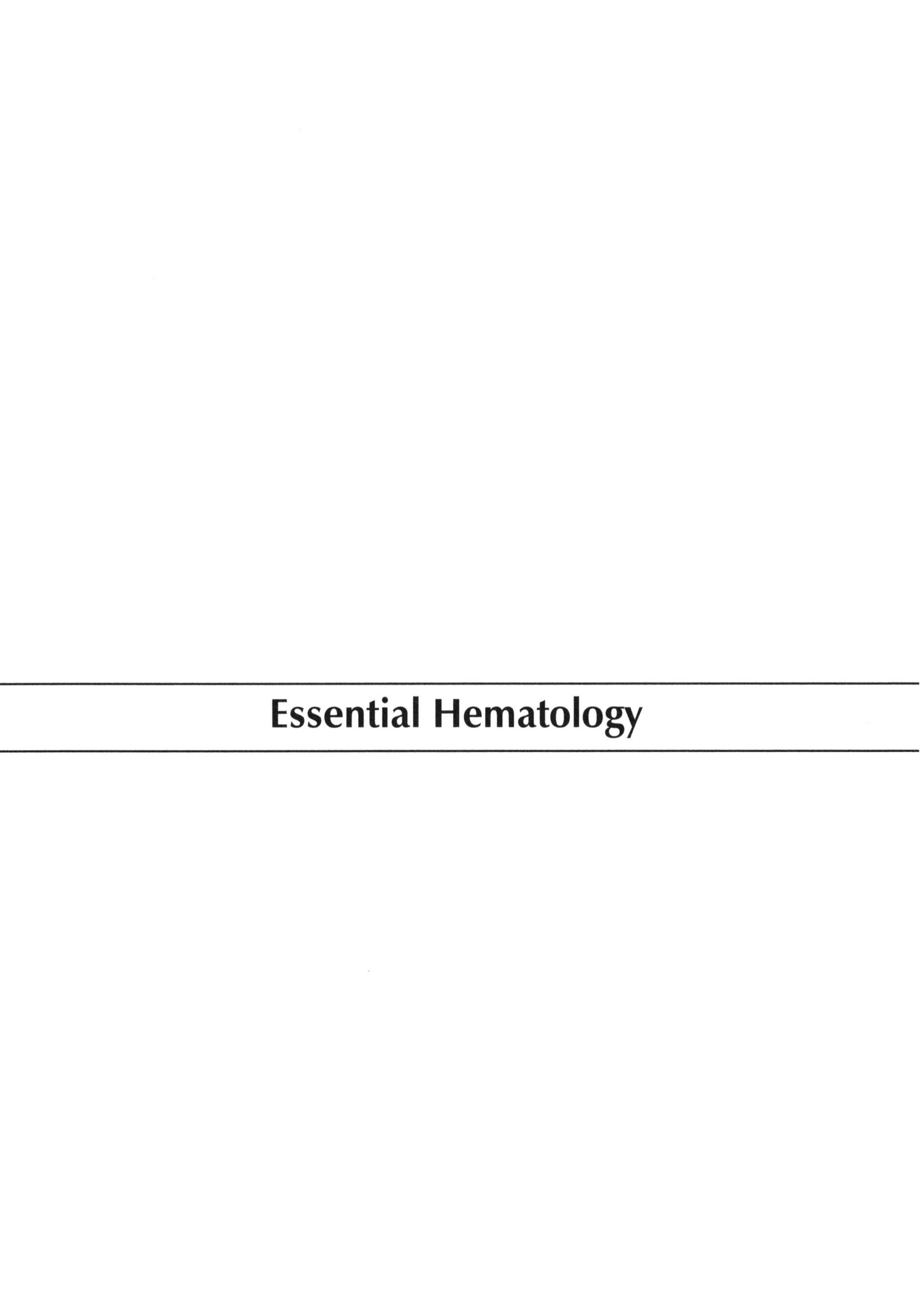

Essential Hematology

Essential Hematology

Editor: Cyril Barnett

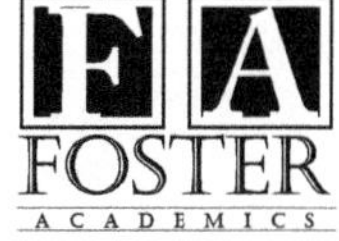

www.fosteracademics.com

www.fosteracademics.com

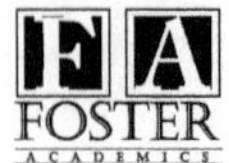

Cataloging-in-Publication Data

Essential hematology / edited by Cyril Barnett.
p. cm.
Includes bibliographical references and index.
ISBN 978-1-63242-676-5
1. Hematology. 2. Blood--Diseases. I. Barnett, Cyril.
RC633 .E87 2019
616.15--dc23

Foster Academics,
118-35 Queens Blvd., Suite 400,
Forest Hills, NY 11375, USA

ISBN 978-1-63242-676-5 (Hardback)

Contents

Preface

Hematology is a branch of medicine. It studies the diseases of blood along with their causes, treatment, prevention and prognosis. Some common blood diseases are blood clots, lymphoma, hemophilia, leukemia, among others. Hematopathologists are pathologists whose expertise lies in the diagnosis of hematological diseases. Blood clotting tests, Coombs test, radioallergosorbent test, Kleihauer–Betke test, live blood analysis, etc. are some of the commonly performed tests to evaluate blood diseases. This book is a valuable compilation of topics, ranging from the basic to the most complex advancements in the field of hematology. It aims to present researches that have transformed this discipline and aided its advancement. This book is a vital tool for all researching or studying hematology as it gives incredible insights into emerging trends and concepts.

Significant researches are present in this book. Intensive efforts have been employed by authors to make this book an outstanding discourse. This book contains the enlightening chapters which have been written on the basis of significant researches done by the experts.

Finally, I would also like to thank all the members involved in this book for being a team and meeting all the deadlines for the submission of their respective works. I would also like to thank my friends and family for being supportive in my efforts.

Editor

1

Use of Valacyclovir for the treatment of cytomegalovirus antigenemia after hematopoietic stem cell transplantation

Shin-Yeu Ong*, Ha-Thi-Thu Truong, Colin Phipps Diong, Yeh-Ching Linn, Aloysius Yew-Leng Ho, Yeow-Tee Goh and William Ying-Khee Hwang

Abstract

Background: Valacyclovir has been used for prophylaxis against cytomegalovirus (CMV) infection after hematopoietic stem cell transplantation (HSCT). We investigated the efficacy and safety of high-dose Valacyclovir as pre-emptive therapy in patients with CMV antigenemia after HSCT.

Methods: In a retrospective single center study of 61 patients, we compared the rates of viral clearance, recurrent antigenemia and adverse events in patients with pp65 CMV antigenemia who received high dose Valacyclovir (n = 15), Valganciclovir (n = 16), and Foscarnet (n = 30).

Results: Overall, 60/61 (98 %) of cases achieved CMV antigenemia clearance by day 28, and no patient developed CMV disease. After adjusting for age, sex, diagnosis, CMV serological status, donor type, CMV antigen level, graft-versus-host disease (GVHD) therapy, and conditioning regimen, there were no significant differences in the rates of viral clearance at day 14 in patients who received Valganciclovir (0.18, 95 % confidence interval (CI) 0.01 to 2.15, p = 0.17) and Foscarnet (OR 0.22, 95 % CI 0.03 to 2.40, p = 0.22), compared with Valacyclovir (assigned OR = 1.00). Recurrent antigenemia by day 180 after clearance of the initial CMV episode occurred in 34/61 (56 %) of patients. Using the multivariate model adjusting for the same covariates, there were also no significant differences in secondary episodes of CMV between treatment groups. With regards to adverse effect monitoring, Foscarnet led to significantly increased creatinine levels ($P = 0.009$), while Valganciclovir led to significant decrease in neutrophil counts ($P = 0.012$).

Conclusion: High dose Valacyclovir is a potential alternative to Valganciclovir and Foscarnet in the stable post-HSCT patient who has cytopenia and is not keen for inpatient treatment of CMV antigenemia.

Background

Cytomegalovirus (CMV) infection poses a serious clinical challenge to hematopoietic stem cell transplant (HSCT) patients as it can result in numerous complications associated with significant morbidity and mortality. These include retinitis, encephalitis, pneumonia, hepatitis and gastrointestinal ulceration. Two approaches for the prevention of CMV infection are currently practiced. The first is universal prophylaxis with routine administration of an antiviral agent to all patients after transplant. Benefits of prophylaxis is that monitoring may not be required if an effective antiviral is used, but some patients are exposed to drug-related toxicities unnecessarily. The second approach is pre-emptive therapy, that is initiated when CMV infection is detected, but before the development of CMV-associated symptoms. Pre-emptive therapy depends on early detection of CMV in blood, which is aided by the ready availability of pp65 antigenemia and DNA PCR-based assays. Both approaches are equally effective in preventing CMV disease.

Ganciclovir, and its modified oral formulation, Valganciclovir (GCV), are first line agents for pre-emptive therapy against CMV [1–3]. When cytopenias are present, Foscarnet is used as an alternative. Although as effective as ganciclovir, Foscarnet is associated with renal toxicity and requires inpatient therapy, hence it is reserved as second

* Correspondence: shinyeu.ong@mohh.com.sg
Department of Hematology, Singapore General Hospital, Singapore, Singapore

line therapy [4, 5]. Valacyclovir satisfies several criteria for an ideal pre-emptive therapeutic agent due to its low toxicity profile, and excellent bioavailability after oral administration [6]. High dose Valacyclovir has already been shown to be safe and effective in CMV prophylaxis after solid organ and stem cell transplantation [7–13], but has not been adequately studied as an antiviral for pre-emptive therapy against CMV antigenemia. Valacyclovir is potentially an important alternative agent in patients with cytopenia who are not eligible for Ganciclovir, and who are unwilling to be hospitalized for intravenous Foscarnet.

We hypothesized that Valacyclovir could be useful as a single agent against CMV antigenemia after HSCT, without significant hematologic or renal toxicity. To evaluate this treatment approach, a retrospective cohort study comparing the use of Valacyclovir, Valganciclovir, and Foscarnet was performed in our institution. The primary outcome was viremia clearance. Secondary outcomes included recurrent antigenemia and adverse events.

Methods

Patients

All consecutive adult patients who underwent allogeneic bone marrow, peripheral blood stem cell, or cord blood transplantation at Singapore General Hospital between January 2008 and September 2011 were included if they had an initial episode of CMV antigenemia before a single antiviral (Valacyclovir, Valganciclovir, or Foscarnet) was started for pre-emptive therapy. Departmental practice guidelines, integrated with patients' preferences, determined the choice of antiviral regimen. Ganciclovir is the first line pre-emptive therapy for CMV in our inpatients, while Foscarnet is used in patients with neutropenia or previous ganciclovir treatment failure. Outpatients with normal gastrointestinal absorption received Valganciclovir, while patients with neutropenia received Valacyclovir. Patients who developed CMV disease before or at the time of the initial detection of CMV antigenemia were excluded. All patients also received acyclovir for prophylaxis against varicella zoster virus and trimethoprim-sulfamethoxazole for *Pneumocystis jirovecii* prophylaxis until immunosuppression was discontinued. Prophylaxis for fungal infections was either posaconazole or itraconazole. Calcineurin-inhibitor-based therapies were the most commonly used GVHD prophylaxis regimens, with the inclusion of anti-thymocyte globulins (ATG) in unrelated donor transplants. All participants gave their informed consent for participation in the research database and the database collection was approved by the institutional review board of the Singapore General Hospital.

Detection of CMV reactivation

All patients were screened for CMV infection using a CMV pp65 antigenemia assay at least twice in the first week after transplant, and at least once a week subsequently. The CMV antigenemia assay was performed as described previously [14], and ≥ 1 CMV antigen positive cell per million leukocytes was used as the threshold for pre-emptive therapy.

Pre-emptive therapy

Patients were treated with either Foscarnet at 90 mg/kg twice daily (BID), or 45 mg/kg BID if creatinine clearance is less than 60 ml/min; Valganciclovir a 900 mg BID or 450 mg BID if creatinine clearance is less than 60 ml/min, or Valacyclovir 2 g four times daily (QID) or 1 g QID in the presence of renal impairment. The median duration of treatment was 14 days. Clearance of CMV antigenemia was defined as 0 positive cells per million leukocytes via the CMV pp65 antigenemia assay. The incidence of recurrent CMV antigenemia after treatment with each agent was recorded for 180 days after the clearance of an initial episode of CMV antigenemia. Patients who relapsed after successful clearance of CMV antigenemia were treated at the discretion of the physician.

Monitoring of adverse events

Patients were monitored for the development of CMV disease as defined previously [15], as well as significant side effects of Valacyclovir, Valganciclovir, or Foscarnet. Haemograms and biochemical panels were performed at least once a week to look for neutropenia, thrombocytopenia and renal impairment. Mortality rates and causes of mortality for up to 6 months post-transplant were recorded.

Statistical analysis

Values are expressed as median (range), and the significance of differences was determined using the chi-square test or analysis of variance, as appropriate. Some analyses compared changes in pre- and post-treatment cell counts and serum creatinine between two groups; these were analyzed using the paired t-test. Multivariable logistic regression models were used to determine the odds of viral clearance at day 14, and of recurrent antigenemia in patients treated with Valganciclovir and Foscarnet, compared with Valacyclovir. Potential confounders considered include age, gender, CMV serological status, donor type, CMV antigen level at diagnosis, conditioning regimen, and graft-versus-host disease therapy.

Results

Patient characteristics

The demographic characteristics of the three groups of patients are shown in Table 1. Comparisons of the three groups for parameters that could influence CMV reactivation showed significant difference with respect to age, but not CMV serological status, sex, donor type, indication for

Table 1 Patient characteristics

	All (n = 61)	Valacyclovir (n = 15)	Valganciclovir (n = 16)	Foscarnet (n = 30)	P[a]
Median age, years (range)	41 (16–66)	47 (18–61)	50 (30–57)	37 (16–66)	0.017
Male, N (%)	31 (50.8)	9 (60.0)	5 (31.3)	27 (56.7)	0.186
Diagnosis, N (%)					0.509
Acute myeloid leukemia	30 (49.2)	7 (46.7)	9 (56.3)	14 (46.7)	
Acute lymphoid leukemia	13 (21.3)	3 (20.0)	1 (6.3)	9 (30.0)	
Non-Hodgkin's lymphoma	2 (3.3)	1 (6.7)	1 (6.3)	0 (0.0)	
Myelodysplastic syndrome	6 (9.8)	1 (6.7)	1 (6.3)	4 (13.3)	
Others	10 (16.4)	3 (20.0)	4 (25.0)	3 (10.0)	
Conditioning regimen, N (%)					0.374
Myeloabalative	32 (53.3)	9 (60.0)	11 (68.8)	12 (41.4)	
Non-Myeloabalative	14 (23.3)	2 (13.3)	3 (18.8)	9 (31.0)	
Reduced Intensity	14 (23.3)	4 (26.7)	2 (12.5)	8 (27.6)	
Donor type, N (%)					0.078
Related	31 (50.8)	11 (73.3)	10 (62.5)	10 (33.3)	
Unrelated	21 (34.4)	2 (13.3)	5 (31.3)	14 (46.7)	
Cord Blood	9 (14.8)	2 (13.3)	1 (6.25)	6 (20.0)	
CMV serologic status, N (%)					0.586
Donor-/recipient+	9 (14.8)	1 (6.7)	3 (18.8)	5 (16.7)	
Donor+/recipient+	52 (85.3)	14 (93.3)	13 (81.3)	25 (83.3)	
GVHD (during study)					0.155
None	27 (44.3)	5 (33.3)	4 (25.0)	18 (60.0)	
Grade I-II	30 (49.2)	9 (60.0)	10 (62.5)	11 (36.7)	
Grade II-IV	4 (6.6)	1 (6.7)	2 (12.5)	1 (33.3)	
GVHD treatment					0.119
None	25 (41.0)	5 (33.3)	3 (18.8)	17 (56.7)	
Steroids	30 (49.1)	9 (60.0)	11 (68.9)	10 (33.3)	
Others	6 (9.8)	1 (6.7)	2 (12.5)	3 (10.0)	
Pre-treatment laboratory results, median (range)					
Creatinine (μM)	78 (40–240)	86 (46–182)	72 (44–240)	78 (40–205)	0.601
ANC (x10^3/mm^3)	2.6 (0.2-22.8)	2.4 (0.2-6.6)	3.6 (1.1-15.6)	1.7 (0.8-22.8)	0.093
Platelet (x10^3/mm^3)	64 (7–260)	98 (15–197)	68 (7–244)	32.5 (8–260)	0.053

CMV, cytomegalovirus; *GVHD*, graft versus host disease; *ANC*, absolute neutrophil count
[a]P value for difference by treatment group, based on chi-square test or analysis of variance

transplant and conditioning regimen. Patients requiring systemic corticosteroids or other agents (e.g. ertanercept, mycophenolate mofetil, tacrolimus) for treatment of GVHD were statistically similar between groups.

CMV antigenemia and pre-emptive treatment

The median number of CMV antigen-positive cells at the initiation of pre-emptive therapy did not differ between groups ($P = 0.77$), and the median viral load for all included patients was 3 (range 1 to 750). Overall, 60/61 (98 %) of cases achieved CMV antigenemia clearance by day 28, with no significant differences between treatment groups (p = 0.591). By day 14, clearance rates among groups who received Valacyclovir, Valganciclovir, and Foscarnet were 14/15 (93 %), 13/16 (81 %), and 22/30 (73 %) respectively. After adjusting for age, sex, diagnosis, CMV serological status, donor type, CMV antigen level, GVHD therapy, and conditioning regimen, there were no significant differences in the rates of viral clearance at day 14 in patients who received Valganciclovir (odds ratio (OR) 0.18, 95 % confidence interval (CI) 0.01 to 2.15, p = 0.17) and Foscarnet (OR 0.22, 95 % CI 0.03 to 2.40, p = 0.22), compared with Valacyclovir (assigned OR = 1.00).

Although high rates of CMV clearance were achieved, recurrent antigenemia by day 180 after clearance of the

Table 2 Response to pre-emptive CMV therapy

	All (n = 61)	Valacyclovir (n = 15)	Valganciclovir (n = 16)	Foscarnet (n = 30)	*P*
Median time to antigenemia (days from transplant, range)	27 (12–387)	39 (16–387)	31.5 (15–119)	24.5 (12–104)	0.084
Median viral load (No. of CMV positive cells per million leukocytes, range)	3 (1–750)	3 (1–40)	3 (2–181)	3.5 (1–750)	0.772
Clearance, N (%)	60 (98.1)	15 (100)	16 (100)	29 (96.7)	0.591
Recurrent antigenemia, N (%)	34 (55.8)	7 (46.7)	11 (68.8)	16 (53.3)	0.434
Median days to recurrence	43.5 (11–173)	59 (27–173)	42 (14–94)	38 (11–163)	0.081

CMV, cytomegalovirus

initial CMV episode occurred in 55.8 % of patients. After adjusting for the same covariates, there were no significant differences in secondary episodes of CMV among patients who received Valganciclovir (OR 3.36, 95 % CI 0.62 to 18.3, p = 0.17) and Foscarnet (OR 1.02, 95 % CI 0.20 to 5.25, p = 0.98, compared with Valacyclovir (OR = 1.00). No patients developed CMV disease during the course of the study. Response to pre-emptive CMV treatment using the three different anti-virals are detailed in Table 2.

Adverse events and survival

The elevation in serum creatinine levels was significantly higher after treatment with Foscarnet, compared to Valacyclovir or Valganciclovir ($P = 0.009$). Treatment with Valganciclovir led to a significant decrease in neutrophil counts, compared to Foscarnet or Valacyclovir ($P = 0.012$). Changes in pre- and post-treatment platelet levels did not differ significantly between groups (Table 3). One patient died of neutropenic enterocolitis on post-transplant day 102 in the Valacyclovir group, one patient died of disease progression on post-transplant day 138 in the Valganciclovir group, and three patients died of disease progression and sepsis on post-transplant days 81, 129, and 131 in the Foscarnet group.

Discussion

In this retrospective study, pre-emptive therapy with Valacyclovir, Valganciclovir and Foscarnet achieved high viral clearance rates in post-HSCT patients with CMV antigenemia (98 %). After adjusting for potential confounders including age, sex, CMV serotype, CMV antigen level at diagnosis, donor type, conditioning regimen and GVHD treatment, the rates of viral clearance and recurrent antigenemia were not significantly different in patients receiving high dose Valacyclovir, compared with Ganciclovir or Foscarnet. Viral clearance with Valacyclovir was achieved with significantly less reduction in neutrophil count or rise in creatinine levels. However, it is important to bear in mind that patients who received Valacyclovir in our study were discharged outpatients who were at least one month post-transplant, had no other active infection, and were not debilitated. Thus our findings may only extend to the stable post-HSCT patient.

Another limitation of our study is the use of a low threshold value of 1 CMV-positive cell per million leukocytes to start pre-emptive therapy. It has been suggested that low positive results may represent transient reactivation [16], or even a rare false positive result [17], hence clearance may in part be spontaneous. However, Boeckh *et al.* showed that the discontinuation of gancyclovir below the threshold of 3 positive cells per 50,000 leukocytes led to a risk of CMV disease [18]. When a single positive cell is used as trigger, the rate of CMV disease was reduced [19]. Other investigators have also used a single positive cell as trigger, recognizing that even low viral loads might be significant in the HSCT patient [16, 20, 21]. Given the rapid doubling time of CMV in immunosuppressed paients [22], withholding anti-CMV therapy may pose significant risks. Future studies applying a higher threshold to begin pre-emptive therapyin a larger group of patients are needed to confirm the therapeutic effect of Valacyclovir in high-level CMV antigenemia.

To our knowledge, no previous report has investigated the use of Valacyclovir for pre-emptive therapy of CMV antigenemia, although several randomized and

Table 3 Hematological and renal toxicity of treatment

	All (n = 61)	Valacyclovir (n = 15)	Valganciclovir (n = 16)	Foscarnet (n = 30)	*P*
Change in parameter (post-treatment − pre-treatment), median (range)					
Creatinine (μM)	14 (−31 to 126)	2 (−31 to 57)	−2.5 (−70 to 73)	31.6 (−65 to 126)	0.009
ANC ($x10^3/mm^3$)	−0.05 (−20.6 to 5.0)	0.19 (−4.2 to 3)	−1.5 (−7.5 to −1.1)	1.1 (−20.6 to 5.0)	0.012
Platelet ($x10^3/mm^3$)	6 (−123 to 196)	6 (−72 to 82)	−7.5 (−123 to 196)	13 (−92 to 150)	0.335

ANC, Absolute neutrophil count

retrospective studies have demonstrated the efficacy of Valacyclovir as prophylactic therapy. For example, results from large randomized multicenter studies have shown that Valacyclovir is more effective in preventing CMV antigenemia than oral acyclovir [11], and has similar efficacy as Ganciclovir in preventing CMV infection and disease [12]. Similarly, retrospective reports have established the potential benefit of Valacyclovir as a prophylactic agent against CMV reactivation, compared with no or other forms of CMV prophylaxis, with significantly reduced rates and delay of CMV reactivation [10, 13]. The small sample size in our study precludes definitive conclusions about the efficacy of Valacyclovir as pre-emptive therapy in HSCT patients, but results are encouraging. Importantly, Valacyclovir represents a cost effective alternative to Valganciclovir [23].

Limitations of this study include its retrospective study design, non-randomized treatment allocation, and small sample size. In recent years, more institutions have switched from pp65 antigenemia assays to quantitative PCR methods to guide pre-emptive therapy. PCR based methods are rapid, more sensitive, provide more precise quantitation of CMV, and can be used in patients with severe neutropenia. Its disadvantage includes inter-assay and inter-laboratory variability in viral load reporting, which has complicated attempts to standardize thresholds for initiating and stopping pre-emtive therapy. Recently, the WHO international reference standard was developed, which enables uniform viral load reporting and interpretation. It remains to be studied if the viral load threshold for preemptive therapy using Valacyclovir is comparable to that using Valganciclovir or Foscarnet.

Conclusions

In conclusion, pre-emptive Valacyclovir, Foscarnet and Valacyclovir led to similar clearance of CMV antigenemia and rates of recurrence. High dose Valacyclovir is potentially a safe and cost-effective option for pre-emptive treatment of CMV antigenemia in the stable post-HSCT patient who has cytopenia or prefers outpatient treatment. These findings must be interpreted in light of limitations inherent to retrospective observational studies. Further prospective randomized studies are needed to validate the efficacy suggested by the results of this retrospective study.

Competing interests

The authors declare that they have no competing interests

Authors' contributions

All authors contributed to the intellectual development of this paper. WHYK had the idea for the study. OSY and HTTT collected data, OSY analyzed the data and wrote the first draft paper. CPD, YCL, AHYL, YTG and WHYK provided patients, and critical corrections to the manuscript. All authors read and approved the final manuscript.

References

1. Akyurekli C, Chan JY, Elmoazzen H, Tay J, Allan DS. Impact of ethnicity on human umbilical cord blood banking: a systematic review. Transfusion. 2014;54:2122–7.
2. Kanda Y, Mineishi S, Saito T, Seo S, Saito A, Suenaga K, et al. Pre-emptive therapy against cytomegalovirus (CMV) disease guided by CMV antigenemia assay after allogeneic hematopoietic stem cell transplantation: a single-center experience in Japan. Bone Marrow Transplant. 2001;27:437–44.
3. Singhal S, Mehta J, Powles R, Treleaven J, Horton C, Carrington D, et al. Three weeks of ganciclovir for cytomegaloviraemia after allogeneic bone marrow transplantation. Bone Marrow Transplant. 1995;15:777–81.
4. Reusser P, Einsele H, Lee J, Volin L, Rovira M, Engelhard D, et al. Randomized multicenter trial of foscarnet versus ganciclovir for preemptive therapy of cytomegalovirus infection after allogeneic stem cell transplantation. Blood. 2002;99:1159–64.
5. Jayaweera DT. Minimising the dosage-limiting toxicities of foscarnet induction therapy. Drug Saf. 1997;16:258–66.
6. Beutner KR. Valacyclovir: a review of its antiviral activity, pharmacokinetic properties, and clinical efficacy. Antiviral Res. 1995;28:281–90.
7. Reischig T, Opatrny Jr K, Bouda M, Treska V, Jindra P, Svecova M. A randomized prospective controlled trial of oral ganciclovir versus oral valacyclovir for prophylaxis of cytomegalovirus disease after renal transplantation. Transpl Int. 2002;15:615–22.
8. Reischig T, Nemcova J, Vanecek T, Jindra P, Hes O, Bouda M, et al. Intragraft cytomegalovirus infection: a randomized trial of valacyclovir prophylaxis versus pre-emptive therapy in renal transplant recipients. Antivir Ther. 2010;15:23–30.
9. Pavlopoulou ID, Syriopoulou VP, Chelioti H, Daikos GL, Stamatiades D, Kostakis A, et al. A comparative randomised study of valacyclovir vs oral ganciclovir for cytomegalovirus prophylaxis in renal transplant recipients. Clin Microbiol Infect. 2005;11:736–43.
10. Vusirikala M, Wolff SN, Stein RS, Brandt SJ, Morgan DS, Greer JP, et al. Valacyclovir for the prevention of cytomegalovirus infection after allogeneic stem cell transplantation: a single institution retrospective cohort analysis. Bone Marrow Transplant. 2001;28:265–70.
11. Ljungman P, de La Camara R, Milpied N, Volin L, Russell CA, Crisp A, et al. Randomized study of valacyclovir as prophylaxis against cytomegalovirus reactivation in recipients of allogeneic bone marrow transplants. Blood. 2002;99:3050–6.
12. Winston DJ, Yeager AM, Chandrasekar PH, Snydman DR, Petersen FB, Territo MC. Randomized comparison of oral valacyclovir and intravenous ganciclovir for prevention of cytomegalovirus disease after allogeneic bone marrow transplantation. Clin Infect Dis. 2003;36:749–58.
13. Mori T, Aisa Y, Shimizu T, Nakazato T, Yamazaki R, Ikeda Y, et al. Prevention of cytomegalovirus infection by valaciclovir after allogeneic bone marrow transplantation from an unrelated donor. Int J Hematol. 2006;83:266–70.
14. Tan BH, Chlebicka NL, Low JG, Chong TY, Chan KP, Goh YT. Use of the cytomegalovirus pp 65 antigenemia assay for preemptive therapy in allogeneic hematopoietic stem cell transplantation: a real-world review. Transpl Infect Dis. 2008;10:325–32.
15. Ljungman P, Griffiths P, Paya C. Definitions of cytomegalovirus infection and disease in transplant recipients. Clin Infect Dis. 2002;34:1094–7.
16. Yanada M, Yamamoto K, Emi N, Naoe T, Suzuki R, Taji H, et al. Cytomegalovirus antigenemia and outcome of patients treated with pre-emptive ganciclovir: retrospective analysis of 241 consecutive patients undergoing allogeneic hematopoietic stem cell transplantation. Bone Marrow Transplant. 2003;32:801–7.
17. Lesprit P, Scieux C, Lemann M, Carbonelle E, Modai J, Molina JM. Use of the cytomegalovirus (CMV) antigenemia assay for the rapid diagnosis of primary CMV infection in hospitalized adults. Clin Infect Dis. 1998;26:646–50.
18. Boeckh M, Gooley TA, Myerson D, Cunningham T, Schoch G, Bowden RA. Cytomegalovirus pp 65 antigenemia-guided early treatment with ganciclovir versus ganciclovir at engraftment after allogeneic marrow transplantation: a randomized double-blind study. Blood. 1996;88:4063–71.
19. Boeckh M, Bowden RA, Gooley T, Myerson D, Corey L. Successful modification of a pp 65 antigenemia-based early treatment strategy for prevention of cytomegalovirus disease in allogeneic marrow transplant recipients. Blood. 1999;93:1781–2.

20. Boivin G, Belanger R, Delage R, Beliveau C, Demers C, Goyette N, et al. Quantitative analysis of cytomegalovirus (CMV) viremia using the pp 65 antigenemia assay and the COBAS AMPLICOR CMV MONITOR PCR test after blood and marrow allogeneic transplantation. J Clin Microbiol. 2000;38:4356–60.
21. Leruez-Ville M, Ouachee M, Delarue R, Sauget AS, Blanche S, Buzyn A, et al. Monitoring cytomegalovirus infection in adult and pediatric bone marrow transplant recipients by a real-time PCR assay performed with blood plasma. J Clin Microbiol. 2003;41:2040–6.
22. Emery VC. Investigation of CMV disease in immunocompromised patients. J Clin Pathol. 2001;54:84–8.
23. Reischig T, Kacer M. The efficacy and cost-effectiveness of valacyclovir in cytomegalovirus prevention in solid organ transplantation. Expert Rev Pharmacoecon Outcomes Res. 2014;14:771–9.

2

Significantly elevated foetal haemoglobin levels in individuals with glucose 6-phosphate dehydrogenase disease and/or sickle cell trait: a cross-sectional study in Cape Coast, Ghana

Patrick Adu[1*], Essel K. M. Bashirudeen[1], Florence Haruna[1], Edward Morkporkpor Adela[2] and Richard K. D. Ephraim[1]

Abstract

Background: Previously published data have demonstrated that sickle red blood cells produce twice as much reactive oxygen species (ROS) suggesting that co-inheritance of sickle cell disease (SCD) and glucose 6-phosphate dehydrogenase (G6PD) enzymopathy could lead to more severe anaemia during sickling crises. Elevated foetal haemoglobin (Hb F) levels have been shown to have positive modulatory effects on sickling crises and disease outcomes. This study sought to assess how inheritance of G6PD enzymopathy affects the level of Hb F and haemoglobin concentration in adults in steady state.

Methods: This cross-sectional study selected 100 out-patients (41 males and 59 females) visiting the University of Cape Coast hospital, between January, 2016 and May, 2016. Cellulose acetate electrophoresis (pH 8.2–8.6), methaemoglobin reductase test, modified Betke alkaline denaturation methods were used to investigate haemoglobin variants, qualitative G6PD status, and %Hb F levels in venous blood samples drawn from these participants. Data was analysed with GraphPad Prism 6 and SPSS and significance set at $p < 0.05$.

Results: Forty one percent of the participants demonstrated qualitative G6PD enzymopathy whereas only 10% demonstrated Hb AS type (Sickle cell trait, SCT). 5% of the participants co-inherited SCT and G6PD enzymopathy. %Hb F levels in G6PD deficient males was significantly higher than in G6PD deficient females [($p = 0.0003$, 2.696% (males) vs 1.975% (females)], although the %Hb F levels was comparable in non-G6PD deficient individuals. %Hb F levels were significantly elevated in males with SCT only ($p < 0.05$), or G6PD enzymopathy only ($p < 0.0001$), or SCT + G6PD enzymopathy ($p < 0.0001$) compared to males with none of these pathologies even though their respective haemoglobin levels were comparable. Male participants with G6PD enzymopathy + SCT co-inheritance had significantly elevated %Hb F when compared to their counterparts with only G6PD enzymopathy ($p < 0.001$). Male gender [($p = 0.001$, OR: 6.912 (2.277–20.984)] partial defective G6PD enzyme [(p = 0.00, OR: 7.567E8 (8.443E7–6.782E9)] SCT [($p = 0.026$, OR: 4.625 (1.196–17.881)] were factors associated with raised %Hb F levels ≥2.5.

Conclusion: The inheritance of G6PD defect and/or SCT significantly elevate %Hb F levels in the steady state even though haemoglobin levels are not affected.

Keywords: Haemoglobinopathy, Sickle cell trait, Glucose 6-phosphate dehydrogenase, Co-inheritance, Foetal haemoglobin

* Correspondence: Patrick.adu@ucc.edu.gh
[1]Medical Laboratory Technology Department, School of Allied Health Sciences, University of Cape Coast, Cape Coast, Ghana
Full list of author information is available at the end of the article

Background

The normal physiologic functions of red blood cells (RBC) may be hampered by inherited haemoglobinopathies (e.g. sickle cell disease), red cell enzymopathy or red cell membrane abnormalities (e.g. G6PD deficiency). Although both G6PD enzymopathy and sickle cell are recessively inherited, whereas G6PD is sex-linked, sickle cell gene is autosomal inherited. SCD occurs due to the substitution of valine for glutamic acid in position 6 in the beta globin [1–3]. This then leads to the production of abnormal haemoglobin Hb S instead of normal haemoglobin Hb A [1, 4, 5]. Heterozygous inheritance leads to sickle cell trait (Hb AS) whereas homozygous inheritance leads to SCD with its consequent vaso-occlusive attacks, reactive oxygen species (ROS) generation, bacterial infections, priapism and chronic visceral complications often associated with ischemia in different organs [4, 6].

On the other hand, about 400 million people are estimated to be G6PD deficient worldwide [6–8]. In G6PD deficiency, terminally differentiated red cells become susceptible to oxidant stress-induced haemolytic anaemia due to absence of NADPH [5, 7, 9–11]. Agents causing oxidant stress in G6PD deficient individuals include fava beans and drugs such as aspirin, primaquine and quinine [4].

As these red cell pathologies are independently inherited, the potential for co-inheritance may be high especially in sub-Saharan Africa where either of these pathologies has been shown to provide protection against malaria infection [12, 13]. Previously published data have demonstrated that sickle red cells produce twice as much ROS such as hydrogen peroxide, superoxides and hydroxyl radicals, compared to normal cells [14]. This means that there is a possibility that SCD individuals with G6PD deficiency will have an increased tendency to frequent acute haemolytic crises as a consequence of ROS generated by sickled red cells. Studies investigating the potential modulatory effect of G6PD enzymopathy on severity of sickle cell anaemia has produced conflicting results. Whereas some studies found lower haemoglobin levels [15, 16], others found no effect on clinical manifestations, haemoglobin level and reticulocyte counts in such co-inherited cases [17]. Besides, in Ghana where co-inheritance of these two red cell pathologies are common [18], there is paucity of such data to inform clinical decisions. Moreover, the endemicity of malaria means that drugs such as quinine, primaquine, and amodiaquine that predispose G6PD deficient to oxidant stress may be routinely prescribed to malaria patients. This necessitates that factors that has the potential to modulate disease pathologies in co-inherited G6PD deficient and SCD ought to be explored. As foetal haemoglobin (Hb F) levels have been demonstrated to positively modulate SCD pathogenesis, we investigated the impact of the inheritance of G6PD enzymopathy and/or SCT on the %Hb F as well as haemoglobin levels in the peripheral blood of these patients in steady state.

Methods

Study design/study site

This cross-sectional study was conducted at the University of Cape Coast hospital in the Central region of Ghana from January to May 2016. The hospital has a bedding capacity of 65, and has an average yearly out-patient department (OPD) attendance and admissions of 61,509 and 2608 respectively. The hospital has OPD, accident and emergency (A & E) unit, Surgical ward, Medical ward, laboratory department, radiography unit and physiotherapy unit.

Participants

A simple convenience sampling technique was used to recruit 100 participants (41 males and 59 females) aged 15–84 years. The rationale for the study was explained to all clients attending the OPD unit of the hospital during the period of the research. Only clients who gave written informed consent were consecutively recruited for the study. Individuals who had been transfused within three months to the period of the research, or pregnant or those taking medications known to cause haemolysis in G6PD deficient individuals [19] were excluded. Only consenting participants who has no history of any chronic disease were recruited for the study.

Sample collection

4mls of whole blood was taken from each participant into an ethylenediaminetetraacetic acid (EDTA) anticoagulated tubes following standard protocols. The blood was used for G6PD screening, haemoglobin concentration, foetal haemoglobin estimation and haemoglobin electrophoresis.

G6PD screening assay

G6PD screening was undertaken using the methaemoglobin reduction assay as described by Cheesbrough [20]. G6PD status was described as full defect (FD), partial defect (PD) or no defect (ND).

Haemoglobin estimation

The haemoglobin levels of each participant was estimated using the URIT-12 haemoglobin meter (URIT Medical Electronic Co. Ltd., Guangxi, China) following manufacturer's protocol [21].

Foetal haemoglobin estimation

The level of foetal haemoglobin in each participant was estimated using the modified Betke alkali denaturation method [22, 23].

Haemoglobin electrophoresis

Haemoglobin variants in the participants were determined using the cellulose acetate electrophoresis (pH 8.2–8.6) in accordance with previously published protocols [24]. Haemoglobin type was described as SCT (AS), or NEG (A).

Statistical analysis

The data was inputted into Microsoft Office Excel 2007 and grouped into various categories and later analyzed using the GraphPad Prism 6 (GraphPad Software Inc., USA). Descriptive analysis was performed and results expressed as numbers and percentages. Data was analysed for normality using D'Agostino-Pearson test. Comparison between two groups were undertaken using two-tailed unpaired t-test (if passed normality test) or Mann–Whitney test (if it did not pass normality test). Multiple comparisons were undertaken either with One-Way ANOVA with Dunn's post-testing (those that passed normality testing) or Kruskal-Wallis test with Tukey's post-testing (those not passing normality testing). The relationship between parameters were explored using Pearson correlation coefficients. However, SPSS version 22 (IBM, USA) was employed to interrogate factors associated with raised %Hb F levels ≥2.5 through logistic regression analysis. *P* value less than 0.05 was considered statistically significant.

Results

The G6PD status and haemoglobin variants of the participants were stratified per gender (Table 1). The mean age of the male and female participants was similar (p = 0.77; 33.5 years vs 34.5 years). Overall, 41% of the study participants demonstrated G6PD defect (31% full defect and 10% partial defect). Whereas 58.5% of the male participants showed G6PD full defect, only 11.9% of the female participants demonstrated G6PD full defect. Additionally, 10% of the study participants also had the SCT (Hb AS type).

Table 1 Qualitative red cell G6PD enzyme test stratified by gender

Parameter	Male (%) N = 41	Female (%) N = 59	Total (%)
Mean age (yrs)	33.50 ± 1.87	34.4 ± 2.43	
G6PD status			
G6PD FD	24 (58.50)	7 (11.90)	31 (31%)
G6PD PD	0 (0.00)	10 (16.90)	10 (10%)
G6PD ND	17 (41.50)	42 (71.20)	59 (59%)
Haemoglobin type			
Hb AS	6 (14.60)	4 (6.80)	10 (10%)
Hb A	35 (85.4.0)	55 (93.20)	90 (90%)

G6PD Glucose-6-phosphate Dehydrogenase, *FD* full defect, *PD* partial defect, *ND* no defect

The prevalence of co-inheritance of G6PD enzymopathy and SCT among the study participants is presented in Table 2. Overall, 5% (4 males vs 1 female) of the study participants co-inherited G6PD enzymopathy and SCT. Whereas 5% (2 males vs 3 females) of the study participants inherited SCT alone, 36% inherited G6PD enzymopathy alone (27 full defect vs 9% partial defect).

Figure 1 shows the %Hb F and haemoglobin levels in participants stratified by their qualitative G6PD and/or SCT status. Participants who demonstrated qualitative G6PD full defect showed significantly higher levels of %Hb F than those with partial defect or normal qualitative G6PD activity [Fig. 1a, p=0.0003; G6PD ND (0.8726%) vs G6PD FD (3.523%); p = 0.0003; G6PD ND (0.8726%) vs G6PD FD + SCT (2.514%)]. However, although inheritance of SCT increased the % Hb F levels compared to those with neither G6PD enzymopathy nor SCT, the increment was not significant ($p > 0.05$). Haemoglobin levels did not significantly differ among the participants irrespective of their G6PD status and/or haemoglobin type ($p > 0.05$, Fig. 1b).

Figure 2 shows the % haemoglobin F among study participants stratified by gender. Overall, male participants had significantly higher %Hb F compared to female participants [Fig. 2a, $p<0.0001$; 1.247% (females) vs 1.973% (males)]. When the data was stratified based on the inheritance of G6PD enzymopathy, the significantly increased %Hb F levels was found only between males and females having G6PD enzymopathy [Fig. 2b, p=0.0003; 1.975% (females) vs 2.696% (males)]. Male and female participants with normal G6PD enzyme activity had comparable %Hb F levels (p = ns, Fig. 2c; 0.9524% (females) vs 0.9518% (males)].

Since the male participants had significantly elevated %Hb F compared to the females, we evaluated the impact of G6PD enzymopathy and/or SCT on %Hb F levels in male participants (Fig. 3). The haemoglobin levels did not significantly differ among the groups (Fig. 3a). However, the inheritance of G6PD enzymopathy and/or SCT was significantly associated with increased %Hb F levels in the male participants (Fig. 3b).

Table 2 G6PD Status + SCT co-inheritance of participants

G6PD status + SCT co-inheritance (N = 100)	Male (%)	Female (%)
G6PD ND + NEG	15 (15)	39 (39)
SCT + G6PD PD	0 (0)	1 (1)
SCT + G6PD FD	4 (4)	0 (0)
SCT + G6PD ND	2 (2)	3 (3)
G6PD FD + NEG	20 (20)	7 (7)
G6PD PD + NEG	0 (0)	9 (9)

G6PD Glucose-6-phosphate Dehydrogenase, *SCT* sickle cell trait, *FD* full defect, *PD* partial defect, *ND* no defect, *NEG* negative

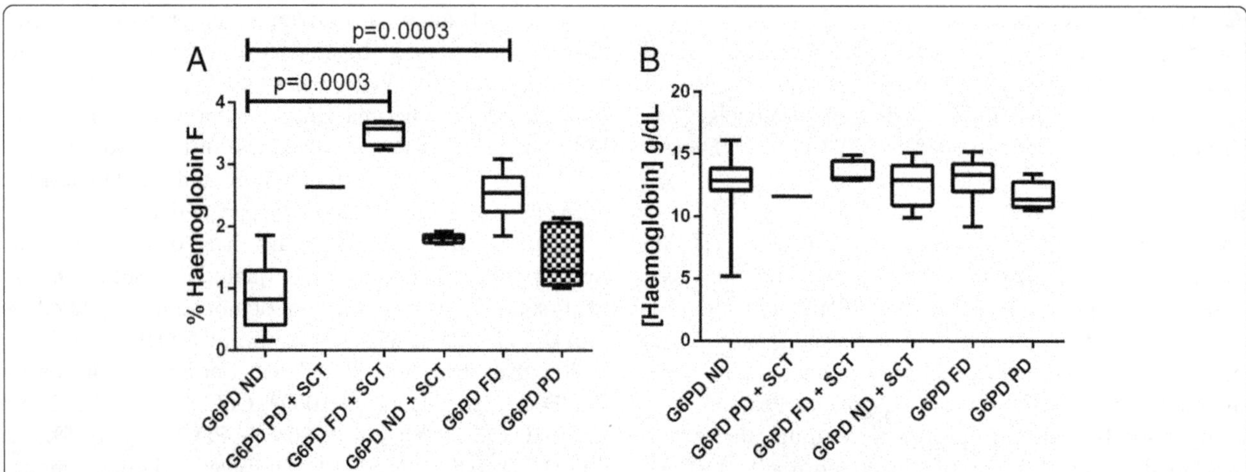

Fig. 1 %Hb F (**a**) and haemoglobin (**b**) levels in participants stratified as per their qualitative G6PD and/or SCT status. [G6PD = Glucose-6-phosphate Dehydrogenase, SCT = Sickle Cell Trait, FD = Full defect, PD = Partial defect, ND = No defect]

The study also explored the relationship between %Hb F, Hb and age of participants through Pearson correlation coefficients (Table 3). Age and %Hb F levels were inversely, but non-significantly correlated to each other (r = −0.022; p = 0.830). However, age and Hb levels as well as Hb and %Hb F levels were positively but non-significantly associated with each other.

Factors associated with raised %Hb F levels ≥2.5% were predicted using binary logistic regression analysis (Table 4). Male gender [p = 0.001, OR: 6.912, 95% CI (2.277–20.984)], partial defective G6PD enzyme [p = 0.00, OR: 7.567E8, 95% CI (8.443E7–6.782E9)] and haemoglobin variant AS [p = 0.026, OR: 4.625, 95% CI (1.196–17.881)] were all significantly associated with raised %Hb F levels ≥2.5.

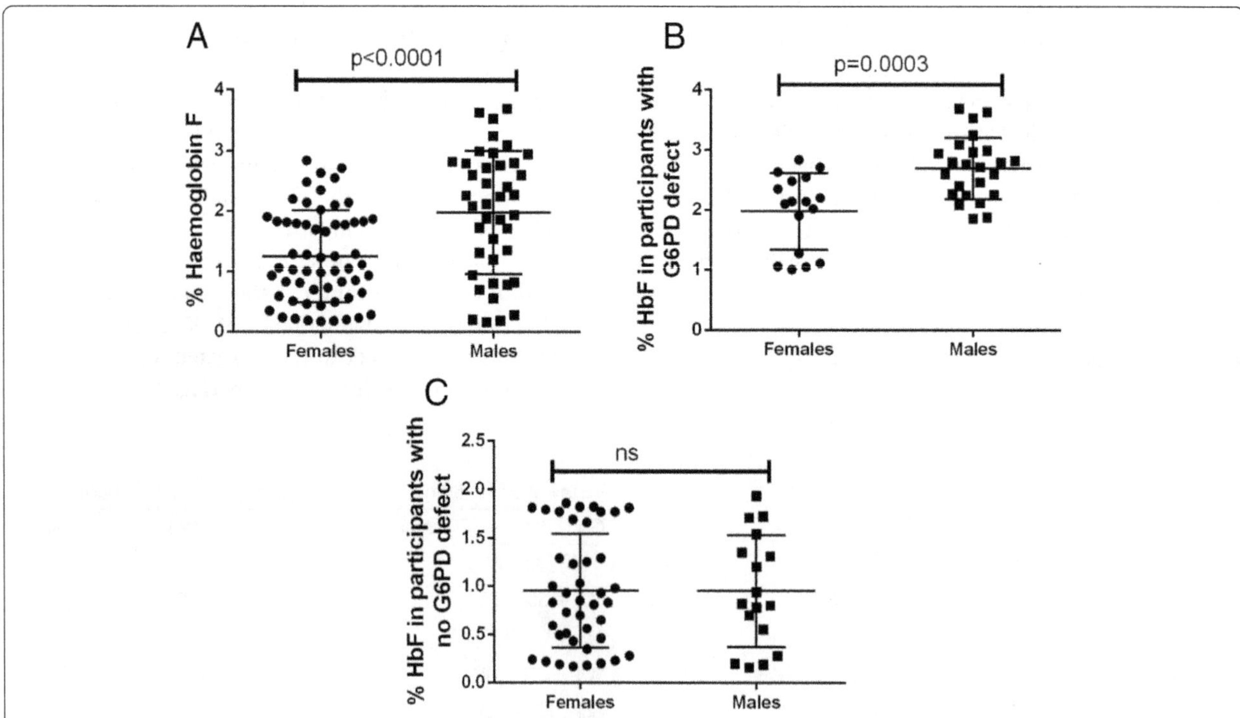

Fig. 2 % Hemoglobin F and G6PD characteristics among study participants stratified by gender. **a** %Haemoglobin F comparison of all participants based on gender; **b** %Haemoglobin F of participants with G6PD defect stratified by gender; **c** %Haemoglobin F of participants with no G6PD defect stratified by gender

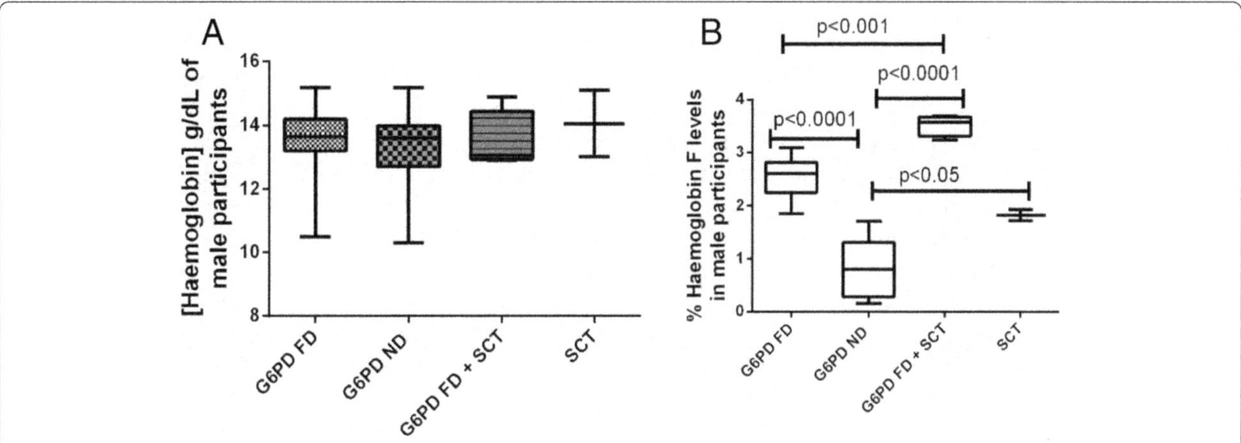

Fig. 3 G6PD enzymopathy and/or SCT on %HbF levels in male participants. **a** compares the haemoglobin levels of male participants; **b** compares the %Hb F levels in male participants

Discussion

We sought to investigate the impact of the inheritance of G6PD enzymopathy and/or SCT on the %Hb F as well as haemoglobin levels in the peripheral blood of these patients in steady state. Our findings showed a 5% co-inheritance of SCT and G6PD enzymopathy and significantly elevated %Hb F levels in individuals with G6PD enzymopathy compared to either individual with SCT or normal G6PD enzyme activity. This suggests that Hb F levels may modulate the severity of G6PD enzymopathy in conditions of oxidant stress.

In the present study, a 41.0% prevalence of G6PD deficiency was recorded among the study population which is higher than the suggested Ghana's 15–26% prevalence by the World Health Organization [25] or the estimated 1.2–30.7% prevalence in Africa [26]. This results is also at variance with a previous cross-sectional study under taken in the Brong-Ahafo region of Ghana which recorded 32% G6PD enzymopathy prevalence among blood donors [27]. Many other studies in the sub-region and beyond have recorded lower prevalence in the past. For example, in a study in Iran, Nabavizadeh and Anushiravani reported a 14.17% prevalence of G6PD enzymopathy among 261 blood donors [28]. Also Omisakin et al., reported a 25.5% G6PD enzymopathy prevalence among blood donors in Nigeria [29]. These differences may be due to the different geographic locations as well as sampling frame employed in the various studies. Our study also found more males with G6PD enzymopathy compared to females [males (24.0% with full defect) vs females (females 7.0% with full defect and 10% with partial defect)]. This is not surprising considering that the genetic locus of the *G6PD* gene is on the X-chromosome and inherited in a recessive manner [30, 31].

The sickle-cell trait is known to be widespread, reaching its highest prevalence in parts of Africa as well as among people with origins in equatorial Africa. Previous studies have recorded high prevalence of SCT for countries such as Democratic Republic of Congo (23.3%) [32], Gabon

Table 3 Correlations between age, Hb and %Hb F levels

Parameter		Age	Hb	%HbF
Age	r	1	0.143	−0.022
	P-value		0.156	0.830
Hb	r		1	0.094
	P-value			0.353
%HbF	r			1

r: Pearson correlation coefficient

Table 4 Factors associated with %Hb F levels ≥2.5

Parameter	OR (95% CI)	*P*-value
Age group		
< 20	0.958 (0.160–5.746)	0.963
20–29	1.420 (0.447–4.506)	0.552
30–09	0.548 (0.121–2.471)	0.433
≥ 40	Reference	–
Sex		
Male	6.912 (2.277–20.984)	**0.001**
Female	Reference	–
Haemoglobin (g/dL)		
< 12	0.610 (0.185–2.014)	0.417
≥ 12	Reference	–
G6PD status		
Normal	Reference	–
PD	7.567E8 (8.443E7–6.782E9)	**< 0.001**
FD	1.238 (1.238E10)	–
Haemoglobin variant		
A	Reference	–
AS	4.625 (1.196–17.881)	**0.026**

(21.1%) [33], and Nigeria (19.68% - 45%) [34, 35], and Uganda (19.8%) [36]. It has been stated that in countries where the trait prevalence is above 20%, the SCD affects about 2% of the population. This study recorded a 10% SCT prevalence among the participants which is lower than the 19.5% SCT recorded among blood donors in Ghana [27]. However, this finding agrees with a previously published 11.3% SCT reported among blood donors in Ghana [37]. This study thus supports the estimated annual prevalence of SCD in Ghana with its associated high rates of morbidity and mortality [38].

Previous studies have indicated the co-existence of G6PD deficiency in patients with sickle cell disease [39, 40]. The prevalence of both diseases are highest in sub-Saharan Africa [41], and the Arabian Peninsula [42]. This study found a 5% prevalence of co-inherited SCT and G6PD enzymopathy which is comparable to the 7% prevalence of co-inherited G6PD enzymopathy and SCT recorded in a previous cross-sectional study in Ghana [27]. Another study in the sub-region by Egesie et al., also recorded a 5.4% coinheritance of SCT and G6PD deficiency among blood donors in Nigeria [43]. This 5% co-inheritance reported herein is however at variance with reported co-inheritance prevalence reported elsewhere. For example Alabdulaali et al., reported SCT and G6PD co-inherited prevalence of 0.35% among blood donors in Riyadh, Saudi Arabia [44]. Another study that investigated the relationship between sickle cell disorders and G6PD deficiency in Central-Eastern India recorded a 0.61% prevalence of SCT and G6PD co-inheritance [45]. The differences in the prevalence reported in this study compared to the previous studies may be a function of the different selective pressures that exists in the different geographic locations where the studies were undertaken.

Studies investigating the potential modulatory effect of G6PD enzymopathy on severity of sickle cell anaemia has produced conflicting results. We report that, in the steady state, the haemoglobin levels of participants with SCT and/or G6PD enzymopathy did not significantly differ from participants with normal G6PD status and/or Hb A. Our study however found significantly raised %Hb F levels in males with G6PD enzymopathy compared to their female counterparts. Additionally, among the G6PD deficient males, the %Hb F levels were significantly elevated irrespective of the SCT status, when compared to the G6PD normal male counterparts. This observation is in agreement with a previous study in India that reported elevated %Hb F levels in G6PD deficient individuals [46]. Hb F has been shown to modulate the severity of haemoglobinopathies. In line with this, hydroxyurea is a pharmaceutical product used clinically to increase Hb F levels. Therefore, we propose that even though the haemoglobin levels did not differ in steady state, it is plausible to suppose that in haemolytic episodes, the elevated %Hb F levels in these defective G6PD and/or SCT may modulate the severity by improving oxygen transport to tissues and organs in the body. It is interesting to note that males who co-inherited SCT and G6PD enzymopathy had significantly elevated %Hb F compared to males who inherited either SCT or G6PD enzymopathy alone. In evaluating the factors associated with increased %Hb F levels ≥2.5%, our study also found male gender, partial defective G6PD enzyme and SCT as predictive of elevated %Hb F levels. This is in agreement with a previous cross-sectional study in Saudi Arabia that also found gender and haemoglobin variants as being associated with increased %Hb F levels [47]. However, whereas that study found age to be associated with elevated %Hb F levels, this study did not. This is not surprising considering that the El-Hazmi et al. study sampled both adults and cord blood taken from day old babies whereas this study recruited only adults (15–84 years).

To our knowledge, this is the first study in the sub-region to clearly demonstrate G6PD enzymopathy to be associated with elevated %Hb F levels. As the %Hb F levels were significantly elevated in those with G6PD enzymopathy compared to those with SCT, it will be interesting to compare the %Hb F levels in those with sickle cell anaemia to those with G6PD defect as well as assess the impact that %Hb F levels on the pathogenesis of oxidant stress in individuals with G6PD enzymopathy. However, the impact of our study was limited by the sample size, and the G6PD screening assay employed which is not as sensitive as the fluorescence method [24]. Additionally, our study did not estimate the reticulocyte count in the participants as reticulocytosis could have confounded the interpretation of the methaemoglobin reductase test.

Conclusion

In the steady state the inheritance of G6PD defect and/SCT significantly elevate %Hb F, but not haemoglobin levels in the peripheral blood. Male gender, SCT and G6PD partial defect are factors associated with elevated %Hb F ≥ 2.5. Therefore, in the management of individuals with G6PD defect and/or SCT, %Hb F levels should be monitored to inform clinical decisions. Further studies employing animal models should be undertaken to understand the modulating effect of %Hb F levels on G6PD defect and/or SCT.

Abbreviations

EDTA: Ethylenediaminetetraacetic acid; G6PD FD: G6PD full defect; G6PD ND: G6PD no defect; G6PD PD: G6PD partial defect; G6PD: Glucose 6-phosphate dehydrogenase; Hb F: foetal haemoglobin; Hb: haemoglobin; ROS: reactive oxygen specie; SCT: Sickle cell trait

Acknowledgements
We would like to thank the staff of laboratory unit of the University of Cape Coast hospital for their assistance during our data collection. We are also indebted to our participants who volunteered to be part of this study.

Funding
This research was self-funded by the researchers.

Authors' contributions
PA and RKDE conceived the study, and participated in the design. EKMB, FH and EMA involved in data acquisition, laboratory work and literature search. PA involved in data analysis and drafted the manuscript. RKDE critically reviewed the manuscript. All authors read and approved the final manuscript.

Competing interests
The authors declare that they have no competing interests.

Author details
[1]Medical Laboratory Technology Department, School of Allied Health Sciences, University of Cape Coast, Cape Coast, Ghana. [2]Haematology unit, Cape Coast Teaching Hospital, Cape Coast, Ghana.

References
1. Lervolino LG, Baldin PEA, Picado SM, Calil KB, Viel AA, Campos LAF. Prevalence of sickle cell disease and sickle cell trait in national neonatal screening studies. Rev Bras Hematol Hemoter. 2011;33(1):49–54.
2. Madegowda C, Rao C. The sickle cell anemia health problems: traditional and modern treatment practices among the Soliga tribes at BR Hills, South India. Antrocom Online J Anthropol. 2013;9(2):243–51.
3. Mavanga NM, Boemer F, Seidel L, Nkebolo A, Malafu AG, Gerard C. Blood groups, hemoglobin phenotypes and clinical disorders of consanguineous YANSI population. 2013.
4. Simpore J, Ilboudo D, Damintoti K, Sawadogo L, Maria E, Binet S, Nitiema H, Ouedraogo P, Pignatelli S, Nikiema J-B. Glucose-6-phosphate dehydrogenase deficiency and sickle cell disease in Burkina Faso. Pak J Biol Sci. 2007;10(3):409–14.
5. Uzoegwu PN, Awah FM. Prevalence of sickle Haemoglobin and glucose–6–phosphate dehydrogenase deficiency genes in the populations of north west and south west provinces, Cameroon. Anim Res Int. 2006;3(3):581–6.
6. Hoffbrand AV, Moss PAH, Pettit JE, editors. Essential hematology, 5th edn. UK: Published by Blackwell Publishing Ltd; 2006.
7. Carter N, Pamba A, Duparc S, Waitumbi JN. Frequency of glucose-6-phosphate dehydrogenase deficiency in malaria patients from six African countries enrolled in two randomized anti-malarial clinical trials. Malar J. 2011;10(1):241.
8. Turgeon ML. Clinical hematology: theory and procedures. 5th ed. Philadelphia: Lippincott Williams & Wilkins; 2012.
9. Beutler E, Duparc S, Group GPDW. Glucose-6-phosphate dehydrogenase deficiency and antimalarial drug development. Am J Trop Med Hyg. 2007; 77(4):779–89.
10. Clark TG, Fry AE, Auburn S, Campino S, Diakite M, Green A, Richardson A, Teo YY, Small K, Wilson J. Allelic heterogeneity of G6PD deficiency in West Africa and severe malaria susceptibility. Eur J Hum Genet. 2009;17(8):1080–5.
11. Monteiro WM, Franca GP, Melo GC, Queiroz A, Brito M, Peixoto HM, Oliveira MRF, Romero GA, Bassat Q, Lacerda MV. Clinical complications of G6PD deficiency in Latin American and Caribbean populations: systematic review and implications for malaria elimination programmes. Malar J. 2014;13(1):70.
12. Santana MS, Monteiro WM, Siqueira AM, Costa MF, Sampaio V, Lacerda MV, Alecrim MG. Glucose-6-phosphate dehydrogenase deficient variants are associated with reduced susceptibility to malaria in the Brazilian Amazon. Trans R Soc Trop Med Hyg. 2013;107(5):301–6.
13. Mehta A, Mason PJ, Vulliamy TJ. Glucose-6-phosphate dehydrogenase deficiency. Baillieres Best Pract Res Clin Haematol. 2000;13(1):21–38.
14. Ali MSM, HMA-b S. glucose 6 phosphate dehydrogenase deficiency screen among males patients with sickle cell disorders in Sudan. Am J Res Commun. 2014;2(10):23–9.
15. Nouraie M, Reading NS, Campbell A, Minniti CP, Rana SR, Luchtman-Jones L, Kato GJ, Gladwin MT, Castro OL, Prchal JT, et al. Association of G6PD with lower haemoglobin concentration but not increased haemolysis in patients with sickle cell anaemia. Br J Haematol. 2010;150(2):218–25.
16. Benkerrou M, Alberti C, Couque N, Haouari Z, Ba A, Missud F, Boizeau P, Holvoet L, Ithier G, Elion J, et al. Impact of glucose-6-phosphate dehydrogenase deficiency on sickle cell anaemia expression in infancy and early childhood: a prospective study. Br J Haematol. 2013;163(5):646–54.
17. Steinberg MH, West MS, Gallagher D, Mentzer W. Effects of glucose-6-phosphate dehydrogenase deficiency upon sickle cell anemia. Blood. 1988;71(3):748–52.
18. Adu P, Simpong DL, Takyi G, Ephraim RK. Glucose-6-phosphate dehydrogenase deficiency and sickle cell trait among prospective blood donors: a cross-sectional study in Berekum, Ghana. Adv Hematol. 2016;2016:7302912.
19. Young DS, Pestaner LC, Gibberman V. Effects of drugs on clinical laboratory tests. Clin Chem. 1975;21(5):1D–432D.
20. Cheesbrough M. District laboratory practice in tropical countries. Cambridge: University press; 2006.
21. Supplier GD, editor. URIT: URIT-12 Hemoglobin meter; easy 3-step operation. China: URIT Electronic (Group) Co. Ltd; 2009.
22. Jonxis J, Huisman T. The detection and estimation of fetal hemoglobin by means of the alkali denaturation test. Blood. 1956;11(11):1009–18.
23. Molden D, Alexander N, Neeley W. Fetal hemoglobin: optimum conditions for its estimation by alkali denaturation. Am J Clin Pathol. 1982;77(5):568–72.
24. Barabara J, Bain IB, Michael A, Laffan S, Lewis M. Dacie and Lewis practical Haematology. Elsevier: Churchill Livingstone; 2011.
25. WHO Working Group WHO. Glucose-6-phosphate dehydrogenase deficiency. Bull World Health Organ. 1989;67(6):601–11.
26. Moradkhani K, Mekki C, Bahuau M, Te VLT, Holder M, Pissard S, Préhu C, Rose C, Wajcman H, Galactéros F. Practical approach for characterization of glucose 6-phosphate dehydrogenase (G6PD) deficiency in countries with population ethnically heterogeneous: description of seven new G6PD mutants. Am J Hematol. 2012;87(2):208–10.
27. Simpong DL, Adu P, Bashiru R, Morna MT, Yeboah FA, Akakpo K, Ephraim RK. Assessment of iodine status among pregnant women in a rural community in ghana - a cross sectional study. Arch Public Health. 2016;74:8.
28. Nabavizadeh SH, Anushiravani A. The prevalence of G6PD deficiency in blood transfusion recipients. Hematology. 2007;12(1):85–8.
29. Omisikan CT, Esan AJ, Ogunleye AA, Ojo-Bola O, Owoseni MF, Omoniyi DP. Glucose-6-phosphate dehydrogenase (G6pd) deficiency and sickle cell trait among blood donors in Nigeria. Am J Pub Health Res. 2014;2(2):51–5.
30. Akanni EO, Oseni BSA, Agbona VO, Tijani BA, Tosan E, Fakunle EE, Mabayoje VO. Glucose-6-phosphate dehydrogenase deficiency in blood donors and jaundiced neonates in Osogbo, Nigeria. J Med Lab Diagn. 2010;1(1):1–4.
31. Minucci A, Moradkhani K, Hwang MJ, Zuppi C, Giardina B, Capoluongo E. Glucose-6-phosphate dehydrogenase (G6PD) mutations database: review of the "old" and update of the new mutations. Blood Cell Mol Dis. 2012;48(3):154–65.
32. Agasa B, Bosunga K, Opara A, Tshilumba K, Dupont E, Vertongen F, Cotton F, Gulbis B. Prevalence of sickle cell disease in a northeastern region of the Democratic Republic of Congo: what impact on transfusion policy? Transfus Med. 2010;20(1):62–5.
33. Delicat-Loembet LM, Elguero E, Arnathau C, Durand P, Ollomo B, Ossari S, Mezui-me-ndong J, Mbang Mboro T, Becquart P, Nkoghe D, et al. Prevalence of the sickle cell trait in Gabon: a nationwide study. Infect Genet Evol. 2014;25:52–6.
34. Jeremiah ZA. Abnormal haemoglobin variants, ABO and Rh blood groups among student of African descent in Port Harcourt, Nigeria. Afr Health Sci. 2006;6(3):177–81.

35. Oludare GO, Ogili MC. Knowledge, attitude and practice of premarital counseling for sickle cell disease among youth in Yaba, Nigeria. Afr J Reprod Health. 2013;17(4):175–82.
36. Ndeezi G, Kiyaga C, Hernandez AG, Munube D, Howard TA, Ssewanyana I, Nsungwa J, Kiguli S, Ndugwa CM, Ware RE, et al. Burden of sickle cell trait and disease in the Uganda sickle surveillance study (US3): a cross-sectional study. Lancet Glob Health. 2016;4(3):e195–200.
37. Antwi-Baffour S, Asare RO, Adjei JK, Kyeremeh R, Adjei DN. Prevalence of hemoglobin S trait among blood donors: a cross-sectional study. BMC Res Notes. 2015;8:583.
38. Antwi-Boasiako C, Frimpong E, Ababio G, Dzudzor B, Ekem I, Gyan B, Sodzi-Tettey N, Antwi D. Sickle cell disease: reappraisal of the role of foetal haemoglobin levels in the frequency of vaso-occlusive crisis. Ghana Med J. 2015;49(2):102–6.
39. Al-Nood H. Thalassaemia and glucose-6-phosphate dehydrogenase deficiency in sickle-cell disorder patients in Taiz, Yemen/Thalassémie et déficit en glucose-6-phosphate déshydrogénase chez des patients atteints de drépanocytose à Taïz (Yémen). East Mediterr Health J. 2011;17(5):404.
40. Benkerrou M, Alberti C, Couque N, Haouari Z, Ba A, Missud F, Boizeau P, Holvoet L, Ithier G, Elion J. Impact of glucose-6-phosphate dehydrogenase deficiency on sickle cell anaemia expression in infancy and early childhood: a prospective study. Br J Haematol. 2013;163(5):646–54.
41. Allison AC. The distribution of the sickle-cell trait in East Africa and elsewhere, and its apparent relationship to the incidence of subtertian malaria. Trans R Soc Trop Med Hyg. 1954;48(4):312–8.
42. Al-Gazali L, Alwash R, Abdulrazzaq Y. United Arab Emirates: communities and community genetics. Public Health Genomics. 2005;8(3):186–96.
43. Egesie OJ, Egesie UG, Jatau ED, Isiguzoro I, Ntuhun DB. Prevalence of sickle cell trait and glucose 6 phosphate dehydrogenase deficiency among blood donors in a Nigerian tertiary hospital. Afr J Biomed Res. 2013;16:143–7.
44. Alabdulaali MK, Alayed KM, Alshaikh AF, Almashhadani SA. Prevalence of glucose-6-phosphate dehydrogenase deficiency and sickle cell trait among blood donors in Riyadh. Asian J Transfus Sci. 2010;4(1):31–3.
45. Balgir RS. Do tribal communities show an inverse relationship between sickle cell disorders and glucose-6-phosphate dehydrogenase deficiency in malaria endemic areas of central-eastern India? Homo. 2006;57(2):163–76.
46. Balgir RS. Hematological profile of twenty-nine tribal compound cases of hemoglobinopathies and G-6-PD deficiency in rural Orissa. Indian J Med Sci. 2008;62(9):362–71.
47. El Hazmi MA, Warsy AS, Addar MH, Babae Z. Fetal haemoglobin level–effect of gender, age and haemoglobin disorders. Mol Cell Biochem. 1994;135(2):181–6.

3

A systematic review of using and reporting survival analyses in acute lymphoblastic leukemia literature

Chatree Chai-Adisaksopha[1,2], Alfonso Iorio[1,2*], Christopher Hillis[2,3], Wendy Lim[1] and Mark Crowther[1,2]

Abstract

Backgrounds: Survival analysis is commonly used to determine the treatment effect among acute lymphoblastic leukemia (ALL) patients who undergo allogeneic stem cell transplantation (allo-SCT) or other treatments. The aim of this study was to evaluate the use and reporting of survival analyses in these articles.

Methods: We performed a systematic review by searching the MEDLINE, EMBASE and Cochrane library databases from inception to April 2015. Clinical trials of patients with ALL comparing allo-SCT compared to another treatment were included. We included only studies that used survival analysis as a part of the statistical methods.

Results: There were 14 studies included in the review. Sample size estimation was described in 4 (29 %) studies. Only 4 (29 %) studies reported the list of covariates assessed in the Cox regression and 6 (43 %) studies provided a description of censorship. All studies reported survival curves using the Kaplan-Meier method. The comparisons between groups were investigated using the log-rank test and Wilcoxon test. Crossing survival curves were observed in 11(79 %) studies. The Cox regression model was incorporated in 10 (71 %) studies. None of the studies assessed the Cox proportional hazards assumption or goodness-of-fit.

Conclusions: The use and reporting of survival analysis in adult ALL patients undergoing allo-SCT have significant limitations. Notably, the finding of crossing survival curves was common and none of the studies assessed for the proportional hazards assumption. We encourage authors, reviewers and editors to improve the quality of the use and reporting of survival analysis in the hematology literature.

Keywords: Acute lymphoblastic leukemia, Mortality, Systematic review, Regression analysis

Background

Survival analysis measures the time from a defined starting point to the occurrence of an interested event where the risk changes over time. The goals of survival analysis serve three purposes: (1) to estimate survival and hazard functions from survival data, (2) to compare survival and hazard functions between groups and (3) to assess the relationship between predictor variables and survival time. The essential components for survival analysis include the time to event and the binary event outcome (success or failure).

* Correspondence: iorioa@mcmaster.ca
[1]Departments of Clinical Epidemiology and Biostatistics, McMaster University, Hamilton, Canada
[2]Departments of Medicine, McMaster University, Hamilton, Canada
Full list of author information is available at the end of the article

The probability of survival can be represented generating a Kaplan-Meier (KM) curve from survival data. Indeed, the KM plot is based on the estimate of the conditional probability of the time to failure [1] calculated at each time point recording an event. The difference in survival between two or more groups (or the treatment effect if treatment is what defines the two groups) can be commonly compared using the log-rank test [2].

The Cox proportional hazard (PH) model is a widely used regression method for survival data. The Cox PH model estimates the effect of predictor variables using the hazard function which does not require specifying a baseline hazard rate [3]. The measure of the effect, unadjusted or adjusted for covariates, is demonstrated as a hazard ratio (HR) which is expressed as an exponent of a regression coefficient in the model. An important property of the Cox PH model is that the PH assumption requires the hazard ratio to be constant over time [4]. Therefore, the Cox PH model is considered to be a semi-parametric model. Other regression models that can be used for survival analysis include an extended Cox PH model or parametric survival model (Weibull, exponential, log-logistic, lognormal, etc.) [5].

A recent systematic review demonstrated that survival analysis was incorporated in only 29 % of internal medicine articles [6]. However, there has been an increasing trend to using survival analysis in all categories of medical journals [6].

Allogeneic stem cell transplantation (allo-SCT) is the most potent post-remission therapy in adult acute lymphoblastic leukemia (ALL). The benefit of allo-SCT in adult ALL remains controversial [7]. Survival analysis is generally used to determine the treatment effect among ALL patients who undergo allo-SCT or other treatments, both in terms of prolongation and increased likelihood of survival. Allo-SCT is associated with high treatment-related mortality. Patients who tolerate the treatment are more likely to have a prolong event free survival and overall survival. On the other hand, non allo-SCT is less intensive treatment but may be associated with lower long-term event free survival. ALL literature were chosen because we expected that the use and report of survival analysis in such articles are complicated. To investigate whether the heterogeneity in study results is at least in part explained by a more or less appropriate use of time to event analysis, we conducted a systematic review of clinical trials which investigated the efficacy and safety of allo-SCT in adult patients with acute ALL. The aim of this study was to evaluate the use and reporting of survival analyses in these articles.

Methods

Data sources

We performed a systematic review by searching in the MEDLINE, EMBASE and The Cochrane library (The Cochrane Register of Controlled Trials and Cochrane Database of Systematic Reviews) databases. The reference lists were searched from the retrieved articles. The search terms were: Bone Marrow Transplantation OR Hematopoietic Stem Cell Transplantation OR Peripheral Blood Stem Cell Transplantation AND nonmyeloblat* OR non-myeloblat* OR Precursor Cell Lymphoblastic Leukemia-Lymphoma OR lymphoblast* OR lymphoid. AND (random* OR RCT OR control* OR trial). The database search was performed from inception to April 2015 with no language restrictions.

Selection criteria

The studies were included if they met the following criteria; were a clinical trial, controlled clinical trial or randomized control trial with allo-SCT compared to autologous SCT or non-transplantation therapy in patients with ALL in first complete remission. We only included studies that used survival analysis as one of the statistical methods.

Study selection and data extraction

Two investigators (CC and CH) independently identified articles using predefined inclusion criteria. Disagreements were resolved by consensus. Two investigators (CC and CH) independently extracted the data using a standardized data extraction from. Disagreements were again resolved by consensus.

We collected the following data: study design, outcome of interest (death, relapse), number of patients and number of events, survival curves estimate, regression method to estimate the hazard rate (Cox PH model or parametric survival model), methods for comparing the survival curves, the shape of the survival curves, variable selection, model building strategy, censoring description, length of follow-up, sample size calculation, test of interaction between variables, test for time dependent covariates, test for proportionality assumption and test for goodness-of-fit.

Analytic criteria

To evaluate the quality of reporting survival analyses, we used the following list of criteria for the proper use and description of the survival analyses.

1. *Sample size:* We evaluated the methods that the investigators described for sample size calculation. In addition, in the studies that used multiple regression analysis we evaluated the number of the events and number of covariates in order to estimate the adequacy of power. According to Peduzzi et al., approximately ten events per covariate is appropriate in PH regression analysis [8].
2. *Censoring description:* We evaluated the description of censoring and whether the investigators reported this adequately, inadequately or there was no mention.
3. *Survival curves:* We evaluated the statistical methods used for generating survival curves. For the comparison of survival between the groups, we documented the reported methods (log-rank test or Wilcoxon test). We also noted the shape of the survival curves (evenly separated or crossing survival curves).
4. *Statistical significance:* The statistical test used to evaluate the difference between two survival curves is determined using a log-rank test or weighted

log-rank test (e.g. Wilcoxon test). The null hypothesis of the test is that there is no difference between the two survival curves. We documented the statistical test reported in the articles.

5. *Regression model:* The statistical methods used for survival regression analysis were evaluated. We were interested in the regression model that the investigators used for calculating the hazard ratio (e.g. Cox PH model, extended Cox PH model or parametric survival model). We were also interested in the other regression models (time-dependent variable, competing risk analysis or repeated event analysis). In addition, the test for interaction of the variable was checked. For the studies that used multivariate regression, we assessed the description of variable selection and the strategy used for model building.
6. *Check for the PH assumption:* We assessed the test for PH assumption described in the articles. The assessment included methods used for checking PH assumption (graphical approach or the goodness-of-fit testing approach).
7. *Model checking:* We evaluated whether the investigators assessed for goodness-of-fit measures. The residual-based diagnostics were also assessed (martingale residuals, Cox-Snell residuals, Schoenfeld residuals or deviance residuals).

Results

Study characteristics

A total of 881 citations were identified by the systematic search strategy. Of these, 325 studies were duplicates. After screening of the titles and abstracts using predefined inclusion criteria, 541 studies were excluded. The reasons for exclusion are summarised in Fig. 1. Of these, we identified 15 potential studies for full-text review. Two studies were identified following manual review of the references. We excluded three studies due to no clinical trials comparing allo-SCT with other treatments. Thus, 14 studies [9–22] were included in our systematic review.

The study characteristics are summarised in Table 1. All of the studies were clinical trials. Patients were randomized to receive either allo-SCT or other treatments (autologous SCT or consolidation chemotherapy). Patients were allocated to undergo allo-SCT if the patient had a human leukocyte antigen (HLA) matched sibling donor, otherwise, the patient received autologous SCT or consolidation chemotherapy according to the study protocols. The median follow-up ranged from 59 to 114 months. The time-to-event outcomes in the included studies were overall survival and disease-free survival.

Analytic criteria

1. *Sample size*
   Sample size estimation was described in 4 of 14 studies (Table 2). The proportion of events per total patients ranged from 36 to 78 %. With respect to the sample size and number of covariates assessed in the regression analysis, only four studies reported the list of covariate assessed in the Cox regression model. Of these, two studies obtained more than ten events-per-covariate (event-per-covariate 20.4 and 23.2, respectively) [11, 13]. However, the other two studies had an event-per-covariate 8.3 [20] and 3.8 [22].
2. *Censoring description*
   There were six studies that provided the censoring description.

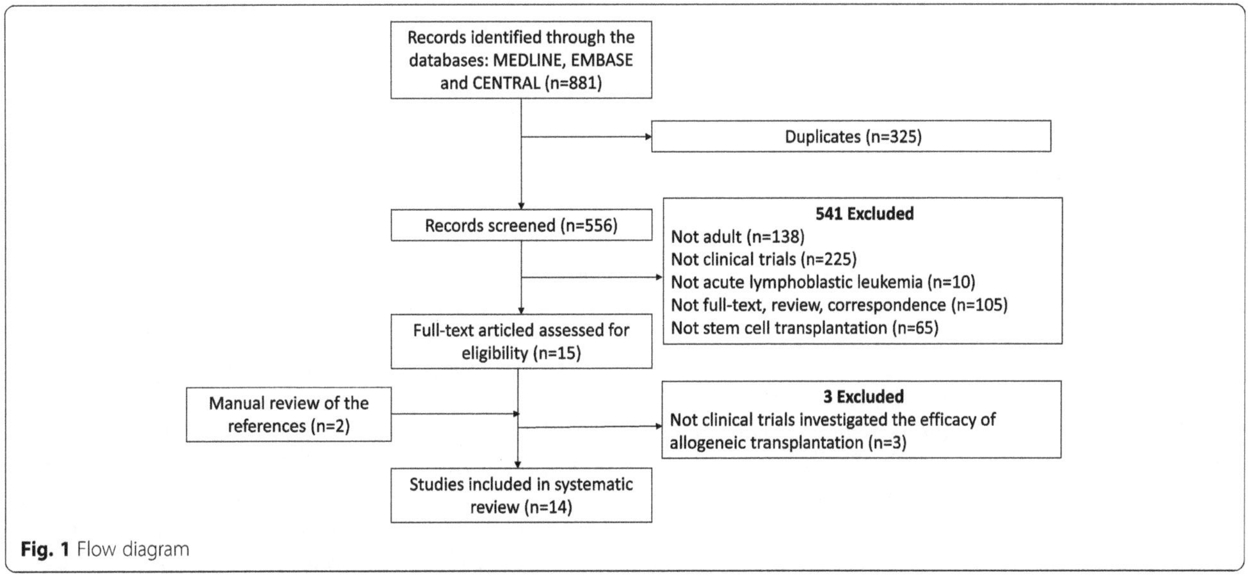

Fig. 1 Flow diagram

Table 1 Study characteristics

Study	Sample size		Median Follow-up (months)	Outcome	Design
	Allo-SCT	Non-allo-SCT			
Attal [9]	41	64	30	DFS	Randomized trial
Bernasconi [10]	11	29	48	DFS	Clinical trial
Cornelissen [11]	96	161	65	OS, DFS	Clinical trial
De Witte [12]	30	33	60	OS, DFS	Clinical trial
Fielding [13]	81	77	98	OS, DFS	Clinical trial
Goldstone [14]	443	588	59	OS, DFS	Clinical trial
Hunault [15]	41	106	61	OS, DFS	Randomized¶ trial
Ifrah [16]	18	32	60	DFS	Clinical trial
Labar [17]	68	116	114	OS, DFS	Clinical trial
Ribera [18]	84	98	70	OS, DFS	Clinical trial
Sebban [19]	116	141	62	OS, DFS	Clinical trial
Thomas [21]	100	159	62	OS, DFS	Clinical trial
Takeuchi [20]	34	108	63	OS, DFS	Clinical trial
Ueda [22]	17	40	62	OS, DFS	Clinical trial

Genetically randomization
Abbreviation: *Allo-SCT* allogeneic-stem cell transplantation, *DFS* disease free survival, *OS* overall survival

3. *Survival curves*
   All studies reported survival curves using the KM method. The comparisons between the groups were investigated using a log-rank test in all studies (two studies used both log-rank test and Wilcoxon test). With regards to the shape of the survival curves, 11 studies reported crossing survival curves [9–15, 17–20] whereas one study reported unevenly separate survival curves [21] and one study reported evenly separated survival curves [22]. The overlapping survival curves were observed in five studies [9, 12, 14, 17, 20]. We were not able to compare survival curves in one study where the graphs were plotted in the separately [16].
4. *Statistical significance*
   All of the studies reported the statistical test used to measure the difference between survival curves. Of these, five studies reported statistical significance for the treatment effect between groups. However, eight studies reported non-statistical significance (one study did not report).
5. *Regression model*
   The regression model was incorporated in 10 of 14 studies. All ten studies used the Cox PH model [9, 11, 14–18, 20–22]. There was no parametric survival analysis used in the included studies. One study mentioned the test for interaction and competing risk analysis [11]. None of the studies described variable selection. Only one study mentioned the strategy used for model building [18].
6. *Check for the PH assumption*
   In studies that used Cox PH model, PH assumption checking was not mentioned in any of the studies that used Cox PH model.
7. *Model checking*
   The summary measures of the regression diagnostic and goodness-of-fit were not mentioned in any of the studies.

Discussion

Our study demonstrates that survival analyses have been used extensively in the landmark trials evaluating all-SCT in adult patients with acute ALL. However, the majority of the trials poorly reported their statistical methods and results. Sample size estimation and censoring description were not routinely described. Almost all the presented survival curves crossed. Moreover, the Cox assumption was not assessed even if the investigators used the Cox PH model. In addition, goodness-of-fit or regression residual analysis were lacking in all of the trials.

Regarding the sample size estimation, according to Consolidated Standards of Reporting Trials (CONSORT), it is important that the authors indicate how sample size was determined [23]. The intent of the sample size estimation is to ensure that a particular study has sufficient statistical power to detect a difference in the treatment effect between groups. Our review demonstrates that only 4 of 14 (29 %) trials described a sample size estimation. With respect to the regression analysis, only four studies provided a full list of covariates. Of these, only two studies

Table 2 Reporting survival analyses in the included studies

Study	Sample size estimation	Event/total	Censoring	Survival curve	Shape of KM-curve	Significance	Regression model	Variable selection	Goodness of fit or PH assumption test
Attal [9]	Yes	86/135 (relapse)	NR	KM method, log-rank test	Crossing, overlapping	S	Cox-PH model	Informal	NR
Bernasconi [10]	NR	NR	NR	KM method, log-rank test	Crossing	NS	N/A	N/A	NR
Cornelissen [11]	NR	102/257 (death), 113/257 (relapse)	Yes	KM method, log-rank test	Crossing	NS	Cox-PH model, interaction, competing risk	Informal	NR
De Witte [12]	NR	32/66 (death)	NR	KM method, log-rank test, Wilcoxon test	Crossing, overlapping	S	N/A	N/A	NR
Fielding [13]	NR	116/165 (death)	NR	KM method, log-rank test	Crossing	NS	N/A	N/A	NR
Goldstone [14]	NR	531/1031 (death)	Yes	KM method, log-rank test	Crossing, overlapping	NS	Cox-PH model	N/A	NR
Hunault [15]	Yes	67/147 (death)	NR	KM method, log-rank test	Crossing	S	Cox-PH model	Informal	NR
Ifrah [16]	Yes	37/50 (relapse)	NR	KM method, log-rank test	Curves were plotted in two different graphs	N/A	Cox-PH model	Informal	NR
Labar [17]	NR	245/340 (death), 131/340 (relapse)	Yes	KM method, log-rank test	Crossing, overlapping	NS	Cox-PH model	Informal	NR
Ribera [18]	Yes	144/182 (death), 88/182 (relapse)	Yes	KM method, log-rank test	Crossing	NS	Cox-PH model	Informal	NR
Sebban [19]	NR	146/255 (death)	NR	KM method, log-rank test	Crossing	NS	N/A	N/A	NR
Thomas [21]	NR	177/259 (relapse)	NR	KM method, log-rank test	Unevenly separate	S	Cox-PH model	Informal	NR
Takeuchi [20]	NR	83/142 (death)	Yes	KM method, log-rank test	Crossing, overlapping	NS	Cox-PH model	Informal	NR
Ueda [22]	NR	38/57 (death)	Yes	KM method, log-rank test, Wilcoxon test	Evenly separate	S	Cox-PH model	Informal	NR

Abbreviation: *PH* proportional hazard, *NR* not reported, *N/A* not applicable; S, statistical significance; NS, non-statistical significance appeared to be sufficiently powered (event-to-covariate ratio more than 10).

In survival analysis, patients who do not experience the relevant outcome over the study period, patients who are lost to follow-up during the study period and patients who withdraw from the study are censored. There are three assumptions regarding censorship in survival analysis: independent, random and non-informative [4]. Thus, the description of censorship is an important aspect to report in publication. However, only 6 of 14 (43 %) trials described their censoring. More importantly, if relapse is the outcome of interest in these studies, patients who die from any cause will be censored. In this circumstance, censoring may be considered informative because patients may die from disease progression or treatment-related causes. Consequently, the results may change based on different censoring descriptions. Providing a definition of censorship is a critical component to reporting these trials in the literature.

All of the studies utilized survival curves. Not surprisingly, crossing survival curves were found in 10 of 14 studies. Allo-SCT is considered the most potent post remission therapy in adult ALL [24]. In long-term follow-up studies, the patients who underwent allo-SCT had a lower relapse rate due to a graft-versus-leukemia effect [11]. However, these patients had a higher early mortality rate from the toxicity of myeloablative chemotherapy when compared with patients who received autologous SCT or consolidation chemotherapy [11, 13]. Therefore, survival curves comparing these two treatments may be expected to cross at some point. Early death from treatment-related complications (commonly found in allo-SCT) and late death from relapsed disease (commonly found in autologous SCT) should be taken into the account in the treatment of ALL. Crossing survival curves make the interpretation of the treatment effects from the interventions much more complicated.

The log-rank test is the most common method used to compare the difference between survival curves based on the chi-square test [25]. It is important to note that the log-rank test may be invalid if the survival curves cross because of an increase of the probability of type II error. Moreover, the log-rank test may lose power in the circumstance of crossing survival curves [26]. Our study reveals that, among ten analyses with crossed survival curves, eight were non-statistically significant and two were statistically significant. We found that five studies had overlapping survival curves that might be explainable for insignificant findings of the interventions. It was difficult to make a conclusion on the rest of the studies based on the log-rank test of crossing over survival curves.

Strategies have been proposed to overcome the limitation of the log-rank test when the survival curves cross. The authors may consider analysing the survival curves at a fixed point in time [27]. Another alternative includes using a weighted log-rank (Harrington-Fleming) test which gives more weight to the later events [28]. Other weighted log-rank tests that may be useful are the methods developed by Gill et al. or Pepe and Fleming [29, 30]. Li et al. recently published a simulation study which investigated several statistical methods in the situation of crossing survival curves. This study showed that adaptive Neyman's smooth tests and the two-stage procedure provided greater stability and higher power as compared to the other methods [29].

Relapse disease and death are the most common outcomes in the ALL literature. Conventional KM method and Cox proportional hazard model convey no information regarding possible competing risks. Competing risk is an event that modifies the chance of the interested outcome [31]. For example, death from any cause is a competing risk for relapse disease. Using the competing risk analysis is therefore considered to be more appropriate in the treatment with high rate of complications. We observed only one study that used competing risk analysis [11]. We encouraged investigators to incorporate competing risk analysis, at least in the sensitivity analysis.

We found that the Cox PH model was commonly used in the collection of articles in our review. There was substantial inadequacy of the description of variable selection, the strategy used for fitting procedure and test for goodness-of-fit. As mentioned above, sample size estimation related to regression analysis was noted in only four studies. Of these, two studies were found to be underpowered based on low event-per-covariate ratio [8]. We strongly encourage authors to describe the process of variable selection, strategy of model building and provide evidence that the sample size is sufficient for regression analysis.

A lack of PH assumption checking may introduce bias to the regression analysis. Our review shows that none of the studies described an assessment of the PH assumption. The Cox PH model assumes that the hazard ratio for comparing any two groups of predictor variables is constant over time [4]. If this assumption is not met, the Cox PH model is not valid for the analysis. We observed that 11 of 14 (79 %) studies had crossing survival curves. A clear violation of the PH assumption occurs if survival curves cross [32, 33]. Therefore, a hazard ratio should not be used to compare the treatment effect between groups. We suggest that authors check for the PH assumption if the Cox PH model is incorporated in the analysis. When the PH assumption is violated, authors may consider using an alternative regression analysis, such as the extended Cox PH model or parametric survival analysis (Weibull, exponential, log-logistic or lognormal model).

Conclusions

Our systematic review evaluating reporting methods for survival analysis in adult ALL patients undergoing allo-SCT show significant shortcomings in the use and reporting of survival analysis. Sample size estimation was not routinely described and studies are frequently statistically underpowered. There was a lack of censoring description. Most notably, crossing survival curves were common and none of the studies checked for the PH assumption. Finally, the description of variable selection, fitting procedure and model checking were neglected.

Survival analysis has been used increasingly in medical research studies [6]. We raise awareness of these limitations and encourage authors, reviewers and editors to improve the quality of the use and reporting survival analysis in the literature.

Abbreviations

ALL, acute lymphoblastic leukemia; CONSORT, Consolidated Standards of Reporting Trials; HLA, human leukocyte antigen; HR, hazard ratio; KM, Kaplan-Meier; PH, proportional hazard; SCT, stem cell transplantation

Acknowledgements

Not applicable.

Funding

Not applicable.

Authors' contributions

CC, AL, MC participated in the design of the study, CC, CH performed study selection, data abstraction, CC performed data analysis, CC drafted the manuscript, CH, WL, AI, MC read and approved the final manuscript.

Authors' information

Not applicable.

Competing interests

MC discloses having sat on advisory boards for Janssen, Leo Pharma, Portola, and AKP America. MC holds a Career Investigator award from the Heart and Stroke Foundation of Ontario, and the Leo Pharma Chair in Thromboembolism Research at McMaster University. MC's institution has received funding for research projects from Leo Pharma. MC has received funding for presentations from Leo Pharma, Bayer, Celgene, Shire and CSL Behring. CC, CH, AI and WL have no relevant conflicts of interest.

Author details

[1]Departments of Clinical Epidemiology and Biostatistics, McMaster University, Hamilton, Canada. [2]Departments of Medicine, McMaster University, Hamilton, Canada. [3]Departments of Oncology, McMaster University, Hamilton, Canada.

References

1. Clark TG, Bradburn MJ, Love SB, Altman DG. Survival analysis part I: basic concepts and first analyses. Br J Cancer. 2003;89(2):232–8.
2. Peto R, Pike MC, Armitage P, Breslow NE, Cox DR, Howard SV, Mantel N, McPherson K, Peto J, Smith PG. Design and analysis of randomized clinical trials requiring prolonged observation of each patient. II. Analysis and examples. Br J Cancer. 1977;35(1):1–39.
3. Cox DR. Regression models and life-tables. J R Stat Soc. 1972;34(2):187–220.
4. Kleinbaum DG, MKlein M. Survival analysis: A self-lerning text, thrid edition. 3rd ed. New York: Springer Sciences + Business Media; 2012.
5. Bradburn MJ, Clark TG, Love SB, Altman DG. Survival analysis part II: multivariate data analysis–an introduction to concepts and methods. Br J Cancer. 2003;89(3):431–6.
6. Abraira V, Muriel A, Emparanza JI, Pijoan JI, Royuela A, Plana MN, Cano A, Urreta I, Zamora J. Reporting quality of survival analyses in medical journals still needs improvement. A minimal requirements proposal. J Clin Epidemiol. 2013;66(12):1340–6. e1345.
7. Ribera JM. Allogeneic stem cell transplantation for adult acute lymphoblastic leukemia: when and how. Haematologica. 2011;96(8):1083–6.
8. Peduzzi P, Concato J, Feinstein AR, Holford TR. Importance of events per independent variable in proportional hazards regression analysis. II. Accuracy and precision of regression estimates. J Clin Epidemiol. 1995;48(12):1503–10.
9. Attal M, Blaise D, Marit G, Payen C, Michallet M, Vernant JP, Sauvage C, Troussard X, Nedellec G, Pico J, et al. Consolidation treatment of adult acute lymphoblastic leukemia: a prospective, randomized trial comparing allogeneic versus autologous bone marrow transplantation and testing the impact of recombinant interleukin-2 after autologous bone marrow transplantation. BGMT Group. Blood. 1995;86(4):1619–28.
10. Bernasconi C, Lazzarino M, Morra E, Alessandrino EP, Pagnucco G, Resegotti L, Locatelli F, Ficarra F, Bacigalupo A, Carella AM, et al. Early intensification followed by allo-BMT or auto-BMT or a second intensification in adult ALL: a randomized multicenter study. Leukemia. 1992;6(2):204–8.
11. Cornelissen JJ, van der Holt B, Verhoef GE, van't Veer MB, van Oers MH, Schouten HC, Ossenkoppele G, Sonneveld P, Maertens J, van Marwijk Kooy M, et al. Myeloablative allogeneic versus autologous stem cell transplantation in adult patients with acute lymphoblastic leukemia in first remission: a prospective sibling donor versus no-donor comparison. Blood. 2009;113(6):1375–82.
12. De Witte T, Awwad B, Boezeman J, Schattenberg A, Muus P, Raemaekers J, Preijers F, Strijckmans P, Haanen C. Role of allogenic bone marrow transplantation in adolescent or adult patients with acute lymphoblastic leukaemia or lymphoblastic lymphoma in first remission. Bone Marrow Transplant. 1994;14(5):767–74.
13. Fielding AK, Rowe JM, Richards SM, Buck G, Moorman AV, Durrant IJ, Marks, DI, McMillan AK, Litzow MR, Lazarus HM, Foroni L, Dewald G, Franklin IM, Luger SM, Paietta E, Wiernik PH, Tallman MS, Goldstone AH. Prospective outcome data on 267 unselected adult patients with Philadelphia chromosome-positive acute lymphoblastic leukemia confirms superiority of allogeneic transplantation over chemotherapy in the pre-imatinib era: results from the International ALL Trial MRC UKALLXII/ECOG2993. Blood. 2009;113(19):4489–96.
14. Goldstone AH, Richards SM, Lazarus HM, Tallman MS, Buck G, Fielding AK, Burnett AK, Chopra R, Wiernik PH, Foroni L, Paietta E, Litzow MR, Marks DI, Durrant J, McMillan A, Franklin IM, Luger S, Ciobanu N, Rowe JM. In adults with standard-risk acute lymphoblastic leukemia, the greatest benefit is achieved from a matched sibling allogeneic transplantation in first complete remission, and an autologous transplantation is less effective than conventional consolidation/maintenance chemotherapy in all patients: final results of the International ALL Trial (MRC UKALL XII/ECOG E2993). Blood. 2008;111:1827–33.
15. Hunault M, Harousseau JL, Delain M, Truchan-Graczyk M, Cahn JY, Witz F, Lamy T, Pignon B, Jouet JP, Garidi R, Caillot D, Berthou C, Guyotat D, Sadoun A, Sotto JJ, Lioure B, Casassus P, Solal-Celigny P, Stalnikiewicz L, Audhuy B, Blanchet O, Baranger L, Bene MC, Ifrah N, Goelams Group. Better outcome of adult acute lymphoblastic leukemia after early genoidentical allogeneic bone marrow transplantation (BMT) than after late high-dose therapy and autologous BMT: a GOELAMS trial. Blood. 2004;104(10):3028–37.

16. Ifrah N, Witz F, Jouet JP, Francois S, Lamy T, Linassier C, Pignon B, Berthou C, Guyotat D, Cahn JY, Harousseau JL. Intensive short term therapy with granulocyte-macrophage-colony stimulating factor support, similar to therapy for acute myeloblastic leukemia, does not improve overall results for adults with acute lymphoblastic leukemia. GOELAMS Group. Cancer. 1999;86(8):1496–505.
17. Labar B, Suciu S, Zittoun R, Muus P, Marie JP, Fillet G, Peetermans M, Stryckmans P, Willemze R, Feremans W, Jaksic B, Bourhis JH, Burghouts JP, Witte T. Allogeneic stem cell transplantation in acute lymphoblastic leukemia and non-Hodgkin's lymphoma for patients < or = 50 years old in first complete remission: results of the EORTC ALL-3 trial. Haematologica. 2004;89:809–17.
18. Ribera JM, Oriol A, Bethencourt C, Parody R, Hernandez-Rivas JM, Moreno MJ, del Potro E, Torm M, Rivas C, Besalduch J, Sanz MA, Ortega JJ, Pethema Group Spain. Comparison of intensive chemotherapy, allogeneic or autologous stem cell transplantation as post-remission treatment for adult patients with high-risk acute lymphoblastic leukemia. Results of the PETHEMA ALL-93 trial. Haematologica. 2005;90(10):1346–56.
19. Sebban C, Lepage E, Vernant JP, Gluckman E, Attal M, Reiffers J, Sutton L, Racadot E, Michallet M, Maraninchi D, et al. Allogeneic bone marrow transplantation in adult acute lymphoblastic leukemia in first complete remission: a comparative study. French group of therapy of adult acute lymphoblastic leukemia. J Clin Oncol. 1994;12(12):2580–7.
20. Takeuchi J, Kyo T, Naito K, Sao H, Takahashi M, Miyawaki S, Kuriyama K, Ohtake S, Yagasaki F, Murakami H, Asou N, Ino T, Okamoto T, Usui N, Nishimura M, Shinagawa K, Fukushima T, Taguchi H, Morii, T, Mizuta S, Akiyama H, Nakamura Y, Ohshima T, Ohno R. Induction therapy by frequent administration of doxorubicin with four other drugs, followed by intensive consolidation and maintenance therapy for adult acute lymphoblastic leukemia: the JALSG-ALL93 study. Leukemia. 2002;16(7):1259–66.
21. Thomas X, Boiron JM, Huguet F, Dombret H, Bradstock K, Vey N, Kovacsovics T, Delannoy A, Fegueux N, Fenaux P, Stamatoullas A, Vernant JP, Tournilhac O, Buzyn A, Reman O, Charrin, C, Boucheix C, Gabert J, Lheritier V, Fiere D. Outcome of treatment in adults with acute lymphoblastic leukemia: analysis of the LALA-94 trial. J Clin Oncol. 2004;22(20):4075–86.
22. Ueda T, Miyawaki S, Asou N, Kuraishi Y, Hiraoka A, Kuriyama K, Minami S, Ohshima T, Ino T, Tamura J, Kanamaru A, Nishikawa K, Tanimoto M, Oh H, Saito K, Nagata K, Naoe T, Yamada O, Urasaki Y, Sakura T, Ohno R. Response-oriented individualized induction therapy with six drugs followed by four courses of intensive consolidation, 1 year maintenance and intensification therapy: the ALL90 study of the Japan adult leukemia study group. [erratum appears in Int J hematol 1998 Dec;68(4):i-ii]. Int J Hematol. 1998;68(3):279–89.
23. Moher D, Hopewell S, Schulz KF, Montori V, Gotzsche PC, Devereaux PJ, Elbourne D, Egger M, Altman DG. CONSORT 2010 explanation and elaboration: updated guidelines for reporting parallel group randomised trials. BMJ. 2010;340:c869.
24. Goldstone AH, Rowe JM. Transplantation in adult ALL. Hematology Am Soc Hematol Educ Program 2009:593–601.
25. Rich JT, Neely JG, Paniello RC, Voelker CC, Nussenbaum B, Wang EW. A practical guide to understanding Kaplan-Meier curves. Otolaryngol Head Neck Surg. 2010;143(3):331–6.
26. Liu K, Qiu P, Sheng J. Comparing two crossing hazard rates by Cox proportional hazards modelling. Stat Med. 2007;26(2):375–91.
27. Klein JP, Logan B, Harhoff M, Andersen PK. Analyzing survival curves at a fixed point in time. Stat Med. 2007;26(24):4505–19.
28. Logan BR, Klein JP, Zhang MJ. Comparing treatments in the presence of crossing survival curves: an application to bone marrow transplantation. Biometrics. 2008;64(3):733–40.
29. Li H, Han D, Hou Y, Chen H, Chen Z. Statistical inference methods for two crossing survival curves: a comparison of methods. PLoS One. 2015;10(1):e0116774.
30. Pepe MS, Fleming TR. Weighted Kaplan-Meier statistics: a class of distance tests for censored survival data. Biometrics. 1989;45(2):497–507.
31. Satagopan JM, Ben-Porat L, Berwick M, Robson M, Kutler D, Auerbach AD. A note on competing risks in survival data analysis. Br J Cancer. 2004;91(7):1229–35.
32. Bouliotis G, Billingham L. Crossing survival curves: alternatives to the log-rank test. Trials. 2011;12 Suppl 1:A137.
33. Seruga B, Amir E, Tannock I. Treatment of lung cancer. N Engl J Med. 2009;361(25):2485. author reply 2486–2487.

4

Sickle-cell disease in febrile children living in a rural village of Madagascar and association with malaria and respiratory infections

Muriel N. Maeder[1], Henintsoa M. Rabezanahary[1], Norosoa J. Zafindraibe[1], Martin Raoelina Randriatiana[2], Tahinamandranto Rasamoelina[1,3], Andry T. Rakotoarivo[3], Philippe Vanhems[4,5], Jonathan Hoffmann[4], Thomas Bénet[4,5], Mala Rakoto Andrianarivelo[1*] and Olivat A. Rakoto-Alson[6]

Abstract

Background: In Madagascar, the last study on sickle cell disease (SCD) was done in the early 1980s. The country is known as endemic for malaria and respiratory infections. The main objective of this study was to estimate the prevalence of SCD; the secondary objective was to evaluate its association with malaria and respiratory infections.

Methods: This is a cross-sectional study which was carried out in a rural village in the south east coast of Madagascar between May 2011 and November 2013. Participants were children aged between 2–59 months presenting with fever measured by axillary temperature ≥37.5 °C at inclusion. Genotyping of haemoglobin S was done by PCR and malaria was diagnosed by Rapid Diagnostic Test. Research for viral and atypical bacterial respiratory pathogens was performed on nasopharyngeal swabs. Uni-and multivariate polytomous logistic regression was done to assess associations between microbiological results and SCD status, with HbAA phenotype as reference.

Results: A total of 807 children were analysed. Prevalence of SCD among febrile children was 2.4% (95% CI, 1.5–3.7%) and that of SCT was 23.8% (95% CI, 20.9–26.9%). There was no difference in the prevalence of malaria infection according to haemoglobin status ($p = 0.3$). Rhinovirus (22.5%), adenovirus (14.1%), and bocavirus (11.6%) were the most common respiratory pathogens detected. After univariate analysis, patients with SCD were more frequently infected by parechovirus ($p = 0.01$), while patients with SCT were more prone to RSV A or B infection ($p = 0.01$). After multivariate analysis, HbAS phenotype was associated with higher risk of RSV A and B infection compared to HbAA (adjusted $OR = 1.9$; 95% CI: 1.2–3.1, $p = 0.009$), while HbSS phenotype was associated with higher risk of parechovirus infection (adjusted $OR = 6.0$; 95% CI: 1.1–31.3, $p = 0.03$) compared to HbAA, independently of age, gender, period per quarter, and the other viruses.

Conclusion: The prevalence of SCD among under-five children presenting with fever was high in the study population. No association was found between SCT and malaria but few viruses, especially parechovirus, seem to play an important role in the occurrence of pneumoniae among SCD patients.

Keywords: Sickle-cell disease, Fever, Malaria, Respiratory Infections, Children, Madagascar

* Correspondence: mala@cicm-madagascar.com
[1]Centre d'Infectiologie Charles Mérieux, Université Antananarivo, P.O. Box 4299, Antananarivo, Madagascar
Full list of author information is available at the end of the article

Background

During its 59th World Health Assembly held in 2006, WHO recognized sickle-cell disease (SCD), an inherited disorder of haemoglobin as a priority of public health. A resolution was adopted to develop and strengthen efforts for its prevention and management. Sickle-cell anaemia, one of the most common forms of SCD, is due to a point mutation within the sixth codon of the β-globin chain. The produced abnormal variant – haemoglobin S (HbS) – is responsible for chronic haemolytic anaemia and vaso-occlusion which are the underlying causes of the clinical presentation of SCD. Individuals who express the homozygous form (HbSS) manifest the disease, while those with the heterozygous form (HbAS), also known as sickle-cell trait (SCT), are usually asymptomatic carriers.

Initially limited to the sub-Saharan Africa, the Middle-East and some parts of India [1], SCD has currently spread to all continents with the migration of populations. The βS-globin gene is found on five common haplotypes in Africa (Bantu, Benin, Cameroon and Senegal) and Asia (Saudi Arab-Indian) [2] that can be used as a marker of genetic diversity and population origin. Approximately 300,000 children with severe haemoglobin disorders are born every year worldwide [3] and over 75% of SCD occur in Africa where carrier frequency ranged from 1% (Central African Republic, Senegal) to 38% (United Republic of Tanzania) [1]. In Madagascar, several studies conducted in 1950s had estimated the general prevalence of SCD from 4% in the Central highlands [4] to 11-13% in the South-eastern coast [5]. Significant ethnical variation and high prevalence in asymptomatic carrier up to 28% were also reported [6]. To our knowledge, the last published study was done in the early 1980s [7]. These studies, however, were based on the detection of sickle red blood cells in hypoxic conditions, also known as "sickling test", and the sickle solubility test [3] now considered as obsolete techniques.

In area where malaria is endemic, its relation with SCT was often studied, in particular the high degree of resistance to severe and complicated malaria in sickle cell trait [8, 9]. Malaria is endemic in Madagascar with strong and persistent transmission in the east coast [10].

From May 2011 to November 2013, a cross-sectional study was conducted in the rural village of Ampasimanjeva in the south east cost of Madagascar aiming to identify blood-borne protein biomarkers that can differentiate the causes of unexplained acute febrile illness in children. The study site is known for its high endemicity to malaria, acute respiratory infections and SCD. The main objective of this study was to estimate the prevalence of SCD; the secondary objective was to evaluate its association with malaria and respiratory infections.

Methods

Study design and population

This is an observational cross-sectional study with prospective data collection of children aged between 2 to 59 months presenting with fever (axillary temperature ≥37.5 °C according to WHO criteria). The study was conducted from May 2011 to November 2013 in the rural village of Ampasimanjeva located in the south east cost of Madagascar. Ampasimanjeva is 320 km away from the capital city Antananarivo with a total inhabitant estimated to be 22,000 according to the last census. The east coast has hot and humid subequatorial climate and an annual high cumulative rainfall of 4,000 mm per year. Transmission of malaria in this region is reported to be strong and intense all over time. A standardized questionnaire on socio-demographic and clinical data was fulfilled for each individual. The Ampasimanjeva community hospital is a Hospital District Centre receiving each year around 950 children between 2 and 5 years old. Acute Respiratory Infections were the main cause of morbidity accounting for 35% of consultation all ages combined.

Ethical approval for the study was obtained from the National Ethical Committee of the Ministry of Health of Madagascar (authorization 019-CE/MINSAN as of 09/04/2010). Individual written informed consent was provided by the parents of all study participants.

Sample collection

For each child, venous blood was collected with safety blood containers on dry and spray-dried EDTA. The samples were transported in a refrigerated container at +4 °C to the Centre d'Infectiologie Charles Mérieux for analysis. Transport of samples was organized twice a week.

Genotyping of haemoglobin

After DNA extraction (QIAamp DNA Mini Kit, Qiagen, Germany) of the EDTA blood samples, the mutation responsible for the generation of HbS was identified by Restriction Fragment Length Polymorphism (RFLP) assay of PCR-amplified DNA (Bio-Rad, USA) [11]. The RFLP pattern of the normal profile (HbAA) of healthy subject is characterized by the presence of the restriction endonuclease Dde*I* site and cleaved in 2 fragments (189 and 93 bp). The homozygous profile (HbSS) responsible of the disease has no restriction site and only one fragment of 282 bp is observed. The heterozygous profile (HbAS) also known as sickle-cell trait combines restriction and no restriction site and reveals 3 fragments (93, 189, and 282 bp).

Malaria assays

Rapid Diagnostic Test (RDT) of malaria was performed on site using CareStart™ Malaria (Access Bio, Inc., New

Jersey, USA) and parasite density was estimated microscopically from the positive samples as previously described [12].

Detection of respiratory pathogens

Bacterial and viral DNAs as well as viral RNA were extracted from the nasopharyngeal swabs using RTP® Pathogen kit (STRATEC Molecular, Germany). A multiplex real-time PCR assay allowing the identification of 22 respiratory pathogens (Fast-track Diagnostics respiratory pathogens kit, FTD Luxembourg) was used as previously described [13]. Following nucleic extraction of EDTA-whole blood samples, another multiplex real-time PCR assay was performed to identify *Staphylococcus aureus, Streptococcus pneumoniae* and *Haemophilus influenzae* type b as previously described [14]. All RNA/DNA amplifications and detections were done using Bio-Rad CFX96 machine (Bio-Rad, USA).

Statistical analysis

Categorical variables were described as number and percentage with their 95% confidence intervals (CI); continuous covariates were described as median and interquartile range (IQR). The Chi2 test or Fisher's exact test was used to compare categorical variables. Continuous covariates were compared by Mann–Whitney *U*-test or Kruskal–Wallis one-way analysis of variance. Univariate and multivariate polytomous logistic regression analysis was done to assess microbiological results associated with haemoglobin status, where the normal phenotype was the reference (HbAA).

Statistical analyses were done using Epi Info™ 7.1.3 (Centers for Disease Control and Prevention, Atlanta, Georgia) and Stat 13.0 (StataCorp). All tests were 2-tailed and a *p*-value of less than 0.05 was considered significant.

Results

Sample size of eligible children

There were 862 children enrolled in the survey. Among them, 55 were excluded because not meeting the age and temperature criteria and because of inadequate blood sample. Subsequently, a total of 807 children were selected for the final analysis.

Demographic and health status

Out of the 807 children participating in the survey, 401 (49.7%) were male and the median age was 20 months (IQR: 10–36 months). The median temperature at inclusion was 38.8 °C (IQR: 38.5–39.4 °C). To assess the weight gain and growth, anthropometric parameters of children were measured [15]. The median upper arm circumference was 140 mm (IQR: 132–146 mm). The median weight-for-height Z-score was–1.5 (IQR:–2,2; 0.7); and 245 (30.5%) had weight-for-height Z-score ≤–2SD. The main reasons for medical consultation were malaria (36.6%), pneumonia (33.2%), acute respiratory infection (28.5%), and asthma (1.6%). Pneumococcal Conjugate Vaccine was introduced in 2012 and the national coverage was 76% in 2013 according to WHO and UNICEF estimates. However no information on the vaccination status against *S. pneumoniae* is available among the study population.

Genotyping of haemoglobin S

To identify the genotype of haemoglobin, the PCR-products from all 807 blood samples were digested and analyzed by the RFLP method. The results of the first 100 genotyping assay were compared to those of the electrophoresis of haemoglobin on alkaline (pH 8.5) agarose gels (Hydragel 7 Hemoglobine, Sebia, Evry, France) and 100% concordant identification was observed (data not shown). Overall, 73.9% (95% CI, 70.7–76.8%) children expressed the normal phenotype HbAA, whereas the prevalence of SCT (heterozygous HbAS) was 23.8% (95% CI, 20.9–26.9%) and that of SCD (homozygous HbSS) was 2.4% (95% CI, 1.5–3.6%).

To classify the nutritional status of the study population, we evaluated the mean weight-for-height Z-score. Individuals with HbSS showed a lower value [–2.2 SD (–3.4;–1.2)] compared to those with HbAS [–1.2 SD (–2.2;–0.5)] or HbAA [–1.5 SD (–2.2; –0.7)] phenotypes ($p = 0.02$), suggesting a state of undernutrition (Table 1). These findings were supported by a significant difference in the values of mid-upper arm circumference between the 3 groups ($p = 0.001$). We also found a higher prevalence of males among individuals with HbSS (68.4%) compared to the HbAS (42.7%) and HbAA (51.3%) groups ($p = 0.03$).

Malaria RDT and microscopy

Out of the 807 children, RDT showed 295 (36.6%; 95% CI, 33.3–39.9%) positive results of which 273 Giemsa-stained thick smear tests were done. The microscopic results showed that 197/273 (72.2%) infections were caused by *Plasmodium falciparum*, 2/273 (0.7%) were due to both *P. falciparum* and *P. vivax*, and the others were negative (74/273, 27.1%). There was no association between haemoglobin status and malaria infection (Table 1). Strikingly, no children with HbS below 2 years of age were infected; however, a trend in an increased detection rate of *P. falciparum* in older children with HbAS and HbSS was observed (Fig. 1).

Respiratory pathogens infection

Overall, 698 (91.4%; 95% CI, 89.1–93.2%) were positive for at least 1 bacterial pathogen and 575 (75.3%; 95% CI, 72.1–78.3%) for at least 1 viral pathogen. Co-detection of at least two viruses or both bacteria and virus was observed in 186 (24.4%; 95% CI, 21.4–27.6%) and 527 (69.0%; 95% CI, 65.5–72.2%) of cases, respectively.

Table 1 Characteristics of study population by haemoglobin phenotype

Characteristics	HbAA ($n = 596$)	HbAS ($n = 192$)	HbSS ($n = 19$)	p
Period, quarter, N (%)				
- January-March	72 (12.1)	31 (16.1)	3 (15.8)	0.19
- April-June	195 (32.7)	57 (29.7)	7 (36.8)	
- July-September	135 (22.6)	54 (28.1)	6 (31.6)	
- October-December	194 (32.5)	50 (26.0)	3 (15.8)	
Age, months, median (IQR)	21.0 (10.5–36.0)	20.0 (9.0–36.5)	17.0 (10.0–33.0)	0.50
Age category, months, n (%)				
- 2–11	160 (26.8)	62 (32.3)	6 (31.6)	0.68
- 12–23	152 (25.5)	45 (23.4)	5 (26.3)	
- 24–59	284 (47.7)	85 (44.3)	8 (42.1)	
Gender, n (%)				
- Male	306 (51.3)	82 (42.7)	13 (68.4)	0.03
- Female	290 (48.7)	110 (57.3)	6 (31.6)	
Temperature, °C, median (IQR)	38.8 (38.6–39.4)	38.8 (38.6–39.4)	38.5 (38.0–38.7)	0.11
Height, cm, median (IQR)	78.0 (71.0–87.0)	77.0 (69.5–86.0)	74.0 (69.0–86.0)	0.18
Weight, kg, median (IQR)	9.5 (8.1–11.6)	9.3 (7.9–11.4)	8.5 (7.2–10.0)	0.61
Mid-upper arm circumference, cm, median (IQR)	140 (133–146)	140 (132–148)	128 (117–136)	0.001
Weight-for-height Z-score ≤2 SD	−1.5 (−2.2; −0.7)	−1.2 (−2.2; −0.5)	−2.2 (−3.4; −1.2)	0.02
Positive RDT malaria, n (%)	227 (38.1)	63 (32.8)	5 (26.3)	0.3
Naso-pharyngeal carriers positive detection, n (%)				
- Parechovirus	9 (1.6)	1 (0.6)	2 (11.1)	0.02
- RSV A and B	56 (9.8)	30 (17.0)	0 (0)	0.01
- Human coronavirus 229E	6 (1.1)	0 (0)	1 (5.6)	0.07
- Viral coinfection	144 (25.3)	34 (19.2)	8 (44.4)	0.03
S. pneumoniae positive from blood, n (%)	11 (1.9)	3 (1.6)	1 (5.3)	0.5

* HbAA, normal phenotype, *HbAS* sickle cell trait, *HbSS* sickle cell disease

Carriage rate of *S. pneumoniae* was very high (88.9%; 95% CI, 86.4–91.0%) and reached all (100%) children in the HbSS group compared to the HbAS (89.8%; 95% CI, 84.4–93.9%) and HbAA (88.2%; 95% CI, 85.2–90.7%) groups.

Out of 764 nasopharyngeal samples tested, rhinovirus (22.5%; 95% CI, 19.7–25.6%; $n = 172$), adenovirus (14.1%; 95% CI, 11.8–16.8%; $n = 108$), bocavirus (11.6%; 95% CI, 9.6–14.1%; $n = 89$), respiratory syncytial virus A or B (11.3%; 95% CI, 9.2–13.7%; $n = 86$), and human metapneumovirus A and B (9.0%; 95% CI, 7.1–11.3%; $n = 69$) were the most common respiratory pathogens detected; *Chlamydia pneumoniae* and *Mycoplasma pneumoniae* accounted for < 2.0% of cases (Fig. 2).

Parechovirus was most frequently detected from respiratory sample in HbSS patients ($n = 2$, 11.1%) compared to the HbAA ($n = 9$, 1.6%) and HbAS ($n = 1$, 0.6%) patients ($p = 0.02$). Similar results were observed with human coronavirus 229E where patients in the HbSS group yielded high positive result ($n = 1$, 5.6%) compared to the HbAA ($n = 6$, 1.1%) and HbAS ($n = 0$) groups ($p = 0.07$) (Table 1). Conversely, respiratory syncytial virus A and B infection were more frequent in HbAS individuals ($n = 30$, 17.0%) compared to HbAA ($n = 56$, 9.8%) and HbSS ($n = 0$) patients ($p = 0.01$). Viral coinfection were frequent in the HbSS group ($n = 8$, 44.4%) compared to the HbAA ($n = 144$, 25.3%) and HbAS ($n = 34$, 19.2%) groups ($p = 0.03$).

Univariate polytomous regression disclosed the risk of respiratory syncytial virus A and B which was 2-fold more higher in HbAS compared to HbAA groups (crude odds ratio [OR] = 1.9; 95% CI: 1.2–3.0, $p = 0.01$), and the risk of parechovirus infection which was higher in HbSS compared to HbAA groups (crude $OR = 7.8$; 95% CI: 1.6–38.9; $p = 0.01$) [Table 2]. After multivariate analysis, HbAS compared with HbAA phenotype remained associated with higher risk of RSV A and B infection (adjusted $OR = 1.9$; 95% CI: 1.2–3.1, $p = 0.01$), independently of age, gender, period per quarter, and parechovirus infection. HbSS compared with HbAA phenotype remained associated with higher risk of parechovirus infection (adjusted $OR = 6.0$; 95% CI: 1.1–

Table 2 Microbiological findings associated with heamoglobin status, univariate polytomous logistic regression

Microorganism	Heterozygous form HbAS ($n = 177$)		Homozygous form HbSS ($n = 19$)	
	Crude odds ratio (95% CI)*	p	Crude odds ratio (95% CI)*	p
> = 1 bacteria from blood	0.8 (0.4–2.0)	0.7	3.8 (1.04–14.2)	0.04
> = 1 bacteria from respiratory sample	1.2 (0.6–2.2)	0.62	NE	–
> = 1 virus from respiratory sample	0.9 (0.6–1.3)	0.57	0.5 (0.2–1.3)	0.15
Coinfection from respiratory sample	0.9 (0.6–1.3)	0.65	0.7 (0.3–1.8)	0.44
Viral coinfection from respiratory sample	0.7 (0.5–1.1)	0.1	2.4 (0.9–6.1)	0.08
Blood				
S. pneumoniae	0.8 (0.2–3.1)	0.8	3.0 (0.4–24.1)	0.31
S. aureus,	0.8 (0.2–3.1)	0.8	3.0 (0.4–24.1)	0.31
H. influenzae	0.4 (0.05–3.6)	0.44	4.7 (0.5–40.0)	0.16
Respiratory sample				
S. pneumoniae	1.2 (0.7–2.0)	0.56	NE	–
S. aureus	1.6 (0.9–2.9)	0.14	1.9 (0.4–8.4)	0.42
H. influenzae	1.0 (0.6–1.7)	0.85	0.4 (0.05–3.0)	0.37
Mycoplasma pneumoniae	0.6 (0.07–5.5)	0.68	NE	–
Chlamydia pneumoniae	2.3 (0.7–7.4)	0.15	NE	–
Respiratory syncytial virus A and B	1.9 (1.2–3.0)	0.01	NE	–
Human metapneumovirus A and B	0.6 (0.3–1.1)	0.11	NE	–
Human rhinovirus	1.0 (0.7–1.5)	0.9	1.8 (0.6–4.8)	0.27
Human parainfluenzavirus 1	0.9 (0.4–2.0)	0.73	NE	–
Human parainfluenzavirus 2	1.2 (0.4–3.5)	0.68	NE	–
Human parainfluenzavirus 3	1.2 (0.5–2.9)	0.7	1.7 (0.2–13.5)	0.6
Human parainfluenzavirus 4	0.5 (0.06–4.5)	0.56	NE	–
Human coronavirus 229E	NE	–	5.5 (0.6–48.4)	0.12
Human coronavirus NL63	1.2 (0.4–3.2)	0.79	NE	–
Human coronavirus OC43	0.5 (0.2–1.4)	0.21	1.1 (0.1–8.5)	0.93
Human coronavirus HKU1	1.2 (0.3–4.6)	0.78	NE	–
Influenza virus A	NE	–	NE	–
Influenza virus A (H1N1)/pdm09	0.2 (0.03–1.7)	0.15	2.3 (0.3–18.8)	0.43
Influenza virus B	0.9 (0.4–2.2)	0.88	NE	–
Human parechovirus	0.4 (0.04–2.8)	0.32	7.8 (1.6–38.9)	0.01
Human adenovirus	1.0 (0.6 (1.7)	0.94	1.8 (0.6–5.5)	0.32
Human bocavirus	0.7 (0.4–1.3)	0.24	1.4 (0.4–5.0)	0.58
Enterovirus	0.5 (0.2–1.1)	0.09	0.7 (0.09–5.4)	0.73

*After polytomous univariate logistic regression, compared with normal form HbAA ($n = 569$)
NE, non estimable

31.3.1, $p = 0.03$), independently of age, gender, period per quarter, and RSV A and B infection.

Out of the 807 whole blood samples tested, invasive pneumococcal disease was reported in 15 patients (1.9%; 95% CI, 1.1–3.3%). All of them recovered well without complication.

Discussion

Our study shows that prevalence of SCD was 2.4% and that of SCT 23.8% among children aged 2–59 months presenting with fever and living in high endemic area for malaria. To our knowledge, this study is the first to document the prevalence of HbSS in febrile young children. Although no similar age group is available for comparison, previous results report high carrier rate of 29.6% to 31.9% [16, 17] from the same ethnic group in which the βS-globin gene frequency was reported to be 0.159 [17]. We cannot certify however the ethnicity of our studied population because it has not been queried during the investigation. In an extensive study of 1,214

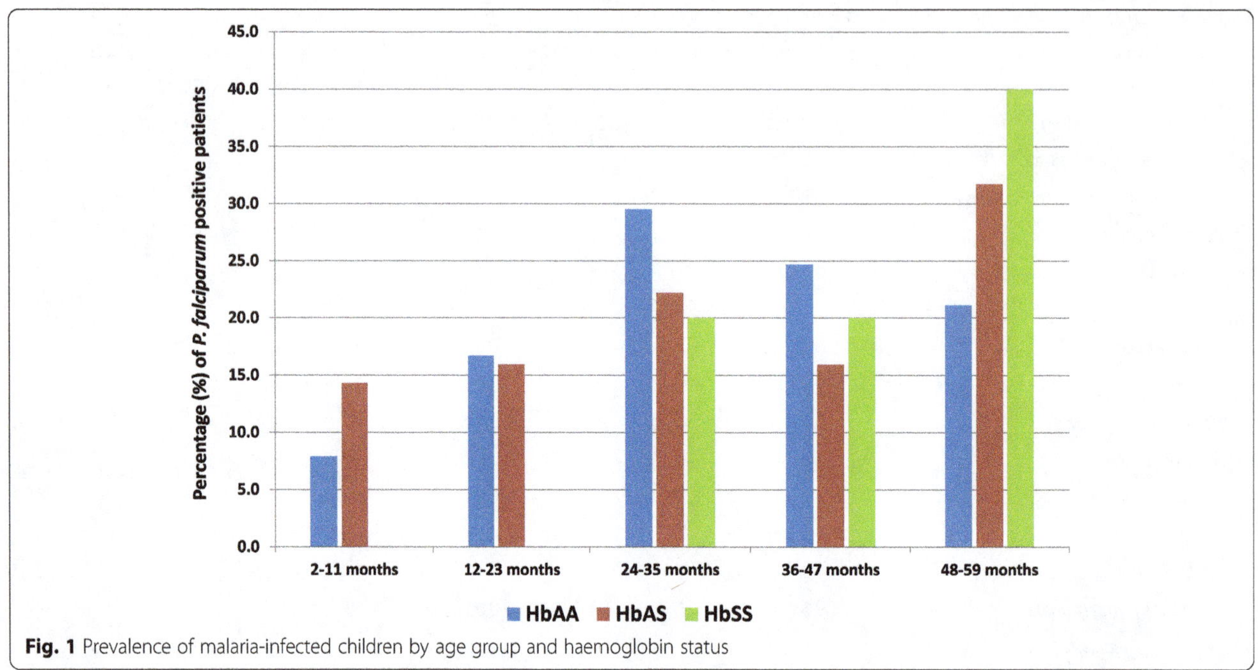

Fig. 1 Prevalence of malaria-infected children by age group and haemoglobin status

individuals of 14 different ethnic groups aged 2–6 years conducted in 2007 (Institut Pasteur de Madagascar, unpublished data), a much lower prevalence of 0.2% for HbSS and 9.4% was found for the heterozygous state compared to our study. When data from the South-east coast only is selected in this later study, the prevalence of HbSS is 0.7% and that of the heterozygous state is 18.7%, slightly lower than that observed in our study. While these data show a higher SCT prevalence among the study population in Madagascar, further study is needed to estimate the real burden among the general population.

Our results demonstrate a significantly lower mean weight-for-height Z-score for patients with SCD than those of normal children and individuals with SCT. Previous studies from other developing countries have reported a state of undernutrition among patients with SCD [18, 19] that may lead to slow growth and maturational abnormality,

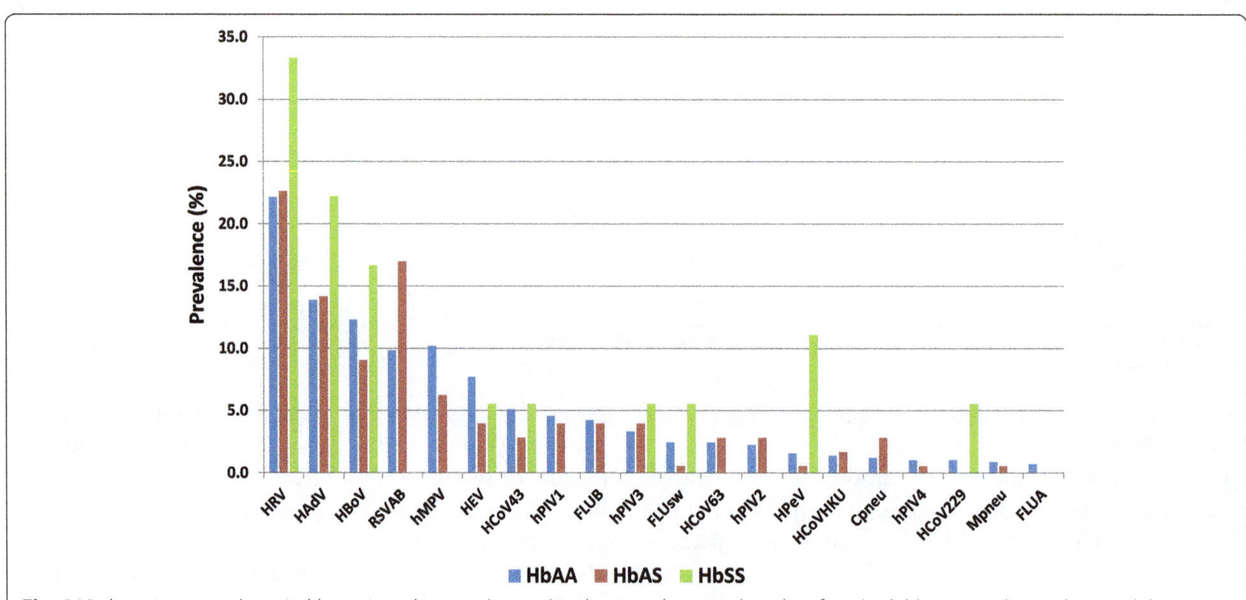

Fig. 2 Viral respiratory and atypical bacteria pathogens detected in the nasopharyngeal swabs of study children according to haemoglobin phenotype. HRV: human rhinovirus; HAdV: human adenovirus; HBoV: human bocavirus; RSV: respiratory syncytial virus A and B; hPIV: human parainfluenzavirus 1, 2, 3 or 4; hMPV: human metapneumovirus A or B; HCoV: human coronaviruses NL63, 229E, OC43 or HKU1; HEV: enterovirus; FLU: influenza viruses A, B or A (H1N1)/pdm09; HPeV: human parechovirus; Cpneu: *Chlamydia pneumoniae*; Mpneu: *Mycoplasma pneumoniae*

amid other complications [20]. These results confirm previous observations that nutritional supplementation is a major component in the management of SCD.

Studies reporting gender differences in SCD incidence are rare and mainly focus on the occurrence of crises or comorbidities [21, 22]. However, in a cross-sectional study carried out over 735 students in India, the prevalence of SCT using the sickling test was higher among male (7.3%) compared to that among female (5.9%) [23]. Our study found higher SCD prevalence among male population, but no significant difference between male and female for SCT prevalence. This should be taken into account in the gender-selective use of medical facilities and management of patients.

Previous studies have shown that SCT protects against severe forms [8] and mild malaria infections [24, 25], although the precise mechanism remains poorly understood. In our study, a high proportion of *P. falciparum* positive result (36.6%) has been found among the studied population. Overall, we did not find any statistical difference between malaria-infected children in the HbAS group compared to the normal phenotype. However, as the age increases, the frequencies of children in the HbAS and HbSS groups who experienced malaria increases. The absence of malaria infection in the patients with SCD up to 2 years of age may have several causes including an early death due to malaria or other infections.

Individuals with SCD are strongly susceptible to encapsulated bacterial organisms such as *S. pneumoniae*, a common colonizer of the nasopharynx in healthy children. Here we report a very high pneumococcal carriage rate among the febrile children studied. Strikingly, all children (100%) with homozygous sickle cell disease in our study were carriers. In previous reports, a much lower rate was found in the US (12%) [26] and Uganda (33%) [27] during study conducted on patients with homozygous sickle cell disease. In our study, pneumonia and acute respiratory infections were the main reasons for medical consultation after malaria. However, the role of *S. pneumoniae* in the development of the disease in the majority of patients is hypothetical due to the absence of healthy matched control group. It should be mentioned that 1.9% of the patients had bacteraemia with *S. pneumoniae* during the course of infection but its causative role has not been proven up as up to 5% of febrile children may also develop asymptomatic or occult bacteraemia [28].

The overall prevalence of viral infection/detection among the study population was high independent of haemoglobin status. However, among the 23 viral and atypical bacteria pathogens studied, there was no statistical difference in prevalence between the three groups for 20 of them and include HRV the most common respiratory virus detected or influenza virus A (H1N1)/pdm09 known to increase disease severity in children with SCD [29]. Parechovirus, a member of the family *Picornaviridae*, was significantly associated with a high risk of infection in SCD patients in our study. Parechovirus infections are usually asymptomatic or lead to a mild gastro-intestinal or respiratory diseases. Only two patients had parechovirus detected, both presenting with symptoms of pneumoniae, suggesting that larger prospective study is required to better describe the real impact of parechovirus infection among SCD population. Conversely, RSV A or B belonging to the family *Paramyxoviridae*, was significantly associated with a high risk of infection in SCT patients compared to the normal population whereas no virus was detected in SCD patients. RSV A and B are a major cause of lower respiratory tract infection during infancy and childhood and were associated with acute chest syndrome similar in severity to influenza infection in febrile children with SCD [30]. The reason why RSV A and B were not detected in our study using a sensitive molecular tool is unknown but it may be linked either to the small number of identified SCD patients, or the possible death of those children. However no follow-up of the study population was carried out to ascertain the latter hypothesis.

Detection of respiratory viruses has been facilitated by the recent widespread availability of nucleic acid amplification techniques. In a study carried out previously in Ampasimanjeva to describe the aetiology of a clinically defined cohort of children with fever and acute respiratory infections, the most representative pathogens were human metapneumovirus (hMPV) for pneumonia, human parainfluenzavirus (hPIV) for other acute lower respiratory infections, respiratory syncytial virus (RSV) for flu-like illnesses and human adenovirus (HAdV) for upper respiratory tract infections [13]. However, the clinical significance of viral detection in biological samples from patients with respiratory infections remains often unclear. For example, when detected in a patient with severe pneumonia, respiratory viruses may represent subclinical infection, persistent shedding after a prior infection, infection restricted to the upper respiratory tract, or infection involving the lower respiratory tract [31–33]. While some pathogens, such as RSV, hMPV and FLU seem to be strict pathogens, other viruses such as HRV are widely identified in both cases and controls. It was beyond the scope of this study to evaluate the viral distribution in asymptomatic patients to study proportion of viral shedding in a control group, or to distinguish between upper and lower respiratory tract infections. Nevertheless, the same study conducted a year ago in the same population has confirmed our findings that a wide range of respiratory viruses might have played a role in escalating respiratory tract viral infections among patients with SCD and SCT.

Our study was limited by the fact that the genotyping method used may not be totally specific to detect haemoglobin S as the presence or the absence of the restriction site Dde*I* may be found in other hemoglobinopathies. However, according to one recent publication [34], HbS seemed to be the most prevalent in Africa where over 700 haemoglobin variants were identified. Additionally, the association between sickle cell trait and malaria is not conclusive for the following reasons: the initial design was probably not optimal to detect this association in the current study, and more accurate methods for detecting HbS should have been used (i.e. hemoglobin electrophoresis). Further independent and well-structured research should be considered in that matter. A second limitation of this study is the absence of long-term follow-up to estimate the outcomes of children and the proportion and causes of death mainly among those living with SCD.

Conclusion

Our findings show that the prevalence of SCD among under-five children presenting with fever was high and a better knowledge of the role and distribution of viral and atypical bacteria pathogens in the study population has been found. This study has helped moving towards a better understanding of the epidemiology of SCD, and we hope it will trigger further research in that direction, for the following reasons. Firstly, as SCD is a major public health concern in Madagascar, a large prospective study on the general population to estimate the true magnitude of the disease should be done. Secondly, it is important to document data about the clinical course and mortality associated to SCD in regions where it is endemic. Thirdly, study involving increasing laboratory capacity should be conducted to help a better understanding of SCD epidemiology, as well as other hemoglobinopathies. Finally, conclusions from these studies will be used for awareness-raising among national authorities in order to strengthen the national control program.

Abbreviations

SCD: Sickle-cell disease; SCT: Sickle-cell trait; HbSS: Homozygous sickle haemoglobin; HbAS: Heterozygous sickle haemoglobin; HbAA: Normal haemoglobin; RFLP: Restriction Fragment Length Polymorphism assay; RDT: Rapid Diagnostic Test

Acknowledgments

This work was supported by grants from the Fondation Mérieux, Lyon, France. The authors thank the children's families for their consent to participate in this study, and the entire medical staff at Medical Foundation of Ampasimanjeva for assistance and cooperation. This paper is dedicated to Doctor Bénédicte Contamin who died in August 2015 for her complete devotion to patients.

Authors' contributions

MNM, JH and ORA contributed to the design of the study, participated in data collection and analysis; MRA, TB, PV, and JH contributed to data analysis and writing of the final manuscript; HMR, NJZ, TR and ATR carried out the experimental work and analyzed the data; MRR acquired data and contributed to the clinical management of patients. All authors read and approved the final version.

Competing interests

The authors declare that they have no competing interests.

Author details

[1]Centre d'Infectiologie Charles Mérieux, Université Antananarivo, P.O. Box 4299, Antananarivo, Madagascar. [2]Fondation Médicale d'Ampasimanjeva, Manakara, Madagascar. [3]UPFR Biochimie-Centre Hospitalier Universitaire Joseph Ravoahangy Andrianavalona, Antananarivo, Madagascar. [4]Laboratoire des Pathogènes Emergents, Fondation Mérieux, Centre International de Recherche en Infectiologie (CIRI), Inserm U1111, CNRS UMR5308, ENS de Lyon, UCBL1 Lyon, France. [5]Service d'Hygiène, Epidémiologie et Prévention, Hôpital Edouard Herriot, Hospices Civils de Lyon, Lyon, France. [6]UPFR Hématologie-Centre Hospitalier Universitaire Joseph Ravoahangy Andrianavalona & Département de Microbiologie, Faculté de Médecine, Antananarivo, Madagascar.

References

1. Weatherall DJ, Clegg JB. Inherited haemoglobin disorders: an increasing global health problem. Bull World Health Organ. 2001;79:704–12.
2. Rumaney MB, Ngo Bitoungui VJ, Vorster AA, Ramesar R, Kengne AP, Ngogang J, et al. The co-inheritance of alpha-thalassemia and sickle cell anemia is associated with better hematological indices and lower consultations rate in Cameroonian patients and could improve their survival. PLoS ONE. 2014;9, e100516.
3. Makani J, Ofori-Acquah SF, Nnodu O, Wonkam A, Ohene-Frempong K. Sickle cell disease: new opportunities and challenges in Africa. Sci World J. 2013;2013:16.
4. Saugrain J. Initial research on sicklemia in Madagascar. Bull Société Pathol Exot Ses Fil. 1954;47:844–84.
5. Chabeuf M, Zeldine G. Blood groups and drepanocytosis on Saint Mary's Island (Madagascar). Médecine Trop Rev Corps Santé Colon. 1962;22:261–7.
6. Saugrain J. New research on drepanocytosis in Madagascar. Bull Société Pathol Exot Ses Fil. 1957;50:480–6.
7. Cerf P, Moyroud J, Coulanges P. Epidemiological survey and sanitary problems in a village in East Central Madagascar. Arch Inst Pasteur Madagascar. 1981;48:151–61.
8. Aidoo M, Terlouw DJ, Kolczak MS, McElroy PD, Ter Kuile FO, Kariuki S, et al. Protective effects of the sickle cell gene against malaria morbidity and mortality. Lancet. 2002;359:1311–2.
9. Luzzatto L. Sickle cell anaemia and malaria. Mediterr J Hematol Infect Dis. 2012;4, e2012065.
10. Mouchet J, Blanchy S, Rakotonjanabelo A, Ranaivoson G, Rajaonarivelo E, Laventure S, et al. Epidemiological stratification of malaria in Madagascar. Arch Inst Pasteur Madagascar. 1993;60:50–9.
11. Kulozik AE, Lyons J, Kohne E, Bartram CR, Kleihauer E. Rapid and non-radioactive prenatal diagnosis of beta thalassaemia and sickle cell disease: application of the polymerase chain reaction (PCR). Br J Haematol. 1988;70:455–8.
12. Woyessa A, Deressa W, Ali A, Lindtjørn B. Evaluation of CareStart™ malaria Pf/Pv combo test for Plasmodium falciparum and Plasmodium vivax malaria diagnosis in Butajira area, south-central Ethiopia. Malar J. 2013;12:218.
13. Hoffmann J, Rabezanahary H, Randriamarotia M, Ratsimbasoa A, Najjar J, Vernet G, et al. Viral and atypical bacterial etiology of acute respiratory infections in children under 5 years old living in a rural tropical area of Madagascar. PLoS ONE. 2012;7, e43666.
14. Picot VS, Bénet T, Messaoudi M, Telles J-N, Chou M, Eap T, et al. Multicenter case–control study protocol of pneumonia etiology in children: Global Approach to Biological Research, Infectious diseases and Epidemics in Low-income countries (GABRIEL network). BMC Infect Dis. 2014;14:635.

15. WHO. WHO child growth standards. Length/height-for-age, weight-for-age, weight-for-length, weight-for-height and body mass index-for-age: methods and development. 2006.
16. Fourquet R, Sarthou JL, Roux J, Acri K. Haemoglobin S and stand origin of Madagascar. New hypothesis on its introduction in Africa. Arch Inst Pasteur Madagascar. 1974;43:185–220.
17. Hewitt R, Krause A, Goldman A, Campbell G, Jenkins T. Beta-globin haplotype analysis suggests that a major source of Malagasy ancestry is derived from Bantu-speaking Negroids. Am J Hum Genet. 1996;58:1303–8.
18. Sadarangani M, Makani J, Komba AN, Ajala-Agbo T, Newton CR, Marsh K, Williams TN. An observational study of children with sickle cell disease in Kilifi, Kenya. Br J Haematol. 2009;146:675–82.
19. Cox SE, Makani J, Fulford AJ, Komba AN, Soka D, Williams TN, et al. Nutritional status, hospitalization and mortality among patients with sickle cell anemia in Tanzania. Haematologica. 2011;96:948–53.
20. Hyacinth HI, Adekeye OA, Yilgwan CS. Malnutrition in sickle cell anemia: implications for infection, growth, and maturation. J Soc Behav Health Sci. 2013;7:1.
21. McClish DK, Levenson JL, Penberthy LT, Roseff SD, Bovbjerg VE, Roberts JD, et al. Gender differences in pain and healthcare utilization for adult sickle cell patients: The PiSCES Project. J Womens Health (Larchmt). 2006;15:146–54.
22. Chang YC, Smith KD, Moore RD, Serjeant GR, Dover GJ. An analysis of fetal hemoglobin variation in sickle cell disease: the relative contributions of the X-linked factor, beta-globin haplotypes, alpha-globin gene number, gender, and age. Blood. 1995;85:1111–7.
23. Akre Charuhas V, Sukhsohale Neelam D, Kubde Sanjay S, Agrawal Sanjay B, Khamgaokar Mohan B, Chaudhary Sanjeev M, et al. Do gender differences influence the prevalence of sickle cell disorder and related morbidities among school children in rural central India? Int J Collab Res Intern Med Public Health. 2013;5:348–58.
24. Migot-Nabias F, Pelleau S, Watier L, Guitard J, Toly C, De Araujo C, et al. Red blood cell polymorphisms in relation to Plasmodium falciparum asymptomatic parasite densities and morbidity in Senegal. Microbes Infect. 2006;8:2352–8.
25. Shim E, Feng Z, Castillo-Chavez C. Differential impact of sickle cell trait on symptomatic and asymptomatic malaria. Math Biosci Eng. 2012;9:877–98.
26. Steele RW, Warrier R, Unkel PJ, Foch BJ, Howes RF, Shah S, et al. Colonization with antibiotic-resistant Streptococcus pneumoniae in children with sickle cell disease. J Pediatr. 1996;128:531–5.
27. Kateete DP, Kajumbula H, Kaddu-Mulindwa DH, Ssevviri AK. Nasopharyngeal carriage rate of Streptococcus pneumoniae in Ugandan children with sickle cell disease. BMC Res Notes. 2012;5:28.
28. Joffe MD, Alpern ER. Occult pneumococcal bacteremia: a review. Pediatr Emerg Care. 2010;26:448–54.
29. Strouse JJ, Reller ME, Bundy DG, Amoako M, Cancio M, Han RN, et al. Severe pandemic H1N1 and seasonal influenza in children and young adults with sickle cell disease. Blood. 2010;116:3431–4.
30. Sadreameli SC, Reller ME, Bundy DG, Casella JF, Strouse JJ. Respiratory syncytial virus and seasonal influenza cause similar illnesses in children with sickle cell disease. Pediatr Blood Cancer. 2014;61:875–8.
31. Jansen RR, Wieringa J, Koekkoek SM, Visser CE, Pajkrt D, Molenkamp R, et al. Frequent detection of respiratory viruses without symptoms: toward defining clinically relevant cutoff values. J Clin Microbiol. 2011;49:2631–6.
32. Jartti T, Jartti L, Peltola V, Waris M, Ruuskanen O. Identification of respiratory viruses in asymptomatic subjects: asymptomatic respiratory viral infections. Pediatr Infect Dis J. 2008;27:1103–7.
33. Lieberman D, Shimoni A, Shemer-Avni Y, Keren-Naos A, Shtainberg R, Lieberman D. Respiratory viruses in adults with community-acquired pneumonia. Chest. 2010;138:811–6.
34. Modell B, Darlison M. Global epidemiology of haemoglobin disorders and derived service indicators. Bull World Health Organ. 2008;86:480–7.

5

A novel fibrinogen mutation: *FGA* g. 3057 C > T (p. Arg104 > Cys) impairs fibrinogen secretion

R. Marchi[1*], M. Linares[1], H. Rojas[2], A. Ruiz-Sáez[3], M. Meyer[4], A. Casini[5] and S.O. Brennan[6]

Abstract

Background: Abnormal fibrinogens can be caused by clinically silent hereditary mutations. A new case was detected accidentally in an 11-year-old girl when routine pre-operative coagulation tests were performed for nasal turbinate surgery.

Methods: The fibrinogen genes FGA, FGG and FGB were sequenced using standard protocols. The kinetics of fibrin formation were followed by turbidity at 350 nm. Purified fibrinogen was incubated with plasmin, and the degradation products analyzed by SDS/PAGE. The formation of fibrinogen-albumin complexes was analyzed by immunobloting. Fibrin structure was examined in a Nikon Eclipse TE 2000-U laser microscope. Secretion of the variant protein was analyzed directly by reverse phase-electrospray time of flight-mass spectrometry (TOF-MS).

Results: DNA sequencing revealed a novel heterozygous g. 3057 C > T mutation in the *FGA* that predicts a p. Arg104 > Cys substitution, in the proband and her father. Both patients were asymptomatic with low functional and antigen fibrinogen concentrations. The proband's plasma fibrinogen polymerization was almost normal, with a 12% decrease in the final turbidity, while, the father's fibrin formation had a diminished slope and final turbidity (2.5× and 40%, respectively). Aα Arg104 is located at a plasmin cleavage site in the coiled-coil region of fibrinogen. However, the father's fibrinogen plasmin degradation was normal. Although the exchanged Cys introduces an unpaired –SH, immunoblotting showed no fibrinogen-albumin complexes. Furthermore, the plasma clot structure observed by confocal microscopy appeared almost normal. TOF-MS showed that the variant Aα chain was underrepresented in plasma and made up only about 25% of the total.

Conclusions: The low expression of the Aα Arg104 > Cys chain in circulation could account for the observed hypodysfibrinogenemia.

Keywords: Abnormal fibrinogen, Hypodysfibrinogenemia, Fibrinogen Aα chain

Background

Fibrinogen is the central protein of blood coagulation. Once the coagulation cascade is initiated, thrombin is formed and catalyzes the conversion of fibrinogen into soluble fibrin monomers that polymerize spontaneously, forming a three-dimensional network that becomes further stabilized by activated factor XIII (FXIIIa). Polymerization is initiated by cleavage of the A and B peptides from the N-terminal of the Aα and Bβ chains [1]. Fibrinogen is a 340 kDa glycoprotein synthetized in the liver and normally circulates in plasma at 160–400 mg/dl [2]. It is composed of two sets of three different polypeptides chains $(A\alpha, B\beta,\gamma)_2$, arranged in three nodules: the N-terminal of the six chains converge at the center forming the globular E region. A coiled coil of all the three chains extends from each side of the E domain to connect with the outer D domains, which form from the C-terminal region of the Bβ and γ chains. The coiled coil is delineated by two disulfide rings and its central region has a kink in

* Correspondence: rmarchi@ivic.gob.ve
[1]Lab. Biología del Desarrollo de la Hemostasia. Instituto Venezolano de Investigaciones Científicas (IVIC), Caracas, Bolivarian Republic of Venezuela
Full list of author information is available at the end of the article

its structure that acts as the primary attack site for plasmin [3].

Inherited fibrinogen disorders can be quantitative (Type I; absence or decreased level of circulating fibrinogen, afibrinogenemia and hypofibrinogenemia, respectively) or qualitative (Type 2; normal or decreased antigenic levels and low fibrinogen activity, dysfibrinogenemia and hypodysfibrinogenemia, respectively) [2, 4].

Dysfibrinogenemia is caused by structural abnormalities that can be inherited (congenital) or acquired [5]. Inherited dysfibrinogenemia is caused by mutations in the coding region of the fibrinogen Aα, Bβ or γ genes and the majority of cases result from heterozygous missense mutations [4]. The prevalence of inherited dysfibrinogenemia in the general population is unknown [5]. The pattern of inheritance is autosomal dominant, and 55% of the patients are asymptomatic, while 25% develop bleeding or thrombosis. Hypodysfibrinogenemia has features of both hypo- and dysfibrinogenemia: the reduced circulating fibrinogen levels confers a hypofibrinogenemia phenotype, and the expression of the mutation that alters functionality, a dysfibrinogenemic phenotype [6]. As with dysfibrinogenemia, in hypodysfibrinogenaemia bleeding extends from mild to moderate, but individuals are more predisposed to thrombosis.

The diagnosis of qualitative fibrinogen disorders is done by the measurement of standard clotting times, whose sensitivity depends upon the methods, reagents and coagulometers used [4]. Usually the thrombin time is prolonged, although with some variants it may be normal [5].

During fibrinogen synthesis, each newly synthetized chain is independently translocated into the endoplasmic reticulum (ER) where chaperones assist in the assembly and folding processes. Molecules are assembled in a step wise manner in the lumen of the ER: first two-chain Aα-γ and Bβ-γ complex are formed. These complexes recruit a Bβ or Aα chain respectively and form half-molecules $(A\alpha\text{-}B\beta\text{-}\gamma)_1$, which in the last step dimerize through N-terminal disulphide bridges to form $(A\alpha\text{-}B\beta\text{-}\gamma)_2$ hexamers [7]. Several studies performed in recombinant systems, using deletion and substitution mutants, indicate that an intact coiled-coil and correct inter- and intrachain disulphide bonds are needed for final molecular assembly [8–10]. In afibrinogenemia mutated molecules are usually absent from circulation. However, in hypofibrinogenemia or hypodysfibrinogenemia if the mutation impairs assembly variant molecules may be secreted, but underrepresented in plasma.

Here we describe a new variant with an Aα Arg104 → Cys mutation in the coiled-coil region that we have named fibrinogen Caracas IX.

Methods

Materials

Bovine thrombin was from Enzyme Research Laboratories (South Bend, IN). Lysine-sepharose 4B was from GE Healthcare (Piscataway, NJ). Pefabloc® SC (4- (2-Aminoethyl) benzenesulfonyl fluoride hydrochloride) was from Fluka, Sigma-Aldrich (Buchs, Switzerland). Tissue-type plasminogen activator and plasmin were from American Diagnostica (Stamford, CT). Human albumin and benzamidine were from Sigma Chemical Company (St Louis, MO). Albumin antibody conjugated to peroxidase was from Dako Corporation (Carpinteria, CA). The substrate 3,3′-diaminobenzidine (DAB) was from Thermo Scientific (Rockford, IL). The LabTek chambers and Alexa Fluor 488 were purchased from Invitrogen, Nalge Nunc International (Rochester, NY).

Blood collection

Blood was collected in citrate (1 volume of 0.13 M trisodium citrate and 9 volumes of blood), the first 3 ml of blood discarded, and centrifuged twice at 2000 g for 10 min. The platelet poor plasma obtained (PPP) was supplemented with benzamidine 10 mM (final concentration), except the plasma to be used for fibrinolysis experiments, aliquoted and kept at −80 °C until use. Routine coagulation tests were performed with citrated plasma on coagulation analyzer STA Compact®, Stago, France. Fibrinogen level was determined by Clauss (Laboratoire Stago, Asnière, France) and clot weight method [11]. Antigenic fibrinogen concentration was measured by a latex immunoassay (Liaphen Fibrinogen, Hyphen BioMed, France).

Mutation analysis

Blood was collected in 0.5 M ethylenediaminetetraacetate tetrasodium salt (EDTA Na_4) (50:1). Genomic DNA was isolated using the Invisorb Spin Blood Mini Kit (Invitek GmbH, Berlin, Germany) according to the manufacturer's protocol. Sequences comprising all exons and exon-intron boundaries from the three fibrinogen genes: FGA, FGB, and FGG were amplified by the polymerase chain reaction (PCR) according to standard protocols. After purification of the PCR products using the Invisorb Spin PCRapid Kit® (Invitek, Berlin, Germany), direct DNA cycle sequencing was performed, applying the Big Dye kit from Applied Biosystems (Foster City, CA), according to the manufacturer's recommendations.

Fibrinogen purification

Fibrinogen was purified essentially as described elsewhere with modifications [12]. Plasma samples were thawed and supplemented with 1 mM Pefabloc® and 5 mM EDTA (final concentrations). Plasma was depleted of plasminogen by passing through a lysine-sepharose 4B column, and then fibrinogen was purified by precipitation (×3) with 25%-saturation ammonium sulphate, pH 7.5. This fibrinogen fraction also contained copurifying fibronectin, factor XIII and vW factor. The precipitate was dissolved in 0.3 M NaCl, dialyzed against the same solution, and stored at −80 °C until used.

The integrity of the purified fibrinogen was analyzed by sodium dodecylsulfate-polyacilamide gel electrophoresis (SDS-PAGE) on 8% gel. The coagulability of the purified fibrinogen was 96% and 93% and the yield 43 and 27%, control and patient, respectively.

Fibrinogen degradation

Fibrinogen was incubated with plasmin as described [13] with minor modifications. Purified fibrinogen (0.9 mg/ml, in TBS) was incubated with plasmin (18 μg/ml, in TBS) in the presence of 1 mM $CaCl_2$ or 5 mM EDTA at 37 °C at different incubation times (15, 30 min and 4 h), quenched with 2% SDS-DTT (v:v) sample buffer and immediately boiled. The zero time sample contained no plasmin. The fibrinogen degradation products were analyzed in a 6% gel SDS-PAGE under non reducing conditions.

Western blotting

In order to detect fibrinogen-albumin complexes, Western blotting was performed under non reduced conditions essentially as described [14]. Briefly, purified fibrinogens (5 μg) and human albumin (5 μg) were loaded in a 5% gel SDS-PAGE, and electroblotted onto nitrocellulose [15]. The membrane was incubated for 2 h with anti-human albumin antibody conjugated to peroxidase (1:1000). The cross-reacting bands were detected with 0.6% 3, 3'diaminobenzidine (DAB), 3% cobalt chloride and 3% hydrogen peroxide.

Activated factor XIII (FXIIIa) fibrin cross-linking

The kinetics of fibrin cross-linking was examined essentially as described elsewhere [14]. Fibrin was cross-linked by the endogenous factor XIIIa that precipitated together with fibrinogen during the purification process. Purified fibrinogen (1 mg/ml) was clotted with 1 U/ml of thrombin and 5 mM $CaCl_2$. The reactions were quenched at different time points (0, 2, 5, 15 min and 1, 4, 24 h) with 2% SDS-DTT and analyzed in a 8% gel SDS-PAGE.

Fibrin polymerization

The kinetics of fibrin formation were studied in plasma and purified fibrinogen [16]. Briefly, 100 μl fresh plasma or 0.5 mg/ml purified fibrinogen in 50 mM Tris, 0.15 M NaCl, pH 7.4 (TBS) were dispensed in a 96-well plate. Then 10 μl of 1 unit/ml bovine thrombin - 20 mM $CaCl_2$ (final) was added to plasma or 5 units/ml bovine thrombin and 5 mM $CaCl_2$ to fibrinogen solution. The changes in optical density (OD) were recorded every 15 s over 1 h at 350 nm in a Tecan Infinite® M 200. The polymerizations were done in three different experiments in triplicate. The lag time (s), slope (mOD/s) and final turbidity (mOD) were calculated from each curve and averaged.

Fibrinolysis

The method was performed as described by Carter et at 2007 [17] with minor modifications. The PPP aliquots without benzamidine were used. Twenty five μl of PPP were aliquoted in a 96-well plate, then 75 μl of tPA 166 ng/ml diluted in 20 mM Hepes, 0.15 M NaCl, pH 7.4 was added. Clotting was initiated by adding 50 μl of thrombin-$CaCl_2$ (0.03 U/ml and 9 mM, respectively).The OD changes were recorded at 350 nm every 15 s over 1.5 h in a TECAN® infinite 2 M microplate reader. The fibrinolysis was done at least three times in triplicate. The time to degrade 50% of the clot (T50%) was calculated from the time elapsed from half the value of the maximum absorbance of the polymerization to half-the value decreased of the maximum absorbance of the lysis curve branch. The rate of clot degradation (slope) was calculated in the descending part of the curve and the absolute value reported.

Direct plasma mass spectrometry

Plasma was precipitated with saturated $(NH_4)_2SO_4$ (25%, final), and the precipitate washed (2×) with 25% saturated $(NH_4)_2SO_4$. The pellet was dissolved in 8 M urea, 30 mM dithiothreitol, 50 mM Tris–HCl, pH 8.0 and left 3 h at 37 °C. The reduced sample was injected into an Agilent 6230 Accurate-Mass electrospray time-of-flight (TOF) mass spectrometry system [18]. A Poroshell 300SB C3 (2.1 × 75 mm) column was used with an acetonitrile gradient and profile data was collected. Multi charged spectral envelopes were deconvoluted using maximum entropy processing and BioConfirm software with an isotope width of 15 Da.

Clots biophysical characterization

In order to characterize some biophysical parameters of the clot structure, the elastic modulus, the Darcy constant (Ks), and fibrin network imaging by confocal microscopy were performed. For these experiments a healthy man with plasma fibrinogen concentration similar to the patient was chosen as a control.

Elastic modulus

The fibrin elastic modulus (EM) was measured in the hemostasis analyzer system (HAS) Hemodyne® (Richmond, VA). Briefly, 700 μL of plasma was placed in the plastic cone and incubated for 1 min at 37 °C. Then 50 μL of a thrombin - $CaCl_2$ solution (1.3 U/ml and 25 mM final concentrations; respectively) was gently and carefully mixed in. The increase in the EM was recorded every 1 min over a 30 min period. Each sample was run in triplicate in three independent experiments. The EM (kdyne/cm^2) reported corresponds to the averaged EM value that was reached at 30 min.

Permeation

Permeation through plasma clots was recorded essentially as described elsewhere [19]. The clotting conditions used were 1 U/ml of thrombin and 20 mM $CaCl_2$ (final concentrations). The clots were left for 2 h in a moist environment at 37 °C in order to fully polymerize. The buffer percolated through the columns was TBS. Nine clots of each sample were run *per* experiment (n = 3) and one measurement *per* clot was taken.

The Darcy constant (Ks) was calculated using the following equation [20]:

$$\mathrm{Ks} = \mathrm{QL}\eta/\mathrm{tAP}$$

Where Q = volume of the buffer (in cm^3), having a viscosity η of 0.01(poise), flowing through the column of height L (cm) and area A (cm^2) in a given time (s) under a hydrostatic pressure P (dyne/cm^2).

Confocal microscopy

The experiments were done essentially as described elsewhere [16]. Briefly, clots were formed inside the eight wells LabTek chambers (Invitrogen, Nalge Nunc International, Rochester, NY). Plasma samples were mixed with Alexa Fluor 488-labeled fibrinogen (10 µg/315 µl final sample volume), then clotted with thrombin-$CaCl_2$ solution (0.3 U/ml and 20 mM, respectively, final concentration). The clots were left for 2 h in a moist environment at 37 °C in order to fully polymerize.

The fibrin clots were observed in a Nikon Eclipse TE 2000 U laser scanning confocal microscopy (LSCM), with an argon ion laser (473 nm excitation and 520/540 nm for emission). The objective used was Plan APO VC 60X water immersion with a work distance of 0.27. The acquisition pinhole was set to 60 µm. Image analyses were done as described [21]. A z-stack of 60 slice was use for construct a 3D projection of 30 µm thick (0.5 µm/slice) were done. Five image by clot (212 × 212 µm) for each experiment (control and patient) were accomplished. Two diagonal lines, a horizontal and a vertical were drawn on the volumetric image of the stack using the Olympus FV10-ASW 2.1 software for obtain the pseudocolor perfil by line. Line graphs were used to calculate density (picks/µ) and diameter of fibers (µm) with Origin Pro 8 software.

Dynamic fibrin clot growth

The spatio temporal dynamics of fibrin clot formation in real time was assessed in plasma by measuring light scattering over 30 min every 15 s using a Thrombodynamics Analyser System (HemaCore, Moscow, Russia) as previously described [21]. Briefly, plasma coagulation is activated when it is brought in contact with tissue factor coated on a plastic cuvette. The clot formation begins on the activator and propagates into the bulk of plasma in which no TF is present. Images are analyzed computationally to measure lag time, initial and stationary growth rate, size at 30 min and clot density. Based on the plots of clot size versus time, the initial velocity of clot growth is measured as the mean slope over the 2–6 min period (characterizing the VIIa-TF pathway) and the stationary velocity of clot growth is measured as the mean slope over the 15–25 min period [22].

Results

Case report

A new abnormal fibrinogen was discovered accidentally in an asymptomatic 11-year-old girl when routine preoperative coagulation tests were performed for nasal turbinate surgery, which proceeded successfully. Her parents reported that when she was 3 years old she had surgery for stenosing tenosynovitis without any complications. Haemostasis work-up showed that the thrombin time was marginally prolonged, and that functional and antigenic fibrinogen levels were decreased without discrepancy in the proband and her father (Table 1). Neither parent report any hemostatic problems. Full DNA sequencing of *FGA*, *FGB* and *FGG* revealed that proband was heterozygous for a novel point mutation in *FGA* g. 3057 C > T that gives rise to an Aα Arg104 > Cys substitution (numbered without the signal peptide). In addition, she was found to be heterozygous for the Aα Ala312/Thr polymorphism. Targeted sequencing of the father showed he was also heterozygous for the novel Aα Arg104 > Cys mutation but his Aα Ala312/Thr status was not explored.

Table 1 Summary of coagulation tests

	Proband	Father	Reference values
TT (s)	18.6	30.8	16–18
PT (s)	15.8	54.6	13–15
aPTT (s)	34.6	42.2	27–34
Fibrinogen (Clauss)	163	122	
(mg/dl)	151		200–400
	158		
Fibrinogen antigen (mg/dl)	177	126	190–400
Factor V (%)	79	-	60–140
Factor II (%)	105	88	60–140
Factor VII (%)	79	69	65–145
Factor X (%)	82	67	65–130

TT thrombin time, *PT* prothrombin time, *aPTT* activated partial thromboplastin time
-: not done

Plasma mass spectrometry

Electrospray TOF MS of purified fibrinogen from the proband and her father showed normal masses and isoforms for the Bβ and γ chain components, with no evidence of any mutations (not shown). Examination of extracted Aα chain spectra from a control, who was homozygous for the AαThr312 polymorphism, showed the expected major peak at 66,136 Da corresponding to the non-phosphorylated form of the Aα chain (theoretical mass 66,132 Da) (Fig. 1). With a peak at 66,134 Da the father appeared to have one normal copy of the AαThr312 allele and one variant copy giving rise to a protein of mass 66,080 Da. This mass decrease of 54 Da was entirely consistent with a point mutation of Arg → Cys (−53 Da). Spectra shows the proband inherited this same variant (theoretical mass 66,079 Da) from her father, together with a copy of the less common AαAla312 allele from her mother. Interestingly the variant chain with the Arg → Cys substitution was under-represented in plasma fibrinogen and contributed only about 25% of the total Aα chain material.

Hereafter, all the studies performed to characterize the new abnormal fibrinogen were performed with the plasma of the proband's father (indicated as patient), except the fibrin polymerisation and the fibrin clot growth assessment performed in both proband and proband's father.

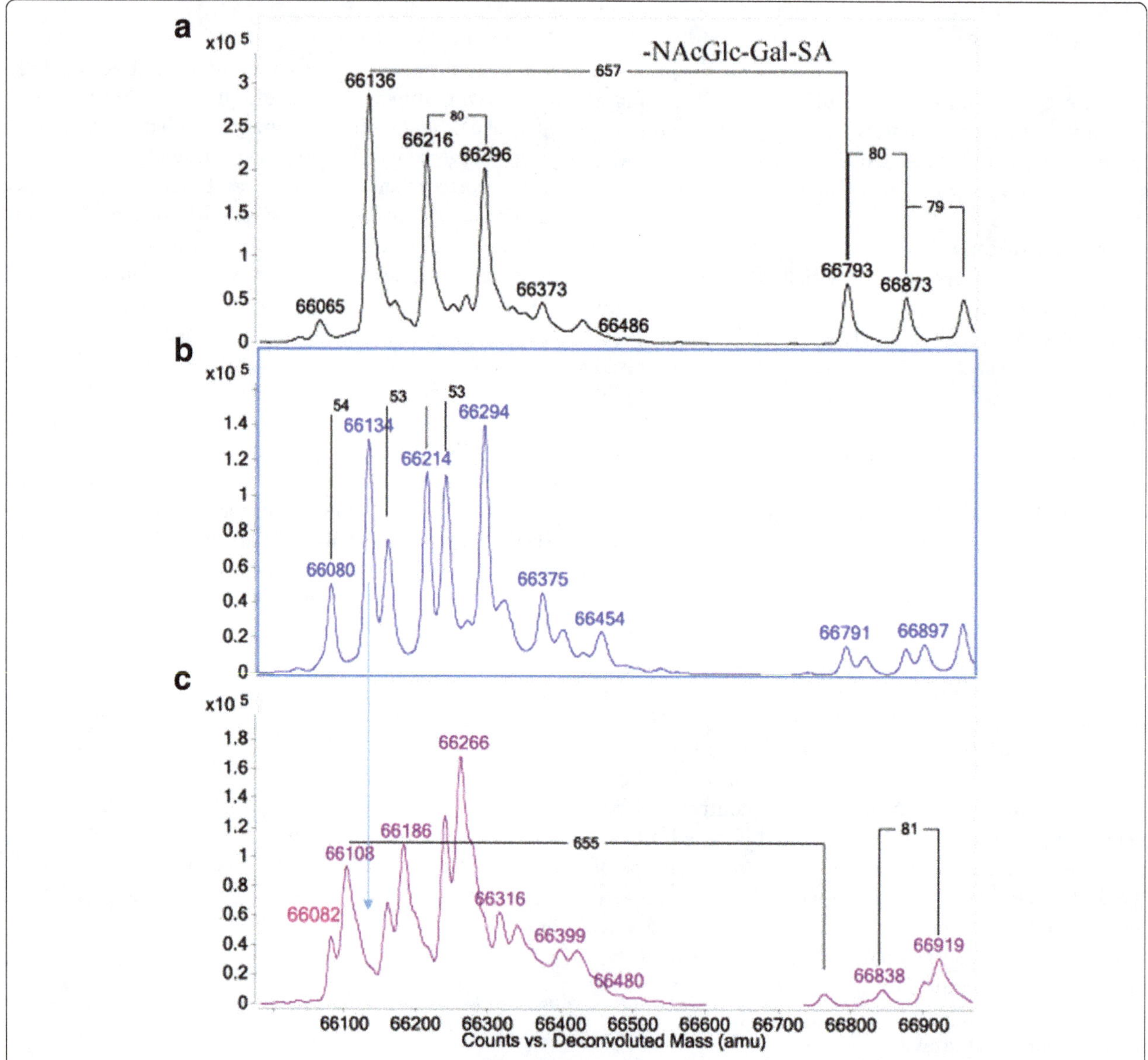

Fig. 1 Transformed electrospray TOF spectra of fibrinogen Aα chains. **a** Normal control homozygote for the Aα Thr312 allele, (**b**) father, (**c**) proband. The father showed a normal Aα312Thr chain at 66,134 Da with a new variant chain at 66,080 Da containing an Arg → Cys mutation (−53 Da). The proband, who had no normal Aα312Thr chains, was heterozygous for the new variant and an Aα312Ala chain (66,108 Da) inherited from her mother. Peaks at +80 Da reflect successive Ser-phosphorylation. The Y- axis depicts a relative voltage response in arbitrary units

Fibrinogen degradation, western blotting and fibrin factor XIIIa cross-linking

Plasmin attacks the middle of the coiled-coil of fibrinogen and generates the degradation products fragments Y and D. Surprisingly, the degradation of patient fibrinogen (Aα Arg104 > Cys) by plasmin was similar to control in the presence of either Ca^{2+} or EDTA (results not shown). In addition, the mutation introduces an unpaired –SH that could potentially form fibrinogen-albumin complexes, although by immunoblotting fibrinogen binding to albumin was negative (results not shown). The patient fibrin α-chain factor XIIIa cross-linking seemed faster compared to control. It can be seen in Fig. 2 that the patient has more intense bands of higher molecular weight corresponding to α-chain factor XIIIa cross-linking at short incubation times (i.e. 2, 5, and 15 min) compared to control.

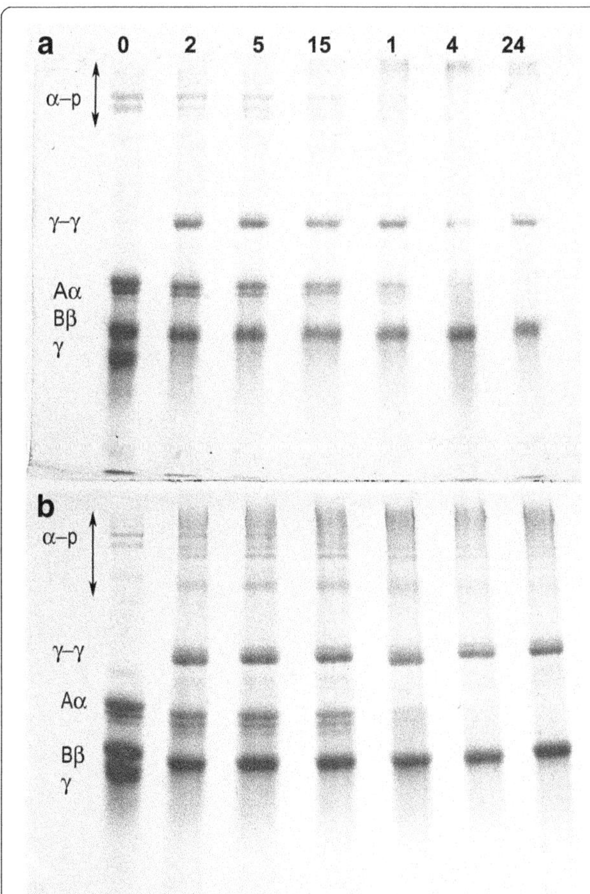

Fig. 2 Fibrin factor XIIIa crosslinking. **a** control fibrinogen, (**b**) fibrinogen from father. Fibrin was cross-linked by the endogenous FXIII co-precipitated with fibrinogen. Polymerisation and crosslinking was initiated by addition of thrombin/$CaCl_2$ and samples removed at different incubation times and run on 8%SDS/PAGE gels under reducing conditions.α-p: α-polymers

Table 2 Plasma fibrin polymerization. Plasma polymerization was done with fresh plasma. The optical density (OD) was multiplied by 1000 (mOD). The results are presented as mean (±SD)

Parameters	Control	Proband	Father	Mother
Fg* [mg/dl]	258	183	168	523
Lag time (s)	0	0	7.5 ± 11	0
Slope (mOD/s)	2.23 ± 0.19	1.66 ± 0.28	0.86 ± 0.24	2.38 ± 0.58
MaxAbs (mOD)	833 ± 18	736 ± 0.6	520 ± 4	970 ± 31

* Fg: fibrinogen, by clot weight method [11]
MaxAbs maximum absorbance

Fibrin polymerization and Fibrinolysis

Fibrin formation in the proband's plasma had a near normal profile with only a slightly decreased final turbidity (~12%), while in the father the fibrin fibers growth (reflected in the slope value) and consequently the final turbidity was decreased approximately 1.3× and 40%, respectively (Table 2, Fig. 3a). With purified fibrinogen,

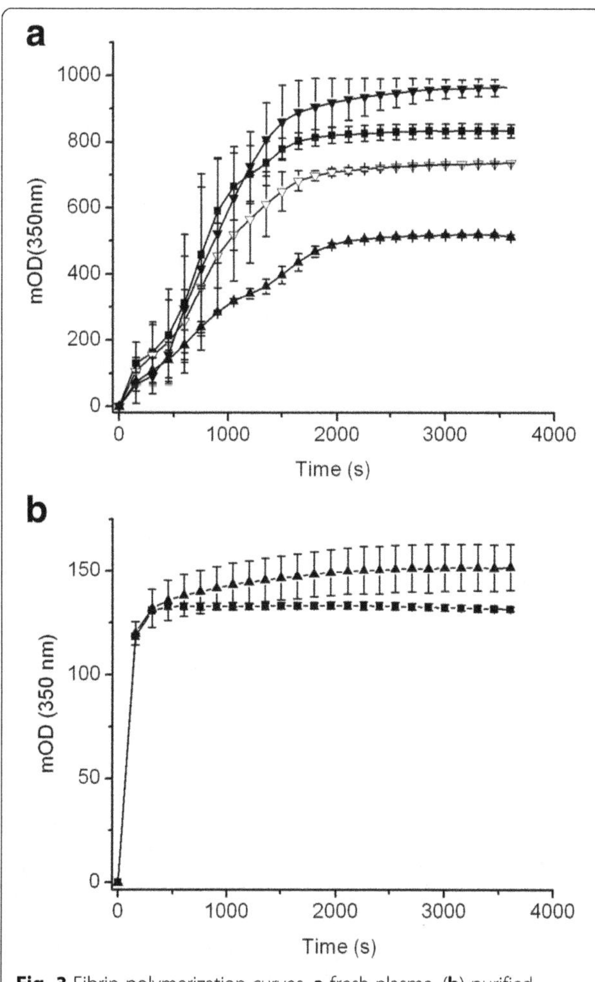

Fig. 3 Fibrin polymerization curves. **a** fresh plasma, (**b**) purified fibrinogen. ■: control, ▼: mother, ▿: proband, ▲: father

the proband's father polymerization was similar to control (Fig. 3b).

The father's fibrin clot dissolution had a slightly shorter T50: 485 ± 33 s compared to 613 ± 62 s in control (p = 0.001), and a slightly delayed fibrinolysis rate: 1.9 ± 0.4 × 10^{-4} OD/s compared to 2.5 ± 0.4 × 10^{-4} OD/s in control (p = 0.008). In Fig. 4a are shown the fibrinolysis curves, the patient area under the curve (AUC) was 1.54 × 10^7 compared to 3.64 × 10^7 control, approximately 2× difference, and in Fig. 4b the T50 s and slopes distribution are represented.

Clots biophysical characterization

The patient fibrin elastic modulus was approximately 500 dyne/cm^2 less than the control, but this was not statistical significant (Table 3). The patient clot's surface available for flux (Ks) was almost 1.8× higher than control (p < <0.001). The confocal microscopy images showed subtle differences between the patient fibrin network and control (Fig. 5). The patient fibrin density and diameter were 0.329 ± 0.016 peaks/μm and 1.150 ± 0.642 μm, respectively, compared to 0.316 peaks/μm ± 0.017 and 1.23 ± 0.02 μm in the control (p < 0.05). In the orthogonal fibrin clot view the patient clot looked more porous, which correlated with the porosity value (Ks) that was approximately 2× higher.

Thrombodynamics

As shown in Table 4, all the values of thrombodynamics parameters were decreased in the proband and her father compared to the healthy control. The lag time, the initial rate and the clot size at 30 min were similar between the proband and her father. The clot density was lower in father compared to the proband (9625.5 versus 11,206 arbitrary unit) reflecting his lower fibrinogen concentration. Videos of dynamic clots growth are

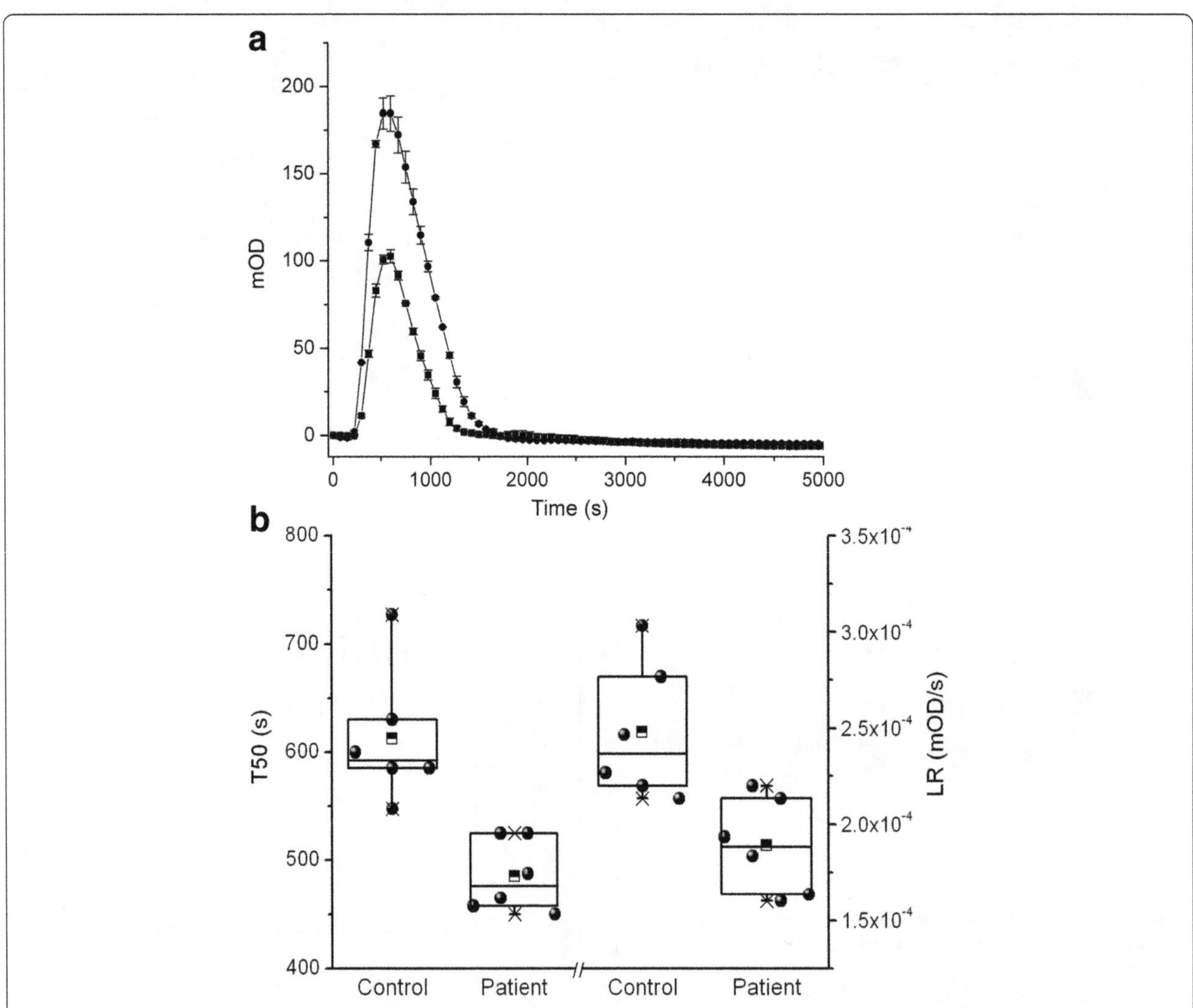

Fig. 4 **a** Fibrinolytic process induced by t-PA. Control (•), father (■). The fathers clot was completely dissolved earlier than control. **b** Box chart of the T50 and lysis rate (LR)

Table 3 Summary of clots biophysical characterization. Results are showed as the mean (±SD). In brackets the number of values averaged

	Control	Father	*p*
Fg (mg/dl)	222	176	
EM (dyne/cm^2)	3239 ± 671 (*n* = 9)	2734 ± 534 (*n* = 7)	0.116
Ks ×10^{-9} (cm^2)	5.1 ± 0.9 (*n* = 20)	9.4 ± 1 (*n* = 22)	1.83 × 10^{-17}

Fg: fibrinogen concentration by clot weight method. EM: elastic modulus. Ks: permeation constant

Table 4 Thrombodynamics data

	Control	Proband	Father
Lag time (min)	1.1	1.45	1.4
Initial rate (μm/min)	57.45	57.5	63.3
Stationary rate (μm/min)	56.4	32.1	33.7
Size at 30 min (μm)	1814	1306.5	1368.6
Density (a.u.)	22,161	11,026	9626.5

Min minutes, *a.u.* arbitrary unit

shown in Additional file 1 (control), Additional file 2 (father) and Additional file 3 (proband).

Discussion

A new fibrinogen mutation was found accidentally in an 11 year-old girl when routine pre-operative coagulation tests were performed. Gene sequencing revealed a missense mutation in *FGA*: g. 3057 C > T that predicts a p. Arg104 > Cys substitution. The low functional and antigenic fibrinogen concentrations in the father and daughter can be explained by the low expression level of the Aα Arg104 → Cys chain in their plasma fibrinogen as the new variant made up only about 25% of the total. Also, because the Aα Arg104 → Cys mutation creates a potential N-glycosylation site (Asn-Asn-Cys) centered on Asn103, mass specters were carefully examined for any new Aα chains with bi-antennary oligosaccharide side chains, but none were observed at or around their expected position at +2202 Da.

The fibrinogen coiled-coil connects the central E nodule with the distal nodule D and is made up of Aα chain

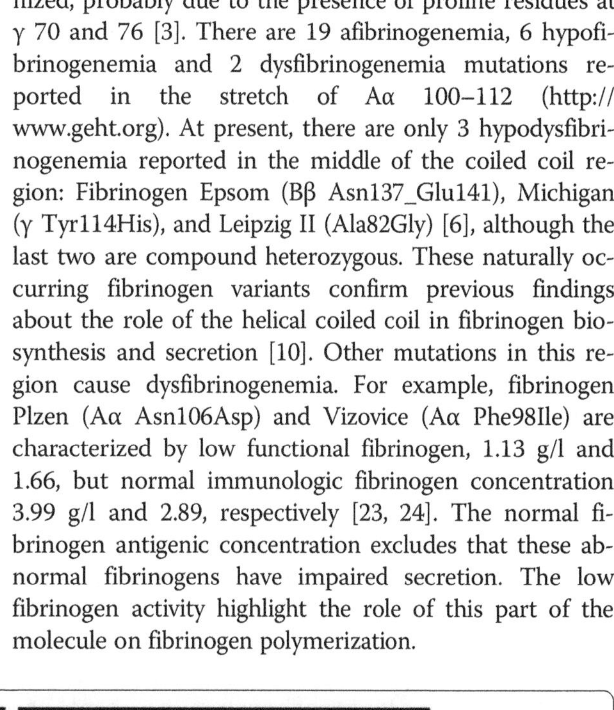

residues 50–160, Bβ 81–191 and γ 24–134 [3]. At the middle of the coiled coil the structure become disorganized, probably due to the presence of proline residues at γ 70 and 76 [3]. There are 19 afibrinogenemia, 6 hypofibrinogenemia and 2 dysfibrinogenemia mutations reported in the stretch of Aα 100–112 (http://www.geht.org). At present, there are only 3 hypodysfibrinogenemia reported in the middle of the coiled coil region: Fibrinogen Epsom (Bβ Asn137_Glu141), Michigan (γ Tyr114His), and Leipzig II (Ala82Gly) [6], although the last two are compound heterozygous. These naturally occurring fibrinogen variants confirm previous findings about the role of the helical coiled coil in fibrinogen biosynthesis and secretion [10]. Other mutations in this region cause dysfibrinogenemia. For example, fibrinogen Plzen (Aα Asn106Asp) and Vizovice (Aα Phe98Ile) are characterized by low functional fibrinogen, 1.13 g/l and 1.66, but normal immunologic fibrinogen concentration 3.99 g/l and 2.89, respectively [23, 24]. The normal fibrinogen antigenic concentration excludes that these abnormal fibrinogens have impaired secretion. The low fibrinogen activity highlight the role of this part of the molecule on fibrinogen polymerization.

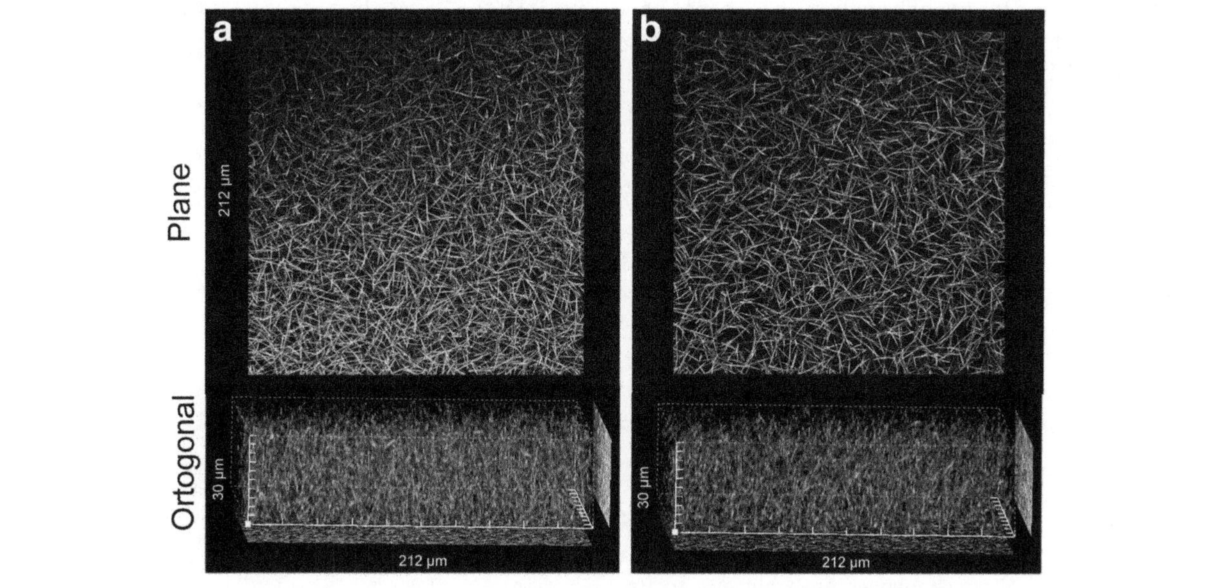

Fig. 5 Confocal microscopy images of plasma clots. **a** Control, (**b**) Father. The fibrin was labeled with Alexa488 coupled to fibrinogen

The kinetics of fibrin formation in plasma studied by turbidity was more impaired in the father compared to the proband. However, by thrombodynamics the father and proband behaved similarly. The results obtained using this last technique seemed more consistent with mass spectrometry. Similar polymerization kinetic would be expected for both individuals as difference of 0.15 g/l in their functional fibrinogen concentrations appeared insufficient to cause major changes polymerization. These discrepant results could result from the fact that the thrombodynamics uses a primarily different principle to initiate the coagulation cascade compared to the turbidity assay. In the former, the clotting is activated by a surface with immobilized tissue factor, which better resembles in vivo clot formation, whereas in the latter the clotting is activated by homogeneously dissolved thrombin. Fibrinogen functional correlations between these two assays require further studies.

We also expected the father would exhibit altered fibrin formation in a purified system, but probably the mutated molecules were underrepresented compared to plasma. In addition, we do not know if the mutated molecules were lost during the purification process. In the future it would be advisable for these cases to choose an immunopurification method.

The proband had higher fibrinogen concentration than her father, despite being about 5 decades younger. Different studies have found that fibrinogen increases with age [25–27]. Hager et al. reported a 25 mg/dl increases per decade [26]. Since fibrinogen is an acute phase reactant protein and CRP was not measured, it cannot be ruled out that the proband at the time of blood withdrawal could have an infectious disease.

When analyzed, an hypofibrinolysis has been observed in most hypodysfibrinogenemia [6]. The Aα Arg104 and Bβ Lys133 are the very first plasmin attack points. However, the fibrinolytic process of fibrinogen Caracas IX was close to normal. In contrast, fibrinogen Epsom with a deletion of the residues Asn137_Glu141 showed hyperfibrinolysis, together with an increased fibrinogen clearance [28]. In fibrinogen Dunedin whose γ82Ala → Gly mutation occurs near the plasmin sensitive site in the coiled coil region also displayed an increased proteolytic sensitivity. It would be interesting in the future to explore the causes of these differences in order to shed light on possibly unknown mechanisms of fibrin(o)gen degradation.

Conclusions

The fibrinogen mutation Aα Arg104 > Cys did not introduce relevant clinical consequences probably due to its low expression levels.

Abbreviations

a.u.: Arbitrary unit; aPTT: Activated partial thromboplastin time; DAB: 3, 3′diaminobenzidine; DTT: Dithiothreitrol; EDTA: Ethylenediaminetetraacetatic acid; EM: Elastic modulus; Fg: Fibrinogen; FXIIIa: Activated factor XIII; HAS: Hemostasis analyzer system; Ks: Permeation constant; MaxAbs: Maximum absorbance; OD: Optical density; PCR: Polymerase chain reaction; PPP: Platelet poor plasma; PT: Prothrombin time; SDS/PAGE: Sodium dodecyl sulfate polyacrylamide gel electrophoresis; TBS: Tris buffered saline; TF: Tissue factor; TOF-MS: Reverse phase-electrospray time of flight-mass spectrometry; tPA: Tissue type plasminogen activator; TT: Thrombin time

Acknowledgements

We are grateful to the patients of the present study for their collaboration.

Funding

The investigation has been partially supported by the government of Bolivarian Republic of Venezuela.

Authors' contributions

MR formulated research goal and aims, performed the analysis of data and wrote the article. LM performed the biochemical and structural fibrinogen variant characterization experiments. RH performed the confocal microscopy experiments, the images data analysis, and figures editing. S-RA performed the clinical evaluation of the patient. MM sequenced the DNA of the patients. CA performed the experiments of dynamic fibrin clot growth, some analytical determinations, analysis of the data, and participated in the writing of the article. BS participated in the formulation of goal and aims, and mass spectrometry studies, analysis of the data, and writing of the article. All authors read and approved the final manuscript and gave their consent for publication.

Competing interests

The authors declare that they have no competing interests.

Author details

Lab. Biología del Desarrollo de la Hemostasia. Instituto Venezolano de Investigaciones Científicas (IVIC), Caracas, Bolivarian Republic of Venezuela. Instituto de Inmunología, Universidad Central de Venezuela and Lab. Fisiología Celular Centro de Biofisica y Bioquímica (IVIC), Caracas, Bolivarian Republic of Venezuela. [3]Banco Municipal de Sangre del Distrito Capital, Caracas, Bolivarian Republic of Venezuela. [4]Medical Engineering and Biotechnology, University of Applied Sciences, Jena, Germany. [5]Division of Angiology and Haemostasis, Faculty of Medicine, University Hospitals of Geneva, Geneva, Switzerland. [6]Molecular Pathology Laboratory, University of Otago, Christchurch, New Zealand.

References

1. Blomback B, Hessel B, Hogg D, Therkildsen L. A two-step fibrinogen–fibrin transition in blood coagulation. Nature. 1978;275:501–5.
2. Asselta R, Duga S, Tenchini ML. The molecular basis of quantitative fibrinogen disorders. J Thromb Haemost. 2006;4:2115–29.
3. Doolittle RF, Goldbaum DM, Doolittle LR. Designation of sequences involved in the "coiled-coil" interdomainal connections in fibrinogen: constructions of an atomic scale model. J Mol Biol. 1978;120:311–25.
4. Neerman-Arbez M, de Moerloose P, Casini A. Laboratory and genetic investigation of mutations accounting for congenital fibrinogen disorders. Semin Thromb Hemost. 2016;42:356–65.
5. Cunningham MT, Brandt JT, Laposata M, Olson JD. Laboratory diagnosis of dysfibrinogenemia. Arch Pathol Lab Med. 2002;126:499–505.

6. Casini A, Brungs T, Lavenu-Bombled C, Vilar R, Neerman-Arbez M, de Moerloose P. Genetics, diagnosis and clinical features of congenital hypodysfibrinogenemia: a systematic literature review and report of a novel mutation. J Thromb Haemost. 2017;15:876–88
7. Maghzal GJ, Brennan SO, Homer VM, George PM. The molecular mechanisms of congenital hypofibrinogenaemia. Cell Mol Life Sci. 2004;61:1427–38.
8. Zhang JZ, Redman CM. Role of interchain disulfide bonds on the assembly and secretion of human fibrinogen. J Biol Chem. 1994;269:652–8.
9. Zhang JZ, Redman C. Fibrinogen assembly and secretion. Role of intrachain disulfide loops. J Biol Chem. 1996;271:30083–8.
10. Xu W, Chung DW, Davie EW. The assembly of human fibrinogen. The role of the amino-terminal and coiled-coil regions of the three chains in the formation of the alphagamma and betagamma heterodimers and alphabetagamma half-molecules. J Biol Chem. 1996;271:27948–53.
11. Ingram IC. The determination of plasma fibrinogen by the clot-weight method. Biochem J. 1952;51:583–5.
12. Niwa K, Takebe M, Sugo T, Kawata Y, Mimuro J, Asakura S, et al. A gamma Gly-268 to Glu substitution is responsible for impaired fibrin assembly in a homozygous dysfibrinogen Kurashiki I. Blood. 1996;87:4686–94.
13. Marchi R, Walton BL, McGary CS, Lin FC, Ma AD, Pawlinski R, et al. Dysregulated coagulation associated with hypofibrinogenaemia and plasma hypercoagulability: implications for identifying coagulopathic mechanisms in humans. Thromb Haemost. 2012;108:516–26.
14. Marchi R, Carvajal Z, Meyer M, Soria J, Ruiz-Saez A, Arocha-Pinango CL, et al. Fibrinogen Guarenas, an abnormal fibrinogen with an Aalpha-chain truncation due to a nonsense mutation at Aalpha 467 Glu (GAA)–>stop (TAA). Thromb Res. 2006;118:637–50.
15. Towbin H, Staehelin T, Gordon J. Electrophoretic transfer of proteins from polyacrylamide gels to nitrocellulose sheets: procedure and some applications. Proc Natl Acad Sci U S A. 1979;76:4350–4.
16. Marchi R, Echenagucia M, Meyer M, Acosta M, Apitz R, Ruiz-Sáez A. Fibrinogen Maracaibo: Hypo-Dysfibrinogenemia Caused by a Heterozygous Mutation in the Gen that Encodes for the Fibrinogen Aα Chain (G.1194G>A: P.Gly13>Glu) with Diminished Thrombin Generation. J Blood Disorders Transf. 2014;5:1–5.
17. Carter AM, Cymbalista CM, Spector TD, Grant PJ. Heritability of clot formation, morphology, and lysis: the EuroCLOT study. Arterioscler Thromb Vasc Biol. 2007;27:2783–9.
18. Brennan SO, Mangos H, Faed JM. Benign FGB (148Lys–>Asn, and 448Arg–>Lys), and novel causative gamma211Tyr–>his mutation distinguished by time of flight mass spectrometry in a family with hypofibrinogenaemia. Thromb Haemost. 2014;111:679–84.
19. Pieters M, Undas A, Marchi R, De Maat MP, Weisel J, Ariens RA. An international study on the standardization of fibrin clot permeability measurement: methodological considerations and implications for healthy control values. J Thromb Haemost. 2012;10:2179–81.
20. Blomback B, Okada M. Fibrin gel structure and clotting time. Thromb Res. 1982;25:51–70.
21. Potze W, Adelmeijer J, Porte RJ, Lisman T. Preserved clot formation detected by the Thrombodynamics analyzer in patients with cirrhosis. Thromb Res. 2015;135:1012–6.
22. Panteleev MA, Ovanesov MV, Kireev DA, Shibeko AM, Sinauridze EI, Ananyeva NM, et al. Spatial propagation and localization of blood coagulation are regulated by intrinsic and protein C pathways, respectively. Biophys J. 2006;90:1489–500.
23. Riedelova-Reicheltova Z, Kotlin R, Suttnar J, Geierova V, Riedel T, Majek P, et al. A novel natural mutation AalphaPhe98Ile in the fibrinogen coiled-coil affects fibrinogen function. Thromb Haemost. 2014;111:79–87.
24. Kotlin R, Reicheltova Z, Maly M, Suttnar J, Sobotkova A, Salaj P, et al. Two cases of congenital dysfibrinogenemia associated with thrombosis - fibrinogen Praha III and fibrinogen Plzen. Thromb Haemost. 2009;102:479–86.
25. Krobot K, Hense HW, Cremer P, Eberle E, Keil U. Determinants of plasma fibrinogen: relation to body weight, waist-to-hip ratio, smoking, alcohol, age, and sex. Results from the second MONICA Augsburg survey 1989–1990. Arterioscler Thromb. 1992;12:780–8.
26. Hager K, Felicetti M, Seefried G, Platt D. Fibrinogen and aging. Aging (Milano). 1994;6:133–8.
27. Spada RS, Toscano G, Chiarenza S, Di Mauro S, Cosentino FI, Iero I, et al. Ischemic stroke and fibrinogen in the elderly. Arch Gerontol Geriatr Suppl. 2004;9:403–6.
28. Brennan SO, Davis RL, Lowen R, Ruskova A. Deletion of five residues from the coiled coil of fibrinogen (Bbeta Asn167_Glu171del) associated with bleeding and hypodysfibrinogenemia. Haematologica. 2009;94:585–8.

6

The expression of embryonic globin mRNA in a severely anemic mouse model induced by treatment with nitrogen-containing bisphosphonate

Hirotada Otsuka[1], Jiro Takito[1], Yasuo Endo[2], Hideki Yagi[3], Satoshi Soeta[4], Nobuaki Yanagisawa[1], Naoko Nonaka[1] and Masanori Nakamura[1*]

Abstract

Background: Mammalian erythropoiesis can be divided into two distinct types, primitive and definitive, in which new cells are derived from the yolk sac and hematopoietic stem cells, respectively. Primitive erythropoiesis occurs within a restricted period during embryogenesis. Primitive erythrocytes remain nucleated, and their hemoglobins are different from those in definitive erythrocytes. Embryonic type hemoglobin is expressed in adult animals under genetically abnormal condition, but its later expression has not been reported in genetically normal adult animals, even under anemic conditions. We previously reported that injecting animals with nitrogen-containing bisphosphonate (NBP) decreased erythropoiesis in bone marrow (BM). Here, we induced severe anemia in a mouse model by injecting NBP injection in combination with phenylhydrazine (PHZ), and then we analyzed erythropoiesis and the levels of different types of hemoglobin.

Methods: Splenectomized mice were treated with NBP to inhibit erythropoiesis in BM, and with PHZ to induce hemolytic anemia. We analyzed hematopoietic sites and peripheral blood using morphological and molecular biological methods.

Results: Combined treatment of splenectomized mice with NBP and PHZ induced critical anemia compared to treatment with PHZ alone, and numerous nucleated erythrocytes appeared in the peripheral blood. In the BM, immature CD71-positive erythroblasts were increased, and extramedullary erythropoiesis occurred in the liver. Furthermore, embryonic type globin mRNA was detected in both the BM and the liver. In peripheral blood, spots that did not correspond to control hemoglobin were observed in 2D electrophoresis. ChIP analyses showed that KLF1 and KLF2 bind to the promoter regions of β-like globin. Wine-colored capsuled structures were unexpectedly observed in the abdominal cavity, and active erythropoiesis was also observed in these structures.

Conclusion: These results indicate that primitive erythropoiesis occurs in adult mice to rescue critical anemia because primitive erythropoiesis does not require macrophages as stroma whereas macrophages play a pivotal role in definitive erythropoiesis even outside the medulla. The cells expressing embryonic hemoglobin in this study were similar to primitive erythrocytes, indicating the possibility that yolk sac-derived primitive erythroid cells may persist into adulthood in mice.

Keywords: Embryonic hemoglobin, Nitrogen-containing bisphosphonate (NBP), Extramedullary erythropoiesis, KLF1, Nucleated erythrocyte

* Correspondence: masanaka@dent.showa-u.ac.jp
[1]Department of Oral Anatomy and Developmental Biology, School of Dentistry, Showa University, 1-5-8 Hatanodai, Shinagawa-ku, Tokyo 142-8555, Japan
Full list of author information is available at the end of the article

Background

Mammalian hematopoiesis occurs in two distinct waves, commonly referred to as primitive and definitive, that originate in the yolk sac and in the fetal liver and bone marrow (BM), respectively [1]. Yolk sac-derived primitive erythroid cells remain nucleated and enucleated terminally in the circulation, whereas definitive erythroid cells produced in the fetal liver are released into circulation after complete maturation [2–5]. The components of the globin tetramer are encoded by the α- and β-globin gene loci. There are 3 functional α-globins (ζ-, α1- and α2) and 4 β-globins (Ey-, βh1-, β1- and β2-) in mice [2, 6, 7]. Primitive erythrocytes express the embryonic complement of globin chains, which initially consist of ζ- and βh1-globins, followed by α1- and α2-, and Ey-globins at the primitive proerythroblast stage [2, 6, 7]. Definitive erythroid cells complete their maturation and enucleation at erythropoietic sites, the fetal liver and BM, where the adult complement of globin chains consists of α1-, α2- β1- and β2- are expressed. All of the globin genes in the α- and β-globin clusters are expressed in primitive erythroid cells, whereas definitive erythroid cells express only the adult globin genes [8].

The expression of globin genes is jointly regulated by elements in the promoter regions and an upstream enhancer region called, the locus control region (LCR) [5]. The TATA, CAAT and CACCC regulatory elements are found within the promoters of all globin genes. A variety of nuclear factors that are involved in transcriptional regulation have been suggested to be related to globin gene expression and switches between them [9, 10]. Members of the KLF (Kruppel-like factor) family are known as an essential transcription factor that bind GC-rich sequences, such as the CACCC element, to regulate the biological dynamic during development [11]. KLF1 (EKLF: erythroid Kruppel-like factor) is a member of the KLF family that plays an essential role in erythropoiesis and is involved in the expression of β-like embryonic globin by binding to its promoter region [12, 13]. KLF2 has been found to regulate biological activity in various tissues and to enhance the expression of β-like embryonic globin [14, 15].

All hematopoietic cells are derived from hematopoietic stem cells (HSC) that develop into mature lineage cells during definitive hematopoiesis [2, 5]. Definitive erythropoiesis requires a specific microenvironment that contacts stromal cells; these groups of cells are called "erythroblastic islands". Macrophages directly contact erythroid progenitors in the BM and fetal liver via several types of adhesion molecules, including EMP, α_V integrin and VCAM-1, which participate in their differentiation, survival and maturation during erythropoiesis [16–19]. These central macrophages may also be an important source of cytokines, particularly erythropoietin (EPO), which supports the maturation of erythroid cells [20, 21]. However, primitive erythropoiesis occurs without macrophages and some cytokines, such as SCF and EPO, are essential for definitive erythropoiesis [3]. These results indicate that erythroblast-macrophage interactions might be specifically essential for definitive erythropoiesis.

Bisphosphonates (BPs) are potent inhibitors of osteoclast-mediated bone resorption and are used as therapeutic agents against bone resorptive disorders such as osteoporosis and metastatic bone diseases [22, 23]. The use of nitrogen-containing bisphosphonates (NBPs) results in strong anti-bone resorptive effects that are much more potent than the effect of non-nitrogen-containing bisphosphonates (non-NBPs). In addition, NBPs have inflammatory side effects including fever, jaw osteomyelitis, osteonecrosis and extramedullary erythropoiesis [24–26]. Our previous study reported that a single injection of a relatively large dose of the NBP into mice inhibited bone resorption by osteoclasts, induced extramedullary erythropoiesis by depleting resident BM macrophages and increased the number of granulocytes in the peripheral blood [26]. Moreover, the injection of an NBP into splenectomized mice induced extramedullary erythropoiesis without anemia and alterations in EPO concentrations in the liver [27]. Phenylhydrazine (PHZ) is used to experimentally induce hemolytic anemia in laboratory animals [28]. The mechanism by which it causes anemia is RBC lipid peroxidation [29]. These results lead to suggest the change of erythropoiesis in the medullary and extramedullary hematopoietic sites by treatment with both NBP and PHZ, which indirectly inhibits erythropoiesis and directly disrupts erythrocytes.

In this study, we established a model of critical anemia in mice through the combined use of NBP with PHZ and analyzed the expression pattern of hemoglobin as well as changes in erythropoiesis and erythropoiesis-regulated factors in medullary and extramedullary erythropoietic sites.

Methods

Animals

Sixty female BALB/c mice (6-week-old) were obtained from Sankyo Laboratories (Tokyo, Japan), and were fed under specific pathogen-free conditions. The mice were anesthetized with an intraperitoneal injection of sodium pentobarbital (50 mg/kg) and performed splenectomies as described in previous reports [27]. The mice were divided into 5 group: a non-treatment group (5 mice), a splenectomized control group (20 mice), a splenectomized and NBP treatment group (10 mice), a splenectomized and PHZ treatment group (5 mice), and a splenectomized and both NBP and PHZ treatment group (20 mice). NBP (40 μmol/kg) or sterile saline was intraperitoneally injected into splenectomized mice 7 days after splenectomy. Two days after NBP injection, the mice were treated with PHZ (50 mg/kg) or saline, and they were killed 3 days after the PHZ or saline treatment (Fig. 1a). The NBP used in this study was 4-amino-1-hydroxybutylidene-1, 1-bisphosphonate (AHBuBP), which was prepared as previously described [24, 26, 27].

All experimental protocols used in this study were reviewed and approved by the Animal Care Committee of Showa University (Permit Number: 14043).

Blood analyses

Peripheral blood samples were collected and centrifuged (10000 × *g*) to determine hematocrit values, and serum was then separated using centrifugation (1000 × *g*). To obtain serum EPO measurements, we used an EPO Mouse ELISA Kit (R & D systems, Minneapolis, MN, USA) according manufacturer's protocol, and whole blood was prepared in blood smears and performed the May-Grünwald Giemsa staining technique.

Antibodies and other materials

The monoclonal antibodies used in this study were as follows: purified anti-mouse TER-119 and anti-mouse CD71, FITC-conjugated anti-mouse TER-119 and PE-conjugated anti-mouse CD71 antibodies were purchased from BD Pharmingen (San Diego, CA, USA). Normal rabbit IgG, biotinylated goat anti-rat IgG antibodies and an avidin-biotin complex kit (ABC Elite standard kit) were purchased from Vector Laboratories (Burlingame, CA, USA). The polyclonal antibodies for ChIP, anti-KLF1 and KLF2 assays were obtained from Abcam (Cambridge, UK), and an alkaline-phosphatase (AP)-conjugated anti-digoxygenin (DIG) antibody was purchased from Roche (Basel, Switzerland). Anti-mouse TER119 antibody microbeads were purchased from Miltenyi Biotec (Bergisch Gladbach, DE).

Tissue preparation

The tissue samples were fixed in 4 % paraformaldehyde prepared in phosphate-buffered saline (PBS). Tibias were demineralized using 10 % ethylenediaminetetraacetic acid (EDTA). Demineralized tibia and soft tissues were washed in 20 % sucrose-PBS, embedded in O.C.T. compound (Sakura Finetek Japan, Tokyo, Japan), and quickly frozen in a mixture of acetone and dry ice. Frozen sections (8 μm thick) were cut, placed on SILANE-coated glass slides, and air dried.

Flow cytometry

The cells isolated from BM, the liver and peripheral blood were obtained as previously described [27, 30], washed using FACS solution (1 mM EDTA, 0.2 % BSA and 0.1 % NaN_3 in PBS), and incubated with FITC-

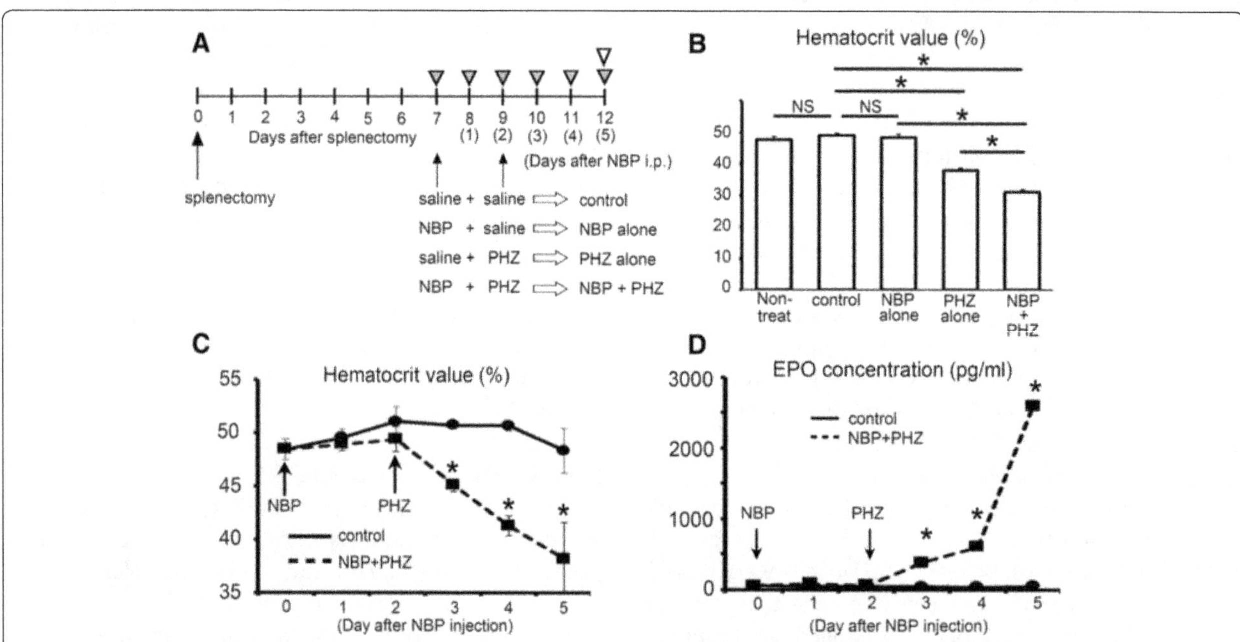

Fig. 1 Experimental schedule and the analysis of peripheral blood. **a** The schema of the experimental schedule. Blood sample were collected every day (gray arrowhead), and tissue samples were obtained at 5 days after NBP injection (white arrowhead). Arrows indicate the time of the treatment (control, NBP alone, PHZ alone or NBP + PHZ). **b** The hematocrit values of all groups at 5 days after treatment. No change was observed by treatment with NBP alone, significant reduction were observed by PHZ treatment. Moreover, serious anemia was induced in the animals treated with both NBP and PHZ (NBP + PHZ). **c** The hematocrit values in the control animals and the animals treated with both NBP and PHZ (NBP + PHZ). Treatment with PHZ and NBP resulted in a significant reduction in hematocrit values after PHZ injection, which occurred 3 days after the NBP injection was detected. **d** The EPO concentration in the serum. The PHZ and NBP group (PHZ + NBP) had significantly increased EPO concentrations compared to the control. The error bars indicate the standard error of the mean (SEM)

conjugated anti-TER-119 and PE-conjugated anti-CD71 antibodies or rat IgG (isotype control) in 1%BSA in PBS. After washing, the cells, they were resuspended in FACS solution and analyzed using a FACS Verse flow cytometer (BD Bioscience, Rockville, MD, USA). The data were collected for 10,000 events, stored in list mode, and subsequently analyzed using the BD FACS Suite software (BD Bioscience, Rockville, MD, USA).

Histology and immunohistochemistry

Some sections were stained with hematoxylin-eosin (HE). The remaining sections were rinsed in PBS and fixed in 0.3 % H_2O_2-methanol for 30 min. After several PBS washes, the sections were incubated in 5 % normal goat serum in PBS. These sections were then incubated with an anti-TER119 or anti-CD71 antibody (1:50). After several rinses with PBS, the sections were incubated with biotinylated goat anti-rat antibodies, followed by a solution containing avidin-biotin-horseradish peroxidase complex. After the sections were washed, they incubated with a mixture of a DAB detection kit (KPL, Gaithersburg, MD, USA). Hematoxylin was used for counterstaining.

In situ hybridization (ISH)

ISH was performed as previously described [31]. Antisense probes were designed to detect murine *hba-x* (ζ-globin, accession no. NM_010405), *hbb-bh1* (βh1-globin, accession no. NM_489729) and *hbb-y* (Ey-globin, accession no. NM_008219). All accession numbers were obtained from the Entrez nucleotide database. The designed probes were labeled using digoxygenin (RNA DIG labeling kit; Roche, Basel, Switzerland). The samples were fixed with 4 % paraformaldehyde and 0.5 % glutaraldehyde and prepared as frozen sections. The frozen sections were washed with PBS, digested with 1 μg/ml Proteinase K, and hybridized in separate buffer solution (50 % deionized formamide, 2 × SSC, 10 % dextran sulfate, and 0.01 % sheared yeast tRNA) containing each probe at 1 μg/ml at 50 °C. After hybridization, the sections were washed in SSC and unreacted probes were ablated using RNase A (Wako, Osaka, Japan). The probes were visualized using an AP-conjugated anti-DIG antibody with NBT/BCIP used as the substrate (Roche, Basel, Switzerland).

RT-PCR, chromatin immune precipitation and quantitative RT-PCR

Mononuclear cells were isolated from BM and the liver as previously described [27], and TER119-positive cells were collected using the MidiMACS system immunomagnetic separation method, (Miltenyi Biotec, Bergisch Gladbach, DE). Total RNA was isolated using an RNeasy Mini kit (QIAGEN K.K., Hilden, DE) and reverse transcribed into cDNA using a PrimeScript RT reagent Kit (Takara, Shiga, Japan). A chromatin immune precipitation (ChIP) was performed according to the manufacturer's instructions (Ez-ChIP; Millipore, Billerica, MA, US). PCR analysis was performed using Takara ExTaq® (Takara, Shiga, Japan). The primer sequences and annealing temperatures used in PCR are listed in Table 1.

Quantitative RT-PCR (qRT-PCR) was performed using an Applied Biosystems7500 Fast Real-time PCR system (Applied Biosystems Inc., Foster City, CA, USA) The following program was used: 50 cycles at 95 °C for 3 sec and 60 °C for 30 sec. The expression of different globin genes was measured using control ct values, and the ct values obtained for actin expression were used for normalization. The primers and probes used for qRT-PCR (TaqMan® gene expression assay, assay ID: *Hba*, Mm00845395_s1, *Hbb1*, Mm01611268_g1, *Hba-x*, Mm00439255_m1, *Hbb-bh1*, Mm00433932_g1 and *Hbb-y*, Mm00433936_g1) were obtained from Applied Biosystems (Foster City, CA, USA).

2D electrophoresis

Hemoglobin was isolated from blood samples, and 2D electrophoresis was performed as previously described [32]. The samples obtained from the hemolytic blood

Table 1 Used primer sequence

Name	Sequence	Annealing(°C) Product size
Actin	F: 5′-GCGTGACATTAAAGAGAAGCTG-3′	60
	R: 5′-CTCAGGAGGAGCAATGATCTTG-3	376 bp
Hba	F: 5′-CTCTCTGGGGAAGACAAAAGCAAC-3′	55
	R: 5′-GGTGGCTAGCCAAGGTCACCAGCA-3′	334 bp
Hbb1	F: 5′-CACAAACCCCAGAAACAGACA-3′	55
	R: 5′-CTGACAGATGCTCTCTTGGG-3′	529 bp
Hba-x	F: 5′- CTGTCTGCTGGTCACAATGG -3′	55
	R: 5′- GGGAGGAGAGGGATCATAGC -3′	165 bp
Hbb-bh1	F: 5′-TGGACAACCTCAAGGAGACC-3′	55
	R: 5′- TGCCAGTGTACTGGAATGGA -3′	231 bp
Hbb-y	F: 5′-CTTGGGTAATGTGCTGGTGA-3′	55
	R: 5′-GTGCAGAAAGGAGGCATAGC-3	183 bp
Klf1	F: 5′-CCTCCATCAGTACACTCACC-3′	55
	R: 5′-CCTCCGATT TCAGACTCACG-3′	150 bp
Klf2	F: 5′-CCAAGAGCTCGCACCTAAAG-3′	55
	R: 5′-GTGGCACTGAAAGGGTCTGT-3′	155 bp
Bcl11a	F: 5′-AACCCCAGCACTTAAGCAAA-3′	55
	R: 5′-ACAGGTGAGAAGGTCGTGGT-3′	122 bp
Gata1	F: 5′- ACCACTACAACACTCTGGCG -3′	60
	R: 5′- CAAGAACTGAGTGGGGCGAT -3′	452 bp
bh1-globin promoter	F: 5′-GGACAGGTCTTCAGCCTCTTGA-3′	56
	R: 5′-CAGATGCTTGTGATAGCTGCCT-3′	123 bp
Ey-globin promoter	F: 5′-TGCTTCTGACACTCCTGTGATCA-3′	56
	R: 5′-GGGTTTTTTCCTCAGCAGTAAAGT-3′	79 bp

solution were treated with a 2D sample kit (ATTO, Tokyo, Japan). The carrier ampholyte isoelectric focusing method was combined with 10 % SDS-PAGE according to instructions in the ATTO Technical Manual (http://www.atto.co.jp/kotsu_series.html), and the gels were then stained using silver. The gel images were observed using chemiDoc (Bio-Rad, Hercules, CA, USA) and analyzed using NIH image software.

Statistical analysis

For quantitative data analysis, a *t*-test was used to determine differences between paired samples. A *p*-value of <0.05 was considered statistically significant.

Results

Blood analyses

We collected peripheral blood to evaluate hematocrit value, to measure the serum EPO concentrations and to observe erythrocytes in blood smears. No changes were observed in hematocrit values and serum EPO levels in animals treated with splenectomy and NBP alone compared to the values in the non-treatment group (Fig. 1b). In splenectomized mice treated with PHZ, a significant reduction in hematocrit values was observed compared to controls and to animals treated with NBP alone (Fig. 1b). However, treating animals with both NBP and PHZ (NBP + PHZ) induced more serious anemia than administering PHZ alone (Fig. 1b). In an analysis of time-dependent changes following NBP injection, the hematocrit values in animals treated with both NBP and PHZ (NBP + PHZ) were significantly reduced compared to control animals at 1-3 days after PHZ-treatment (Fig. 1c). The concentration of EPO in serum samples taken from mice treated with NBP and PHZ was also significantly increased at 1-3days after PHZ-treatment (Fig. 1d).

The blood smears showed that only normal enucleated erythrocytes were observed in the control and NBP-only groups (Fig. 2a). In contrast, numerous nucleated erythrocytes and reticulocytes were observed in the peripheral blood of mice treated with both NBP and PHZ (Fig. 2a).

Flow cytometric analysis showed that the number of TER119 and CD71 double-positive cells was markedly increased in the mice treated with both NBP and PHZ, while almost erythrocytes were single-positive for TER119 in the other groups (Fig. 2b). In the blood vessel, some CD71-positive nucleated erythroid cells were observed in addition to CD71-positive reticulocytes (Fig. 2c).

These results indicate that splenectomized mice treated with both NBP and PHZ become critically anemic and display a significant increase in EPO levels, which enhances erythropoiesis. The results from the blood smears suggest the induction of abnormal erythropoiesis because nucleated erythrocytes are not normally observed in

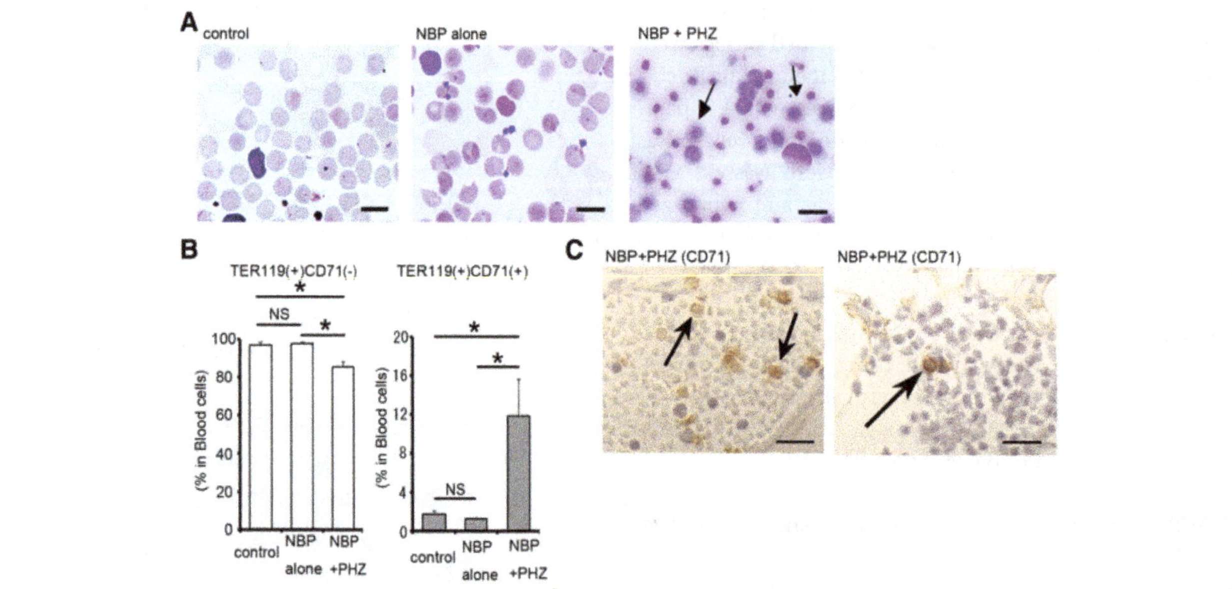

Fig. 2 Morphological analysis of peripheral blood. **a** Blood smears stained with May-Grünwald Giemsa stain in control animals and the animals treated with NBP-alone (at 5 days after the NBP) and both NBP and PHZ (at 3 days after PHZ). Nucleated erythroid cells were easily detected in the NBP + PHZ mice (arrows). **b** Flow cytometry analysis of erythroid lineage cells in the peripheral blood at 5 days after NBP injection. The majority of cells in the control and NBP-alone groups were single-positive TER119 cells at 5 days after NBP injection, whereas the number of TER119 and CD71 double-positive cells was significantly increased by treatment with NBP and PHZ (NBP + PHZ) at 3 days after PHZ injection. **c** Immunohistochemical detection of CD71-positive cells in peripheral blood of splenectomized mice treated with NBP and PHZ (3 days after PHZ). CD71-positive reticulocytes were observed (arrows in left panel), and CD71-positive nucleated cells also existed in the blood vessel (arrows in right panel). Asterisks indicate statistical significance, and NS denote no significance versus the control. Bars indicate 10 m (**a**) and 25 m (**c**). The error bars indicate the SEM

the blood in mammals except during the early embryonic stages.

Detection of erythropoiesis in the BM

In the control BM samples, appropriately 20 % of all BM cells were TER119-positive, and three-fourth of the TER119-positive population of cells was TER119/CD71 double-positive (Fig. 3a). The TER119-positive erythroid lineage was significantly decreased by the injection of NBP (NBP alone) as a result of the elimination of resident BM macrophages, as previously described [26, 27]. However, the proportion of TER119-/CD71- double-positive cells in the NBP and PHZ group (NBP + PHZ) was significantly increased despite the use of NBP (Fig. 3a). The enhanced granulopoiesis and relative reduction of B-lymphopoiesis were observed in the BM of the animals treated with both NBP and PHZ (Additional file 1).

Many of the TER119-positive cells formed clusters in the control mice, as shown by immunohistochemistry (Fig. 3c). In the NBP-treated mice (NBP alone), fewer TER119-positive cells appeared to form into clusters in the BM (Fig. 3c). However, more TER119-positive cells were detected in the BM of the mice treated with both NBP and PHZ (Fig. 3c).

These results suggest that elevated levels of EPO supports the maturation of the erythroid lineage in the absence of BM macrophages and inhibits apoptosis during erythropoiesis in BM.

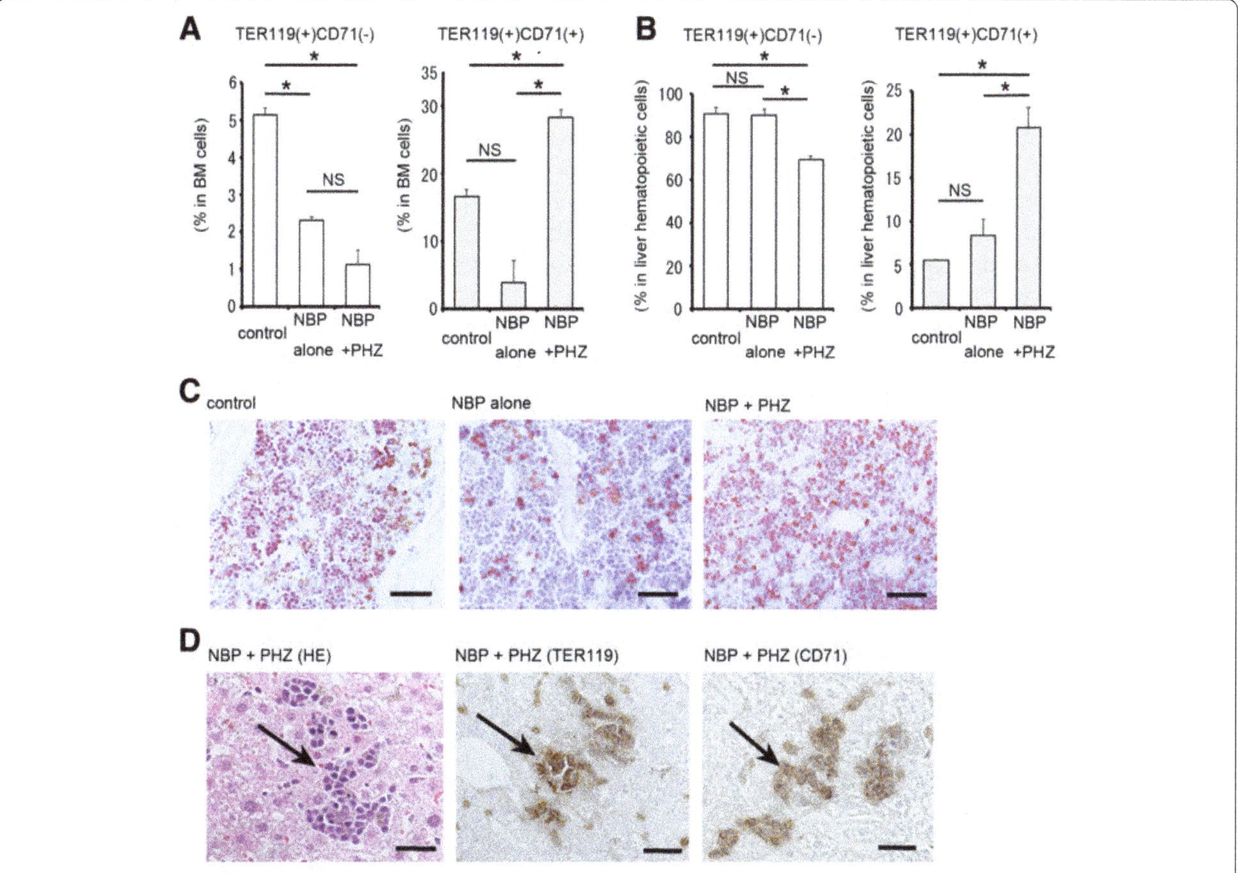

Fig. 3 Erythropoiesis in the BM and liver. **a** Flow cytometric analysis of erythroid cells in the BM at 5 days after the treatment. In the controls animals, TER119 single-positive and TER119 and CD71 double-positive erythroid lineage cells comprised the majority of the cells. A significant decrease in the number of TER119-positive cells was induced by the NBP injection. In the animals treated with both NBP and PHZ (NBP + PHZ), the number of TER119 and CD71 double-positive (erythroid lineage) cells was markedly increased despite treated with NBP. **b** Flow cytometric analysis of erythroid cells in the liver at 5 days after the treatment. The number of TER119 single-positive cells was decreased in animals treated with both NBP and PHZ. TER119 and CD71 double-positive cells were rare in the control animals but were increased by treatment with NBP. The number of TER119/CD71-double-positive erythroblasts was decreased with the NBP treatment. The number of TER119/CD71 double-positive erythroblasts was higher in the group treated with both NBP and PHZ. **c** Immunohistochemical detection of TER119-positive cells in the BM at 5 days after the treatment. TER119-positive cells were significantly decreased by NBP treatment alone, but a decline in erythropoiesis was not detected in the group treated with both NBP and PHZ (NBP + PHZ). **d** Histological analysis of the livers of mice treated with NBP and PHZ at 5 days after NBP injection. The left panel shows HE staining. Mononuclear cells accumulated in the liver and formed numerous clusters (arrow). The middle and right panel show immunohistochemistry for TER119 and CD71, respectively. The cells that formed clusters in the liver were TER119- and CD71-positive erythroblasts (arrow). Bars indicated 50 m (**c**) and 25 m (**d**). The error bars indicate the SEM (**a** and **b**)

Detection of erythropoiesis in the liver

In splenectomized mice, the liver is the main site of extramedullary erythropoiesis. Therefore, we next evaluated hepatic erythropoiesis using histological and immunohistochemical methods and flow cytometry. In control mice, TER119 single-positive cells were the most abundant, and CD71 double-positive cells were very rare (Fig. 3b). After the injection of NBP alone, the number of TER119 and CD71 double-positive cells was slightly increased (Fig. 3b). These results indicate that extramedullary erythropoiesis was induced in the liver. Furthermore, treatment with both NBP and PHZ induced a significant increase in TER119 and CD71 double-positive cells in the liver (Fig. 3b).

Histological analysis indicated the clusters of mononuclear cells in the livers of splenectomized mice treated with PHZ and NBP (Fig. 3d). These cells were TER119-positive and/or CD71-positive erythroblasts (Fig. 3d). Immunohistochmically, the clusters of granulocytes and lymphocytes could not be detected in the liver.

The injection of NBP and PHZ therefore induced extramedullary erythropoiesis in the liver and significantly increased the formation of erythroblast clusters compared to results in the control and NBP-only groups.

Expression of embryonic globin mRNAs at hematopoietic sites

To determine the expression pattern of hemoglobin subunits, we performed RT-PCR analysis on TER119-positive hematopoietic cells isolated from BM and the liver and collected using MACS (Miltenyi Biotec, Bergisch Gladbach, DE). The embryonic globins ζ-, βh1- and Ey- (*Hba-x, Hbb-bh1* and *Hbb-y*) and the adult globins α- and β major (*Hba* and *Hbb1*) were expressed in BM and the liver in the PHZ- and NBP-treated mice, whereas the TER119-positive cells in the control mice expressed only the adult globins (Fig. 4a). The expression level of embryonic globins in the liver was higher than the level in the BM, and *Hbb-y* was not detected in the control mice (Additional file 2). These results suggest that abnormal erythropoiesis may occur in this critical anemic model and that embryonic globins may be activated as a response to hypoxemia.

We next performed *in situ* hybridization to identify the cell clusters that expressed the embryonic globins ζ-, βh1- and Ey- (*Hba-x, Hbb-bh1* and *Hbb-y*) in the BM and liver of mice treated with both NBP and PHZ. We observed the expression of embryonic globins in the BM (Fig. 4b), but only a small number of cells expressed embryonic globin in the BM.

These results show that both embryonic-type and adult-type hemoglobin are co-expressed in clusters of cells in the BM and livers in splenectomized mice that were treated with NBP and PHZ and that definitive erythropoiesis could be of primary importance in the BM under these conditions.

Hemoglobin fraction in the peripheral blood

We performed qRT-PCR to detect embryonic globins in the peripheral blood but did not detect the globins of embryonic-type in the control mice (Additional file 3). Therefore, we analyzed the pattern of hemoglobin expression in peripheral blood using 2D electrophoresis.

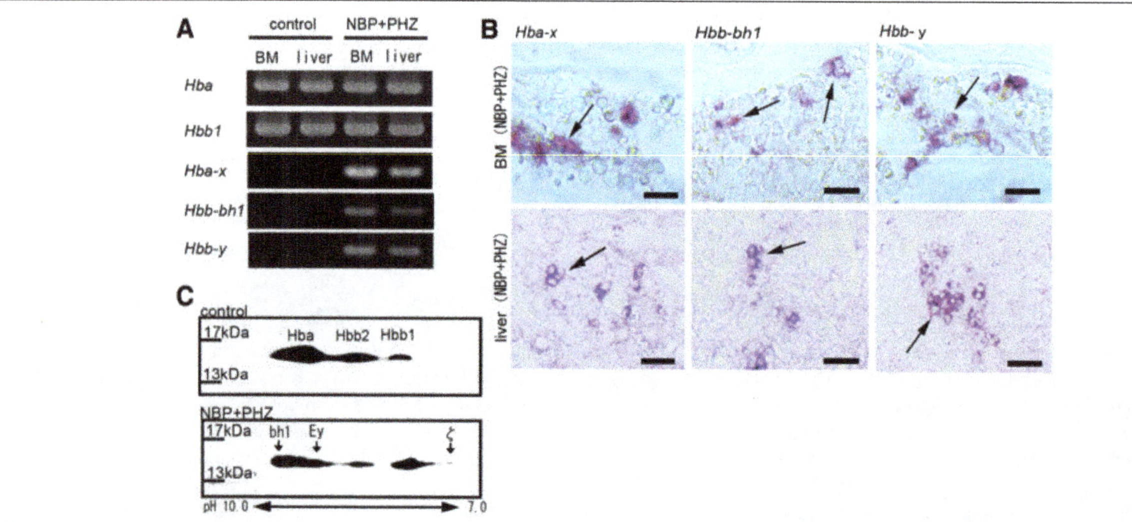

Fig. 4 Expression of embryonic globins in the BM and liver. **a** RT-PCR analysis of globin mRNAs in the BM and liver. In control animals, only adult globins were expressed in the BM. Embryonic globins (*Hba-x*: -, *Hbb-bha1*: βh1- and *Hbb-y*: Ey-globin) were expressed after treatment with both NBP and PHZ (NBP + PHZ) in the BM and liver. **b** *In situ* hybridization to detect embryonic globin. Some of hematopoietic cells in the BM and some cells that formed clusters in the liver expressed embryonic globins. These cells were diffuse in the BM. Bars indicate 20 m. **c** 2D electrophoresis in the peripheral blood. The control showed three spots approximately 16 kDa in size. Three additional spots (arrows) appeared in the analysis of the blood of splenectomized mice that were treated with both NBP and PHZ (NBP + PHZ), with represented -, βh1- and Ey-embryonic globin

While the molecular weights of embryonic and adult globins are very similar, the isoelectric points of embryonic globins differ from those of adult globins (Additional file 4). Control erythrocytes showed only 3 adult globin spots: α (α1 and α2 are the same), β major and β minor (Fig. 4c). The molecular weight of these globins were approximately 15.5-16.5 kDa, and the isoelectric points were different (Fig. 4c). However, erythrocytes from the NBP- and PHZ-treated mice showed 6 spots corresponding to 3 definitive globins and 3 embryonic globins (Fig. 4c).

These results indicate that embryonic globins were induced at both the mRNA and protein levels by treatment with both NBP and PHZ and that these globins can form embryonic or semi-embryonic type hemoglobin subunits.

Expression of embryonic globin transcription factors

The expression of several embryonic globin transcription factors was analyzed using RT-PCR. The expression levels of *Klf1, Klf2* and *Gata1* were up-regulated, but the level of *Bcl11a* was unchanged in control animals and animals treated with NBP and PHZ (NBP + PHZ) (Fig. 5a). Because the expression of *Klf1* and *Klf2* was markedly increased, we used ChIP and PCR (ChIP-PCR) targeting of the embryonic globin promoters with anti-KLF1 or anti-KLF2 antibodies. DNA fragments that bound to KLF1 or KLF2 were used for globin promoter PCR. The results showed that binding of the βh1- and Ey-globin promoters bound KLF1 and KLF2 in the BM and livers of mice treated with NBP and PHZ (Fig. 5b). These results indicate that KLF1 and/or KLF2 regulate the transcription of embryonic β-like globins in the BM and liver. The expression patterns of *Bcl11a* suggests that the globin switching mechanism observed in this study might be different from the mechanism used during embryogenesis because Bcl11a plays an essential role in globin switching in normal ontogenic development of eythropoiesis.

Extramedullary erythropoiesis in newly identified structures

Extramedullary erythropoiesis occurs in various organs, including the lungs, heart, thymus, and hemal nodes, under abnormal conditions.

In this study, we unexpectedly observed the formations of wine-colored miliary structures in the abdominal cavities of several mice that were treated with both NBP and PHZ (Fig. 6a). In histological examination, these structures were capsule-shaped and filled with many hematopoietic cells, including megakaryocytes (Fig. 6b). Immunohistochemical analysis showed that many of the mononucleated cells were TER119-positive erythroblasts (Fig. 6c). Moreover, the embryonic globin mRNA was detected in these structure (Fig. 6d). These results indicated that these structures were the site of induction for extramedullary erythropoiesis in this critically anemic mouse model.

Discussion

Primitive and definitive erythroid cells display many differences that are consistent with the notion that they constitute distinct erythroid lineages. The two sequences of erythropoietic events that lead to the development of these cells never occur simultaneously in adults; therefore, embryonic globin is not expressed in adult mammals under normal conditions [2, 5, 9, 31]. However, in this study, we detected the expression of embryonic globins in genetically normal adult splenectomized mice under specific conditions including the the elimination of BM resident macrophages and the induction of critical anemia. Moreover, numerous nucleated erythrocytes appeared in the peripheral blood, and some erythroid cells were found to be CD71-positive. These cells were very similar to primitive erythrocytes [32]. Although certain diseases such as thalassemia and some knockout models that contain deletions in some important hemoglobin switching genes are associated with the expression of embryonic globins

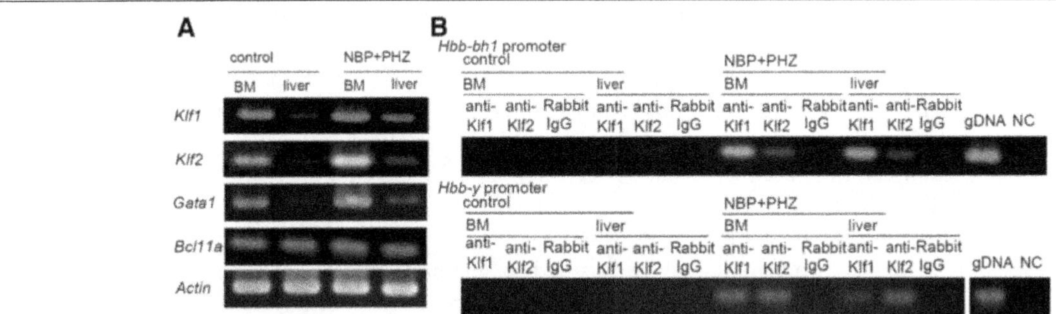

Fig. 5 The expression of erythropoiesis-related transcription factors in the BM and liver. **a** The expression levels of erythropoiesis-related factors (*Gata1, Klf1* and *Klf2*) were up-regulated in the BM and liver after treatment with both NBP and PHZ (NBP + PHZ), but no change was observed in the expression of *Bcl11a*. **b** ChIP-PCR analysis of KLF1 and KLF2 promoter-binding region. KLF1 and KLF2 promoter-binding regions were detected using PCR amplification in splenectomized mice that were treated with NBP and PHZ but not in control animals. Genomic DNA (gDNA) was used as a positive control. NC indicates results of PCR performed without primers. Rabbit IgG was used as a negative control for ChIP

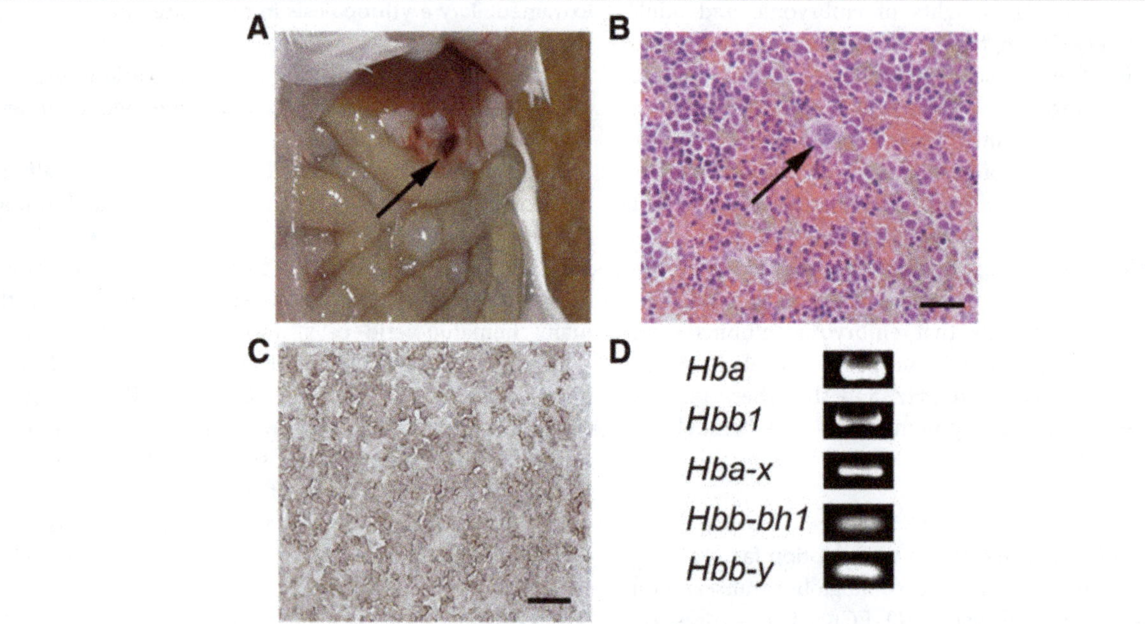

Fig. 6 Extramedullary erythropoiesis in newly identified structures. **a** Macroscopic observation of the abdominal cavity. Wine-colored structures were observed in the omentum in splenectomized mice that were treated with both NBP and PHZ (arrow). **b** The histological analysis stained with H-E. Numerous hematopoietic cells including megakaryocytes (arrow), were observed in these structures. **c** Immunohistochemical detection of TER119-positive cells. Most of the cells in this structure were TER119-positive erythroblasts. **d** RT-PCR analysis to determine globin mRNA levels in these newly identified structures. Both adult and embryonic globin mRNAs were expressed. Bars show 25 m (**b, c**)

after birth, there are no reports showing that wild type adult mice express embryonic globins [32–34]. Therefore, the present study contributes a novel experimental model that can be used to analyze the expression of embryonic globins and the results of this study suggests that yolk sac-derived primitive erythroid precursors are maintained in adult mammals in this model.

Various transcription factors related to erythropoiesis and the regulation of hemoglobin expression have been identified [5, 11]. In this study, the up-regulation of *Klf1* and *Klf2* was detected in the BM and liver. Moreover, we also confirmed KLF1 and KLF binding to the promoter region of β-like embryonic globin. These results indicate that KLF1 and KLF2 regulate the expression of β-like embryonic globin. We detected the expression of *Gata1* and *Bcl11a* mRNAs in the BM and liver in splenectomized mice that were treated with both NBP and PHZ. A recent study has shown that *Bcl11a* expression is regulated by KLF1, suggesting an intricate mechanism in which the developmental regulation of β-like globin genes is coordinated by KLF1 and Bcl11a [35]. In fact, the conditional knock out of *Bcl11a* in mice resulted in a decrease in the expression levels of embryonic globins in the BM compared to levels in the E18.5 fetal liver [36]. In this study, *Bcl11a* was constitutively expressed in the BM and liver under normal conditions, and its expression levels were unchanged even in animals with anemia. These results suggest that Bcl11a may not be associated with the expression of embryonic globin in this study because the cells expressing embryonic globin contained decreased levels of Bcl11a and the cells that expressed adult globin showed no change in the expression of Bcl11a. In addition, Bcl11a is essential for normal lymphocyte development mice.

During embryogenesis, the embryo is exposed to hypoxemia. Therefore, primitive hemoglobin has a higher affinity for oxygen than adult hemoglobin because it must provide all oxygenation to the body, and changes in the partial pressure of oxygen has been associated with globin switching [37, 38]. Our data suggest that the expression of embryonic globins might be more effectively rescuing the hypoxemia that is associated with critical anemia than the enhanced production of normal definitive erythroid cells. The hypoxic response is controlled by two transcriptional regulatory complexes called hypoxia inducible factors (HIFs). These link iron homeostasis and erythropoiesis by targeting EPO [5, 39]. Although a direct association between the HIFs and the expression of embryonic globins has not been described, EPO has been suggested to support primitive hematopoiesis and to increase the expression of embryonic globin during embryogenesis [40, 41]. Therefore, the high EPO concentration caused by hypoxia might be partially responsible for the expression of embryonic globins in this study.

We confirmed that there were differences in expression patterns between the BM and liver, suggesting that cells in the liver originate in a different microenvironment, via a different mechanism and/or from a cell origin that is different from that in the BM. In fact, some hematopoiesis-related factors show different expression patterns between the E18.5 fetal BM and liver [42]. Our ISH data indicate that a relatively large number of cells expressed embryonic globins in the liver whereas only a few cells expressed these mRNAs in the BM. qRT-PCR analysis also showed that the expression level of embryonic globin in the liver was higher than level in the BM (Additional file 2). Erythropoiesis in the BM may primarily produce definitive erythroid cells, and the primitive-type may originate from a small population of hematopoietic cells. The liver is associated with fetal hematopoiesis, including primitive erythropoiesis [43]. These results may be related to the availability for quick induction of extramedullary hematopoiesis and the formation of a niche for primitive erythropoiesis in the liver.

Resident macrophages act as pivotal stromal cells during definitive erythropoiesis. In fact, erythropoiesis was inhibited by the elimination of BM resident macrophages in our previous studies [26, 27]. In addition, macrophages perform essential roles even in extramedullary erythropoiesis and abnormal erythropoiesis, such as that observed in β-thalassemia, whereas primitive erythroid cells do not require macrophages in the stroma [44]. An ISH study indicated that some TER119-positive colonies were composed of both embryonic globin-expressing and -non-expressing cells. In the early stage of the transition from primitive to definitive hematopoiesis, primitive hematopoietic cells migrate to the fetal liver, contact macrophages, and continue to express embryonic type globins within a short period of time. In our experiments, some of the TER119-positive cells did not express embryonic globin mRNAs. These results did not clearly indicate the origin of the hematopoietic cells expressing embryonic globins, but they do suggest that the expression of embryonic globins in this study could have been caused by both the depletion of macrophages and stimulation with an acute hypoxemia.

In this study, we were unable to define the origin of the erythroid cells that expressed embryonic globins. Because some tissue macrophages originate in the yolk sac and then proliferate in peripheral tissues [45, 46], we were unable to eliminate the possibility that these cells were derived from primitive hematopoietic cells and that these primitive erythroid precursor cells might be reactivated by the elimination of stroma cells and the presence of hypoxic stress. Further studies will be necessary to determine the origin of these cells.

New structures were unexpectedly induced in the peritoneum and/or omentum of some of the splenectomized mice that were treated with both NBP and PHZ (Fig. 6). These were wine-colored structures that resembled hemal nodes and showed active hematopoiesis. Extramedullary erythropoiesis is induced in various organs by certain conditions such as acute anemia, NBP injection, myelofibrosis, and blood cancer [26–28]. The induction of hemal node-like structures could be caused by insufficient hematopoiesis in the BM and the liver. Further study is required to clarify the mechanism that cause the induction of these newly hematopoietic organs.

The results showing that a relatively large number of erythroblasts form clusters and nucleated erythrocytes in the peripheral blood suggest the existence of primitive erythroid cells in the mice. These cells were large, nucleated erythrocytes. The presence of embryonic or fetal hemoglobin has been suggested in hematopoietic progenitors in human peripheral blood, but this does not explain the expression of these hemoglobin in hematopoietic sites [47, 48]. Several reports have also demonstrated the expression of embryonic or fetal globins *in vitro* [49, 50]; however, our study has shown for the first time, the simultaneous expression of embryonic and adult globins in erythrocytes in genetically normal mice. These results contribute to our understanding of normal and disease-related hematopoiesis.

Conclusions

We established a severely anemic mice model by the sequential treatment with NBP and PHZ. This model showed the emergence of nucleated erythrocytes in peripheral blood and the expressions of embryonic types of hemoglobin in hematopoietic sites. Our results might indicate the flexible property of hematopoiesis and the possibility that yolk sac-derived primitive erythroid cells may persist into adulthood in mice.

Abbreviations

NBP: nitrogen-containing bisphosphonate; PHZ: phenylhydrazine; BM: bone marrow; EPO: erythropoietin; AP: alkaline-phosphatase; PBS: phosphate-buffered saline; EDTA: ethylenediaminetetraacetic acid; HE: hematoxylin-eosin; ISH: in situ hybridization; qRT-PCR: quantitative RT-PCR; ChIP: chromatin immunoprecipitation.

Competing interests

The authors declare that they have no competing interests.

Authors' contributions

HO, NY and NN carried out all experiments: blood analyses, histology, immunohistochemistry, ISH, RT-PCR, ChIP, flow-cytometry and electrophoresis, SS handled animals and prepared samples, and HY analyzed and reconstructed image data. YE produced NBP used in this study; and JT and MN provided this study and wrote the paper. All authors read and approved the final manuscript.

Acknowledgments

We thank to kind advices from Dr Kuraoka, M. and Dr Hyzewicz, J., Department of Molecular Therapy, National Institute of Neuroscience, National Center of Neurology and Psychiatry; and Dr. Tanaka, J., Irie, T. and Mishima, K., Department of Oral Pathology, School of Dentistry, Showa University.

Funding

The part of this study was supported by the Grant-in-Aid for Scientific Research (20592148, 21592342 and 15K11022), Research Activity start-up (24890237) and Young Scientists (15K20367) from the Ministry of Education, Culture, Sports, Science and Technology of Japan. This study was also in part supported by High-Tech Research Center Project for Private Universities from Ministry of Education, Culture, Sports, Science and Technology, Japan.

Author details

[1]Department of Oral Anatomy and Developmental Biology, School of Dentistry, Showa University, 1-5-8 Hatanodai, Shinagawa-ku, Tokyo 142-8555, Japan. [2]Division of Molecular Regulation, Graduate School of Dentistry, Tohoku University, 4-1 Seiryo-machi, Aoba-ku, Sendai 980-8575, Japan. [3]Faculty of Pharmacy, International University of Health and Welfare, 2600-1 Kitakanamaru, Otawara-shi, Tochigi 324-8501, Japan. [4]Department of Veterinary Anatomy, Nippon Veterinary and Animal Science University, 1-7-1 Kyonan-cho, Musashino-shi, Tokyo 180-8602, Japan.

References

1. Palis J, Yoder MC. Yolk-sac hematopoiesis: the first blood cells of mouse and man. Exp Hematol. 2001;29(8):927–36.
2. McGrath KE, Palis J. Hematopoiesis in the yolk sac: more than meets the eye. Exp Hematol. 2005;33(9):1021–8.
3. McGrath K, Palis J. Ontogeny of erythropoiesis in the mammalian embryo. Curr Top Dev Biol. 2008;82:1–22.
4. Kingsley PD, Malik J, Fantauzzo KA, Palis J. Yolk sac-derived primitive erythroblasts enucleate during mammalian embryogenesis. Blood. 2004;104(1):19–25.
5. Palis J. Molecular Biology of Erythropoiesis. In: Wickrema A, Kee B, editors. Molecular Basis of Hematopoiesis. New York: Springer; 2009. p. 73–93.
6. Baron MH, Isern J, Fraser ST. The embryonic origins of erythropoiesis in mammals. Blood. 2012;119(21):4828–37.
7. Kingsley PD, Malik J, Emerson RL, Bushnell TP, McGrath KE, Bloedorn LA, et al. "Maturational" globin switching in primary primitive erythroid cells. Blood. 2006;107(4):1665–72.
8. McGrath KE, Frame JM, Fromm GJ, Koniski AD, Kingsley PD, Little J, et al. A transient definitive erythroid lineage with unique regulation of the beta-globin locus in the mammalian embryo. Blood. 2011;117(17):4600–8.
9. Sankaran VG, Xu J, Orkin SH. Advances in the understanding of haemoglobin switching. Br J Haematol. 2010;149(2):181–94.
10. Tsiftsoglou AS, Vizirianakis IS, Strouboulis J. Erythropoiesis: model systems, molecular regulators, and developmental programs. IUBMB Life. 2009;61(8):800–30.
11. McConnell BB, Yang VW. Mammalian Kruppel-like factors in health and diseases. Physiol Rev. 2010;90(4):1337–81.
12. Hodge D, Coghill E, Keys J, Maguire T, Hartmann B, McDowall A, et al. A global role for EKLF in definitive and primitive erythropoiesis. Blood. 2006;107(8):3359–70.
13. Drissen R, von Lindern M, Kolbus A, Driegen S, Steinlein P, Beug H, et al. The erythroid phenotype of EKLF-null mice: defects in hemoglobin metabolism and membrane stability. Mol Cell Biol. 2005;25(12):5205–14.
14. Basu P, Lung TK, Lemsaddek W, Sargent TG, Williams Jr DC, Basu M, et al. EKLF and KLF2 have compensatory roles in embryonic beta-globin gene expression and primitive erythropoiesis. Blood. 2007;110(9):3417–25.
15. Alhashem YN, Vinjamur DS, Basu M, Klingmuller U, Gaensler KM, Lloyd JA. Transcription factors KLF1 and KLF2 positively regulate embryonic and fetal beta-globin genes through direct promoter binding. J Biol Chem. 2011; 286(28):24819–27.
16. Bessis M, Mize C, Prenant M. Erythropoiesis: comparison of in vivo and in vitro amplification. Blood Cells. 1978;4(1-2):155–74.
17. Seshi B, Kumar S, Sellers D. Human bone marrow stromal cell: coexpression of markers specific for multiple mesenchymal cell lineages. Blood Cells Mol Dis. 2000;26(3):234–46.
18. Manwani D, Bieker JJ. The erythroblastic island. Curr Top Dev Biol. 2008;82:23–53.
19. Chasis JA, Mohandas N. Erythroblastic islands: niches for erythropoiesis. Blood. 2008;112(3):470–8.
20. Rich IN, Heit W, Kubanek B. Extrarenal erythropoietin production by macrophages. Blood. 1982;60(4):1007–18.
21. Rich IN. A role for the macrophage in normal hemopoiesis. II. Effect of varying physiological oxygen tensions on the release of hemopoietic growth factors from bone-marrow-derived macrophages in vitro. Exp Hematol. 1986;14(8):746–51.
22. Body JJ. Rationale for the use of bisphosphonates in osteoblastic and osteolytic bone lesions. Breast. 2003;12 Suppl 2:S37–44.
23. Cremers SC, Eekhoff ME, Den Hartigh J, Hamdy NA, Vermeij P, Papapoulos SE. Relationships between pharmacokinetics and rate of bone turnover after intravenous bisphosphonate (olpadronate) in patients with Paget's disease of bone. J Bone Miner Res. 2003;18(5):868–75.
24. Endo Y, Shibazaki M, Yamaguchi K, Nakamura M, Kosugi H. Inhibition of inflammatory actions of aminobisphosphonates by dichloromethylene bisphosphonate, a non-aminobisphosphonate. Br J Pharmacol. 1999; 126(4):903–10.
25. Yamaguchi K, Oizumi T, Funayama H, Kawamura H, Sugawara S, Endo Y. Osteonecrosis of the jawbones in 2 osteoporosis patients treated with nitrogen-containing bisphosphonates: osteonecrosis reduction replacing NBP with non-NBP (etidronate) and rationale. J Oral Maxillofac Surg. 2010;68(4):889–97.
26. Nakamura M, Yagi H, Endo Y, Kosugi H, Ishi T, Itoh T. A time kinetic study of the effect of aminobisphosphonate on murine haemopoiesis. Br J Haematol. 1999;107(4):779–90.
27. Otsuka H, Yagi H, Endo Y, Nonaka N, Nakamura M. Kupffer cells support extramedullary erythropoiesis induced by nitrogen-containing bisphosphonate in splenectomized mice. Cell Immunol. 2011;271(1):197–204.
28. Perry JM, Harandi OF, Paulson RF. BMP4, SCF, and hypoxia cooperatively regulate the expansion of murine stress erythroid progenitors. Blood. 2007;109(10):4494–502.
29. Josef B. Phenylhydrazine haematotoxicity. J Appl Biomed. 2007;5:125–30. Zhu X, Liu J, Feng Y, Pang W, Qi Z, Jiang Y, Shang H, Cao Y. Phenylhydrazine administration accelerates the development of experimental cerebral malaria. *Exp Parasitol* 2015; 156:1-11.
30. Esteghamat F, Gillemans N, Bilic I, van den Akker E, Cantu I, van Gent T, et al. Erythropoiesis and globin switching in compound Klf1::Bcl11a mutant mice. Blood. 2013;121(13):2553–62.
31. McConnell SC, Huo Y, Liu S, Ryan TM. Human globin knock-in mice complete fetal-to-adult hemoglobin switching in postnatal development. Mol Cell Biol. 2011;31(4):876–83.
32. D'Amici GM, Rinalducci S, Zolla L. An easy preparative gel electrophoretic method for targeted depletion of hemoglobin in erythrocyte cytosolic samples. Electrophoresis. 2011;32(11):1319–22.
33. Wen L, Zhu P, Liu Y, Pan Q, Qu Y, Xu X, et al. Development of a fluorescence immunochromatographic assay for the detection of zeta globin in the blood of (–(SEA)) alpha-thalassemia carriers. Blood Cells Mol Dis. 2012;49(3-4):128–32.
34. Laing EL, Brasch HD, Steel R, Jia J, Itinteang T, Tan ST, et al. Verrucous hemangioma expresses primitive markers. J Cutan Pathol. 2013;40(4):391–6.
35. Zhou D, Liu K, Sun CW, Pawlik KM, Townes TM. KLF1 regulates BCL11A expression and gamma- to beta-globin gene switching. Nat Genet. 2010;42(9):742–4.
36. Sankaran VG, Xu J, Ragoczy T, Ippolito GC, Walkley CR, Maika SD, et al. Developmental and species-divergent globin switching are driven by BCL11A. Nature. 2009;460(7259):1093–7.
37. He Z, Lian L, Asakura T, Russell JE. Functional effects of replacing human alpha- and beta-globins with their embryonic globin homologues in defined haemoglobin heterotetramers. Br J Haematol. 2000;109(4):882–90.

38. Bichet S, Wenger RH, Camenisch G, Rolfs A, Ehleben W, Porwol T, et al. Oxygen tension modulates beta-globin switching in embryoid bodies. FASEB J. 1999;13(2):285–95.
39. Shah YM, Xie L. Hypoxia-inducible factors link iron homeostasis and erythropoiesis. Gastroenterology. 2014;146(3):630–42.
40. Malik J, Kim AR, Tyre KA, Cherukuri AR, Palis J. Erythropoietin critically regulates the terminal maturation of murine and human primitive erythroblasts. Haematologica. 2013;98(11):1778–87.
41. Kieran MW, Perkins AC, Orkin SH, Zon LI. Thrombopoietin rescues in vitro erythroid colony formation from mouse embryos lacking the erythropoietin receptor. Proc Natl Acad Sci U S A. 1996;93(17):9126–31.
42. Ciriza J, Hall D, Lu A, De Sena JR, Al-Kuhlani M, Garcia-Ojeda ME. Single-cell analysis of murine long-term hematopoietic stem cells reveals distinct patterns of gene expression during fetal migration. PLoS One. 2012;7(1):e30542.
43. Isern J, Fraser ST, He Z, Baron MH. The fetal liver is a niche for maturation of primitive erythroid cells. Proc Natl Acad Sci U S A. 2008;105(18):6662–7.
44. Chow A, Huggins M, Ahmed J, Hashimoto D, Lucas D, Kunisaki Y, et al. CD169(+) macrophages provide a niche promoting erythropoiesis under homeostasis and stress. Nat Med. 2013;19(4):429–36.
45. Ginhoux F, Greter M, Leboeuf M, Nandi S, See P, Gokhan S, et al. Fate mapping analysis reveals that adult microglia derive from primitive macrophages. Science. 2010;330(6005):841–5.
46. Schulz C, Gomez Perdiguero E, Chorro L, Szabo-Rogers H, Cagnard N, Kierdorf K, et al. A lineage of myeloid cells independent of Myb and hematopoietic stem cells. Science. 2012;336(6077):86–90.
47. Lau ET, Kwok YK, Chui DH, Wong HS, Luo HY, Tang MH. Embryonic and fetal globins are expressed in adult erythroid progenitor cells and in erythroid cell cultures. Prenat Diagn. 2001;21(7):529–39.
48. Luo HY, Liang XL, Frye C, Wonio M, Hankins GD, Chui DH, et al. Embryonic hemoglobins are expressed in definitive cells. Blood. 1999;94(1):359–61.
49. Qiu C, Olivier EN, Velho M, Bouhassira EE. Globin switches in yolk sac-like primitive and fetal-like definitive red blood cells produced from human embryonic stem cells. Blood. 2008;111(4):2400–8.
50. Yang CT, French A, Goh PA, Pagnamenta A, Mettananda S, Taylor J, et al. Human induced pluripotent stem cell derived erythroblasts can undergo definitive erythropoiesis and co-express gamma and beta globins. Br J Haematol. 2014;166(3):435–48.

7

Coagulation profile of Sudanese children with homozygous sickle cell disease and the effect of treatment with omega-3 fatty acid on the coagulation parameters

Shiekh Awoda[1,3], Ahmed A. Daak[1,2,4*], Nazik Elmalaika Husain[3], Kebreab Ghebremeskel[4] and Mustafa I. Elbashir[1]

Abstract

Background: It has been reported that patients with SCD do have an abnormal coagulation profile. Coagulopathy is thought to be one of the key factors that contribute to the vaso-occlusive crisis that characterises sickle cell disease (SCD). In this study, we investigated whether Sudanese sickle cell patients have an abnormal coagulation profile. In addition, the effect of treatment with either omega-3 fatty acids or hydroxyurea on coagulation profile was assessed.

Methods: Homozygous SCD patients untreated ($n = 52$), omega-3 treated ($n = 44$), hydroxyurea (HU) treated ($n = 8$) and healthy (HbAA) controls ($n = 52$) matched for age (4–20 years), gender and socioeconomic status were enrolled. Patients on omega-3 fatty acids, according to age, received one to four capsules containing 277. 8 mg DHA and 39.0 mg eicosapentnoic. Patients on Hydroxyurea were in on dosage more than 20 mg/kg/day. The steady state levels of the coagulation parameters and the effect of the treatments with either HU or omega-3 fatty acids on markers of coagulation were investigated.

Results: Compared to the healthy controls, treated and untreated HbSS patients had lower hemoglobin, plasma Protein C, proteins S and higher white blood cell count (WBC), platelets count (PLTs) and plasma D-dimer levels,($p < 0.05$). In comparison to untreated HbSS, treatment with neither omega-3 nor HU had effect on the WBC, plasma proteins C and S, ($p > 0.05$). HU treated group had a lower PLTs count compared to HbSS untreated group ($p < 0.5$). The prothrombin and activated partial thromboplastin times and international normalized ratio (INR) of untreated patients are significantly higher than n-3 treated, HU-treated patients and health controls, ($p < 0.05$). Patients treated with omega-3 had lowered D-dimer levels in comparison to HU-treated and untreated HbSS patients, ($p < 0.001$).

Conclusion: This study provides evidence that Sudanes patients have abnormal coagulation profile and treatment with either HU or omega-3 fatty acids might partially ameliorate SCD-associated chronic coagulopathic state.

Keywords: Sickle cell disease, Coagulation, Omega-3 fatty acids, D-dimer, Protein C, Protein S

* Correspondence: ahmed.malik@meduofk.net; malikdaak@hotmail.com
[1]Department of Medical Biochemistry, Faculty of Medicine, University of Khartoum, Alghasr Street, Khartoum, Sudan
[2]Center of Molecular Biology and Biotechnology (CMBB), Florida Atlantic University (FAU), Boca Raton, USA
Full list of author information is available at the end of the article

Background

Chronic hypercoagulable or prothrombotic state is generally known to be one of the factors that contribute to vaso-occlusion and progressive end-organ damage in sickle cell disease (SCD) [1, 2]. Studies on SCD patients at steady state patients from different geographic and demographic origins have shown elevated level of markers of coagulation activation [3, 4], and decreased natural anticoagulant proteins [5, 6]. Agents that physiologically activate platelets and coagulation in vivo include adenosine diphosphate (ADP), collagen, epinephrine, thrombin, serotonin, arachidonic acid and thromboxane A2 [7]. Interestingly, blood cell membranes of patients with SCD have an abnormal fatty acid profile which is characterised by low levels of omega-3, namely eicosapentaenoic (EPA) and docosahexaenoic acids (DHA), and a high level of omega-6, particularly arachidonic acid (AA) [8, 9]. A high intake of omega-3 fatty acids is inversely associated with thromboxane level and prothrombotic activity [10, 11]. Consequently, it has been postulated that regular intake of n-3 fatty acids in patients with SCD may modulate markers of coagulation.

On the other hand, Hydroxyurea (hydroxycarbamide) is currently the only approved drug to prevent the acute complications of the disease [12], and has several well-defined beneficial effects that might involve mitigation of the hypercoagulability state in patients with SCD [13]. In this study we investigated whether (1) Sudanese sickle cell patients have an abnormal profile of coagulation parameters; (2) the coagulation parameter are modified by omega-3 fatty acids or hydroxyurea.

Methods

Subjects

In this study, steady state homozygous sickle cell patients (HbSS) on high DHA omega-3 treatment (n = 44), hydroxyurea treatment HbSS (HU, n = 8), steady HbSS patients not treated either with HU or omega-3 fatty acids (n = 52) controls and healthy sibling controls (HbAA, n = 52), matched one to one by age (4–20 years), gender and socioeconomic status were included. "Steady state" is defined as being free from acute painful crisis or other medical condition for at least one month before the enrolment. The patients and healthy controls, who were mostly siblings of the patients, were enrolled from Abnaof Paediatric Hospital, Khartoum, Sudan, between February and May 2014. We selected the patients' healthy HbAA siblings as controls in order to minimise the potential effect of dietary background and genetic factors on the variables under investigation. Haemoglobin phenotypes were confirmed using cellulose acetate electrophoresis at pH 8.5. The exclusion criteria for participation in the study were other chronic disorder and conditions (defined as the one that lasting 3 months or more), blood transfusion in the previous four-months. The patients on n-3 fatty acids received a daily dosage of one, two, three or four capsules according to the patient's age (< 5), (5–10), (11–16) and (>17) years, respectively. The n-3 capsule contains 277.8 mg docosahexaenoic (DHA) and 39.0 mg eicosapentnoic (EPA) and (1.5 mg) of vitamin E to prevent fatty acids peroxidation. The n-3 fatty acid group was on same dosage of n-3 fatty acids for minimum of three years. The hydroxyurea group was treated daily with a dose of 20 mg per kilogram body weight orally for minimum of at least one year. The patients participated in this study were on regular folate supplement. The healthy control subjects did not receive folate or any other nutritional supplement.

The equation ($n = (Z_{\alpha/2} + Z_{\beta})^2 * 2 * \sigma^2 / d^2$) was employed to calculate the sample size, and the assumption that the mean difference of D-dimer between the omega-3 treated and untreated patients 1 μg/ml compared to untreated. The population variance was assumed to equal to 2 μg/ml. To detect the assumed mean difference with 95% power at a 5% significance level, minimum of 43 patients is required in each arm.

Blood sample collection and processing

Blood was drawn under sterile conditions into EDTA coated (2.5 ml) and tri-sodium citrate (2.5 ml) containing vacutainer tubes. The EDTA blood was used for hematological tests. The citrate blood was immediately fractionated into plasma and red blood cells by cold centrifugation at 3000 rpm for 15 min. The resulting top plasma layer was carefully siphoned off, without contaminating with buffy coat, and transferred into another tube and stored at–80 °C. The stored plasma was subsequently used for the determination of coagulation profile and anticoagulation proteins.

Hematological parameters

Haemoglobin concentration (Hb), haematocrit (Ht), mean corpuscular volume (MCV), mean corpuscular haemoglobin (MCH), mean corpuscular haemoglobin concentration (MCHC), total white blood cell count (TWBC), platelet count (PLTs) and total red blood cell count were measured with the use of Sysmex KX-21 N Automated Hematology Analyzer (Sysmex Corporation, Kobe, Japan).

Coagulation profile

Prothrombin time (PT) and activated partial thromboplastin time (aPTT) were determined by an automated micro-computer controlled coagulometer, DiaMed-CD2 (DIaMed, GmbH, Cressier, Switzerland). International normalized ratio (INR) was also assessed.

D-dimer

The concentration of D-dimer was measured by enzyme-linked immune-sorbent assay using i-Chroma hsCRP test kits and i-CHROMA Reader (BodiTech Med Inc., Gang-won do, Korea).

Anticoagulation proteins C and S

Proteins C and S concentrations were determined by enzyme linked immune-sorbent assay kit (Asys Hitech GmbH, Austria).

Data analysis

According to the parametric or non-parametric distribution, the data were expressed as mean ± SD or median and interquartile range (IQR) as pertinent. The groups were compared for haematological profile, coagulation profile, anticoagulant proteins and D-dimer levels by using one-way an ANOVA on ranks (Kruskal-Wallis H test). When statistical differences were indicated, Dunn's non-parametric comparison for post-hoc tests were obtained. The statistical significance was assumed at a "p" value of less than 0.05. The data were analysed with SPSS for Windows, Version 19 (SPSS Ltd., Surrey, UK).

Results

Demographic and haematological characteristics

The baseline demographic and haematological values of the omega-3 fatty acid treated and untreated patients and healthy controls were described in Table 1. The mean age of the patients on HU was significantly higher than that of the other three groups ($p < 0.05$).

Haematological parameters

The hematological values of the groups studied were shown in Table 2. Apart from PLT count, neither treatment with omega-3 nor HU resulted in significant change in haematological profile in comparison to HbSS untreated patients. The haematological parameters MCV, MCH and MCHC values of the patients and healthy controls were not different ($p > 0.05$).

Table 1 Baseline demographic and hematological characteristics of the patients and healthy controls

	HbSS Omega −3 treated	HbSS Omega −3 untreated	HbSS HU-treated	HbAA Healthy controls
Number of patients (*n*)	44	52	8	52
Male	22	28	6	28
Female	22	24	2	24
Age (years, mean ± SD)	9.8 ± 2.9	10.8 ± 4.0	17.4 ± 0.9*	11.3 ± 4.0

*$P < 0.05$ hydroxyurea group compared with groups

Coagulation profile (PT, aPTT and INR)

In comparison with the healthy controls, the omega-3 fatty acid treated, HU-treated and untreated patients had increased PT, aPTT and INR ($p < 0.01$, Table 3). The omega-3 treated and, HU-treated patients had significantly lower coagulation parameters when compared with Untreated patients ($p < 0.05$, Table 3).

Plasma D-dimer levels

The healthy control subjects had a lower level of plasma D-dimer concentration than the omega-3 fatty acid treated, HU-treated and un-treated patients ($p < 0.001$). The omega-3 fatty acid treated group compared with HU-treated (Median = 1.14 (IQR = 0.74) µg/ml vs Median = 2.33.0 (IQR = 3.17) µg/ml, ($p < 0.001$)) and untreated (Median = 1.4 (IQR = 0.74) µg/L vs Median = 1.75 (IQR = 1.16) µg/ml, ($p < 0.001$) patients had a lower plasma D-dimer level. Patients treated with HU had a higher levels of plasma D-dimer compared to HbSS untreated ($p < 0.01$, Fig. 1).

Plasma proteins C and S levels

The untreated patients had reduced level of plasma protein C compared with the healthy controls (Median = 90.5 (IQR = 20.0) µg/mL, ($p < 0.001$). The omega-3 fatty acid (Median = 60.5 (IQR = 19) µg/mL) and HU (Median = 59.5 (IQR = 13) µg/mL), ($p > 0.05$) treated and the untreated (Median = 60.0 (IQR = 23.0) µg/mL) patients had comparable concentration of protein C ($p > 0.05$, Fig. 2).

Plasma protein S concentration was lower in the treated (omega-3 and HU) and untreated patients than in the healthy controls (Median = 139.5 (IQR = 28.0) µg/mL, ($p < 0.001$)). There was no difference in protein S level between the unntreated (Median = 42.5 (IQR = 18.0) µg/mL), omega-3 treated (Median = 45.5 (IQR = 14.0) µg/mL) and HU-treated (Median = 40.5 (IQR = 11) µg/mL) patients ($p > 0.05$, Fig. 3).

Discussion

Hydroxyurea, which is a cytotoxic, antimetabolic and antineoplastic agent, is the only disease-modifying therapy approved for sickle cell disease [14]. Hydroxyurea has been shown to be partially effective in reducing the frequency of vaso-occlusive events; but, there is no evidence that it prevents organ damage [15]. One of the factors which restricts HU usage is that it undergoes renal clearance, and hence there is a need for careful dose adjustment and close monitoring of myelotoxicity in individuals with renal impairment [16]. This vital requirement is hardly possible to undertake in most developing countries where SCD is highly prevalent because of lack of functional facilities and expertise. Therefore, there is a need for safe, effective and easily manageable treatment(s) for children and adult patients with sickle cell disease. Clinical trials have provided

Table 2 Mean (±sd) hematological parameter values of omega-3 fatty acid treated, hydroxyurea treated and untreated patients (HbSS) and healthy controls

	Omega-3 FA Treated Patients	Untreated patients	HU Treated	Healthy Controls
Hb (g/l)	75.6 ± 16.2***	75.9 ± 10.3^{+++}	79.5 ± 10.3	126.0 ± 10.9
HCt	22.9 ± 4.7***	22.9 ± 3.0^{+++}	23.8 ± 2.8	38.0 ± 3.5
RBC	2.8 ± 0.7***	2.7 ± 0.5^{+++}	2.8 ± 0.6	4.6 ± 0.5
MCV (fl)	84.3 ± 8.6	86.5 ± 7.1	87.8 ± 11.6	82.3 ± 4.7
MCH (pg)	27.9 ± 3.4	28.6 ± 3.0	29.5 ± 4.4	27.6 ± 1.9
MCHC	33.3 ± 2.0	33.1 ± 1.4	33.4 ± 0.9	33.5 ± 1.5
PLT	489.5 ± 121.1***	533.6 ± 98.7^{+++}	414.5 ± 109.9^{x}	330.3 ± 72.5
WBC	12.4 ± 4.3***	13.3 ± 3.4^{+++}	13.6 ± 3.7	6.3 ± 1.3

***$p < 0.001$ Omega 3 treated versus healthy controls
++$p < 0.01$, +++$p < 0.001$ Untreated patients versus healthy controls
$^{x}p < 0.05$, HU treated versus untreated patients

evidence that omega-3 fatty acids are effective in reducing frequency and severity of vaso-occlusive episodes, severe anemia, blood transfusion rate, markers of inflammation and oxidative stress [17–21]. In the current study, patients treated with omega-3 showed a significant reduction in D-dimer. The findings of this study indicate that treatment with omega-3 may partially ameliorate SCD-associated coagulopathy.

The SCD patients and healthy controls who participated in this study were homogenous with respect to ethnicity and socio-economic background and the patients received similar quality of care under regular management protocols. The samples were collected in one clinic and at the same time of the year. Therefore, the observed findings are likely to be due to the effect of intervention with omega-3 fatty acids or hydroxyurea treatment rather than of extraneous confounding factors.

Consistent with previous studies, both the omega-3 fatty acid treated and untreated patients had elevated steady state white blood cell and platelet counts confirming that sickle cell disease is a chronic inflammatory disorder [22]. Similarly, Tomer et al. [18] have reported that treatment with omega-3 fatty acids do not effect significantly the blood cell count, MCV or MCHC.

There is evidence which indicates that HU mediates its beneficial effects in SCD, partially, by lowering leukocyte, reticulocyte and platelet counts [23]. In the current study, HU treatment reduced platelet count significantly but had no noticeable effect on WBC. This unexpected effect of HU on WBC among Sudanese children with SCD might be a reflection of the fact that HU is generally being administered mostly to the severely ill children with SCD [24], or a response peculiar to Sudanese SCD patients that warrant further research.

The PT, aPTT and INR levels of the untreated patients were significantly higher than the n-3 fatty acid and hydroxyurea treated groups. Similar findings have been observed on Americans [25] and Nigerians children [26] and adult Jamaicans [6] with sickle cell disease. The prolongation of PT in the adult patients was not as remarkable as in the children. In contrast, another study investigated 17 subjects did not find a difference in mean PT between SCD and healthy children [27]. These controversial findings might be a reflection of the study small sample size.

Table 3 Mean (±sd) coagulation profile parameter values of omega-3 fatty acid and hydroxyurea treated and untreated sickle cell patients (HbSS) and healthy contols

	Omga-3 treated	untreated	HU treated	Healthy controls
PT (sec)	17.2 ± 1.8†††	31.3 ± 11.1^{+++}	18.2 ± 1.8^{xxx}	14.5 ± 0.7
aPTT (sec)	38.3 ± 4.2†††	57.0 ± 11.3^{+++}	42.8 ± 2.7^{xxx}	37.0 ± 3.8
INR	1.2 ± 0.14†††	2.3 ± 0.90^{+++}	1.3 ± 0.12^{xxx}	1.01 ± 0.05

†††$p < 0.001$ omega-3 treated versus untreated patients
$^{+++}p < 0.001$ untreated patients versus healthy controls
$^{xxx}p < 0.001$ HU treated versus untreated patients

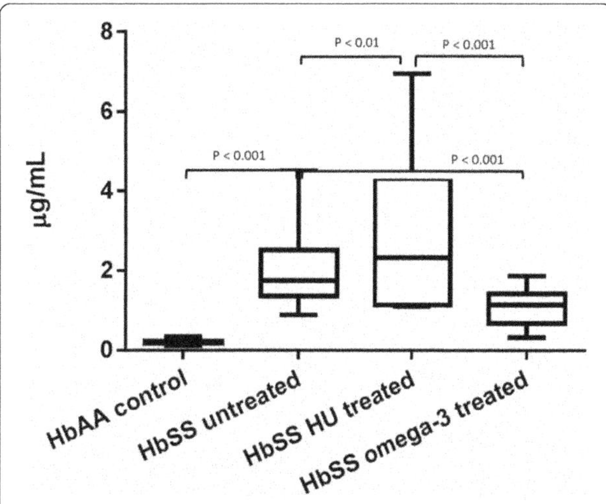

Fig. 1 Plasma D-dimer levels of omega-3 fatty acid treated, hydroxyurea treated and untreated patients with homozygous sickle cell disease (HbSS)

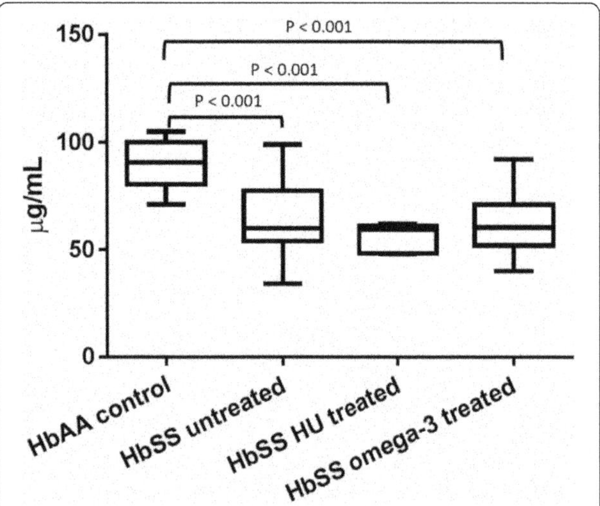

Fig. 2 Plasma Protein C levels of omega-3 fatty acid treated, hydroxyurea treated and untreated patients with homozygous sickle cell disease (HbSS) .*There were no significant differences ($p > 0.05$) between the HbSS untreated, HbSS HU treated and HbSS omega-3 treated

The mechanism behind the prolongation of PT in children with SCD is not fully understood. It is suggested that impaired liver function [25] and depletion of coagulation factors [28] play a role in the prolongation process. However, it is worth pointing out that a relationship between an abnormal liver function and coagulation prolongation is yet to be established.

In contrast to the findings of the current study, high omega-3 fatty acid intake did not have a significant effect on PT and aPTT in adult patients with sickle cell disease

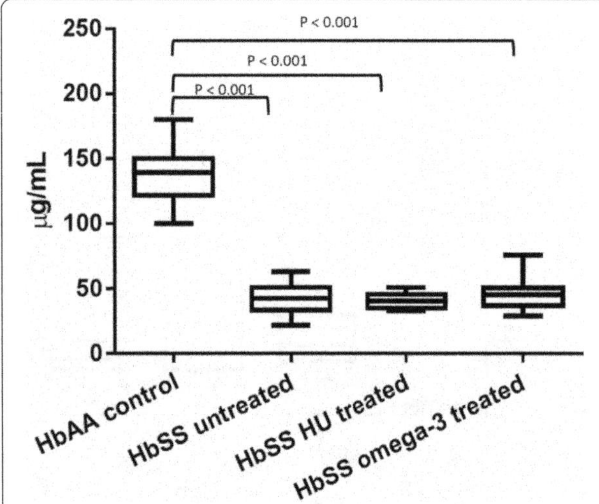

Fig. 3 Plasma Protein S levels of omega-3 fatty acid treated, hydroxyurea treated and untreated patients with homozygous sickle cell disease (HbSS). *There were no significant differences ($p > 0.05$) between the HbSS untreated, HbSS HU treated and HbSS omega-3 treated

[18], and in adult carcinoma patients undergoing elective surgery [29]. The subjects in the latter two studies, [18, 29], were adults from different ethnic background clinical complications and normal coagulation parameter values at baseline. In addition, the n-3 fatty acids composition of the oil/supplement used in these two studies were different from the high DHA capsules given to the children in the current study. The observed reduction of coagulation parameters in treated SCD patients in this study could be the result of increased availability of the coagulation factors and the possible concomitant reduction in coagulation activation that could surpass its potential detrimental hypo-coagulant effect [30, 31]. HU treatment had a similar effect as n-3 fatty acids on PT and aPTT suggesting that children with abnormal coagulation profile are responsive to either therapy.

The low level steady-state proteins C and S in the Sudanese children with SCD, which agrees with previous findings [6, 32], is in line with the hypothesis that the chronic activation of both the inflammatory and coagulant pathways in SCD are partially due to the disease associated down regulation of anti-coagulant pathway [33]. Protein C, activated by thrombin in the presence of protein S, inhibits the clotting ability of factor V and VIII [34]. The underlying cause of the natural anti-coagulant deficiency is yet to be elucidated. However, it has been generally attributed to the known SCD-associated hemostatic abnormalities and hepatic dysfunction [27]. An earlier study [35] reported a decrease in proteins C in children with sickle cell disease treated with hydroxyurea. That study included 11 children, 5 of them were homozygous SCD patients. The discrepancy of HU effect on proteins C and S between this study and the previous study could be due to the fact that Koc et al. study [35] was relatively underpowered to detect the true HU effect on natural anti-coagulant system.

Despite the observed improvement in coagulation parameters and hypercoagulable state, treatment with n-3 fatty acids did not result in a significant change on the level of the natural anti-coagulant proteins C and S. These findings may indicate that the liver role on low natural anticoagulant in SCD might outweigh the effect of over-consumption due to SCD-associated hypercoagulable state.

The high levels of D-dimer in patients in the current study confirm that hypercoagulability state is one of the major elements of pathophysiology of the disease [33, 36]. Previous studies have reported that omega-3 fatty acid intake is inversely associated with the level of fibrinogen, factor VIII and von Willebrand factor (VWF) [37] and D-dimer [18]. Consistent with the latter study, the current investigation demonstrates high DHA omega-3 fatty acid, but not HU, treatment reduces plasma D-dimer concentration in patients with SCD. The decrease of D-dimer by omega-3 fatty acids has implications for clinical management of patients because plasma D-dimer level is associated with a history of stroke in SCD [36].

This study did not attempt to elucidate the mechanism through which omega-3 fatty acids, particularly DHA and EPA, mediate their anti-coagulant effect. Nevertheless, it is well established that some of the metabolites of these fatty acid are antithrombotic, antiaggregatory, antiinfalammrory and vasodilatory. EPA by competing with arachidonic acid (AA) for cyclooxygenase and lipooxygenase enzymes [38] inhibits the synthesis of the prothrombotic proaggregatory, pro-inflammatory and vasoconstrictor metabolites of AA. Recent animal and human studies suggest that DHA is more potent anti-aggregatory agent than EPA at high doses [39–41]. Interestingly, studies in SCD have demonstrated that endothelial tissue factor expression is specifically dependent upon the nuclear factor-kappa B (NFκB) component of blood mononuclear cells [42]. Our group and others have shown that treatment with high DHA omega-3 fatty acid was associated with down regulation of NFκB gene expression in mononuclear cell and amelioration of SCD-associated chronic inflammatory state [20, 43]. Hence, it is justifiable to attribute the observed improvements in the patient's hypercoagulable state after high DHA intervention to its suppressive effect on NFκB gene expression and partial resolution of the chronic inflammatory state [44].

Besides the limitations of the observational studies, the current study did not assess liver function in order to have a better understanding of the observed abnormalities of coagulation system and the responses to HU and omega-3 treatments. In addition, the effect of omega-3 fatty acids and HU treatments on markers of thrombin generation such as prothrombin fragment F1, 2 and thrombin-anti-thrombin complexes, was not investigated. Due to the fact that only patients above 10 years of age are treated with HU and generally small fraction of patients were treated with HU in Sudan, we did not manage to recruit enough number of patients on HU matched by age and gender.

Conclusion

In conclusion, this study provides an evidence that Sudanese children with sickle cell disease have an abnormal coagulating profile which characterized by prolonged PT and aPTT compared to heathy controls. These two parameters were significantly reduced by treatment with either HU or omega-3 fatty acids. With the exception of the D-dimer, treatment with neither omega-3 fatty acids nor HU resulted in a significant change in markers of coagulation compared to the untreated group. To elucidate the putative effects of omega-3 fatty acids on SCD-associated coagulopathy, a well-designed, prospective, randomized trial with an extended panel of hemostaticis is warranted.

Abbreviations

AA: Arachidonic acid; aPTT: Activated thromboplastin time; DHA: Doxosahexaenoic acid; EPA: Eicosapentaenoic acid; Hb: Hemoglobin; HbAA: Hemoglobin AA; HbSS: Hemoglobin SS; Ht: Haematocrit; HU: Hydroxyurea; MCH: Mean cporpuscular haemoglobin; MCHC: Mean corpuscular haemoglobin concentration; MCV: Mean corpuscular volume; PLt: Platelet count; PT: Prothrombin time; SCD: Sickle Cell Disease; TWBC: Total white blood cell count

Acknowledgements

We are grateful to Dr. Bakhita Attallah who established the Sickle Cell Referral Clinic in Ibn-Aoaf Paediatric Hospital, Khartoum and devoted her professional life caring for the patients with the disease. Particular thanks go to the to the staff of the Sickle Cell Disease Referral Clinic, and Khartoum Teaching Hospitals (Sudan), and to Peter Clough, Efamol Limited UK, for his expert advice on the selection of the supplements used and for support throughout the duration of this study.

Funding

Efamol Lt, UK and Faculty of Medicine University of Khartoum.

Authors' contributions

AD conceptualized, designed the study and wrote the manuscript. SA collated the data and performed the laboratory analysis. AD and SA conducted the statistical analysis. ME and SA contributed to writing the manuscript. ME, NH and KG contributed to reviewing the manuscript. All authors approved the final version of the manuscript.

Competing interests

The funding bodies (Efamol Limited UK and University of Khartoum) had no influence on the study design, collection and analysis of data, interpretation of results or writing. The authors declare that they have no competing interests.

Author details

[1]Department of Medical Biochemistry, Faculty of Medicine, University of Khartoum, Alghasr Street, Khartoum, Sudan. [2]Center of Molecular Biology and Biotechnology (CMBB), Florida Atlantic University (FAU), Boca Raton, USA. [3]College of Medical Laboratory Sciences, Sudan University of Science& Technology, Khartoum, Sudan. [4]Lipidomics and Nutrition Research Centre, London Metropolitan University, London, UK.

References

1. Stuart MJ, Setty BN. Hemostatic alterations in sickle cell disease: relationships to disease pathophysiology. Pediatr Pathol Mol Med. 2001;20(1):27–46.
2. Ataga KI, Orringer EP. Hypercoagulability in sickle cell disease: a curious paradox. Am J Med. 2003;115(9):721–8.
3. Tomer A, et al. Thrombogenesis in sickle cell disease. J Lab Clin Med. 2001;137(6):398–407.
4. Francis RB Jr. Elevated fibrin D-dimer fragment in sickle cell anemia: evidence for activation of coagulation during the steady state as well as in painful crisis. Haemostasis. 1989;19(2):105–11.

5. Westerman MP, et al. Antiphospholipid antibodies, proteins C and S, and coagulation changes in sickle cell disease. J Lab Clin Med. 1999;134(4):352–62.
6. Wright JG, et al. Protein C and protein S in homozygous sickle cell disease: does hepatic dysfunction contribute to low levels? Br J Haematol. 1997; 98(3):627–31.
7. Zhou L, Schmaier AH. Platelet aggregation testing in platelet-rich plasma: description of procedures with the aim to develop standards in the field. Am J Clin Pathol. 2005;123(2):172–83.
8. Connor WE, et al. Abnormal phospholipid molecular species of erythrocytes in sickle cell anemia. J Lipid Res. 1997;38(12):2516–28.
9. Ren H, et al. Blood mononuclear cells and platelets have abnormal fatty acid composition in homozygous sickle cell disease. Ann Hematol. 2005; 84(9):578–83.
10. Singer P, Wirth M. Can n-3 PUFA reduce cardiac arrhythmias? Results of a clinical trial. Prostaglandins Leukot Essent Fatty Acids. 2004;71(3):153–9.
11. Gao LG, et al. Influence of omega-3 polyunsaturated fatty acid-supplementation on platelet aggregation in humans: a meta-analysis of randomized controlled trials. Atherosclerosis. 2013;226(2):328–34.
12. Steinberg MH, et al. Effect of hydroxyurea on mortality and morbidity in adult sickle cell anemia: risks and benefits up to 9 years of treatment. JAMA. 2003;289(13):1645–51.
13. Colella MP, et al. Hydroxyurea is associated with reductions in hypercoagulability markers in sickle cell anemia. J Thromb Haemost. 2012; 10(9):1967–70.
14. McGann PT, Ware RE. Hydroxyurea for sickle cell anemia: what have we learned and what questions still remain? Curr Opin Hematol. 2011;18(3): 158–65.
15. Wang WC, et al. Hydroxycarbamide in very young children with sickle-cell anaemia: a multicentre, randomised, controlled trial (BABY HUG). Lancet. 2011;377(9778):1663–72.
16. Yan JH, et al. The influence of renal function on hydroxyurea pharmacokinetics in adults with sickle cell disease. J Clin Pharmacol. 2005; 45(4):434–45.
17. Daak AA, et al. Effect of omega-3 (n-3) fatty acid supplementation in patients with sickle cell anemia: randomized, double-blind, placebo-controlled trial. Am J Clin Nutr. 2012;97(1):37–44.
18. Tomer A, et al. Reduction of pain episodes and prothrombotic activity in sickle cell disease by dietary n-3 fatty acids. Thromb Haemost. 2001;85(6): 966–74.
19. Daak AA, et al. Docosahexaenoic and eicosapentaenoic acid supplementation does not exacerbate oxidative stress or intravascular haemolysis in homozygous sickle cell patients. Prostaglandins Leukot Essent Fatty Acids. 2013;89(5):305–11.
20. Daak AA, et al. Omega 3 (n-3) fatty acids down-regulate nuclear factor-kappa B (NF-kappaB) gene and blood cell adhesion molecule expression in patients with homozygous sickle cell disease. Blood Cells Mol Dis. 2015; 55(1):48–55.
21. Okpala I, et al. Pilot study of omega-3 fatty acid supplements in sickle cell disease. APMIS. 2011;119(7):442–8.
22. Curtis SA, et al. Elevated steady state WBC and platelet counts are associated with frequent emergency room use in adults with sickle cell anemia. PLoS One. 2015;10(8):e0133116.
23. Ballas SK, et al. Erythropoietic activity in patients with sickle cell anaemia before and after treatment with hydroxyurea. Br J Haematol. 1999;105(2):491–6.
24. Tripathi A, Jerrell JM, Stallworth JR. Clinical complications in severe pediatric sickle cell disease and the impact of hydroxyurea. Pediatr Blood Cancer. 2011;56(1):90–4.
25. Raffini LJ, et al. Prolongation of the prothrombin time and activated partial thromboplastin time in children with sickle cell disease. Pediatr Blood Cancer. 2006;47(5):589–93.
26. Chinawa JM, et al. Coagulation profile of children with sickle cell anemia in steady state and crisis attending the university of Nigeria teaching hospital, Ituku-Ozalla, Enugu. Niger J Clin Pract. 2013;16(2):159–63.
27. Bayazit AK, Kilinc Y. Natural coagulation inhibitors (protein C, protein S, antithrombin) in patients with sickle cell anemia in a steady state. Pediatr Int. 2001;43(6):592–6.
28. De Franceschi L, Cappellini MD, Olivieri O. Thrombosis and sickle cell disease. Semin Thromb Hemost. 2011;37(3):226–36.
29. Heller AR, et al. Impact of n-3 fatty acid supplemented parenteral nutrition on haemostasis patterns after major abdominal surgery. Br J Nutr. 2002; 87(Suppl 1):S95–101.
30. Vanschoonbeek K, et al. Variable hypocoagulant effect of fish oil intake in humans: modulation of fibrinogen level and thrombin generation. Arterioscler Thromb Vasc Biol. 2004;24(9):1734–40.
31. Nieuwenhuys CM, et al. Vitamin K-dependent and vitamin K-independent hypocoagulant effects of dietary fish oil in rats. Thromb Res. 2001; 104(2):137–47.
32. Piccin A, et al. Circulating microparticles, protein C, free protein S and endothelial vascular markers in children with sickle cell anaemia. J Extracell Vesicles. 2015;4:28414.
33. Hebbel RP, Vercellotti G, Nath KA. A systems biology consideration of the vasculopathy of sickle cell anemia: the need for multi-modality chemo-prophylaxsis. Cardiovasc Hematol Disord Drug Targets. 2009;9(4):271–92.
34. Marlar RA, Kleiss AJ, Griffin JH. Mechanism of action of human activated protein C, a thrombin-dependent anticoagulant enzyme. Blood. 1982; 59(5):1067–72.
35. Koc A, Gumruk F, Gurgey A. The effect of hydroxyurea on the coagulation system in sickle cell anemia and beta-thalassemia intermedia patients: a preliminary study. Pediatr Hematol Oncol. 2003;20(6):429–34.
36. Ataga KI, et al. Association of coagulation activation with clinical complications in sickle cell disease. PLoS One. 2012;7(1):e29786.
37. Shahar E, et al. Associations of fish intake and dietary n-3 polyunsaturated fatty acids with a hypocoagulable profile. The atherosclerosis risk in communities (ARIC) study. Arterioscler Thromb. 1993;13(8):1205–12.
38. Nomura S, Kanazawa S, Fukuhara S. Effects of eicosapentaenoic acid on platelet activation markers and cell adhesion molecules in hyperlipidemic patients with type 2 diabetes mellitus. J Diabetes Complicat. 2003;17(3):153–9.
39. Cottin SC, Sanders TA, Hall WL. The differential effects of EPA and DHA on cardiovascular risk factors. Proc Nutr Soc. 2011:1–17.
40. Woodman RJ, et al. Effects of purified eicosapentaenoic acid and docosahexaenoic acid on platelet, fibrinolytic and vascular function in hypertensive type 2 diabetic patients. Atherosclerosis. 2003;166(1):85–93.
41. Adan Y, et al. Effects of docosahexaenoic and eicosapentaenoic acid on lipid metabolism, eicosanoid production, platelet aggregation and atherosclerosis in hypercholesterolemic rats. Biosci Biotechnol Biochem. 1999;63(1):111–9.
42. Kollander R, et al. Nuclear factor-kappa B (NFkappaB) component p50 in blood mononuclear cells regulates endothelial tissue factor expression in sickle transgenic mice: implications for the coagulopathy of sickle cell disease. Transl Res. 2010;155(4):170–7.
43. Kalish BT, et al. Dietary omega-3 fatty acids protect against vasculopathy in a transgenic mouse model of sickle cell disease. Haematologica. 2015; 100(7):870–80.
44. Esmon CT. The interactions between inflammation and coagulation. Br J Haematol. 2005;131(4):417–30.

8

Anaemia and its association with month and blood phenotype in blood donors in Fako division, Cameroon

Tebit Emmanuel Kwenti[1,2,3*] and Tayong Dizzle Bita Kwenti[3]

Abstract

Background: Anaemia is one of the main factors in the deferral (disqualification) of blood donors following haematological screening. There is paucity of data on the prevalence of anaemia in blood donors in Sub-Saharan Africa. This study was undertaken to determine the prevalence of anaemia and its association with month and blood phenotype in blood donors in Fako division of Cameroon.

Methods: Blood donors were recruited between the 1st of January and 31st of December 2014, and their haemoglobin concentration (Hb) was determined using a haemoglobinometer. Anaemia was considered as Hb < 12 g/dl for females and Hb < 13 g/dl for males. The ABO and Rhesus blood groups were determined using standard techniques with monoclonal antibodies and the Coombs' test. The Pearson's chi-square, Pearson's correlation, student T test, ANOVA, univariate and multivariable logistic regression analyses adjusting for gender and age as categorical variable were all performed as part of the statistical analysis.

Results: A total of 1896 blood donors predominantly males (91.35%) took part in the study. The mean age of the donors was 32 ± 7.81 years. On average, donors had donated blood 5.07 ± 3.54 times in their lifetime. The prevalence of anaemia observed in this study was 31.44% (95% CI: 29.35–33.58). The prevalence of anaemia was higher in females ($p \leq 0.0001$) and in participants of age 20 years and below ($p = 0.001$). A marginal association was observed between prevalence of anaemia and season ($p = 0.051$). Furthermore, a significant association was observed between prevalence of anaemia and the blood group AB ($p = 0.001$). The risk of developing anaemia was higher in females compared to males (OR = 2.7, $p < 0.0001$). The mean Hb observed in this study was 13.42 ± 1.65; the mean Hb was not observed to be associated with the month or season adjusting for age and gender.

Conclusion: This study revealed a high prevalence of anaemia which translates to a high rate of donor deferral as a result of anaemia in the study area. The prevalence of anaemia was observed to be associated with the blood phenotype and the month, but not the season (dry or rainy). Further studies will be needed to ascertain the aetiology and associated factors for anaemia in blood donors in the study area.

Keywords: Anaemia, Blood donors, Prevalence, Association, Blood phenotype, Season, Fako Division, Cameroon

* Correspondence: kwentitebit@yahoo.com
[1]Regional Hospital Buea, P.O. Box 32, Buea, South West Region, Cameroon
[2]Department of Medical laboratory Sciences, Faculty of Health Sciences, University of Buea, P.O. Box 63, Buea, Cameroon
Full list of author information is available at the end of the article

Background

Anaemia is a condition where there is a decrease in the amount of red blood cells or less than the normal quantity of haemoglobin in the blood. It is the most common disorder of the blood and it symbolizes both poor nutrition and poor health [1]. The causes of anaemia are multifactorial and may result from blood loss, decreased red blood cell production or increased red blood cell breakdown [2]. Anaemia is a global public health problem affecting nearly a quarter of the world's population [3]. Although its effect is felt in both developing and developed countries, developing countries are the most affected [4]. The management of anaemia commonly involves the use of iron pills, intravenous iron, and erythropoiesis-stimulating medications or by blood transfusion on a case-by-case basis.

The impact of anaemia on maternal and child health is well recognised. Severe anaemia has been linked to increased risk of maternal and child mortality [1, 5, 6]. Anaemia has also been linked to impaired psychological and physical development, behaviour, and work performance of the population [7]. In Cameroon, like most countries in Sub-Saharan Africa, the prevalence of anaemia is very high. In 2011, the prevalence was estimated at 63.3% in children and 49.5% in pregnant women [8]. Malnutrition is one of the main culprit for anaemia in Africa [9]. In addition to malnutrition, there are also infectious causes of anaemia in Cameroon including malaria and intestinal parasitic infections [10–12].

The impact of anaemia on a country's blood banking services has received relatively little attention. Anaemia is one of the main reasons for deferral (disqualification) of potential blood donors [13]. In countries where the prevalence of anaemia is high, this will have a profound effect on the blood stock, eventually compromising the quality of health care. This is not very unusual in developing countries like Cameroon where shortages of blood and blood products are frequent due to the high demand driven by the high rate of anaemia.

The prevalence of anaemia doesn't seem to be constant all year round. In one study, Bondevik et al. [14] had observed a clear seasonal variation of the risk of anaemia in pregnant Nepali women, associated with rainfall and temperature. An earlier study by Palva and Salokannel [15] had also reported a seasonal variation in megaloblastic anaemia. Studies on the seasonal variation of anaemia among blood donor are not readily available.

In Cameroon, data on the prevalence of anaemia among blood donors is lacking in the scientific literature. It was against this drawback that we conducted this study to determine the prevalence of anaemia among blood donors in the Fako Division of Cameroon. The association between anaemia and blood phenotype, and between anaemia and month were also determined. This will generate baseline data which hopefully will be useful in the planning and implementation of blood transfusion services in the country.

Methods

Study design and duration

This was a cross-sectional study which started on the 1st of January and concluded on the 31st of December 2014. The study participants were donors who came to donate blood in the Regional Hospital of Buea during the study period.

Study area

The study was performed in Fako Division (4°10'00"N, 9° 10'00"E) of the South West Region of Cameroon. The department covers an area of 2093 km^2 with an elevation of 2707 m above sea level. Fako Division has an estimated population of 534,854 [16]. The major towns in Fako Division include Buea, Idenau, Limbe (Divisional headquarter), Muyuka and Tiko. The climate of Fako division is generally hot and dry with the exception of Buea where the climate tends to be humid because of its location at the foot of Mount Cameroon. Fako division has two seasons, the rainy and the dry seasons. The rainy season is usually between April and September, and the dry season is between October and March.

Study population

Blood donors (males or females) in the Regional Hospital of Buea were approached to take part in the study. Participants were to be between the ages 17 and 52 years and of weight ≥ 50 kg. All participants were expected to provide a signed informed consent which was duly explained to them in English, French or the local broken English language. Excluded from the study were individuals who did not meet the criteria for blood donation (unfit) such as donors on any medication, women who were breastfeeding or those on menstruation, and donors who had donated blood within 3 months prior to the study.

Participants were consecutively recruited into the study as they came to donate. Participants were enrolled just once and a single blood sample was collected from the participants.

Measurement of blood haemoglobin concentration (Hb)

Participants' Hb was measured using a haemoglobinometer (ACON Mission Plus Hb, ACON Laboratories, Inc., USA). Briefly, about 10 μl of capillary blood from a finger prick was placed on the sample pad on the test strip in the haemoglobinometer using a capillary tube and the haemoglobin concentration (Hb) was read within 20 s. The haemoglobinometer was recalibrated on a daily bases using the control strip supplied by the manufacturer. In this study, anaemia was defined according to the WHO definition of Hb level lower than 12.0 g/dl for females and 13.0 g/dl for males [4]. The severity of anaemia was classified based on the WHO scheme as mild (Hb ≥ 11 but less than normal), moderate (Hb between 8 and 10.9 g/dl) and severe (Hb < 8) [17].

Blood group determination

The ABO and Rhesus (D) blood groups were determined using a commercially available kit for blood grouping (HUMAN DIAGNOSTIC, Germany). In determining ABO and Rhesus blood group, 4 spots of 30 μl of washed red cells were placed on a clean plate and anti-A, anti-B, anti-AB and anti-D grouping sera were added, mixed and rocked for 2mins on a mixer. Positive results were shown by haemagglutination.

Reverse ABO blood grouping was performed to confirm the blood groups of the participants by determining the reaction of the participants' serum to known ABO washed red cells.

Statistical analysis

Statistical analysis was performed using Stata® version 12.1 (StataCorp LP) statistical package. Statistical tests performed included univariate and multivariable logistic regression analyses adjusting for gender and age as categorical variable and the Pearson's chi-square for qualitative variables, the student T test, ANOVA, and Pearson's correlation analysis for quantitative variables. All quantitative variables were normally distributed. Statistical significance was set at $p < 0.05$.

Results

By the end of the study, 1896 potential blood donors were enrolled. Among them were 1,732 (91.35%) males and 164 (8.65%) females. The participants were between 17 and 52 years of age (mean ± SD = 32 ± 7.81). The donors had donated blood on the average 5.07 ± 3.54 times (range: 1–19) in their lifetime.

Five hundred and ninety six (596) of the 1896 donors were anaemic giving a prevalence of 31.44% (95% CI: 29.35–33.58). The prevalence of anaemia was higher in females 87/164 (53.1%) compared to males 509/1732 (29.4%). A significant association was observed between anaemia and gender ($\chi^2 = 38.91$, $p \leq 0.0001$). Overall, the prevalence of anaemia was highest in participants of age 20 years and below (62.5%), and lowest in participants between 30 and 39 years of age (28.6%) (See Table 1). A significant association was observed between prevalence of anaemia and age ($\chi^2 = 17.32$, $p = 0.001$) (See Table 1). The association between prevalence of anaemia and age

Table 1 Prevalence of anaemia stratified according to age

Age category	Males		Females		Total	
	N	Anaemic (%)	N	Anaemic (%)	N	Anaemic (%)
≤20	25	15 (60.0)	7	5 (71.4)	32	20 (62.5)
21–29	702	200 (28.5)	93	51 (54.8)	795	251 (31.6)
30–39	611	165 (27.0)	39	21 (53.9)	650	186 (28.6)
≥40	394	129 (32.7)	25	10 (40.0)	419	139 (33.2)
Total	1732	509 (29.4)	164	87 (53.1)	1896	596 (31.4)

was significant among males ($\chi^2 = 15.369$, $p = 0.002$) but not among females ($\chi^2 = 2.788$, 0.424) (See Table 1).

Overall, the prevalence of anaemia was highest in the month of February (39.7%) and lowest in October (25.2%) (See Table 2). A marginal association was observed between the prevalence of anaemia and month ($\chi^2 = 19.62$, $p = 0.051$). Among females, the prevalence was highest in March (66.7%) and lowest in July (33.3%), while among males, the prevalence was highest in February (39.5%) and lowest in October (20%) (See Table 2).

The prevalence of anaemia in the Rainy season was 32.3% (318/986) and in the Dry season, it was 30.6% (278/910). No significant association was observed in the prevalence of anaemia with season ($\chi^2 = 0.64$, $p = 0.425$).

The risk of becoming anaemic was higher in females compared to males [OR = 2.7 (95% CI: 1.96–3.75), $p \leq 0.0001$]. Univariate analysis (with January as the reference month) revealed that the risk of becoming anaemic was higher in the month of February (OR = 1.75, $p = 0.038$) and December (OR = 1.73, $p = 0.036$) (see Table 2). Furthermore univariate analysis (with February as the reference month) revealed that the risk of becoming anaemic was lower in the months of January (OR = 0.57, $p = 0.038$), March (OR = 0.55, $p = 0.029$) and October (OR = 0.48, $p = 0.003$). However multivariate analysis adjusting for age and gender revealed that the risk of becoming anaemic was comparable across the different months of the year (see Table 2).

In all, 457 (76.7%) of the participants had mild anaemia, 129 (21.6%) had moderate anaemia and 10 (1.7%) had severe anaemia (see Table 3). No significant association was observed between the degree of anaemia and month ($\chi^2 = 27.26$ $p = 0.202$) or season ($\chi^2 = 2.23$ $p = 0.328$).

Overall, the mean Hb in the study population was 13.42 ± 1.65 (range: 6.9–18.9). The mean Hb in females was 11.78 g/dl ± 1.44 (range: 6.9–15), while it was 13.57 ± 1.59 (range: 7.2–18.9) in males. The mean Hb was highest in the month of October and lowest in December (see Fig. 1). In males the mean Hb was highest in October, meanwhile in females, it was highest in May. In males, the mean Hb was lowest in February while in females, it was lowest in December (see Fig. 1). Multivariate analysis adjusting for gender and age

Table 2 Prevalence of anaemia stratified according to month and gender in the study population

Month	Males		Females		Total		Univariate analysis	Multivariate analysis
	N	Anaemic (%)	N	Anaemic (%)	N	Anaemic (%)	OR (95% CI)	OR (95% CI)
Jan	120	32(26.7)	8	3(37.5)	128	35(27.3)	1.00	0.91 (0.55–1.51), $p = 0.716$
Feb	124	49(39.5)	12	5(41.7)	136	54(39.7)	1.75 (1.04–2.94), $p = 0.038$	1.54 (0.96–2.47), $p = 0.077$
Mar	133	33(24.8)	6	4(66.7)	139	37(26.6)	0.96 (0.56–1.66), $p = 0.894$	0.90 (0.55–1.48), $p = 0.677$
Apr	172	46(26.7)	20	10(50.0)	192	56(29.2)	1.04 (0.67–1.8), $p = 0.723$	0.92 (0.59–1.45), $p = 0.729$
May	161	53(32.9)	12	3(25.0)	173	56(32.4)	1.16 (0.7–1.9), $p = 0.548$	1.13 (0.72–1.79), $p = 0.591$
Jun	113	36(31.9)	10	5(50.0)	123	41(33.3)	1.33 (0.77–2.28), $p = 0.302$	1.16 (0.71–1.91), $p = 0.555$
Jul	111	32(28.8)	6	2(33.3)	117	34(29.1)	1.09 (0.62–1.9), $P = 0.765$	1.01 (0.6–1.69). $p = 0.973$
Aug	119	31(26.1)	9	5(55.6)	128	36(28.1)	1.04 (0.6–1.8), $p = 0.889$	0.91 (0.55–1.50), $p = 0.700$
Sep	155	43(27.7)	22	12(54.6)	177	55(31.1)	1.2 (0.73–1.98), $p = 0.48$	1.00
Oct	160	32(20.0)	20	11(55.0)	180	43(25.2)	0.83 (0.5–1.4), $p = 0.492$	0.71 (0.44–1.14), $p = 0.154$
Nov	233	73(31.3)	28	20(71.4)	261	93(35.6)	1.47 (0.93–2.34), $p = 0.102$	1.29 (0.85–1.96), $p = 0.226$
Dec	131	49(37.4)	11	7(63.6)	142	56(39.4)	1.73 (1.04–2.89), $p = 0.036$	1.54 (0.96–2.47), $p = 0.071$
Total	1732	509(29.39)	164	87(53.05)	1896	596(31.44)		

revealed no significant association between mean Hb and month ($p = 0.079$).

In this study, no significant difference was observed in the mean Hb between the rainy and the dry season ($p =$ 0.350) adjusting for age and gender (see Fig. 2).

In the current study, no significant correlation was observed between Hb and age ($r = 0.043$, $p = 0.062$).

The prevalence of anaemia was highest in participants with blood group AB 16(64%) (see Table 4). A significant association was observed between anaemia and blood group ($\chi^2 = 15.63$, $p = 0.001$).

In all, 1827 (96.4%) of the participants were Rhesus (D) positive while 69 (3.6%) were Rhesus (D) negative.

Table 3 Severity of anaemia with respect to month in the study population

Month	Degree of anaemia			Total
	Mild (%)	Moderate (%)	Severe (%)	
Jan	30(85.7)	5(14.3)	0(0)	35
Feb	45(83.3)	9(16.7)	0(0)	54
Mar	30(81.1)	6(16.2)	1(2.7)	37
Apr	44(78.6)	12(21.4)	0(0)	56
May	50(89.3)	6(10.7)	0(0)	56
Jun	31(75.6)	10(24.4)	0(0)	41
Jul	29(85.3)	5(14.7)	0(0)	34
Aug	23(63.9)	12(33.3)	1(2.8)	36
Sep	39(70.9)	15(27.3)	1(1.8)	55
Oct	34(79)	7(16.3)	2(4.7)	43
Nov	63(67.7)	27(29)	3(3.2)	93
Dec	39(69.6)	15(26.8)	2(3.6)	56
Total	457(76.7)	129(21.6)	10(1.7)	596

The prevalence of anaemia was higher among participants that were Rhesus (D) positive 575 (31.5%) compared to those that were Rhesus (D) negative 21 (30.4%). However no significant difference was observed between prevalence of anaemia and the Rhesus (D) antigen ($\chi^2 =$ 0.033, $p = 0.855$).

Discussion

Anaemia is one of the main factors of clinical deferral of blood donors in developing countries including Cameroon. In this study, we investigated the prevalence of anaemia and its association with blood phenotypes as well as month among blood donors in Fako division of Cameroon. A high prevalence of 31.44% was observed in this study. The prevalence was higher compared to the 16% reported in Nigeria [18], 4.2% in Brazil [13], and 1.8% in India [19]. The difference between the prevalence of anaemia in these studies compared to ours could be attributed to the differences in the nutritional habits of these populations. Malnutrition and infectious diseases (such as malaria, intestinal parasitic infections, HIV) are some of the main factors contributing to the high prevalence of anaemia especially in children in Cameroon [12]. The high prevalence of anaemia implies 31.44% of the donors were deferred as a result of the anaemia over the year thereby constituting a huge loss of blood stock. Low supply of blood in a country with a high prevalence of anaemia like Cameroon will compromise the blood supply and therefore have an adverse effect on the quality of health care. In this study, the prevalence of anaemia was significantly higher in females compared to males, which is in line with studies performed elsewhere [19, 20]. Females were also observed to be at increased risk of anaemia in comparison to their

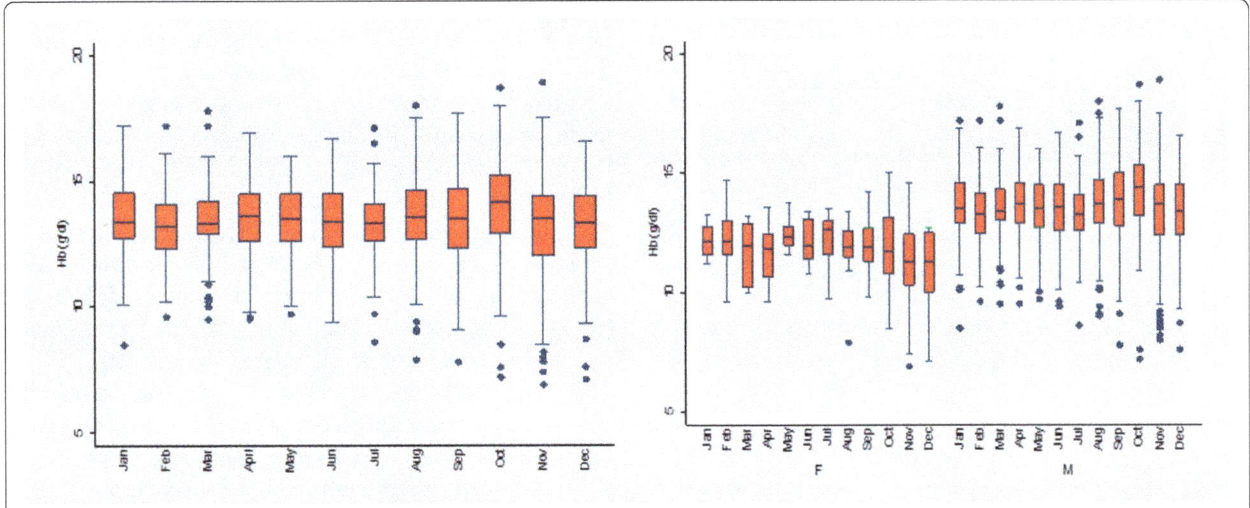

Fig. 1 Monthly distribution of Hb in the study population overall (*left*), and stratified according to gender (*right*). No significant association was observed between Hb and month adjusting for age and gender

male counterparts (OR = 2.7, $p \leq 0.0001$). This is not unusual owing to the fact that women often fail to compensate their menstruational blood loss. In this study, 8.65% of the donors were females. Pregnancy, lactation and menstruation are some of the causes preventing blood donation in females. This may have resulted in a selection bias against females consequently influencing the true representation of the prevalence of anaemia in this group. The finding of fewer female donors in this study corroborate with work done by Silva et al. [13]. In this study, the prevalence of anaemia was observed to be higher in participants of 20 years and below irrespective of gender. A significant association was observed between prevalence of anaemia and age ($p = 0.001$). The finding of higher prevalence of anaemia among younger donors could be attributed to the fact that many of them were students who undergo a lot of stress with their study and hardly feed well. The association between prevalence of anaemia and age was significant among males but not among females. This difference could be

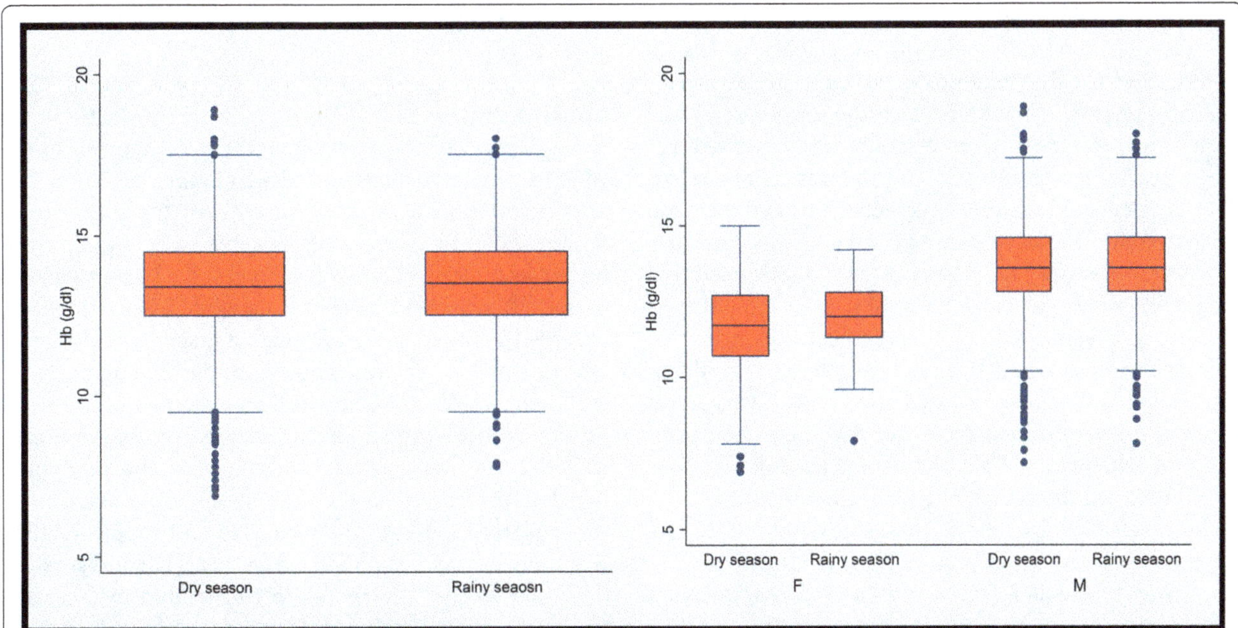

Fig. 2 Distribution of mean Hb according to season in the study population. The mean Hb was observed to be higher in the rainy season overall (*left*) and in both males and females (*right*). The difference in the mean Hb between the two seasons was not observed to be significant ($p = 0.350$) adjusting for age and gender

Table 4 The distribution of anaemia with respect to blood phenotype

Blood group	N	Anaemic (%)	χ^2	*P*-value
A	231	73(31.6)	15.63	0.001
AB	25	16(64)		
B	216	78(36.1)		
O	1424	429(30.1)		
Total	1896	596		

due to the observation that the prevalence of anaemia was generally high among females irrespective of the age.

In this study, it was observed that the donors had donated blood on the average of 5 times in their lifetime. Studies have shown that there is an increasing depletion of the iron stores with increasing number of blood donation [21–23]. The high frequency of blood donation observed in this study could have also contributed to the high prevalence of anaemia observed in this study.

We also observed the prevalence of anaemia to be highest in February and lowest in October. In the study area, the dry season is usually between October and March meanwhile the rainy season is between April and September. February which has the highest rate of anaemia falls in the heart of the dry season during which there is scarcity of foodstuffs including vegetables, which are also very expensive where available. This negatively affects the feeding habit of the population of Fako hence the high rate of anaemia. October which has the lowest prevalence of anaemia falls in the transition between the dry and the rainy season. During this period there is abundance of foodstuffs especially vegetables, which are also cheaper. At this time of the year, vegetables constitute a large part of the diet hence the lower prevalence of anaemia. A marginal association was observed between prevalence of anaemia and months in this study. The prevalence of anaemia was higher in the dry season compared to the rainy season which is not unusual. However no significant association was observed between prevalence of anaemia and season. The risk of developing anaemia was also observed to be higher in February and December but multivariate analysis adjusting for age and gender revealed similar risk of anaemia across the different months of the year. Like the prevalence of anaemia, no significant association was observed between the degree of anaemia and month.

The mean Hb observed in this study was 13.42 g/dl and ranged between 6.9 and 18.9 g/dl. The mean Hb was lower in females (11.78 g/dl) compared to males (13.57 g/dl). This is not unusual owing to the fact that the Hb of females is generally always lower than the Hb in males for reasons highlighted above. The mean Hb was highest in October and lowest in December. In this study, no significant association was observed between Hb and month ($p = 0.079$) adjusting for age and gender. The variation in the mean Hb with month could be attributed to the same factors associated with the prevalence of anaemia highlighted above. In females, the mean Hb was highest in the month of May and lowest in December, which is contrary to males in which mean Hb was observed to be highest in October and lowest in February. Like with the prevalence of anaemia in this study, no significant association was observed between Hb and season ($p = 0.350$), neither was there any significant association between Hb and age ($p = 0.062$).

In this study, it was observed that anaemia was significantly associated with blood group AB ($p = 0.001$). Not many studies have associated a particular blood group with anaemia in the literature. A previous study in 1956 had linked pernicious anaemia to blood group A [24]. In this study we did not determine the aetiology of anaemia which prevented us from knowing the exact type of anaemia associated with blood group AB. The prevalence of anaemia was higher in donors who were Rhesus (D) positive (31.5%) compared to Rhesus (D) negative (30.4%) donors. However this difference was not observed to be significant ($p = 0.855$). This difference could be attributed to the fact that the majority of donors were Rhesus (D) positive (96.4%).

In the current study, we did not determine the aetiology and risk factors for anaemia in the study population and this constitutes a major limitation. Studies are therefore required to ascertain the aetiology of anaemia in the study population as well as make prepositions to reduce the high rate of anaemia in blood donors in the study area.

Conclusion

A high prevalence of anaemia (31.44%) was observed which translates to an equivalent number of blood donors deferred as a result of anaemia in the study timeframe. The prevalence of anaemia was significantly higher in females compared to males and in participants of age 20 years and below. A marginal association was observed between the prevalence of anaemia and month but not with the season. The risk of developing anaemia was comparable across the different months of the year. Female blood donors and donors with the blood group AB were the most at-risk of developing anaemia compared to the others. In the current study, no association was observed between the mean Hb and month neither was there any association between mean Hb and season.

Further studies will therefore be required to ascertain the aetiology and risk factors for anaemia in the study population as well as make prepositions aimed at reversing the current high rate of anaemia in the study population.

Abbreviations
CI: Confidence interval; Hb: Haemoglobin concentration; OR: Odd ratio

Acknowledgements
The authors wish to thank the director, doctors, nurses and laboratory staff of the Regional Hospital of Buea for allowing us to use their donors and for their help in the data collection. Our sincere gratitude also goes to the blood donors who took part in this study.

Funding
This study was funded by the authors.

Authors' contributions
TEK conceived and designed the study, participated in data collection, took part in the analysis and interpretation, conducted the literature search and review and critically revised the paper. TDBK participated in the statistical analysis, conducted the literature search and review and wrote the first draft of the paper. All authors read and approved the final paper.

Competing interest
The authors declare that they have no competing interest.

Author details
[1]Regional Hospital Buea, P.O. Box 32, Buea, South West Region, Cameroon. [2]Department of Medical laboratory Sciences, Faculty of Health Sciences, University of Buea, P.O. Box 63, Buea, Cameroon. [3]Department of Microbiology and Parasitology, Faculty of Science, University of Buea, P.O. Box 63, Buea, Cameroon.

References
1. WHO. Iron Deficiency Anemia: assessment, prevention and control. Geneva: WHO; 2001. http://apps.who.int/iris/bitstream/10665/66914/1/WHO_NHD_01.3.pdf?ua=1. Accessed 22 Oct 2015.
2. Kumar V, Abbas AK, Fausto N, Mitchell R. Robbin's basic pathology. 8th ed. Philadelphia: Saunders; 2007. ISBN 1-4160-2973-7.
3. Janz TG, Johnson RL, Rubenstein SD. Anemia in the emergency department: evaluation and treatment. Emerg Med Pract. 2013;15 Suppl 11:1–15. quiz 15–6.
4. WHO. Worldwide prevalence of anaemia 1993 – 2005: WHO global database on anaemia. Geneva: World Health Organisation; 2008. http://whqlibdoc.who.int/publications/2008/9789241596657_eng.pdf. Accessed 22 Oct 2015.
5. Anorlu RI, Odum CU, Essien EE. Asymptomatic malaria parasitaemia in pregnant women at booking in a primary health care facility in a periurban community in Lagos, Nigeria. Afr J Med Sci. 2001;30:39–41.
6. Aimakhu CO, Olayemi O. Maternal haematocrit and pregnancy outcome in Nigerian women. West Afr J Med. 2003;22:18–21.
7. Sandstead HH. Causes of iron and zinc deficiencies and their effects on brain. J Nutr. 2000;130:347S–9S.
8. Stevens GA, Finucane MM, De-Regil LM, Paciorek CJ, Flaxman SR, Branca F, et al. Global, regional, and national trends in haemoglobin concentration and prevalence of total and severe anaemia in children and pregnant and non-pregnant women for 1995–2011: a systematic analysis of population-representative data. Lancet Glob Health. 2013;1 Suppl 1:e16–25.
9. Korenromp EL, Armstrong-Schellenberg JR, Williams BG, Nahlen BL, Snow RW. Impact of malaria control on childhood anaemia in Africa – a quantitative review. Trop Med Int Health. 2004;9:1050–65.
10. Richardson DJ, Richardson KR, Richardson KE, Gross J, Tsekeng P, Dondji B, Foulefack S. Malaria, intestinal parasitic infection, anemia, and malnourishment in Rural Cameroonian Villages with an assessment of early interventions. J Ark Acad Sci. 2011;65:72–97.
11. Zeukeng F, Tchinda VHM, Bigoga JD, Seumen CHT, Ndzi ES, Abonweh G, et al. Co-infections of malaria and geohelminthiasis in two Rural Communities of Nkassomo and Vian in the Mfou Health District, Cameroon. PLoS Negl Trop Dis. 2014;8 Suppl 10:e3236.
12. Njunda AL, Fon SG, Assob JCN, Nsagha DS, Kwenti TZB, Kwenti ET. Coinfection with malaria and intestinal parasites, and its association with anaemia in children in Cameroon. Infect Dis Poverty. 2015;4:43.
13. Silva MA, de Souza RA, Carlos AM, Soares S, Moraes-Souza H, Pereira GA. Etiology of anemia of blood donor candidates deferred by hematologic screening. Rev Bras Hematol Hemoter. 2012;34 Suppl 5:356–60.
14. Bondevik GT, Lie RT, Ulstein M, Kvale G. Seasonal variation in the risk of anaemia among pregnant Nepali women. Int J Gynaecol Obstet. 2000;69(3): 215–22.
15. Palva IP, Salokannel SJ. Seasonal variation in megaloblastic anaemia. Br J Nutr. 1972;27:593–5.
16. Statoids. Annuaire Statistique du Cameroun 2006. Obtained from Institut National de la Statistique du Cameroun. http://www.statoids.com/ycm.html. 2009. Accessed 25 Oct 2015.
17. WHO. Haemoglobin concentrations for the diagnosis of anaemia and assessment of severity. Geneva: WHO; 2011. http://www.who.int/vmnis/indicators/haemoglobin.pdf. Accessed 22 Oct 2015.
18. Erhabor O, Imrana S, Buhari H, Abubakar W, Abdulrahaman Y, Isaac IZ, et al. Prevalence of anaemia among Blood Donors in Sokoto, North Western, Nigeria. Int J Clin Med Res. 2014;1 Suppl 3:85–9.
19. Bahadur S, Pujani M, Jain M. Donor deferral due to anemia: A tertiary care center-based study. Asian J Transfusion Sci. 2011;5:53–5.
20. Gupta AK, Agarwal SS, Kaushak R, Jain A, Gupta VK, Khare N. Prevalence of anemia among rural population living in and around of rural health and training center, Ratua village of Madhya Pradesh. Muller J med Sci Res. 2014;5:15–8.
21. Badar A, Ahmed A, Ayub M, Ansari AK. Effect of frequent blood donations on iron stores of non anaemic male blood donors. J Ayub Med Coll Abbottabad. 2002;14 Suppl 2:24–7.
22. Cançado RD, Chiattone CS, Alonso FF, Langhi Júnior DM, Alves Rde C. Iron deficiency in blood donors. Sao Paulo Med J. 2011;119 Suppl 4:132–4.
23. Addullah SM. The effect of repeated blood donations on the iron status of male Saudi blood donors. Blood Transf. 2011;9:167–71.
24. Aird I, Bentall HH, Bingham J, Blackburn EK, Mackay MS, Swan HT et al. An association between blood group A and pernicious anaemia: a collective series from a number of centres. BMJ 1956;2:723–724.

9

Prevalence and determinants of anemia among pregnant women in Ethiopia; a systematic review and meta-analysis

Getachew Mullu Kassa[1*], Achenef Asmamaw Muche[2], Abadi Kidanemariam Berhe[3] and Gedefaw Abeje Fekadu[4]

Abstract

Background: Anemia during pregnancy is one of the most common indirect obstetric cause of maternal mortality in developing countries. It is responsible for poor maternal and fetal outcomes. A limited number of studies were conducted on anemia during pregnancy in Ethiopia, and they present inconsistent findings. Therefore, this review was undertaken to summarize the findings conducted in several parts of the country and present the national level of anemia among pregnant women in Ethiopia.

Methods: Preferred Reporting Items for Systematic Reviews and Meta-Analyses (PRISMA) guideline was followed for this systematic review and meta-analysis. The databases used were; PUBMED, Cochrane Library, Google Scholar, CINAHL, and African Journals Online. Search terms used were; anemia, pregnancy related anemia and Ethiopia. Joanna Briggs Institute Meta-Analysis of Statistics Assessment and Review Instrument (JBI-MAStARI) was used for critical appraisal of studies. The meta-analysis was conducted using STATA 14 software. The pooled Meta logistic regression was computed to present the pooled prevalence and relative risks (RRs) of the determinate factors with 95% confidence interval (CI).

Results: Twenty studies were included in the meta-analysis with a total of 10, 281 pregnant women. The pooled prevalence of anemia among pregnant women in Ethiopia was 31.66% (95% CI (26.20, 37.11)). Based on the pooled prevalence of the subgroup analysis result, the lowest prevalence of anemia among pregnant women was observed in Amhara region, 15.89% (95% CI (8.82, 22.96)) and the highest prevalence was in Somali region, 56.80% (95% CI (52.76, 60.84)). Primigravid (RR: 0.61 (95% CI: 0.53, 0.71)) and urban women (RR: 0.73 (95% CI: 0.60, 0.88)) were less likely to develop anemia. On the other hand, mothers with short pregnancy interval (RR: 2.14 (95% CI: 1.67, 2.74)) and malaria infection during pregnancy (RR: 1.94 (95% CI: 1.33, 2.82)) had higher risk to develop anemia.

Conclusions: Almost one-third of pregnant women in Ethiopia were anemic. Statistically significant association was observed between anemia during pregnancy and residence, gravidity, pregnancy interval, and malaria infection during pregnancy. Regions with higher anemia prevalence among pregnant women should be given due emphasis. The concerned body should intervene on the identified factors to reduce the high prevalence of anemia among pregnant women.

Keywords: Prevalence of anemia, Anemia during pregnancy, Short birth interval, Malaria during pregnancy, Ethiopia, Meta-analysis, Systematic review

* Correspondence: gechm2005@gmail.com
[1]College of health Sciences, Debre Markos University, Debre Markos, Ethiopia
Full list of author information is available at the end of the article

Background

World health organization (WHO) defines anemia as a low blood hemoglobin concentration. It is one of the major public health problems globally with diverse consequences [1, 2]. It affects the physical health and cognitive development of individual causing low productivity and poor economic development of a country [1, 3]. The problem is also related to high maternal and infant morbidity and mortality especially in developing countries [4, 5].

WHO report showed that anemia affects more than half a billion reproductive age women globally. From this, 38% of the anemic women were pregnant [5]. Anemia is the most common complication related to pregnancy, which affects almost half of pregnant women globally [6–10]. It usually results due to the normal physiological changes of pregnancy resulting in hemoglobin concentration [6, 11]. The problem is more common in developing countries where there is inadequate diet and poor prenatal vitamins and iron and folic acid intake [1, 6, 12]. The most common type of anemia is iron deficiency anemia which mainly affects women of reproductive age group, particularly pregnant women [4, 13].

Several studies have shown that anemia during pregnancy has several adverse effects. Based on the type and severity of anemia, the pregnancy may have poor maternal and fetal outcomes. The most common obstetric problems of anemia include; abortion, prematurity, intrauterine fetal death, low birth weight and perinatal mortality [4, 6, 14–16].

Even though studies have been conducted on the magnitude of anemia among pregnant women in Ethiopia, they present inconsistent and inconclusive findings. So, this systematic review and meta-analysis was conducted to determine the prevalence and determinants of anemia among pregnant women in Ethiopia using the available published evidence. The study will be important to design appropriate interventions to reduce the high burden of the disease.

Methods

Study design and search strategy

A systematic review of published studies was used to determine the prevalence of anemia and its determinant factors among pregnant women in Ethiopia. Review of all published studies was done in the following major databases; PubMed, Cochrane Library, Google Scholar, CINAHL, and African Journals Online. The search for published studies was not restricted by time, and all published articles up to January 01/2017 were included into the review. Search of the reference list of already identified studies to retrieve additional articles was done. The search terms used were; "anemia OR anemia during pregnancy OR determinants of anemia AND Ethiopia". Preferred Reporting Items for Systematic Reviews and Meta-Analyses (PRISMA) guideline was strictly followed when conducting this review [17].

Study selection and eligibility criteria

This review included studies that were conducted and published on anemia among pregnant women in Ethiopia. All studies conducted at the community or health institution level were included. Studies that provide the prevalence of anemia in pregnant women using the WHO definition (hemoglobin level less than 11 g/dl), and published in the English language were included. Studies conducted among pregnant women but who had comorbidities like; like HIV/AIDS, renal disease, and other medical or surgical conditions were excluded from this study. Articles were assessed for inclusion using their title, abstract and then a full review of papers was done before inclusion to the final review.

Outcome of interest

The primary outcome of this study was magnitude of anemia during pregnancy. The WHO defines anemia in pregnany as low blood hemoglobin concentration, below 11 g/dl or hematocrit level less than 33% [1]. The determinant variables included in this review were; residence (urban vs rural), pregnancy interval (less than two years, greater than or equal to two years), malaria infection during pregnancy and total number of pregnancy (primigravida or multigravida). Primigravida refers to women who are pregnant for the first time and multigravida refers to women who are pregnant two or more times [18, 19].

Quality assessment and data collection

Joanna Briggs Institute Meta-Analysis of Statistics Assessment and Review Instrument (JBI-MAStARI) was used for critical appraisal of studies [20]. Two reviewers independently assessed the articles for overall study quality and for inclusion in the review. Any unlear information and disagreement which arises between the reviewers was resolved through discussion and by involving a third reviewer. The researchers developed a data extraction tool. The tool included information on the name of the author/s, publication year, study period, study design, sample size, study area, age of study participants, response rate, mean hemoglobin level, and the prevalence of anemia. Inaddition, the tool contains questions on the prevalence of anemia by residence, number of pregnancy, malaria infection during pregnancy and pregnancy gap.

Publication bias and heterogeneity

Publication bias and heterogeneity were assessed using the Egger's and Begg's tests [21, 22]. A *p*-value less than 0.05 were used to declare statistical significance of publication bias. The heterogeneity of studies was also checked using I^2 test statistics. The I^2 test statistics of 25%, 50%, and 75% was declared as low, moderate and high heterogeneity respectively [23]. A p-value less than 0.05 was used to declare heterogeneity. For the test result which indicates the presence of heterogeneity, random effect model was used as a method of analysis, since it reduces the heterogeneity of studies [23].

Statistical methods and analysis

Data were entered into Microsoft Excel and then exported to STATA 14 software for further analysis. Forest plot was used to present the combined estimate with 95% confidence interval (CI) of the meta-analysis. Subgroup analysis was conducted by regions of the country and type of study design. The effect of selected predictor variables which include; number of pregnancy, malaria infection during pregnancy, pregnancy gap, and residence on the anemia during pregnancy was analyzed using separate categories of meta-analysis. The findings of meta-analysis were presented using forest plot and relative risk (RR) with its 95% CI.

Results

Study selection

This review included published studies on anemia among pregnant women in Ethiopia. The electronic search was done on several databases, which include; PUBMED, Cochrane Library, Google Scholar, CINAHL, and African Journals Online. The review found a total of 1592 published articles. From this, 86 duplicate records were removed and 1467 records were excluded after screening by title and abstracts. A total of 39 full-text articles were screened for eligibility. From this, 19 articles were excluded since they included non-pregnant women and the outcome variables was not reported. Finally, 20 studies were included in the final quantitative meta-analysis (Fig. 1).

Characteristics of included studies

All included studies were cross-sectional conducted among pregnant women. The minimum sample size was 150 participants in a study conducted in Nekemte [24]. While, the higher sample size was 1678, conducted in Haramaya district of Oromia region [25]. Overall, this

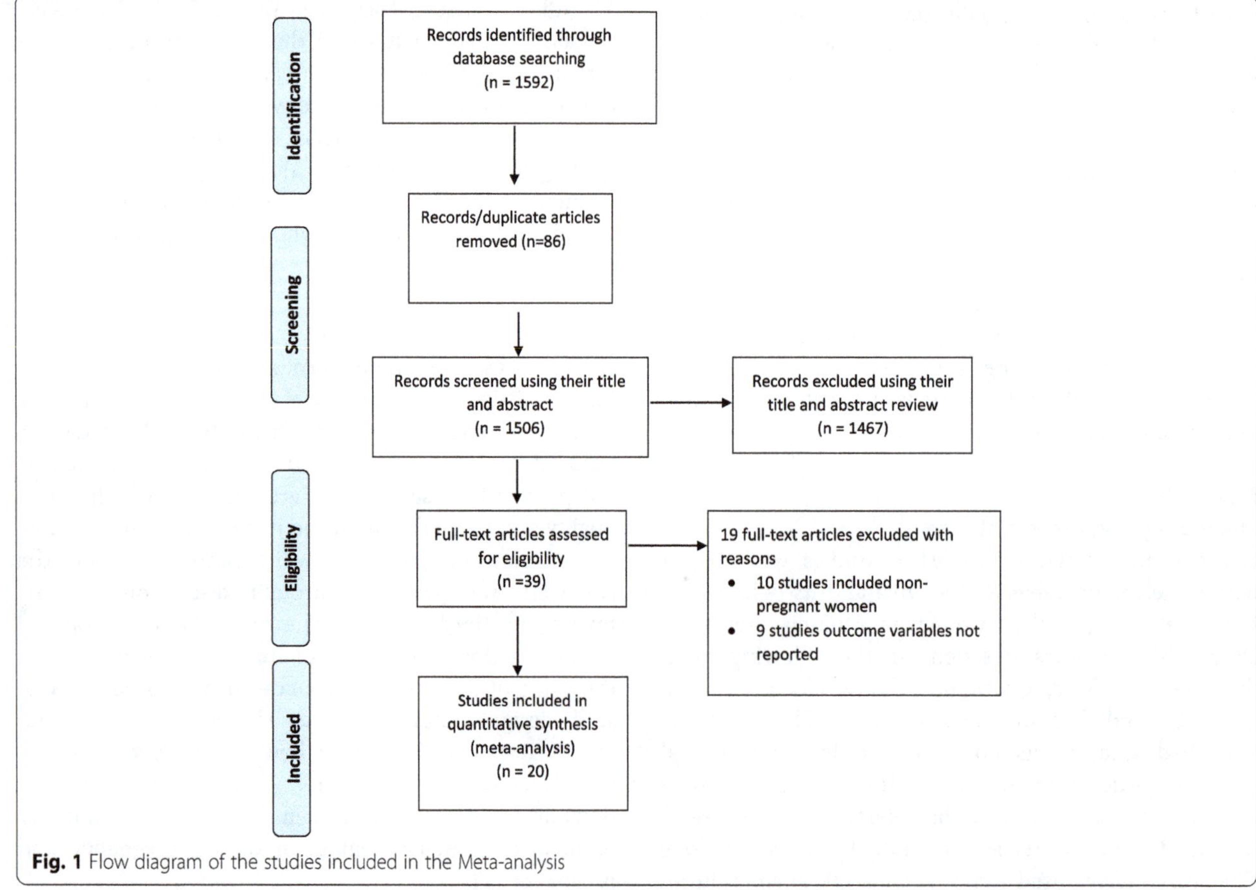

Fig. 1 Flow diagram of the studies included in the Meta-analysis

meta-analysis included a total of 10, 281 pregnant women. All studies used the WHO definition of anemia during pregnancy [1]. The minimum and maximum age of pregnant women included in this review were 14 years and 42 years respectively. Thirteen, 65% of the included studies were conducted at health institution [24, 26–37] and 7(35%) of studies were community-based studies [25, 38–43]. Most of the regions in Ethiopia were represented in this review. One of the study was conducted in Addis Ababa, capital city of Ethiopia [34], 3 were from Amhara region [27, 28, 36], 6 from Oromia region [24, 25, 30, 35, 37, 42], 1 from Somali region [38], 5 from SNNPR [29, 32, 33, 40, 43], 2 from Tigray region [26, 31], and 2 were nationwide studies [39, 41] (Table 1).

Prevalence of anemia among pregnant women

The minimum prevalence of anemia was 9.7% observed in a study conducted in North Shoa zone [28]. The highest, 56.8% was observed in a study conducted in Eastern Ethiopia [38]. The I^2 test result showed high heterogeneity (I^2 97.7%, p = <0.001). Using the random effect analysis, the pooled prevalence of anemia among pregnant women in Ethiopia was 31.66% (95% CI (26.20, 37.11)) (Fig. 2).

A subgroup analysis by region in Ethiopia was computed to compare the prevalence of anemia acroos different participants characterstics. Based on this analysis, the lowest prevalence of anemia among pregnant women was observed in Amhara region, 15.89% (95% CI (8.82, 22.96)) and the highest prevalence was in Somali region; 56.80%(95% CI (52.76, 60.84)). A higher prevalence (39.49%) of anemia among pregnant women was observed in studies conducted at community level than facility based studies (27.31%) (Table 2).

Association of malaria infection and anemia during pregnancy

Women who had malaria infection during pregnancy were almost two times more likely to develop anemia during pregnancy than women had no such infection, RR: 1.94 (95% CI (1.33, 2.82)). The heterogeneity test showed statistical evidence of heterogeneity, p = <0.001. As a result, weights were calculated using the random-effects analysis. The Begg's and Egger's test for publication bias showed no statistical evidence of publication bias, p-value = >0.05 and p-value = 0.543 respectively (Fig. 3).

Association of number of pregnancy with anemia during pregnancy

The meta-analysis showed that premigravida women were 61% less likely to develop anemia during pregnancy compared tomultigravida women, RR: 0.61 (95% CI (0.53, 0.71)). The heterogeneity test showed no statistical evidence of heterogeneity, p = 0.530. The Begg's and Egger's test for publication bias also showed no statistical evidence of publication bias, p-value = 0.36 and p-value = 0.397 respectively (see Additional file 1).

Association of short pregnancy interval with anemia during pregnancy

Women who had short pregnancy interval were more than two times more likely to develop anemia during the current pregnancy than women who had more than two years pregnancy interval, RR: 2.14 (95% CI (1.67, 2.74)). The heterogeneity test showed no statistical evidence of heterogeneity, p = 0.108. The Begg's and Egger's test for publication bias also showed no statistical evidence of publication bias, p-value = 0.266 and p-value = 0.112 respectively (see Additional file 2).

Association of residence with anemia during pregnancy

Women living in urban areas were 73% less likely to be anemic during pregnancy than women in the rural area, RR: 0.73 (95% CI (0.60, 0.88)). The heterogeneity test showed statistical evidence of heterogeneity, p = 0.003. But, the Begg's and Egger's test for publication bias showed no statistical evidence of publication bias, p-value = 0.602 and p-value = 0.581 respectively (**see** Additional file 3).

Discussion

This review was conducted to determine the pooled prevalence and determinants of anemia among pregnant women in Ethiopia using published studies. Anemia during pregnancy is associated with increased risk of obstetric problems [44]. Studies have shown that anemia is associated with maternal physical and psychological comorbidity, and with an increased risk of perinatal and maternal morbidity and mortality [45–47].

The pooled meta-analysis of this review found that the prevalence of anemia among pregnant women in Ethiopia was 31.66% (95%CI: (26.20, 37.11)). The 2016 Ethiopian demographic and health survey (EDHS) report showed a lower (24%) prevalence of anemia among reproductive-aged women, and 29% among pregnant women [48]. This showed a higher prevalence of anemia among pregnant women than non-pregnant reproductive age women. This could be explained by an extra demand of iron by the pregnant women for fetal growth and development during pregnancy. This report is lower than the current finding. The possible explanation for the difference could be related to the sampling and study period. The EDHS was conducted in a nationally representative sample across all regions of the country,

Table 1 Summary characteristics of included studies in the meta-analysis

Author, year of publication	Study area	Study year	Type of cross sectional study	Sample size	Response rate (%)	Mean hemoglobin level (in g/dl)	Prevalence of anemia among pregnant women
Alene KA. and Dohe AM., 2014 [38]	Gode town, Somali Region	2013	Community based	581	99.3	10.79	56.8
Abriha A. et al., 2014 [26]	Mekele town, Tigray Region	2014	Facility based	632	97.9	11.7	19.7
Alem M. et al., 2013 [27]	Azezo Health Center, Gondar, Amhara Region	2011	Facility based	384	100	–	21.6
Alemu T. & Umeta M., 2015 [39]	Data from 2011 EDHS	2011	Community based	1212	–	–	23
Ayenew F. et al., 2014 [28]	Debre Birhan, Amhara region	2013	Facility based	330	89.4	–	9.7
Bekele A.et al., 2016 [29]	Arba Minch, SNNPR	2015	Facility based	332	100	–	32.8
Ejeta E. et al., 2014 [30]	Nekemte Referral Hospital, Oromia Region	2014	Facility based	286	100	12.67	29
Gebre A. & Mulugeta A., 2015 [31]	Northwestern zone, Tigray Region	2014	Facility based	714	97.7	11.21	36.1
Gebremedhin S. et al., 2014 [41]	Eight rural woredas of Tigray, Amhara, Oromia and SNNP regions	2012	Community based	445	93	11.5	33.2
Gebremedhin S, Enquselassie F., & Umeta M., 2014 [40]	Sidama, SNNPR	2011	Community based	700	93.1	11.4	31.6
Gedefaw L.et al., 2015 [32]	Wolayita Soddo Otona Hospital, SNNPR	2014	Facility based	363	100	11.55	39.9
Getachew M. et al., 2012 [42]	Districts around Gilgel Gibe Dam area, Oromia Region	2011	Community based	388	98.7	10.9	53.9
Gies S. et al., 2003 [33]	Awassa, SNNPR	2001	Facility based	403	100	12.3	15.1
Jufar AH. & Zewde T., 2014 [34]	Tikur Anbesa Specialized Hospital, Addis Ababa	2013	Facility based	395	100	12	21.3
Kedir H.et al., 2013 [25]	Haramaya district, Oromia Region	2010	Community based	1678	94.7	11	43.9
Kefiyalew F. et al., 2014 [35]	Bisidimo Hospital, Babile Woreda, Somalie	2013	Facility based	258	100	11.4	27.9
Melku M.et al., 2014 [36]	Gondar University hospital, Amhara region	2012	Facility based	302	100	11.96	16.6
Mihiretie H. et al., 2015 [24]	Nekemte, Oromia region	2011	Facility based	150	100	–	52
Nega D.et al., 2015 [43]	Arba Minch Town, SNNPR region	2013	Community based	354	96.3	11.73	34.6
Obse N.et al., 2013 [37]	Shara woreda, West Arsi zone, Oromia region	2011	Facility based	374	100	12.05	36.6

while this study included only few regions of the country. The current review also included studies conducted since 2001.

A meta-analysis on global trend of anemia showed that 38% of pregnant women were anemic in 2011 [3]. The review also showed that 36% prevalence of anemia among pregnant women in East Africa and 22% prevalence in high-income regions [3]. The East African finding is relatively higher than the findings of this review. A possible explanation could be the time difference between the two reviews in which the current review also included recent studies and the difference in the sociodemographic characteristics of participants included in the review.

Subgroup analysis based on the regions of the country showed a lower and higher prevalence of anemia in Amhara region (15.89%) and Somali region (56.8%) respectively. The difference in the prevalence between the regions in Ethiopia could be attributed due to the difference in the sociodemographic, socioeconomic, iron-folic acid intake and the difference in the magnitude of the communicable and non-communicable diseases. The difference in the number of studies included in each category of analysis could also be the reason for the difference.

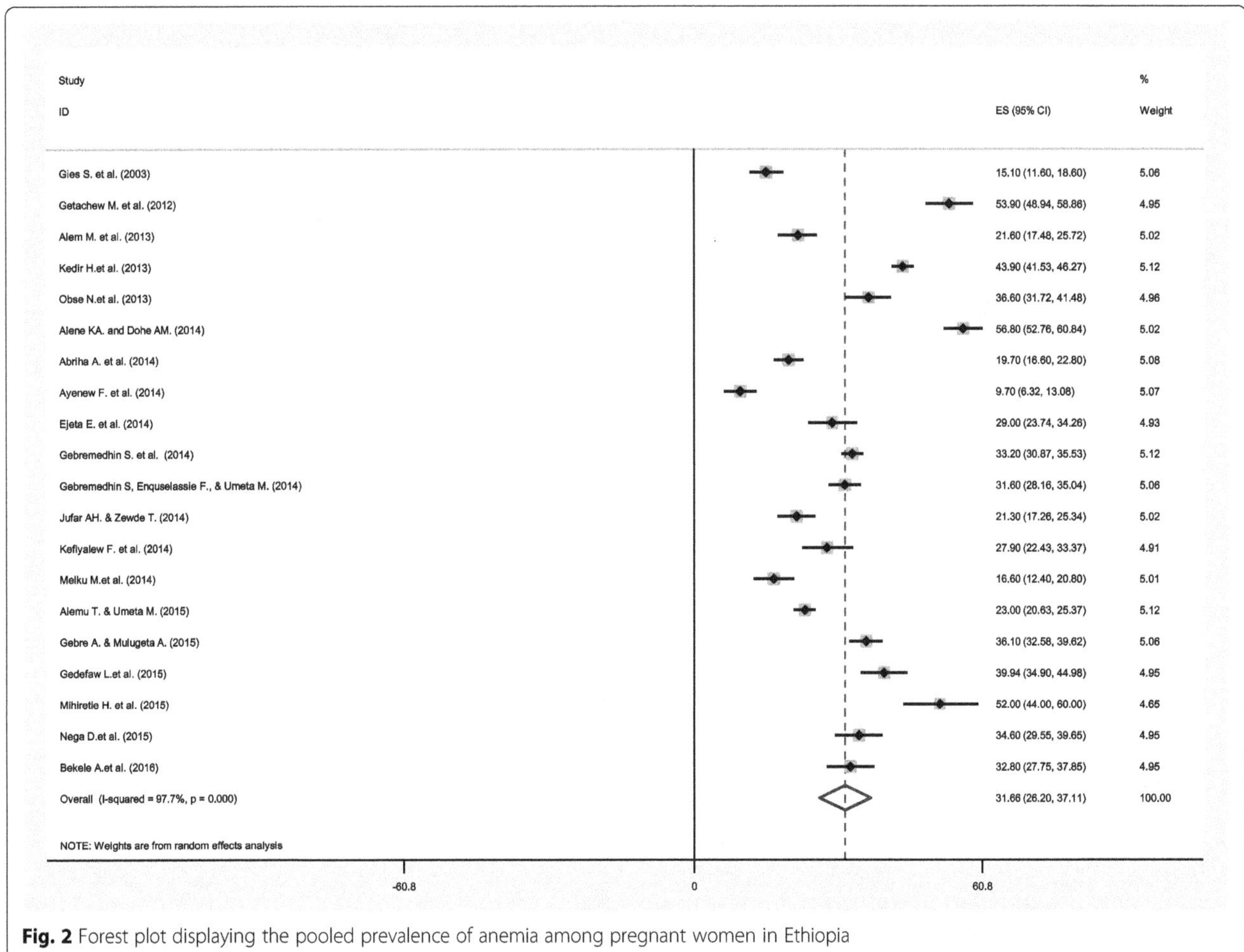

Fig. 2 Forest plot displaying the pooled prevalence of anemia among pregnant women in Ethiopia

The result of the meta-analysis showed that primigravida women were 61% less likely to develop anemia during pregnancy compared to multigravida women. This could be because of the effect of repeated pregnancy in depleting the iron store of a pregnant woman [49, 50]. A study conducted in Malaysia also found a higher proportion of anemia (66.7%) among grand multigravida women [51].

A shorter interpregnancy interval increases the risk of adverse obstetric outcomes [52]. Short birth interval is associated with preterm births, low birth weight, stillbirth and early neonatal death [52]. The current study also found that pregnant women with short pregnancy interval were more than two times more likely to develop anemia during the current pregnancy than

Table 2 Sub-group analysis of prevalence of anemia among pregnant women in Ethiopia

Sub group	No. of included studies	Prevalence (95% CI)	Heterogeneity statistics	*p*-value	I^2
By region					
Addis Ababa City	1	21.30 (17.26, 25.34)	–	–	–
Amhara region	3	15.89 (08.82, 22.96)	19.89	<0.001	89.9
Oromia region	6	40.44 (32.67, 48.20)	83.85	<0.001	94.0
SNNPR	5	30.71 (21.74, 39.68)	87.75	<0.001	95.0
Somali region	1	56.80 (52.76, 60.84)	–	–	–
Tigray region	2	27.88 (11.81, 43.95)	46.91	<0.001	97.9
Nationwide study	2	28.10 (18.11, 38.10)	36.12	<0.001	97.2
By study type					
Community based study	7	39.49 (30.84, 48.14)	321.93	<0.001	98.1
Institutional based study	13	27.31 (21.51, 33.10)	289.66	<0.001	97.7

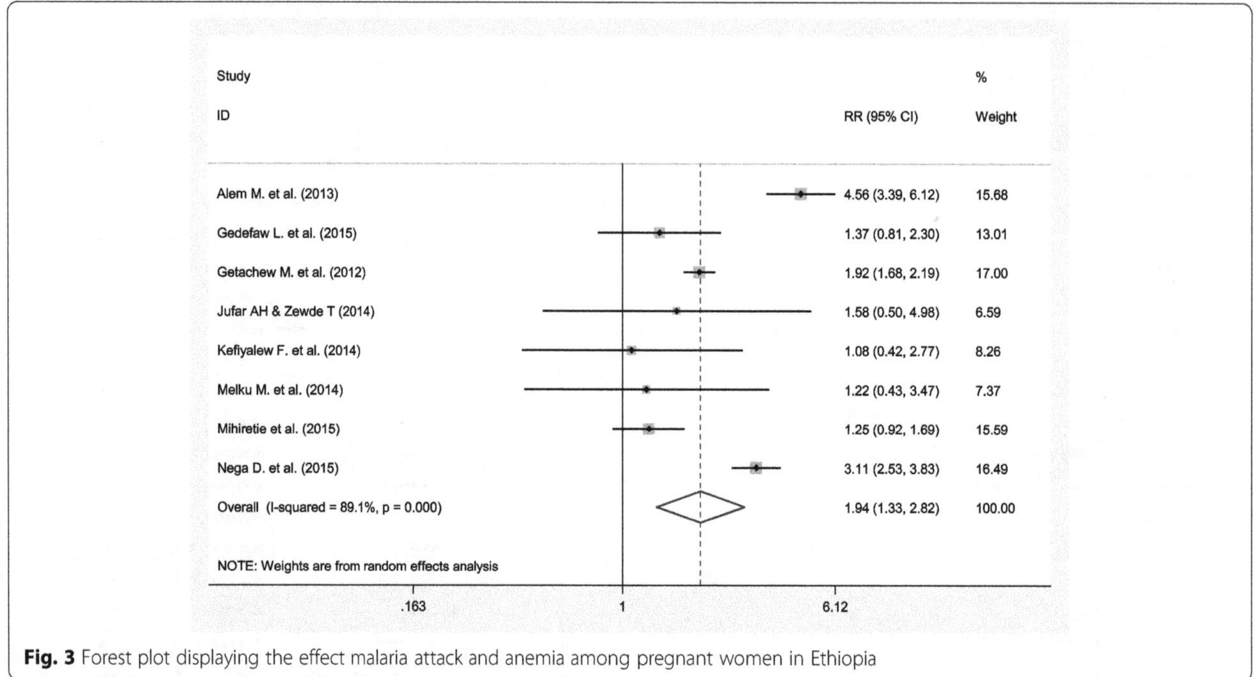

Fig. 3 Forest plot displaying the effect malaria attack and anemia among pregnant women in Ethiopia

women who had more than two years pregnancy interval. This could be explained by the effect of repeated and short interpregnancy interval and breastfeeding on the overall physiologic status of the mother. The woman will not get enough time to recover from the depleted nutrients [50]. A systematic review of the effect of birth spacing on the maternal and child nutritional status found that short birth intervals are related to maternal anemia [49]. Similar findings were also observed in a study conducted in Tanzania [53].

Pregnant women living in urban areas are 73% less likely to be anemic during pregnancy than women in the rural area. The difference in the socioeconomic status, educational and occupational status of pregnant women, difference in the health service access between rural and urban areas could be the justification for the difference. Additionally, inadequate counselling by health professionals in resolving the wrong beliefs and myths regarding the iron supplementation could contribute to higher prevalence of anemia among pregnant women in rural areas [54, 55]. A study conducted in India also showed that pregnant women from the rural areas are more likely to develop anemia than women from the urban area [54].

WHO recommends early diagnosis and effective treatment of malaria infections and the use of long-lasting insecticidal nets (LLINS) during pregnancy [56]. The result of this meta-analysis showed that women who had malaria attack during pregnancy are almost two times more likely to develop anemia during pregnancy. A review of studies conducted in Sub-Saharan African countries also found that there is a higher (26%) risk of severe anemia in pregnant women secondary to malaria infection. Malaria infection is responsible for one in ten cases of severe anemia in pregnant women [46]. Similar findings was also observed in a study conducted in Kenya [57].

This review used a comprehensive search strategy and more than one reviewer was involved in each step of the review process. PRISMA guideline was strictly followed during the review process. This review has certain limitations. Studies included were cross-sectional and the outcome variable may be affected by other confounding variables. Some studies included in this review didn't consider respondents' residential altitude above sea level to define anemia. Studies have shown that there is an increase in the hemoglobin level when people's live at high altitude [58, 59]. These limitations could affect the overall prevalence of anemia in the country presented in this review.

Conclusions

Almost one-third of pregnant women in Ethiopia were anemic. Statistically significant association was observed between anemia during pregnancy and residence, gravidity, pregnancy interval and malaria infection during their pregnancy. Regions with higher anemia prevalence among pregnant women should be given due attention. Further studies should be conducted to better understand the determinant factors in these regions.

The government and non-governmental organizations should focus on strengthening iron and folic acid supplementation for all pregnant women as part of the routine antenatal care. The use of long-lasting insecticidal nets during pregnancy, early diagnosis and appropriate treatment of malaria in pregnant women, and the use of long-acting family planning methods to prevent short pregnancy intervalsis important and should be stengtehend in areas of higher anemia prevalence in Ethiopia. Health extension workers should be involved in the promotion of antenatal follow-ups and community-based awareness programs, especially in rural areas. Further nationwide studies are needed to understand the determinant factors for anemia in pregnant women.

Additional files

Additional file 1: Forest plot displaying the effect of gravidity in a pregnant woman and anemia among pregnant women in Ethiopia. Description of figure: This figure presents the effect of gravdity on anemia during pregnancy. Multigravida women are more likely to develop anemia during pregnancy than primigravida. (DOCX 18 kb)

Additional file 2: Forest plot displaying the effect of short pregnancy interval and anemia among pregnant women in Ethiopia. Description of figure: This figure presents the effect of short pregnancy interval on anemia during pregnancy. Women who have shorter pregnancy interval are more likely to develop anemia during pregnancy than women with pregnancy interval of more than two years. (DOCX 17 kb)

Additional file 3: Forest plot displaying the effect residence of pregnant woman and anemia among pregnant women in Ethiopia. Description of figure: This figure presents the effect of residence on anemia during pregnancy. Women who are residing in rural areas are more likely to develop anemia during pregnancy than pregnant women in urban areas. (DOCX 18 kb)

Abbreviations

CI: Confidence Interval; EDHS: Ethiopian Demographic and Health Survey; LLINS: Long-lasting insecticidal nets; RR: Relative Risk; SNNPR: Southern Nations, Nationalities, and Peoples' Region of Ethiopia; WHO: World Health Organization

Acknowledgements

We would like to acknowledge to authors of studies included in this review.

Funding

No funding was obtained for this study.

Authors' contributions

GMK involved in the design, selection of articles, data extraction, statistical analysis and manuscript writing. AAM, AKB, and GAF also involved in data extraction, analysis, and manuscript editing. All authors read and approved the final draft of the manuscript.

Competing interest

The authors declare that they have no competing interest.

Author details

[1]College of health Sciences, Debre Markos University, Debre Markos, Ethiopia. [2]Department of Epidemiology and Biostatistics, Institute of Public Health, University of Gondar, Gondar, Ethiopia. [3]Department of Nursing, College of Medicine and Health Science, Adigrat University, Tigray, Ethiopia. [4]School of Public Health, College of Medicine and Health Sciences, Bahir Dar University, P.O.Box 79, Bahir Dar, Ethiopia.

References

1. WHO. The global prevalence of anaemia in 2011. Geneva: World Health Organization; 2015.
2. Black RE, Allen LH, Bhutta ZA, Caulfield LE, De Onis M, Ezzati M, Mathers C, Rivera J, Maternal and child undernutrition study group. Maternal and child undernutrition: global and regional exposures and health consequences. The lancet. 2008;371(9608):243–60.
3. Stevens GA, Finucane MM, De-Regil LM, Paciorek CJ, Flaxman SR, Branca F, et al. Global, regional, and national trends in haemoglobin concentration and prevalence of total and severe anaemia in children and pregnant and non-pregnant women for 1995–2011: a systematic analysis of population-representative data. Lancet Glob Health. 2013;1(1):e16–25.
4. Huch R. Anemia in pregnancy. Praxis. 1999;88(5):157–63.
5. WHO. Global nutrition targets 2025: anaemia policy brief (WHO/NMH/NHD/14.4). Geneva: World Health Organization; 2014.
6. Sifakis S, Pharmakides G. Anemia in pregnancy. Ann N Y Acad Sci. 2000;900:125–36.
7. Schwartz WJ 3rd, Thurnau GR. Iron deficiency anemia in pregnancy. Clin Obstet Gynecol. 1995;38(3):443–54.
8. McClure EM, Goldenberg RL, Dent AE, Meshnick SRA. Systematic review of the impact of malaria prevention in pregnancy on low birth weight and maternal anemia. Int J Gynaecol Obstet. 2013;121(2):103–9.
9. Lee AI, Okam MM. Anemia in pregnancy. Hematol Oncol Clin North Am. 2011;25(2):241–59. vii
10. Karaoglu L, Pehlivan E, Egri M, Deprem C, Gunes G, Genc MF, et al. The prevalence of nutritional anemia in pregnancy in an east Anatolian province, Turkey. BMC Public Health. 2010;10:329.
11. Olubukola A, Odunayo A, Adesina O. Anemia in pregnancy at two levels of health care in Ibadan, south west Nigeria. Annals of African medicine. 2011;10(4):272–7.
12. Ouedraogo S, Koura GK, Bodeau-Livinec F, Accrombessi MM, Massougbodji A, Cot M. Maternal anemia in pregnancy: assessing the effect of routine preventive measures in a malaria-endemic area. The American journal of tropical medicine and hygiene. 2013;88(2):292–300.
13. Kazmierczak W, Fiegler P, Adamowicz R, Muszer M, Kaminski K. Prevention of iron deficiency anemia–influence on the course of pregnancy, delivery and the infant's status. Wiadomosci lekarskie. 2004;57(Suppl 1):144–7.
14. Scholl TO, Reilly T. Anemia, iron and pregnancy outcome. J Nutr. 2000; 130(2S Suppl):443S–7S.
15. Lops VR, Hunter LP, Dixon LR. Anemia in pregnancy. Am Fam Physician. 1995;51(5):1189–97.
16. Kalenga MK, Mutach K, Nsungula K, Odimba FK, Kabyla I. Anemia in pregnancy. Clinical and biological study. Apropos of 463 cases seen in Lubumbashi (Zaire). Revue francaise de gynecologie et d'obstetrique. 1989;84(5):393–9.
17. Moher D, Liberati A, Tetzlaff J, Altman DG. Preferred reporting items for systematic reviews and meta-analyses: the PRISMA statement. Ann Intern Med. 2009;151(4):264–9.
18. Danish N, Fawad A, Abbasi N. Assessment of pregnancy outcome in primigravida: comparison between booked and un-booked patients. Journal of Ayub Medical College, Abbottabad : JAMC. 2010;22(2):23–5.
19. Woman to Woman Childbirth Education. Primigravida, primiparous, multigravida. https://womantowomancbe.wordpress.com/. Accessed 29 June 2017.
20. The Joanna Briggs Institute. Joanna Briggs institute reviewers' manual: 2008.
21. Begg CB, Mazumdar M. Operating characteristics of a rank correlation test for publication bias. Biometrics. 1994;50(4):1088–101.
22. Egger M, Smith GD, Schneider M, Minder C. Bias in meta-analysis detected by a simple, graphical test. BMJ. 1997;315(7109):629–34.
23. Higgins JP, Thompson SG, Deeks JJ, Altman DG. Measuring inconsistency in meta-analyses. BMJ: British Medical Journal. 2003;327(7414):557.
24. Mihiretie H, Fufa M, Mitiku A, Bacha C, Getahun D, Kejela M, Sileshi G, Wakshuma B. Magnitude of anemia and associated factors among pregnant women attending antenatal care in Nekemte health center, Nekemte, Ethiopia. Journal of Medical Microbiology & Diagnosis. 2015;4(3):1–4.
25. Kedir H, Berhane Y, Worku A. Khat chewing and restrictive dietary behaviors are associated with anemia among pregnant women in high prevalence rural communities in eastern Ethiopia. PLoS One. 2013;8(11):e78601.
26. Abriha A, Yesuf ME, Wassie MM. Prevalence and associated factors of anemia among pregnant women of Mekelle town: a cross sectional study. BMC research notes. 2014;7(1):1.

27. Alem M, Enawgaw B, Gelaw A, Kenaw T, Seid M, Olkeba Y. Prevalence of anemia and associated risk factors among pregnant women attending antenatal care in Azezo health center Gondar town, Northwest Ethiopia. Journal of Interdisciplinary Histopathology. 2013;1(3):137–44.
28. Ayenew F, Abere Y, Timerga G. Pregnancy anaemia prevalence and associated factors among women attending ante Natal Care in north Shoa zone, Ethiopia. Reproductive System & Sexual Disorders. 2014;3(135):1–7.
29. Bekele A, Tilahun M, Mekuria A. Prevalence of anemia and its associated factors among pregnant women attending antenatal Care in Health Institutions of Arba Minch town, Gamo Gofa zone, Ethiopia: a cross-sectional study. Anemia. 2016;2016:9. doi:10.1155/2016/1073192.
30. Ejeta E, Alemnew B, Fikadu A, Fikadu M, Tesfaye L, Birhanu T, Nekemte E. Prevalence of anaemia in pregnant womens and associated risk factors in Western Ethiopia. Food Science and Quality Management. 2014;31:82–91.
31. Gebre A, Mulugeta A. Prevalence of anemia and associated factors among pregnant women in north western zone of Tigray, northern Ethiopia: a cross-sectional study. Journal of nutrition and metabolism. 2015;2015:7. doi:10.1155/2015/165430.
32. Gedefaw L, Ayele A, Asres Y, Mossie A. Anaemia and associated factors among pregnant women attending antenatal care clinic in Walayita Sodo town, southern Ethiopia. Ethiopian journal of health sciences. 2015;25(2):155–64.
33. Gies S, Brabin BJ, Yassin MA, Cuevas L. Comparison of screening methods for anaemia in pregnant women in Awassa, Ethiopia. Tropical Med Int Health. 2003;8(4):301–9.
34. Jufar AH, Zewde T. Prevalence of anemia among pregnant women attending antenatal care at tikur anbessa specialized hospital, Addis Ababa Ethiopia. Journal of Hematology & Thromboembolic. Diseases. 2014;2014:2–125. doi:10.4172/2329-8790.1000125.
35. Kefiyalew F, Zemene E, Asres Y, Gedefaw L. Anemia among pregnant women in Southeast Ethiopia: prevalence, severity and associated risk factors. BMC research notes. 2014;7(1):1.
36. Melku M, Addis Z, Alem M, Enawgaw B. Prevalence and predictors of maternal anemia during pregnancy in Gondar, Northwest Ethiopia: an institutional based cross-sectional study. Anemia. 2014;2014:9. doi:10.1155/2014/108593.
37. Obse N, Mossie A, Gobena T. Magnitude of anemia and associated risk factors among pregnant women attending antenatal care in Shalla Woreda, west Arsi zone, Oromia region, Ethiopia. Ethiopian journal of health sciences. 2013;23(2):165–73.
38. Addis Alene K, Mohamed Dohe A. Prevalence of anemia and associated factors among pregnant women in an urban area of eastern Ethiopia. Anemia. 2014;2014:7. doi:10.1155/2014/561567.
39. Alemu T, Umeta M. Reproductive and obstetric factors are key predictors of maternal anemia during pregnancy in Ethiopia: evidence from demographic and health survey (2011). Anemia. 2015;2015:8. doi:10.1155/2015/649815.
40. Gebremedhin S, Enquselassie F, Umeta M. Prevalence and correlates of maternal anemia in rural Sidama, southern Ethiopia. Afr J Reprod Health. 2014;18(1):44–53.
41. Gebremedhin S, Samuel A, Mamo G, Moges T, Assefa T. Coverage, compliance and factors associated with utilization of iron supplementation during pregnancy in eight rural districts of Ethiopia: a cross-sectional study. BMC Public Health. 2014;14(1):1.
42. Getachew M, Yewhalaw D, Tafess K, Getachew Y, Zeynudin A. Anaemia and associated risk factors among pregnant women in Gilgel gibe dam area, Southwest Ethiopia. Parasit Vectors. 2012;5(1):1.
43. Nega D, Dana D, Tefera T, Eshetu T. Anemia associated with asymptomatic malaria among pregnant women in the rural surroundings of Arba Minch town, South Ethiopia. BMC research notes. 2015;8(1):1.
44. Central Statistical Agency/Ethiopia, ICF International. Ethiopia demographic and health survey 2011. Addis Ababa, Ethiopia: Central Statistical Agency/ Ethiopia and ICF International; 2012.
45. Shulman CE. Malaria in pregnancy: its relevance to safe-motherhood programmes. Annals of Tropical Medicine & Parasitology. 1999;93(sup1):S59–66.
46. Guyatt HL, Snow RW. The epidemiology and burden of plasmodium falciparum-related anemia among pregnant women in sub-Saharan Africa. The American journal of tropical medicine and hygiene. 2001;64(1_suppl):36–44.
47. Desai M, ter Kuile FO, Nosten F, McGready R, Asamoa K, Brabin B, et al. Epidemiology and burden of malaria in pregnancy. Lancet Infect Dis. 2007;7(2):93–104.
48. Central Statistical Agency (CSA) [Ethiopia] and ICF. Ethiopia demographic and health survey 2016. Addis Ababa, Ethiopia, and Rockville, Maryland, USA: CSA and ICF; 2016.
49. Dewey KG, Cohen RJ. Does birth spacing affect maternal or child nutritional status? A systematic literature review. Maternal & child nutrition. 2007;3(3):151–73.
50. Merchant K, Martorell R. Frequent reproductive cycling: does it lead to nutritional depletion of mothers? Progress in food & nutrition science. 1988; 12(4):339–69.
51. Nik Rosmawati N, Mohd Nazri S, Mohd II. The rate and risk factors for anemia among pregnant mothers in Jerteh Terengganu, Malaysia. J Community Med Health Educ. 2012;2(150):2161–0711.1000150.
52. Wendt A, Gibbs CM, Peters S, Hogue CJ. Impact of increasing inter-pregnancy interval on maternal and infant health. Paediatr Perinat Epidemiol. 2012;26(s1):239–58.
53. Lilungulu A, Matovelo D, Kihunrwa A, Gumodoka B. Spectrum of maternal and perinatal outcomes among parturient women with preceding short inter-pregnancy interval at Bugando medical Centre, Tanzania. Maternal health, neonatology and perinatology. 2015;1(1):1.
54. Gowri D, Sakthi D, Palanivel C. Influence of awareness and attitude about anemia and iron supplements on anemic status of pregnant women attending a tertiary care centre in South India. Journal of contraceptive studies. 2017;2:1. doi:10.21767/2471-9749.100026.
55. Adamu AL, Crampin A, Kayuni N, Amberbir A, Koole O, Phiri A, et al. Prevalence and risk factors for anemia severity and type in Malawian men and women: urban and rural differences. Popul Health Metrics. 2017;15(1):12.
56. World Health Organization. Malaria in pregnant women. Last update: 25 May 2017. retrived on 29/06/2017, from; http://www.who.int/malaria/areas/high_risk_groups/pregnancy/en/.
57. Shulman C, Marshall T, Dorman E, Bulmer J, Cutts F, Peshu N, et al. Malaria in pregnancy: adverse effects on haemoglobin levels and birthweight in primigravidae and multigravidae. Tropical Med Int Health. 2001;6(10):770–8.
58. Dirren H, Logman MH, Barclay DV, Freire WB. Altitude correction for hemoglobin. Eur J Clin Nutr. 1994;48(9):625–32.
59. Dallman PR, Siimes MA, Stekel A. Iron deficiency in infancy and childhood. Am J Clin Nutr. 1980;33(1):86–118.

10

Diagnostic predictive value of platelet indices for discriminating hypo productive versus immune thrombocytopenia purpura in patients attending a tertiary care teaching hospital in Addis Ababa, Ethiopia

Mikias Negash[1*], Aster Tsegaye[1] and Amha G/Medhin[2]

Abstract

Background: Bone marrow examination may be required to discriminate causes of thrombocytopenia as hypoproductive or hyperdestructive. However, this procedure is invasive and time consuming. This study assessed the diagnostic value of Mean Platelet Volume (MPV), Platelet Distribution Width (PDW) and Platelet Large Cell-Ratio (P-LCR) in discriminating causes of thrombocytopenia as hypoproductive or hyperdestructive (Immune thrombocytopenia purpura).

Method: A prospective cross-sectional study was conducted on 83 thrombocytopenic patients (Plt < 150×10^9/L). From these, 50 patients had hypoproductive and the rest 33 Immune Thrombocytopenia Purpura (ITP). Age and sex matched 42 healthy controls were included as a comparative group. Hematological analysis was carried out using Sysmex XT 2000i 5 part diff analyzer. SPSS Version16 was used for data analysis. A two by two table and receiver operating characteristic (ROC) curve was used to calculate sensitivity, specificity, positive and negative predictive values, for a given platelet indices (MPV, PDW and P-LCR). Student *t* test and Mann Whitney *U* test were used to compare means and medians, respectively. Correlation test was used to determine associations between continuous variables.

Results: All Platelet indices were significantly higher in ITP patients ($n = 33$) than in hypoproductive thrombocytopenic patients ($n = 50$) ($p < 0.0001$). In particular MPV and P-LCR have larger area under ROC curve (0.876 and 0.816, respectively), indicating a better predictive capacity, sensitivity and specificity in discriminating the two causes of thrombocytopenia. The indices were still significantly higher in ITP patients compared to 42 healthy controls ($p < 0.0001$). A significant negative correlation was observed between platelet count and platelet indices in ITP patients, ($p < 0.001$).

Conclusion: MPV, PDW and P-LCR help in predicting thrombocytopenic patients as having ITP or hypoproductive thrombocytopenia. If these indices are used in line with other laboratory and clinical information, they may help in delaying/ avoiding unnecessary bone marrow aspiration in ITP patients or supplement a request for bone morrow aspiration or biopsy in hypoproductive thrombocytopenic patients.

Keywords: Bone marrow, Platelet indices, Immune thrombocytopenia purpura (hyperdestructive thrombocytopenia), Hypoproductive thrombocytopenia

* Correspondence: mikiasn2@gmail.com
[1]College of Health Science, Department of Medical Laboratory Science, Addis Ababa University, Addis Ababa, Ethiopia
Full list of author information is available at the end of the article

Background

Platelets play a pivotal role in the first steps of clot formation by adhering to damaged blood vessel as well as donating their membrane phospholipids for the activation of coagulation factors [1]. A platelet count of less than 150×10^9/L is considered to be thrombocytopenic. The two main causes of thrombocytopenia excluding pseudo thrombocytopenia are increase destruction or peripheral consumption (hyper-destructive thrombocytopenia), such as immune thrombocytopenic purpura (ITP), disseminated intravascular coagulation (DIC), and thrombotic thrombocytopenic purpura (TTP). Whereas decreased platelet productions (hypo-production thrombocytopenia) are associated with a number of bone marrow diseases [2].

The gold standard method for discriminating these two causes is bone marrow examination. No consensus is reached regarding the necessity of a bone marrow examination in the evaluation of idiopathic thrombocytopenic purpura. Due to its invasiveness and being unfriendly for the patients, this procedure is not recommended as first line diagnosis. ITP still remains a diagnosis by exclusion due to lack of accurate clinical and laboratory parameters [3].

Studies conducted elsewhere showed that platelet indices like Mean Platelet Volume (MPV) are sensitive, specific and have diagnostic predictive value in discriminating ITP (hyper-destructive thrombocytopenia) from hypoproductive [4–7]. However, many of these studies either evaluated a single parameter like MPV or compared patients with one type of disease category. These platelet indices such as MPV (average size of platelet), Platelet Distribution Width (PDW; the width measured at 20 % of the platelet histogram) and Platelet Large Cell-Ratio (P-LCR; percentage of platelets with size more than 12 fl) are usually available as part of hematology outputs of many of the automated analyzers. A study in Ethiopia reported that majority of the hematological parameters including platelet indices are underutilized in clinical patient management [8]. This hospital based prospective study was conducted to demonstrate the discriminating potential of the three platelet indices between Immune thrombocytopenia purpura versus hypoproductive thrombocytopenia and determine a cut of value with the highest prediction in Ethiopian patients.

Methods

Study site

The study was conducted at Tikur Anbessa Specialized Teaching Hospital of Addis Ababa University, Ethiopia. This is a pioneer tertiary hospital which manages patients with hematological disorders in our country. Suspected or confirmed hematological patients with platelet count below150 x 10^9/L who volunteered to participate were enrolled in to the study.

Laboratory analysis

Blood sample for complete blood count (CBC) analysis was collected into 5 ml EDTA anti-coagulated tubes. CBC analysis was performed using Sysmex XT 2000i fully automated hematology analyzer (Kobe, Japan) based on the manufacturer's protocol. All blood samples were analyzed in less than 4 h of blood collection. This analyzer measures white blood cells (WBC) and reticulocytes with an optical detector block based on the flow cytometry principle, red blood cells (RBC) and platelet counts are analyzed via the impedance method. The performance of the instrument was monitored by running quality control materials. A peripheral blood smear was also reviewed to estimate platelet counts, rule out pseudo thrombocytopenia and fragments of cells like shistocytes.

Study participants

Based on clinical and laboratory information, including preceding and follow-up laboratory data, the patients were divided into two groups; those with marrow disease (hypoproductive) and those with ITP (hyperdestructive). Suspected and confirmed hematological patients with platelet counts below 150×10^9/L were traced from wards and follow up hematology clinic. Patients' medical records were reviewed and any newly diagnosed patients were followed to find out the cause of their thrombocytopenia. The presence of bone marrow disease was diagnosed based on bone marrow examination and it was performed by residents and senior pathologists at Tikur Anbessa pathology laboratory. In this study 83 thrombocytopenic patients were enrolled; 50 had hypoproductive thrombocytopenia while the rest 33 were ITP patients. Bone marrow examination was performed in all 50 hypoproductive patients and in 10 of the 33 ITP patients as part of their medical follow up and diagnosis. ITP Patients who did not have bone marrow examination were monitored during their follow up period to ascertain the diagnosis (for a minimum of 6–8 months). Patients living with the human immunodeficiency virus (HIV) and who had been transfused with platelet concentrate or whole blood in the previous 9 days were excluded from the study. As a control group, 42 age and sex matched apparently healthy individuals were included. Ethical approval was obtained from department of medical laboratory and department of internal medicine of Addis Ababa University. Verbal consent was obtained from adults and parents/guardians of children. In addition assent was secured from children aged 12–17 years provided their parents/guardians consented for their participation.

Statistical analysis

The data was entered and analyzed using SPSS Version 16 (SPSS INC, Chicago, IL, USA). A two by two table and receiver operating characteristic (ROC) curve was used to calculate sensitivity, specificity, positive predictive value (PPV), negative predictive value (NPV), for a given platelet indices (MPV, PDW and P-LCR). Student *t* test and Mann Whitney *U* test were used to compare means and medians, respectively; Correlation test was used to see the association between continuous variables. A *P*-value of < 0.05 was considered as statistically significant.

Result

A total of 83 patients were enrolled in this study. Among these patients, 50 had hypoproductive thrombocytopenia (bone marrow disease) and 33 were ITP patients. The mean age (± standard deviation) of the patients was 41 ± 17.8 and 27 ± 16.3) years, respectively. Females were the predominant study participants in ITP patients, while males were predominant in the hypo productive group ($p = 0.008$). For comparison, 42 apparently healthy controls were included. This is summarized in Table 1.

Comparison of platelet count and Platelet indices between study participants

The platelet count and the platelet indices were compared between ITP, hypoproductive patients and healthy controls. The platelet count was not significantly different between hypoproductive and ITP patients. However, all the platelet indices MPV, PDW and P-LCR were significantly higher ($P < 0.0001$) in patients with ITP than in patients with hypoproductive thrombocytopenia. All the platelet indices were significantly higher in ITP patients as compared to healthy controls (Table 2), but no such significant difference was observed between the healthy controls and patients with hypo-productive thrombocytopenia except for their MPV ($P = 0.01$).

Thrombocytopenia causes

The different causes of thrombocytopenia were analyzed for the two patient groups along with the respective platelet count and platelet indices. The main cause of thrombocytopenia in hypoproductive patients was bone marrow toxicity secondary to chronic myelogenous leukemia (CML) chemotherapy (Table 3). In patients with ITP, the predominant cause was chronic ITP which accounted 28 out of the 33 cases. The remaining acute ITP patients had an average low platelet count of 12.6 × 10^9/L with an MPV of 16.6 fl, PDW 19 fl and P-LCR 51.5 %.

Table 1 Socio-demographic characteristics of patients and apparently healthy controls

Variable	Number	Sex		Age in years Mean (SD)
		Male	Female	
Hypoproductive	50	33	17	41 (17.8)
ITP	33	12	21	27 (16.3)
Healthy controls	42	26	16	25 (6.8)
Total	125	71	54	

Correlation between platelet parameters

There was statistically significant negative correlation between platelet count and the platelet indices in ITP patients (Fig. 1). However, the platelet count and platelet indices did not show significant correlation in Hypoproductive patients (the correlation coefficient between the platelet count and MPV, PDW, and P-LCR was 0.09, -0.13 and -0.01 respectively). A significant negative correlation between the platelet count and the indices was observed in the 42 healthy controls with a correlation coefficient of -0.38, -0.37 and -0.39 for MPV, PDW, and P-LCR respectively.

ROC Curve for analysis of sensitivity and specificity

The area under the curve (AUC) gives the probability that a patient with bone marrow disease has lower values of the measurement (here MPV, PDW and P-LCR). The AUC in Fig. 2 shows lines shifting towards the left upper corner particularly for MPV and P-LCR giving an area of .876 (87.6 %) and .816 (81.6 %), respectively.

Sensitivity and specificity were extrapolated from different coordinate points of the ROC curve. The platelet indices, MPV and P-LCR in particular have better sensitivity, specificity and predicative value in discriminating the two types of thrombocytopenia (Tables 4 and 5). An MPV of <10.75 fl can identify thrombocytopenic patients as hypoproductive with 74 % sensitivity, 70 % specificity, 79 % PPV and 64 % NPV. These indices can also identify patients with ITP, such that an MPV of >11.05 fl can identify patients as having ITP with 67 % sensitivity, 95 % specificity, 88 % PPV and 81 % NPV.

Discussion

Simple, inexpensive and non invasive tests like MPV have been reported to identify causes of thrombocytopenia as hyperdestructive or hypoproductive with sufficient predictive capacity, sensitivity and specificity [4, 5, 7]. In the study reported herein, three platelet indices MPV, PDW and P-LCR were analyzed for their diagnostic predictive capacity in different patients with thrombocytopenia. Consistent with the above studies [4, 5, 7], there was a significant difference in MPV between hypoproductive and ITP patients. Moreover, PDW and P-LCR had significant differences between the two patient groups and better discriminating potential.

Table 2 Comparison of mean platelet count and mean platelet indices between hypo-productive, ITP patients and healthy controls

Variable	Hypo-Production	P-value	95 %CI	ITP	P-value	95 %CI	Healthy Controls
Plt10^9/L	70.4(32)	0.8	-21.4 to 17.3	72.4(49)	<0.001	147 to191.5	241 (47)
MPV(fl)	9.7(0.9)	<0.001	-3.1 to -1.3	12.4(3.6)	<0.001	-3.7 to-0.7	10.3(0.8)
PDW(fl)	13.2(2.3)	<0.001	-3.5 to -1.1	15.5(3.2)	<0.001	-4.3 to-1.8	12.5(1.7)
PLCR(%)	25 (7)	< 0.001	-17 to -7	36.8(13)	<0.001	-14.5 to-4.6	27.2(5.2)

MPV mean platelet volume, *PDW* platelet distribution width, *P-LCR* platelet larger cell ratio; results are presented as mean, values in bracket are standard deviation; *P* value was considered significant at level of 0.05

Niethammer et al. reported that maximum of the histogram, that is the highest peak of the platelet volume distribution curve, has better efficiency than MPV in identifying thrombocytopenia caused by ITP and that resulted from decreased platelet production secondary to receiving chemotherapy [9]. MPV was able to predict the presence of bone marrow metastasis in solid tumor patients with 85 % PPV and 90 % NPV [10]. There is a growing interest in the use of platelet markers in discriminating different forms of thrombocytopenia. Monteagudo et al. measured reticulated platelets by using flow cytometry and showed this parameter has high sensitivity and specificity in identifying thrombocytopenia with increased thrombopoietic activity [11].

Studies showed immature platelet fraction (IPF) measured by Sysmex XE2100 had better sensitivity and specificity in the diagnosis of hyperdestructive thrombocytopenia like ITP and TTP [12, 13]. Though this IPF is one of the out puts from the Sysmex XE2100, such kind of automated analyzer is not available in our country for routine hematology analysis. Sysmex XT 2000i is the model currently available in our country which was also used in this study.

The most common cause of thrombocytopenia in hypoproductive patients was bone marrow suppression secondary to CML chemotherapy. This could be due to the predominance of CML as the leading type of leukemia in Ethiopia which accounts for more than 57.8 % of all the leukemia causes [14].

There was uneven distribution of sex among the study subjects, where females were almost twice than males in ITP, on the other hand males were twice in hypoproductive patients. This may be due to some epidemiological differences in the incidence and prevalence of chronic ITP which is more common in females (in particular in women of child bearing age) compared to males with ratio of 2–3 to 1 [15, 16], while CML is more common in old ages and in males than females with ratios of 1.5–1.8 to 1 [17, 18].

MPV values of 9.7 fl for the hypoproductive group and 12.4 fl for ITP patients observed in our study is much higher than those reported from UK [5], Taiwan [6] and India [19]. In all these studies, they showed that MPV was significantly different between hypoproductive and hyperdestructive patients. However, the reported mean MPV values are 8.1 fl and 9.8 fl in the UK study [5], 7.2 fl and 8.8 fl in the Taiwan [6] and 7.3 fl and 8.62 fl in the Indian study [19] in hypoproductive and hyperdestructive patients, respectively.

The first possible explanation for such differences between this and the above studies could be the kind of automated hematology analyzers that is used for enumerating the platelets. A study conducted by Kaito et al.

Table 3 Causes of thrombocytopenia in hypoproductive patients and respective average platelet count and platelet indices

Diagnosed causes of thrombocytopenia	Number	Pltx10^9/L	MPV (fl)	PDW (fl)	P-LCR (%)
BM toxicity secondary to CML chemotherapy	27	72	9.5	12.3	23
ALL on chemotherapy	5	57	10	13.7	27.5
ALL chemotherapy naïve	2	12	11	13	34
Myelodysplastic syndrome	1	88	8.8	15.3	17
AML on chemotherapy	3	77	8.5	14.4	18
Myelofibrosis	2	44.5	9.5	16.5	24
Erythroid hyperplasia	2	77	10.4	14	31
CLL chemotherapy naïve	4	79	10.4	16.2	34
BM toxicity to lymphoma chemotherapy	4	56	9.9	13	25
Total/average	50	70.4	9.7	13.2	25

CML chronic myelogenous leukemia, *BM* bone marrow, *ALL* acute lymphocytic leukemia, *AML* Acute myeloid leukemia, *CLL* chronic lymphocytic leukemia

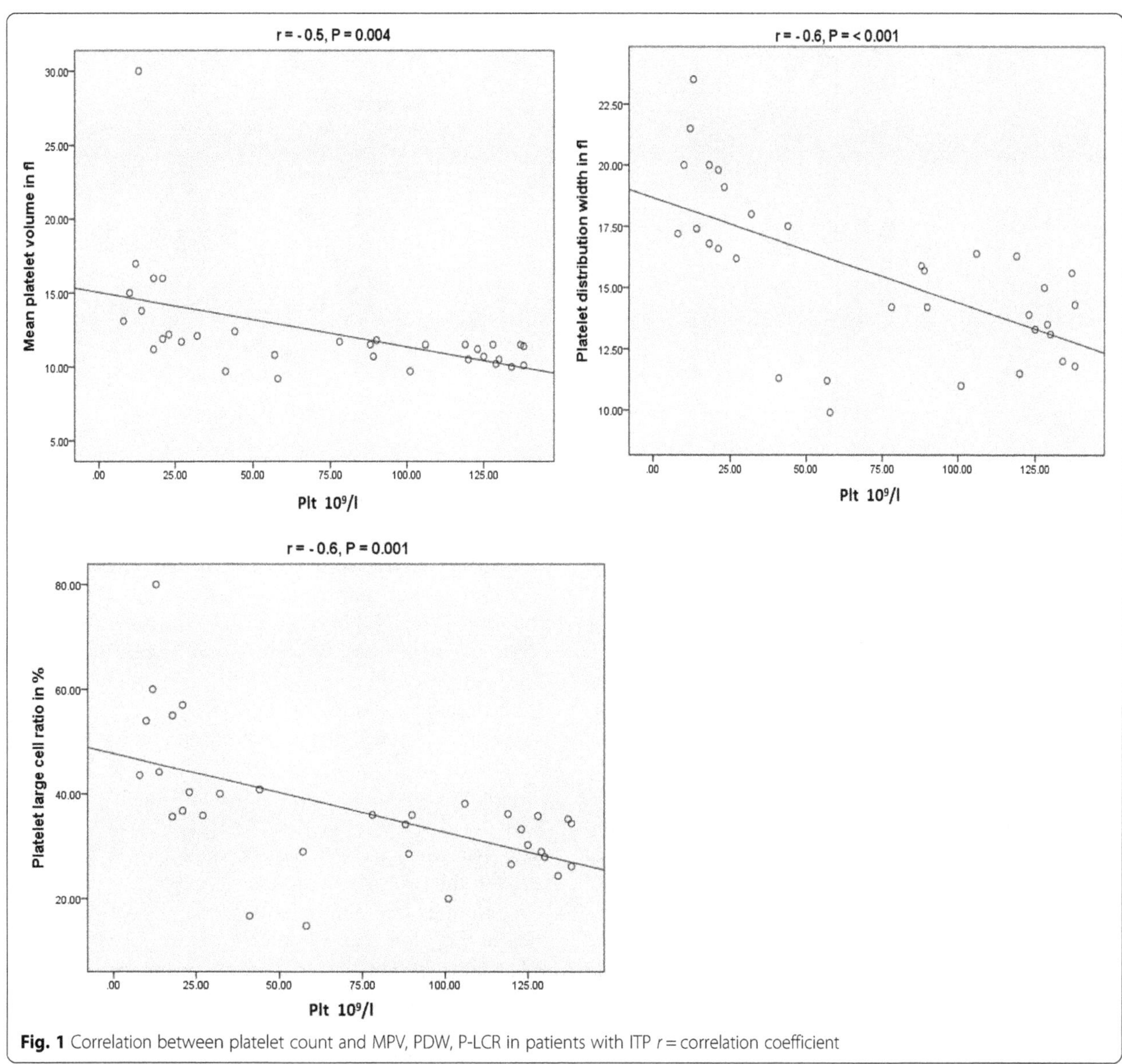

Fig. 1 Correlation between platelet count and MPV, PDW, P-LCR in patients with ITP r = correlation coefficient

In Japan using Sysmex-XE2100 analyzer (Kobe, Japan) reported a mean MPV of 10.2 fl in aplastic anemia and 12.2 fl in ITP patients [7], whose values are closer to our finding for ITP. A similar finding was also reported from a study conducted by Ntaios et al. who also used sysmex-XE2100 automated analyzer [4]. Ntaios et al. emphasized that the higher values of the platelet indices in their study compared to others could be due to a difference in hematology analyzers. Large or giant platelets could be excluded from the platelet count with instruments which use impedance method like coulter STKS [6] and coulter Gen-S [5] used by the above studies, but the Sysmex XT2000i and XE2100 series also employ optical fluorescence detection method [20].

The second possible reason could be an actual difference in the platelet indices among population from country to country. A study by Hong et al. in healthy Chinese adults using Sysme XT 2100 indeed confirmed variations of platelet indices between regions. The reported value of MPV for example ranged from 10.30 ± 0.80 to 12.36 ± 1.34 [21]. In another study by Maluf et al. a statistically significant difference in MPV, PDW, and P-LCR according to self-declared race/skin color was demonstrated, where mean MPV, PDW, and P-LCR values of white individuals were lower than those of individuals self-declared black or pardo (mixed skin color/brown) [22]. An earlier study by Barbara J to evaluate ethnic and sex differences in hematological profiles including platelet count and MPV reveled an MPV of 8.9 fl in Caucasians (eastern Europe), 9.1 fl in Afro-Caribbean's and 9.4 fl in Sub-Saharan Africans (including few Ethiopians) [23]. It is evident that Africans have

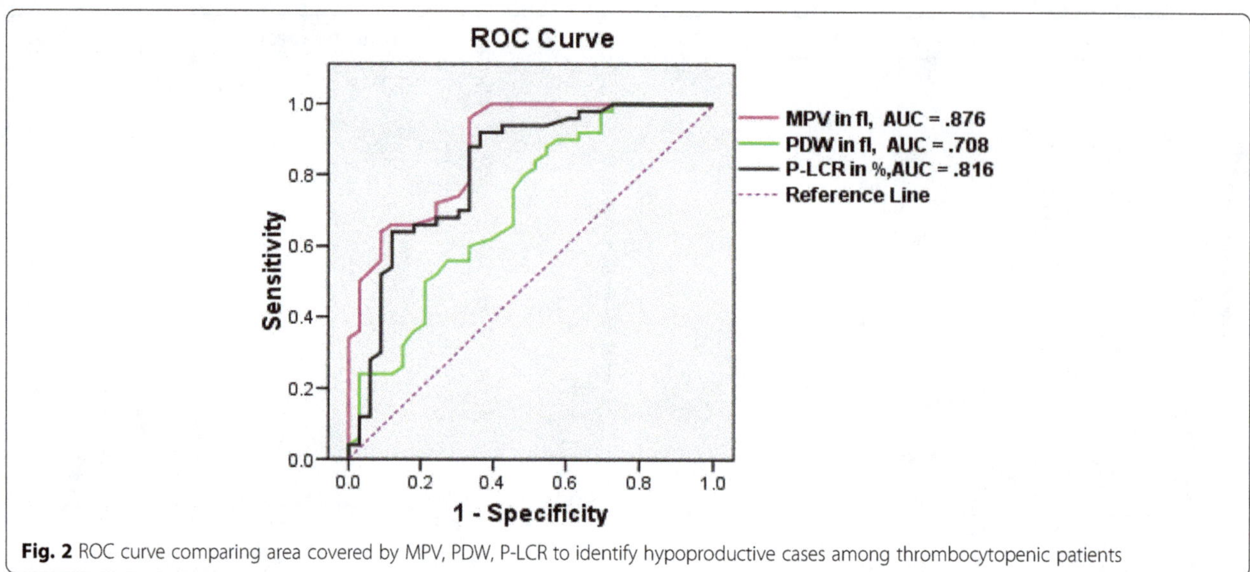

Fig. 2 ROC curve comparing area covered by MPV, PDW, P-LCR to identify hypoproductive cases among thrombocytopenic patients

higher MPV as compared to the other groups. Though we have analyzed 42 healthy controls, the mean MPV was 10.3 fl which suggest that the actual size of the platelet in our study subjects could be higher.

The mean MPV of the healthy controls (10.3 fl) in the current study can identify ITP patients with 82 % sensitivity, 66 % specificity, 61.4 % positive predictive value and 85 % negative predictive value. In a similar study conducted by T. Numbenjapon et al. in healthy Thais, the mean MPV was 7.9 fl. This identified hyperdestructive thrombocytopenic patients with a sensitivity of 82.3 %, a specificity of 92.5 %, a PPV of 94.4 %, and a NPV of 77.1 % [6]. Kaito et al. analyzed the role of MPV, PDW and P-LCR in the diagnosis of ITP and reported somewhat an improved sensitivity and specificity where an MPV of >11 fl has a sensitivity of 87.2 % and a specificity of 80.0 % [7].

This variation in sensitivity, specificity and predictive values could be due to differences in the type of study participants, where some have compared only one patient group, bone marrow disease due to aplastic anemia against ITP [4, 7]. However, in our study more than 8 causes of bone marrow disease were identified. The other reason could be the predominance of chronic ITP which accounts 28 out of 33 ITP patients. These patients have relatively stable platelet count, on average 88×10^9/L and a mean MPV of 11.6 fl with a range of 9.2 to 17. On the other hand hypoproductive patients have a mean MPV of 9.7 fl with arrange of 7.1 to 11.2; hence it is evident that some platelet indices values are overlapping between the two patient groups.

Supporting the above explanation in vitro studies showed that plasma auto antibodies from ITP patients not only are involved in platelet destruction, but may also contribute to the inhibition of platelet production by affecting megakaryocyte production and maturation [24, 25]. It suggests that a similar effect may occur in vivo. This may partly explain the lower platelet indices in our chronic

Table 4 Sensitivity and specificity of the platelet indices for diagnosis of hypoproductive thrombocytopenia (bone marrow disease) at different cut off points from ROC curve coordinate

MPV (fl)	Sensitivity %	Specificity %	P-LCR (%)	Sensitivity %	Specificity %
<10.75	74	70	<31.4	76	67
<10.95	90	67	<33.15	88	67
<11.05	95	67	<33.7	90	64
<11.3	100	61	<34.3	92	61
PDW (fl)					
<15.5	76	55			
<15.65	80	52			
<15.75	82	49			
<15.85					

Table 5 Sensitivity and specificity of the platelet indices for diagnosis of ITP at different cut off points from ROC curve coordinates

MPV (fl)	Sensitivity %	Specificity %	P-LCR (%)	Sensitivity %	Specificity %
>11.05	67	95	>33.15	67	88
>10.75	70	74	>30.05	70	70
>10.15	85	66	>28	82	66
>9.95	91	64	>26.15	88	64
PDW (fl)					
>14.25	61	62			
>14.1	67	40			
>13.05	79	50			

MPV mean platelet volume, *PDW* platelet distribution width, *P-LCR* platelet larger cell ratio, *ROC* receiver operating characteristics curve, *ITP* immune thrombocytopenia purpura

ITP patients compared to the acute ITP cases. Despite hyper-destructive thrombocytopenia which is characterized by higher MPV, these chronic patients may have normal or even suppressed platelet production rate.

The significant negative correlation between the platelet count and the platelet indices in ITP patients seems to be mainly contributed by acute ITP patients who had a mean platelet count of $12.6x10^9$/L and mean MPV of 16.6 fl, PDW 19 fl and P-LCR of 51.5 %. This shows the platelet indices in particular MPV and P-LCR could have a better discriminating or prediction capacity for ITP where they are needed the most, during the early investigation and diagnosis of thrombocytopenic patients. Among the 33 ITP patients, 10 of them had bone marrow examination with result of no primary or secondary bone marrow disease. If not in all these 10 patients, the platelet indices could have assisted in predicting most patients to have ITP and could prevent them from undergoing this invasive procedure.

Conclusion

In conclusion these indices in particular MPV and P-LCR can discriminate ITP from hypoproductive thrombocytopenia and they may help in avoiding or delaying ITP patients from undergoing unnecessary, invasive bone marrow aspiration or prevent undesirable platelet transfusion. The mean platelet indices are relatively higher in our study groups. Therefore, cut off values need to be established on the given laboratory setup and place for the indices to be used as a discriminating tool for thrombocytopenia. Future studies comparing impedance and impedance with optical method and inclusion of more types of hyper-destructive thrombocytopenia may enable us to use these indices for broader patient groups.

Limitation of the study

When there is abnormal distribution of platelets or fragments of RBCs and blasts, the analyzer may not display the values of platelet indices; thus, interpreting the result from the histogram and reviewing the smear could be necessary. Relatively the smaller sample size and limited disease categories in particular in hyper destructive thrombocytopenia group may limit application of this finding in broader patient groups.

Abbreviations

ALL, acute lymphocytic leukemia; AML, acute myelocytic/myelogenous leukemia; BM, bone marrow; CBC, complete blood count; CLL, chronic lymphocytic leukemia; CML, chronic myolegenous leukemia; DIC, disseminated intravascular coagulation; EDTA, ethylene diamine tetra-acetic acid; fL, femto liter (10^{-15} litre); Hb, hemoglobin; HIV, human immunodeficiency virus; IPF, immature platelet fraction; IPU, information processing unit; ITP, immune thrombocytopenic purpura; IVIg, intravenous Immunoglobulin; MCH, mean cell hemoglobin; MCV, mean cell volume; MPV, mean platelet volume; NPV, negative predictive value; PCT, platecrit; PDW, platelet size distribution width; P-LCR, platelet large cell ratio; PPV, positive predictive value; RDW, red cell distribution width; RNA, ribonucleic acid; ROC, receiver operating curve; RP, reticulated platelets; TTP, thrombotic thrombocytopenic purpura

Acknowledgment

This work was financially supported by Addis Ababa University. We would like to thank the patients attending Tikur Anbessa Specialized Hospital and healthy controls without whom this study would not be possible and special thanks goes to staffs from hematology follow up clinic and hematology laboratory. Finally we would like to thank Haramaya University who supported the principal investigator in all possible ways during his study and research period.

Authors' contributions

MN (MSc in Clinical laboratory science) has conducted the research and analyzed it. AGM and AT have contributed in the shaping of the research design, revising the paper and its final approval. All authors read and approved the final manuscript.

Competing interests

The authors declare that they have no competing interests.

Author details

[1]College of Health Science, Department of Medical Laboratory Science, Addis Ababa University, Addis Ababa, Ethiopia. [2]Department of Internal Medicine, Addis Ababa University, Addis Ababa, Ethiopia.

References

1. Di Paola JA, Buchanan GR. Immune thrombocytopenic purpura. Pediatr Clin North Am. 2002;49(5):911–28.
2. Sekhon SS, Roy V. Thrombocytopenia in adults: a practical approach to evaluation and management. South Med J. 2006;99(5):491–8.
3. Guidelines for the investigation and management of idiopathic thrombocytopenic purpura in adults, children and in pregnancy. Br J Haematol. 2003;120(4):574-596.
4. Ntaios G, Papadopoulos A, Chatzinikolaou A, Saouli Z, Karalazou P, Kaiafa G, et al. Increased values of mean platelet volume and platelet size deviation width may provide a safe positive diagnosis of idiopathic thrombocytopenic purpura. Acta Haematologica. 2008;119(3):173–7.
5. Bowles K, Cooke L, Richards E, Baglin T. Platelet size has diagnostic predictive value in patients with thrombocytopenia. Int Clin & Lab Hematol. 2005;27(3):70–373.
6. Numbenjapon T, Mahapo N, Pornvipavee R, Sriswasdi C, Mongkonsritragoon W, Leelasiri A, et al. A prospective evaluation of normal mean platelet volume in discriminating hyperdestructive thrombocytopenia from hypoproductive thrombocytopenia. Int J Lab Hematol. 2008;30(5):408–14.
7. Kaito K, Otsubo H, Usui N, Yoshida M, Tanno J, Kurihara E, et al. Platelet size deviation width, platelet large cell ratio, and mean platelet volume have sufficient sensitivity and specificity in the diagnosis of immune thrombocytopenia. Br J Haematol. 2005;128(5):698–702.
8. Birhaneselassie M, Birhanu A, Gebremedhin A, Tsegaye A. How useful are complete blood count and reticulocyte reports to clinicians in Addis Ababa hospitals, Ethiopia? BMC Hematology. 2013;13(1):11.
9. Niethammer AG, Forman EN. Use of the platelet histogram maximum in evaluating thrombocytopenia. Am J Hematol. 1999;60(1):19–23.
10. Aksoy S, Kilickap S, Hayran M, Harputluoglu H, Koca E, Dede D, et al. Platelet size has diagnostic predictive value for bone marrow metastasis in patients with solid tumors. Int J Lab Hematol. 2008;30(3):214–9.
11. Monteagudo M, Amengual MJ, Muñoz L, Soler J, Roig I, Tolosa C. Reticulated platelets as a screening test to identify thrombocytopenia aetiology. QJM. 2008;101(7):549–55.
12. Abe Y, Wada H, Tomatsu H, Sakaguchi A, Nishioka J, Yabu Y, et al. A simple technique to determine thrombopoisis level using immature platelet fraction (IPF). Thromb Res. 2006;118(4):463–9.
13. Briggs C, Kunka S, Hart D, Oguni S, Machin SJ. Assessment of an immature platelet fraction (IPF) in peripheral thrombocytopenia. Br J Haematol. 2004; 126(1):93–9.
14. Shamebo M. Leukemia in adult Ethiopians. Ethiop Med J. 1990;28(1):31–7.
15. Marieke Schoonen W, Kucera G, Coalson J, Li L, Rutstein M, Mowat F, et al. Epidemiology of immune thrombocytopenic purpura in the General Practice Research Data base. Br J Hematol. 2009;145(2):235–44.
16. Gernsheimer T. Epidemiology and pathophysiology of immune thrombocytopenic purpura. Eur J Hematol. 2008;80 Suppl 69:3–8.
17. Rodriguez-A breu D, Bordoni A, Zucca E. Epidemiology of hematological malignancies. Ann Oncol. 2007;18 suppl 1:i3–8.
18. Siegel R, Naishadham D, Jemal A. Cancer statistics. CA Cancer J Clin. 2013; 63(1):11–30.
19. Chandra H, Chandra S, Rawat A, Verma S. Role of mean platelet volume as discriminating guide for bone marrow disease in patients with thrombocytopenia. Int J Lab Hematol. 2010;32(5):498–505.
20. Ntaios G, Papadopoulos A, Chatzinikolaou A, Girtovitis F, Kaiafa G, Savopoulos C, et al. Evaluation of mean platelet volume in the differential diagnosis of thrombocytopenia. Int J Lab Hematol. 2009;31(6):688–9.
21. Hong J, Min Z, Bai-shen P, Jie Z, Ming-ting P, Xian-zhang H, et al. Investigation on reference intervals and regional differences of platelet indices in healthy Chinese Han adults. J Clin Lab Anal. 2015;29(1):21–7.
22. Maluf CB, Barreto SM, Vidigal PG. Standardization and reference intervals of platelet volume indices: Insight from the Brazilian longitudinal study of adult health (ELSA-BRASIL). Platelets. 2015;26(5):413–20.
23. Bain BJ. Ethnic and sex differences in the total and differential white cell count and platelet count. J Clin Pathol. 1996;49(8):664–6.
24. McMillan R, Wang L, Tomer A, Nichol J, Pistillo J. Suppression of invitro megakaryocyte production by antiplatelet autoantibodies from adult patients with chronic ITP. Blood. 2004;103(4):1364–9.
25. Chang M, Nakagawa PA, Williams SA, Schwartz MR, Irnfeld KL, Buzby JS, et al. Immune thrombocytopenic purpura (ITP) plasma and purified ITP monoclonal auto antibodies inhibit megakaryocytopoiesis in vitro. Blood. 2003;102(3):887–95.

11

Numerical analysis of in vivo platelet consumption data from ITP patients

Ted S. Strom[1,2]

Abstract

Background: Numerical methods have recently allowed quantitative interpretation of in vivo murine platelet consumption data in terms of values for the random destruction rate constant (RD), intrinsic lifespan (LS), and the standard deviation of ln LS (SD), as well as the platelet production rate (PR) and age distribution (AD). But application of these methods to data obtained in thrombocytopenic patients is problematic for two reasons. First, such data has in all cases been obtained with radiolabeled platelets, and uptake of the radio-isotope by long lived cells complicates the analysis. Second, inferred values of the platelet production rate (PR) and random destruction rate (RD) are difficult to interpret, since increased RD can occur either as a cause or a consequence of thrombocytopenia.

Methods: We used a numerical method to analyze in vivo platelet consumption data from a series of *41* patients with immune thrombocytopenic purpura (ITP). An additional parameter, the fraction of labeled long-lived cells (LL), was evaluated concurrently with RD, LS, and SD. To provide a basis for interpreting these values, we used an iterative interpolation process to predict their response to different pathophysiologic mechanisms. The process also generates predicted effects on the widely used immature platelet fraction (IPF).

Results: Optimal parameter value sets were identified in 76 % (31 of 41) of the data sets. 27 of 31 ITP patients showed no substantial homeostatic increase in platelet production, with the remaining 4 showing both augmented platelet consumption and a compensatory increase in PR. Up to 1/3 of the patients showed the degree of increased RD expected to result from reduced thrombopoiesis only. "Jacknife" resampling yielded CV values of <0.5 in over 75 % of the evaluable data sets. Predicted platelet age distributions indicate that interpretation of the IPF and absolute IPF (aIPF) is a complex function of platelet count. We found, counter-intuitively, that reduced PR can *increase* the IPF, and increased RD can *reduce* the aIPF.

Conclusions: Our findings support the feasibility of using numerical analysis to quantitatively interpret in vivo platelet consumption data, to identify likely etiologies of thrombocytopenias, and to assess the utility of IPF measurements in that context.

Keywords: Platelets, Thrombocytopenia, Immune thrombocytopenic purpura, Numerical analysis

Background

In vivo platelet consumption studies have often been used to quantify the rates of both random and lifespan-dependent consumption processes, and to evaluate production rate, but their interpretation can be problematic. The aim of the present study is to demonstrate that a numerical analysis method can reliably quantify these rates, and thereby identify fundamental pathophysiologic features, in thrombocytopenic patients.

Methods which have been used to interpret such studies include a simple exponential decay model [1], a weighted mean method that applies an empirical mixture of separately optimized linear and exponential decay processes [2], a purely lifespan-dependent model [3], the Mills-Dornhorst equation (which includes but does not solve for a random (exponential) consumption rate constant) [4, 5], the widely used multiple hit model (based on a unique consumption mechanism for which

Correspondence: tstrom@uthsc.edu
[1]Department of Pathology and Laboratory Medicine, Memphis Veterans Administration Medical Center, 1030 Jefferson Ave, Memphis, TN 38104, USA
[2]Department of Pathology and Laboratory Medicine, University of Tennessee Health Sciences Center, Memphis, TN, USA

there is little experimental support) [6, 7], and combined use of the latter two approaches [8, 9].

None of these methods allow concurrent modeling of the random (hemostatic and phagocyte-mediated) and lifespan-dependent processes known to result in most in vivo platelet consumption. Numerical analysis models have been designed for that purpose, and their utility for the analysis of murine platelet consumption data has been demonstrated [10, 11].

It is not clear, however, whether these methods can be adapted to evaluate existing clinical data, since the latter in all cases involves tracking of radiolabeled platelets and includes contributions from uptake of the radioisotope by other, longer-lived cell types. It is also unclear how to translate the resultant kinetic parameter values into useful conclusions about how individual patients became thrombocytopenic. Here we have modified a previously described numerical model [10] to successfully analyze and interpret published data from a series of patients with immune thrombocytopenic purpura (ITP) [12].

Methods

Patients

Entry criteria for the ITP patients have been described previously [12]. The study, including informed consent procedures, was performed according to the principles outlined in the Declaration of Helsinki of 1975. Briefly, ^{111}Indium-labeled autologous platelet consumption data from 41 consecutive adult patients with prednisone non-responsive primary ITP was reviewed. The data was obtained either (A) at the time of diagnosis, or (B) after failure to sustain a platelet count response to prednisone treatment. Diagnostic criteria for all patients included exclusion of other malignant, metabolic, or pharmacologic causes, as well as causes of "secondary" ITP such as hepatitis C virus (HCV) infection. For those in group (A), rapid consumption of autologous ^{111}Indium-labeled platelets (interpreted via the multiple hit model [6]) was an additional diagnostic criterion. For those in group (B), demonstration of antiplatelet antibodies on the platelet surface via indirect immunofluorescence [13] was used for this purpose.

All of the patients in this study underwent splenectomy after failing to respond adequately to prednisone treatment. Patients were deemed to have had a complete response to splenectomy if their platelet count persistently exceeded 100×10^9/L thereafter, with no significant bleeding episodes. They were considered "non-responders" if their subsequent platelet count did not exceed either 30×10^9/L, or twice their baseline count, or if they had persistent significant bleeding episodes.

Platelet kinetics studies

These have been described in detail previously [12]. Briefly, platelet rich plasma was prepared by differential centrifugation, and platelets prepared by a subsequent high speed centrifugation were labeled with ^{111}Indium oxine by standard methods. Peripheral blood specimens obtained at 30 min after injection were considered "baseline" measurements (for patient 30, a 1.5 h time point was used), and all subsequent measurements were normalized to these for each patient. Equilibration with a pool of splenic platelets is thought to be complete well within this initial time frame [14]. All post-injection specimens for each patient were evaluated in a gamma counter at the same time to eliminate decay-related effects on recovery.

Numerical analysis

Data analysis was performed on desktop computers using Microsoft Excel. Baseline (initial) parameter ranges searched were RD 0–19 (resolution 1 %) %/h, LS 0–15.2 % (resolution 0.8 %), and SD 20–267 h (resolution 13 h). LL and RD ranges and resolutions were then empirically optimized to the values shown in Table 1. The equilibration metric was calculated as the net platelet count produced by the model at the midpoint of the equilibration phase divided by the net platelet count at the end of the equilibration phase, as described previously [10]. All searches achieved an equilibration metric value of > 0.997 (1000 interval equilibration phase, 0.5 h per interval). Searches of resampled data sets were performed over the same parameter ranges shown in Table 1. For cases in which all resampled data sets yielded the same parameter values as the complete data set at resolution "R", the upper limit of the standard deviation was estimated by the value obtained had one resampled data set yielded a parameter value one "R" range removed from that of the complete data set.

Results and discussion

Modeling in vivo platelet turnover

The numerical model used here [10] posits that an in vivo platelet population can be visualized in a spreadsheet as a series of small platelet cohort concentrations. The cohorts are assumed to be produced at a constant rate (PR, K/ul/h) in short sequential time periods, and individually consumed, by both random and lifespan-dependent processes, at the end of each such time period. The consumption curve for individual cohorts is determined by a random destruction rate constant (RD, %/h), by the lognormally distributed cohort lifespan (LS, hr), and by the standard deviation of ln LS (SD). Population platelet consumption curves are generated by summing the cohort values at sequential time points. Optimal theoretical consumption curves generated by a

Table 1 Patient characteristics, search parameter ranges, and optimal parameter values

Patient characteristics		Search parameter ranges			Optimal parameter values and residuals (SS/n)								
Patient	Platelets (x 10e9/L)	n (data points)	RD (%/h)	LL (%)	RD (%/h)	CV	LS (hr)	CV	LL (%)	CV	SD (of ln LS)	PR (K/ul/h)	SS/n
1	30	6	0–4.75	0–15.2	2.5	0.08	189	0.39	6.4	0.44	0.2	0.77	0.43
2	119	9	0–4.75	0–15.2	0.75	0.39	228	0.2	12.8	0.3	0.2	0.89	6..92
3	165	9	0–4.75	0–15.2	2	0.15	176	0.2	8.8	0.11	0.3	3.55	1.81
4	24	9	4.5–9.25	0–15.2	6.75	0.13	267	na*	4.8	0.31	0.2	1.62	8.26
5	80	9	3.5–8.25	0–15.2	5.5	0.06	215	na*	4.8	0.23	0.2	4.4	2.61
7	41	9	1.0–5.75	0–15.2	3.5	0.06	176	0.51	6.4	< 0.13**	0.1	1.44	12
8	58	8	0–4.75	15.2–30.4	2	0.43	202	0.36	23.2	0.44	0.1	1.64	42.5
11	10	5	9.5–14.75	0–15.2	12.5	0.02	267	na*	7.2	1.81	0.2	1.25	19.3
13	44	6	0–4.75	0–15.2	1.5	0.28	189	0.39	9.6	0.63	0.1	0.71	15.8
14	17	5	9.5–15.25	0–15.2	12.25	0.11	72	2.94	0	(sd < 0.06**)	0.3	2.08	7.02
17	8	9	0–4.75	0–15.2	1.75	0.2	215	0.56	10.4	1.05	0.1	0.14	36.3
18	88	7	0–4.75	0–15.2	2	0.2	150	0.77	8	0.34	0.2	1.92	3.3
20	45	9	2.5–7.25	0–15.2	5.25	0.11	228	0.4	6.4	0.42	0.2	2.36	22.1
21	143	9	0–4.75	8.8–24.0	0	(sd < 0.22**)	124	< 0.12**	11.2	0.16	0.2	1.34	5.82
22	85	8	0–4.75	0–15.2	1.25	0.32	111	0.14	5.6	0.43	0.3	1.61	1.49
23	119	9	0–4.75	15.2–30.4	0	(sd = 0.22)	124	0.09	22.4	0.07	0.3	1.2	4.03
24	20	6	0–4.75	0–15.2	2.5	0.8	33	0.66	1.6	0.42	0.3	1.04	21.4
25	39	9	2.0–6.75	0–15.2	4.5	0.09	228	0.75	4.8	0.2	0.2	1.76	8.2
27	2	9	5.5–10.25	0–15.2	8.25	0.06	176	0.73	11.2	0.18	0.1	0.17	4.77
28	22	9	0–4.75	0–15.2	2.25	0.2	254	0.35	13.6	0.25	0.1	0.5	24.4
29	34	9	2.0–6.75	0–15.2	4.5	0.23	189	0.85	6.4	0.4	0.1	1.53	18.1
30	13	6	0–4.75	0–15.2	1.75	0.24	137	0.25	6.4	1.05	0.2	0.26	6.28
32	36	5	3.0–7.75	0–15.2	7.25	0.04	72	0.53	2.4	0.27	0.1	2.63	0.38
33	238	7	0–4.75	13.6–28.8	0.25	2.56	163	0.47	20.8	0.39	0.2	2.33	10.2
34	77	6	2.0–6.75	16.8–32.0	4.5	0.27	124	0.35	24	0.23	0.1	3.49	5.51
35	37	9	0.5–5.25	0–15.2	3	0.48	137	1.02	5.6	0.36	0.3	1.17	13.4
36	32	6	4.5–9.25	0–15.2	5.75	0.15	111	0.58	6.4	0.95	0.2	1.85	5.88
37	102	6	0–4.75	11.2–26.4	3	0.58	228	0.31	17.6	0.43	0.1	3.07	49.5
38	170	7	0–4.75	17.6–32.8	0.25	1.2	150	0.07	24.8	0.05	0.1	1.45	2.81
39	21	6	3.0–7.75	0–15.2	5.25	0.35	111	1.27	12.8	0.39	0.2	1.12	27.3
40	43	6	2.5–7.25	0–15.2	5	0.35	124	na*	14.4	0.41	0.2	2.16	15.8
Normalized	191	23	0.05–1.0	na	0.5		140		na		0.2	2.12	57.3

Platelet counts were obtained at the time of the study. Patients 1,2, and 3 showed a major subsequent response to splenectomy (see text). Resolution is equal to 5 % of the search ranges shown. The *"normalized"* data set is pooled data from the three patients (3, 33, and 38) whose platelet counts transiently exceeded 150 K/ul in response to prednisone. CV values were obtained by "jackknife" resampling (see text). "na*" denotes cases for which one or more of the resampled or complete data sets yielded LS values at the high end of the search range. Values marked by ** were for cases in which all of the resampled data sets yielded the same optimal parameter value (see Methods)

large range of possible parameter values are identified via quantitative comparison to each data set (summed squared residual values, or SS).

For the 41 patient studies analyzed here, each patient's platelet consumption data was normalized to the first (baseline) measurement of circulating ^{111}In. Visual inspection of the data strongly suggests that many of the labeled platelet preparations contained long lived species, as others have described in similar studies [15, 16]. This is evident in the plateau phase seen at late times in the consumption data (for example, patients 35 and 27, Fig. 4). To take this into account, we evaluated a fourth parameter: the fraction of the labeled cells/platelets consisting of long lived (species (LL, %). This parameter simply "shrinks" the scope of the analysis to the consumption of platelets from 100 % of the time zero value to an optimizable minimum percentage

(LL). For modeling purposes, lifespans of these long lived species are assumed to be infinite.

Optimal parameter value search process

Optimal parameter value searches were performed as shown schematically in Fig. 1. For a given data set, SS values are determined for each possible set of parameter values in a four-dimensional parameter space defined by RD, LS, SD, and LL. The core component of the search is an evaluation of SS for each point in a 20 × 20 plane of possible LS and LL values at fixed values of RD and SS. The resultant minimum "planar" SS values are visually identifiable (see examples in Fig. 2). This process is repeated over a range of 20 RD values, yielding in most cases single "volume" SS minima as shown in Fig. 3a. Finally, the entire process is repeated at a series of SD values, and the resultant volume minima are compared in order to identify a "global" minimum SS value and its associated parameter values. Distinguishable alternative volume minima showing SS values greater than those of the global minima were also seen in some data sets (see below). Searches were performed for only three SD values, as this generated a plausible range of distribution widths for the resultant lifespan-dependent consumption rates (see examples in Fig. 3b) while significantly reducing computation time. Examples of the consumption curves generated by the optimal parameter values are shown in Fig. 4.

Data quality evaluation and optimal parameter value search results

This process is outlined in Fig. 5. Of the 41 originally reported ITP patient data sets, one was excluded due to lack of initial time point data. One patient demonstrated an initial platelet clearance rate of 46 % in the first 1.5 h of the study (>4 standard deviations faster than the mean). Because this value suggests the type of platelet activation during labeling/processing that we have on occasion seen in murine platelet clearance studies (TS, unpublished), this data was also excluded. For the remainder, quality of parameter value optimization was evaluated in terms of the ratio of SS to n (the number of data points per patient data set), where n ranged from 5 to 9 (Table 1). One case (patient 31) with an SS/n value of 143 (over four standard deviations from the mean value of 18.5) was then excluded. No other SS/n values fell beyond two sd from the mean.

A single "global" minimum SS value, with its associated (optimal) parameter values, was identified in 24 of the 39 evaluable data sets. The optimal consumption curves show a large amount of inter-patient variation, as the examples in Fig. 4a demonstrate. Of those showing more than one minimum, convincing global minima were identified in four data sets on the basis of goodness-of-fit. Specifically, the global minima in these cases showed SS values which were less than 50 % of those defining the alternative (local) minima. Three data sets showed global minima for which comparison of absolute vs. squared residuals provided additional support for their significance (see Additional file 1). Seven data sets, however, showed local minima that could not be distinguished from the global minima on these bases. In sum, we were able to identify convincing global minima in 31 of the 39 evaluable data sets (79 %) shown in Table 1.

Data quality was further evaluated by performing "jackknife" resampling studies on each of the patient data sets in Table 1 [17]. Optimal parameter values were obtained for each of the n subsets for each data set via the same process

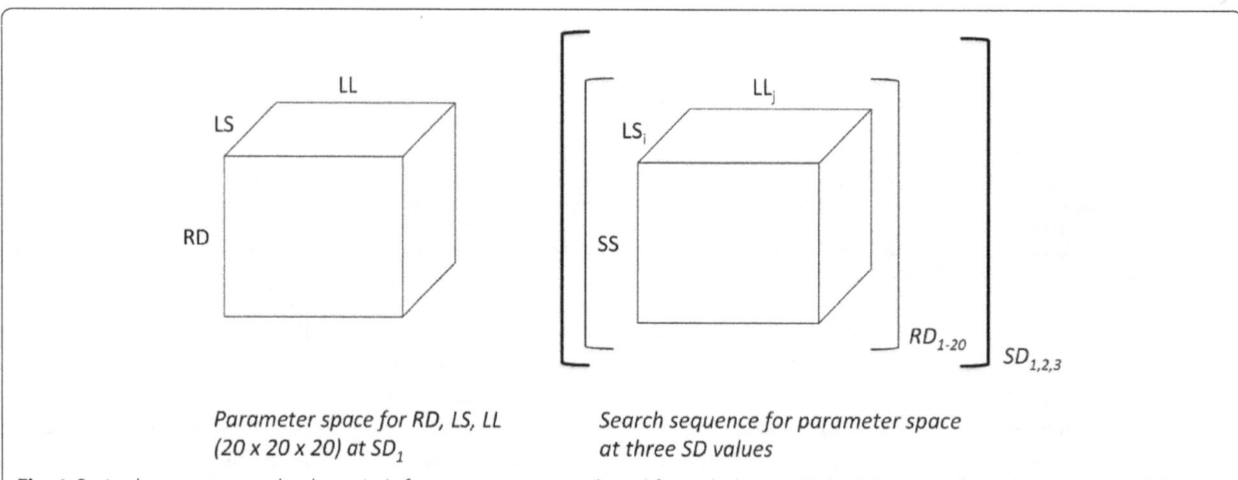

Fig. 1 Optimal parameter search schematic. Left: parameter space evaluated for each data set. Right: Schematic of search sequence used. For each data set, SS values were calculated for each point in each RD-defined plane in parameter space. Minimal SS values were identified for each plane; each plane was evaluated at 20 RD values; and each RD value was evaluated at 3 SD values

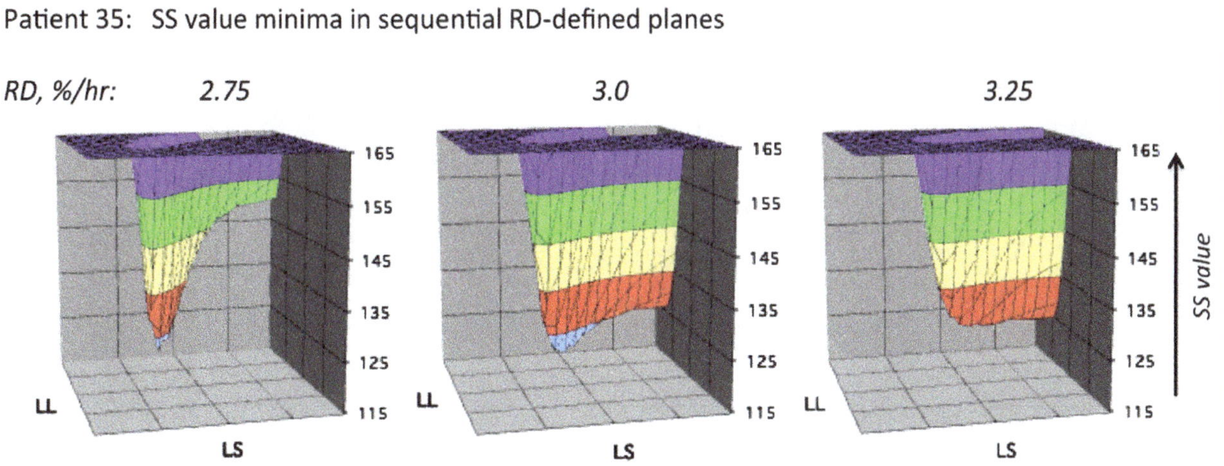

Fig. 2 Identifying optimal parameter values. The graphs demonstrate three 'planar' SS value minima, of which the minimum in the plane defined by RD = 3.0 %/h is the 'volume' minimum at this SD value (0.3). The parameter values associated with this SS minimum yield the consumption curve for this patient shown in Fig. 4. Horizontal axis scales are as follows: For LL, 0 to 15.2 %, resolution 0.8 %. For LS, 20 to 267 h, resolution 13 h. See Table 1 for additional data

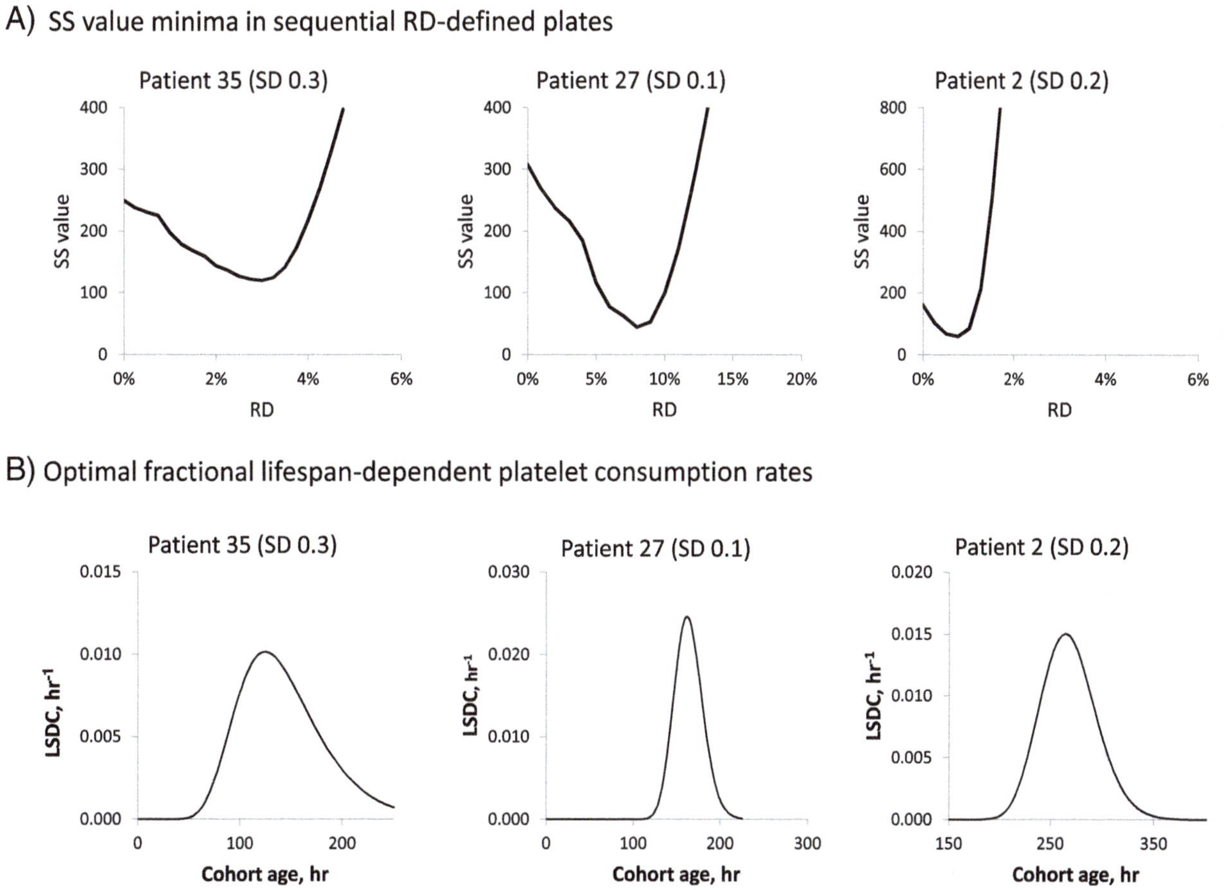

Fig. 3 Optimal parameter value searches and lifespan distributions. Top: The examples shown yielded optima in three different SD-defined parameter spaces. The low points on the SS value curves define the optimal parameter value sets. Resolution is 0.25 %/h (patients 35, 2), 1 %/h (patient 27). Bottom: the optimal fractional lifespan dependent consumption rate (LSDC) distributions for these optima are shown. For example, the optimal parameter values for patient 35 demonstrate the distribution of lifespan-dependent consumption rates per cohort (peaking at 1 %/h) shown at left. Resolution is 0.5 hr

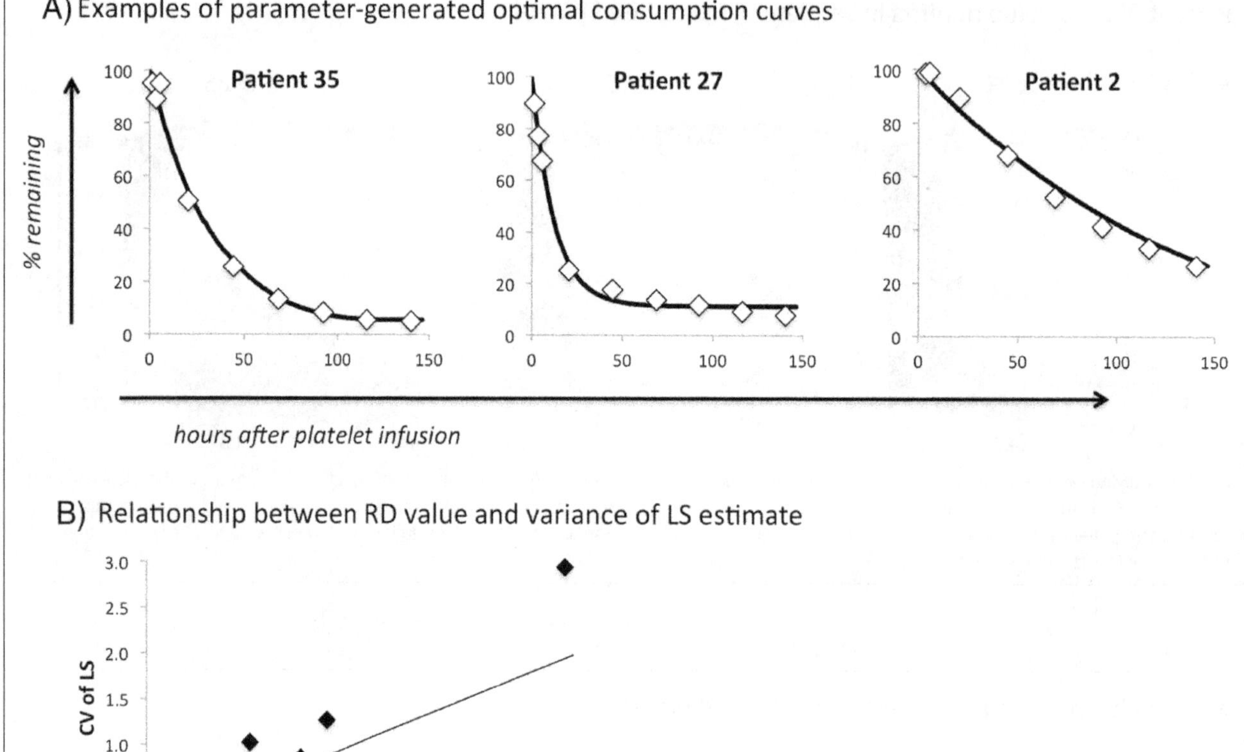

Fig. 4 Modeled consumption curves, LS variance. **a** Examples of parameter-generated optimal modeled consumption curves. The data points shown for each patient were used to infer optimal parameter values (RD, LS, SD, and LL; Table 1) predictive of the consumption curves shown. **b** Relationship between RD value and variance of LS. Values are from Table 1

used to analyze each complete data set (at the SD value of the complete data set's global minimum). We found CV values for calculated RD and LL parameters to be under 0.5 for over 75 % of these cases (Table 1). Quantification of platelet lifespan was more difficult, with only 52 % of our cases showing CV values for the LS parameter of under 0.5. That is expected, however, because LS value estimates showed a larger variance in cases where random destruction predominated (Fig. 4b).

Predicting the effects of reduced platelet production and increased random destruction

As a guide to interpreting the parameter values in Table 1, we used the model to predict how a normal platelet population's consumption parameter values might shift in response to A) impaired production, B) increased consumption, or C) increased consumption in association with a homeostatic increase in platelet production. Our assumptions were:

i) The optimal parameter values (RD_0, LS_0, and SD_0) and the associated platelet production rate (PR_0) obtained for the three patients in the study whose platelet counts transiently normalized in response to prednisone (patients 3, 33, and 38, Table 1) are representative of normal.
ii) RD is comprised of two component processes: Hemostatic RD (HRD) and non-hemostatic RD (NHRD) (i.e. RD = HRD + NHRD). Substantial hepatic NHRD is a well characterized phenomenon [18].
iii) The absolute HRD value at a normal platelet count ($aHRD_0$) makes up a given normal fraction ("f") of absolute RD (i.e. $aHRD_0/RD_0 = f$). We do not know the normal value of f.
iv) $aHRD_0$ is maintained, as platelet count declines, via an increase in HRD and a resultant increase in RD, as suggested by earlier studies of platelet turnover [8].

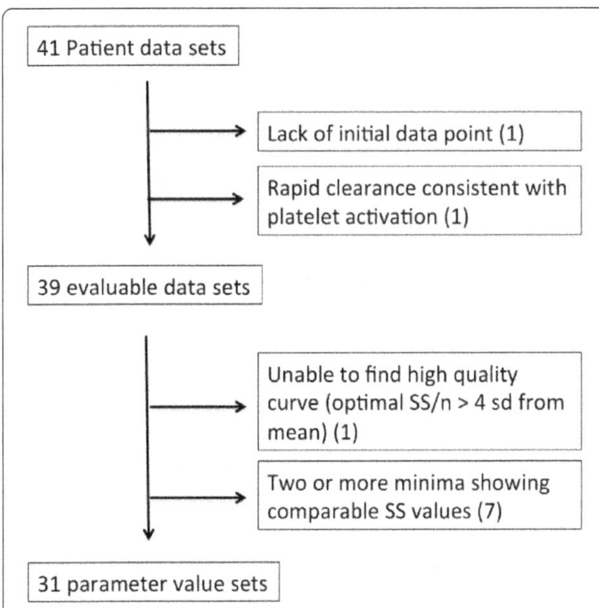

Fig. 5 Data quality evaluation. Schematic showing criteria used to remove non-evaluable data sets from evaluation. The first data point obtained for the patient lacking an initial data point was obtained at 6 h after infusion of labeled platelets

v) LS is not affected by reduced platelet production. Studies of the genetic basis of platelet lifespan support this assumption [3].

The effect of reduced platelet production (PR) on RD and platelet count was modeled as shown in Fig. 6. The process begins (step A) with the optimal (baseline) parameter values for pooled data from the three patients who transiently normalized their platelet counts (Table 1), using an initial "f" value of 1.0. From this set, a "target" reduced platelet production rate (PR_1) is generated, corresponding to 90 % of PR_0. Using that value, the model generates the expected (reduced) aHRD value ($aHRD_1$). We then (step B) incrementally increase HRD until the model generated value of aHRD ($aHRD_i$) = $aHRD_0$. The associated RD_i value (=HRD_i + $NHRD_0$) and platelet count values are those predicted to occur at PR_1. Finally (step C), we repeat steps A and B with a series of reduced platelet production rates (PR_i). This generates predicted HRD and platelet count values for each PR_i value. We then repeated this analysis at f values of 0.5 and 0.2.

We note that for our baseline parameter values, aRD_0 (RD × platelet count) is equal to 45 % of PR_0. We make no quantitative predictions for the effect of reducing PR

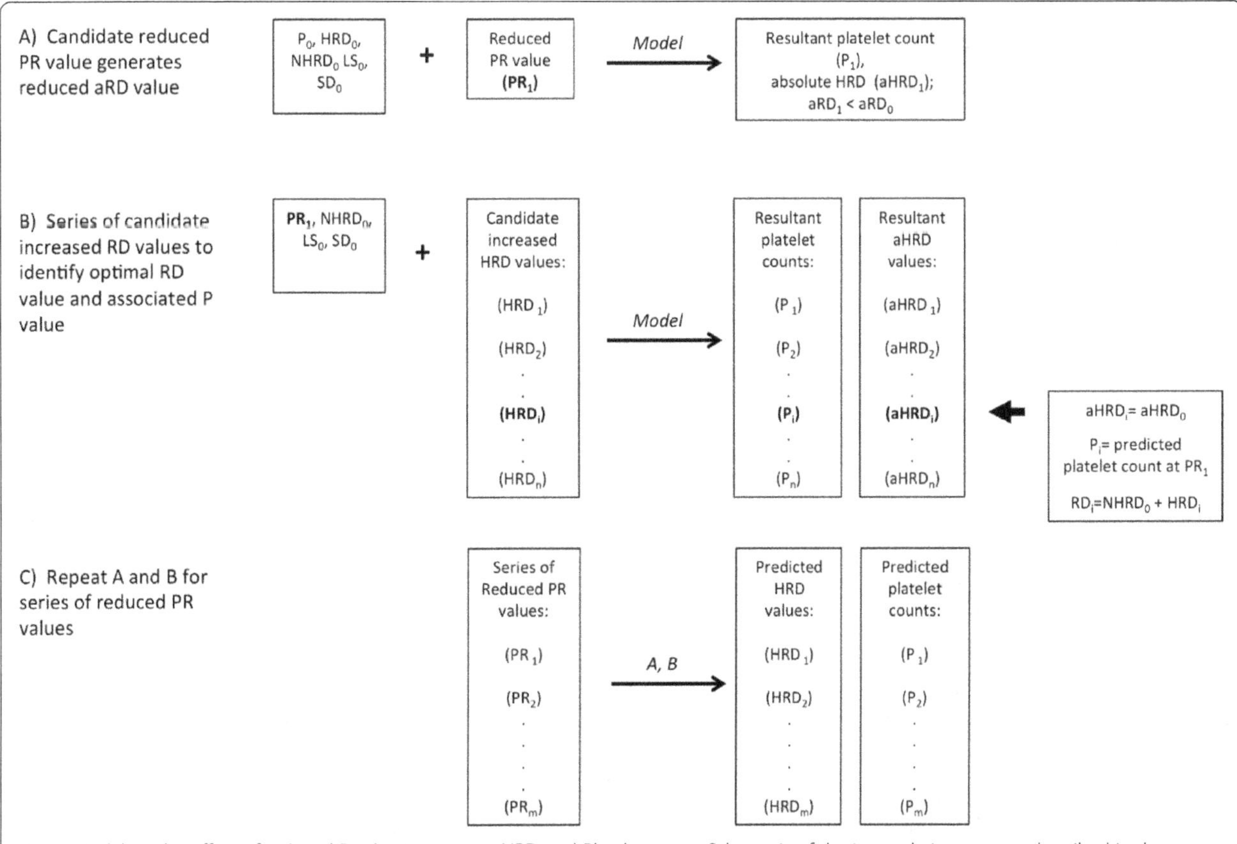

Fig. 6 Modeling the effect of reduced Production rate on HRD and Platelet count. Schematic of the interpolation process described in the text

below aRD_0 because the assumptions underlying the current numerical analysis model may not hold in that case. This is because the number of hemostatic targets is expected to increase below platelet counts at which hemostasis begins to be impaired. That in turn would invalidate the assumption of a constant absolute HRD rate, which is one of the bases for our iterative predictive method (Fig. 5). A model incorporating a dynamic hemostatic target population will be needed to predict platelet consumption rates in these circumstances.

To model the effect of increased random platelet consumption (RD), we generated a series of incrementally reduced target platelet counts (P_i)(range: 90 % to 10 % of baseline), and to achieve each we incrementally increased RD from its baseline value until the model generated value of P (P_m) was equal to P_i. To model the concurrent effects of increased RD and homeostatically increased PR, we used the same series of target platelet counts (P_i), and for each we increased PR in a manner proportional to the reduction in platelet count (to a maximum of twice the baseline PR value, a conservative theoretical starting point) before, again, empirically identifying RD_i.

The results of these three modeling approaches are plotted with the values obtained for the patients in Fig. 7.

Optimal patient parameter values in comparison to modeled values

Surprisingly, only four patients in the study showed a platelet production rate that is even modestly increased (>50 %) in comparison to the presumed normals (Fig. 7c). The latter showed a mean platelet production rate (2.12 K/ul/h) comparable to the 1.7 K/ul/h rate estimated for normals in a previous study [8]. The finding of predominantly low to normal production rates in the thrombocytopenic cases (Fig. 7a) is corroborated by the distribution of random destruction rates (Fig. 7b), where

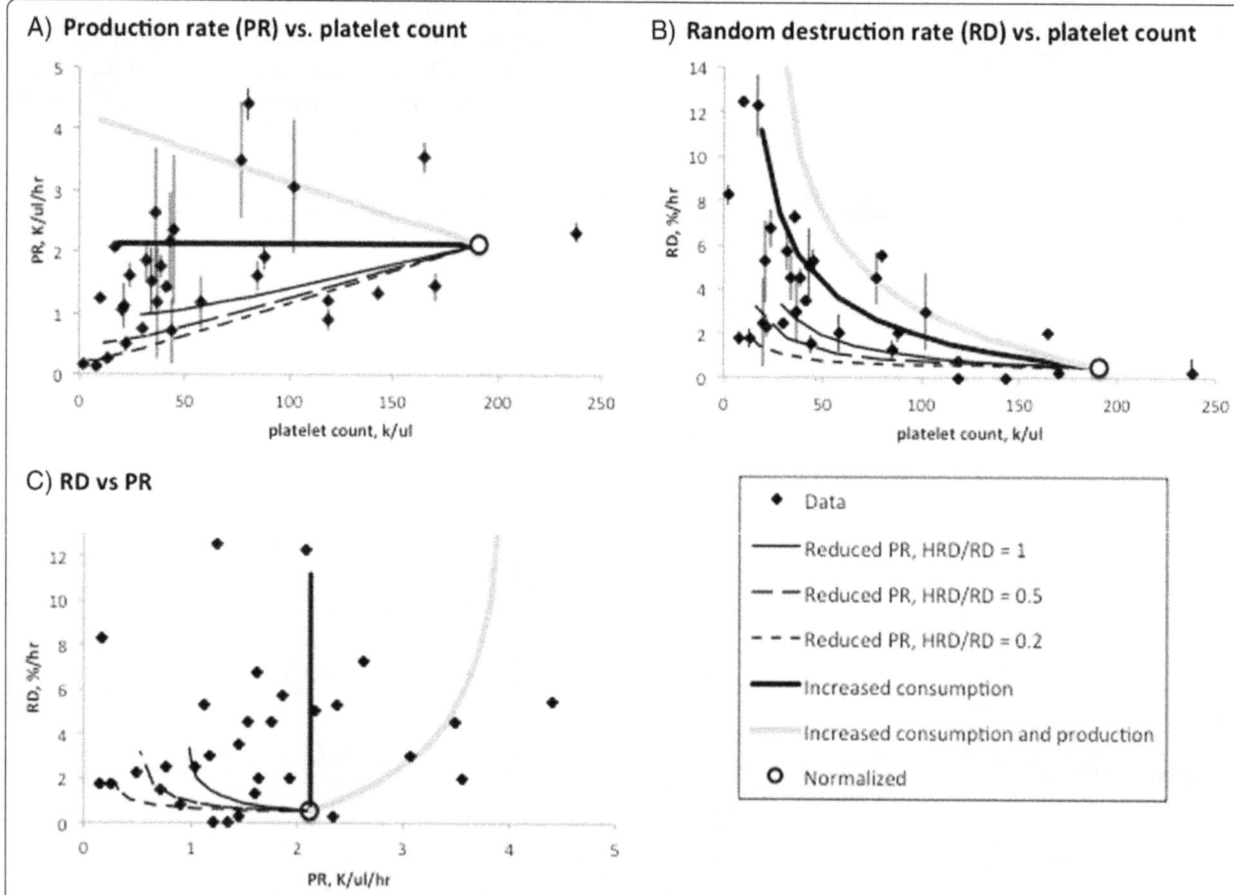

Fig. 7 Platelet production and consumption, observed and predicted parameter values. Optimal RD and PR values from Table 1 are plotted for each of the patients in the study. Projected values for thrombocytopenias due to reduced production (at three values of HRD/RD), increased consumption with no homeostatic increase in production, and increased consumption with a compensatory increase in production rate, were interpolated as described in the text. **a** Population turnover rate, which at equilibrium equals platelet production rate, vs. platelet count. **b** Random destruction rate (RD) vs. platelet count. **c** RD and PR values from **a** and **b**. Error bars are standard deviations arrived at via jacknife resampling (see text)

rates consistent with no increase in platelet production are seen for, again, all but a handful of the patients. A surprisingly large number of cases (at least 12 of 31) fall near the RD rates predicted to result solely from impaired platelet production. The predicted rates vary significantly, however, as a function of $aHRD_0/RD_0$ ('f').

Because we don't know the normal value of 'f', our ability to predict the increase in RD at low platelet counts is limited. Future studies in patients with thrombocytopenias due to impaired platelet production could resolve that problem.

Modeling of immature platelet fraction values

An ability to take up fluorescent marker dyes such as thiazole orange (a marker of "reticulated platelets", RP) or the proprietary dyes used in Sysmex hematology analyzers (marking the "immature platelet fraction", IPF) is thought to be characteristic of those platelets which have recently been released into the bloodstream. The age threshold (T) at which "young' platelets stop taking up these marker dyes is not known. Because the numerical analysis model generates a platelet age distribution for any given set of parameter values, it can be used both to estimate T and to predict the effect of altered production and consumption rates on the fraction of platelets of age less than T (i.e. the IPF).

Specifically, the normal range for the IPF is approximately 4.5 % (each clinical laboratory typically establishes its own range; this is the value in use at the Memphis VA Medical Center). Per the age distribution predicted by the model for our normalized controls (Fig. 8a), the youngest 4.5 % of platelets corresponds to those aged less than 4 h (i.e. T = 4 h). Application of that cutoff to the age distributions generated during modeling of the effects of altered production and/or consumption (Fig. 7), generates the predicted IPF and absolute IPF (aIPF) for thrombocytopenias induced by those mechanisms, as shown in Fig. 8b.

We note that this analysis depends on the assumption that *all* nascent platelets below a given age (T) take up the fluorescent markers used in the RP and IPF assays. Our measurements of mass turnover for mature and reticulated murine platelets suggest that this may not be the case [19].

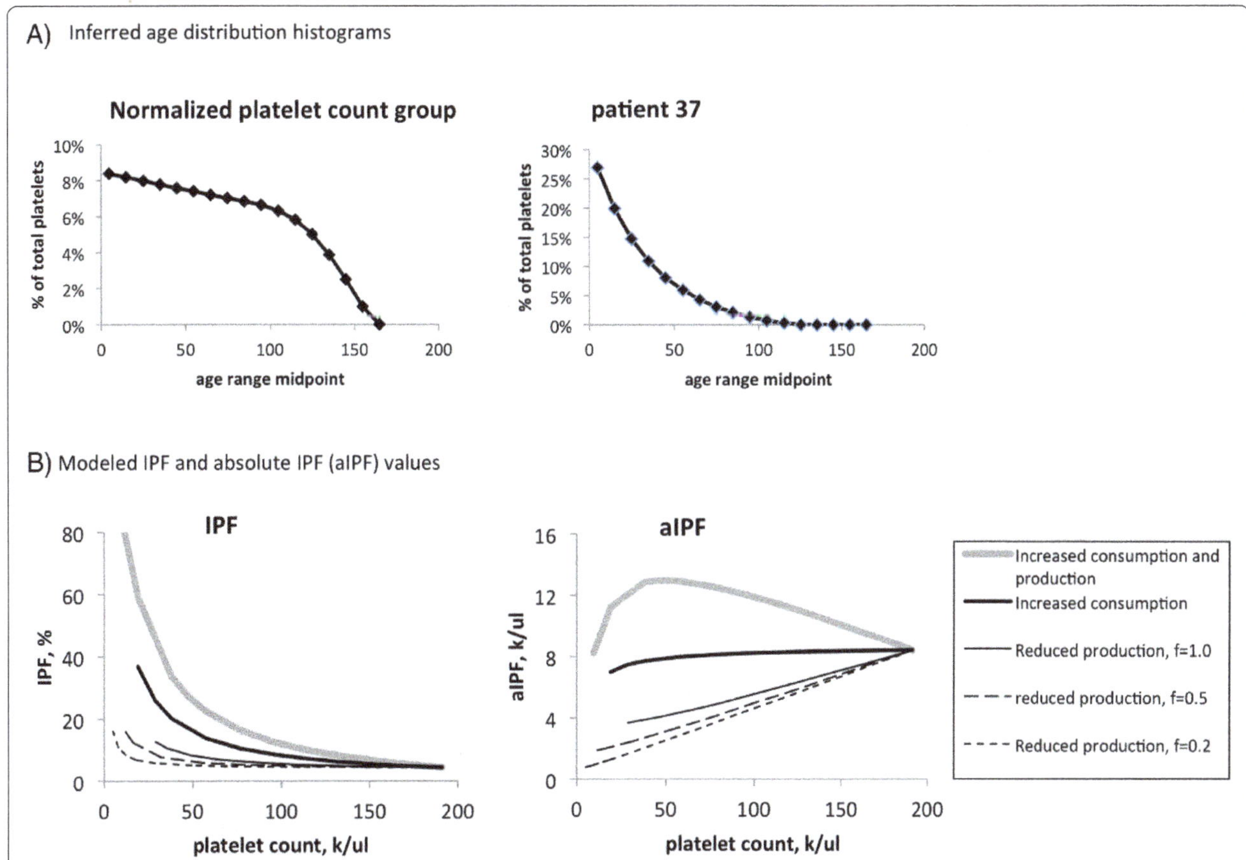

Fig. 8 Age distribution histograms and IPF modeling. **a** Histograms were generated from the optimal kinetic parameter values shown in Table 1, using bin sizes of 10 h. **b** Projected IPF and absolute IPF (aIPF) were generated from the parameter values for the normalized platelet count group (Table 1), as described in the text

Conclusions

Here we have shown the feasibility of quantifying platelet consumption and production rate parameters via numerical analysis of clinical autologous ^{111}In-labeled platelet consumption data. Although in some cases more than one set of rate parameters yields a consumption curve that closely fits the in vivo platelet consumption data, we were able to identify a single "global" optimum parameter set for 79 % of the evaluable data sets. We have shown that the technical challenges associated with quantifying the variable amount of long-lived labeled cells in these studies are tractable. It would however be preferable to avoid the need for such calculations via the use of fluorescently labeled, rather than radiolabeled, platelets in this type of study.

Only a small fraction of the prednisone-refractory ITP patients in this study (4 of 39 evaluable patients) showed evidence of a compensatory increase in platelet production rate. Platelet production rates below those of the presumed normals were frequent, and for several patients a thrombocytopenia due solely to impaired platelet production could not be ruled out. More data from normal controls would be needed to confirm these conclusions, as would studies aimed at quantifying the normal (absolute) rate of random hemostatic platelet consumption. Also, it remains possible that a strong homeostatic increase in platelet production rate is characteristic of those ITP patients who demonstrate a durable response to prednisone. If they can be correlated with other types of study (such as evaluation of the immunologic effects on megakaryocyte function that others have reported [20]) [21]), our findings would be consistent with the normal serum thrombopoietin (TPO) levels seen in most ITP patients [22–25]. That observation remains difficult to explain.

Finally, our modeling of the impact of changes in platelet production and consumption rates on the platelet age distribution suggest that there is no simple correlation between the aIPF and the etiology of a given thrombocytopenia. Despite the fact that the platelet count is used to calculate the aIPF, the aIPF can only be interpreted in the context of the platelet count (Fig. 8b). But if the predicted curves in Fig. 8b can be verified by comparison of IPF values to measured clinical platelet production and consumption rates in bone marrow failure patients, the IPF and platelet count could subsequently be used to infer the kinetic bases for most thrombocytopenias.

Abbreviations

RD: Random destruction (%/h); LS: Intrinsic lifespan (hr); SD: Standard deviation of ln LS; PR: Production rate (K/ul/h); AD: Age distribution; ITP: Immune thrombocytopenic purpura; CV: Coefficient of variation (stdev/mean); IPF: Immature platelet fraction (%); aIPF: Absolute immature platelet fraction (K/ul/h); LL: Long lived species (%); SS: Sum of squared residuals value; SS/n: SS value normalized to the number of data points in a given data set; RD_0, LS_0, SD_0: Optimal parameter values for the "normalized" subset of patients; HRD: Hemostatic random destruction (%/h); NHRD: Non-hemostatic random destruction (%/h); aHRD, aNHRD: Absolute values of HRD and NHRD (K/ul/h); HRD_0, RD_0: Values of HRD and RD for the "normalized" subset of patients; "f": Ratio of $aHRD_0$ to RD_0; P_i: Platelet count at rank "I" in the interpolation process (Fig. 6); RP: Reticulated platelets; T: Threshold age below which platelets are identified as "immature".

Competing interests

The numerical analysis model is disclosed in a patent application filed in the USPTO December 2012, naming the author (T.S. Strom) as inventor.

Authors' contributions

TS designed the numerical analysis model, performed the data analysis, and wrote the paper.

Acknowledgements

We thank Dr. Manel Roca (Department of Nuclear Medicine, Hospital Universitari de Bellvitge, L'Hospitalet de Llobregat, Spain) and Dr. Nuria Pujol-Moix (Platelet Pathology Unit, Hospital de la Santa Creu I Sant Pau, Universitat Autonoma de Barcelona, Spain) for sharing of clinical and laboratory data and assisting in the data analysis. Model development by TS (as previously applied to animal studies) was supported by R01AI071163 (David J. Rawlings, Principal Investigator), by NIAID 1R21AI079757-01A1 (TS), and by the Department of Veterans Affairs.

References

1. Recommended methods for radioisotope platelet survival studies: by the panel on Diagnostic Application of Radioisotopes in Hematology, International Committee for Standardization in Hematology. Blood 1977;50(6):1137–1144.
2. Lotter MG, Heyns AD, Badenhorst PN, Wessels P, Martin van Zyl J, Kotze HF, et al. Evaluation of mathematic models to assess platelet kinetics. J Nucl Med. 1986;27(7):1192–201.
3. Dowling MR, Josefsson EC, Henley KJ, Hodgkin PD, Kile BT. Platelet senescence is regulated by an internal timer, not damage inflicted by hits. Blood. 2010;116(10):1776–8.
4. Dornhorst AC. The interpretation of red cell survival curves. Blood. 1951;6(12):1284–92.
5. Mills J. The life-span of the erythrocyte. J Physiol Soc. 1946;105 (16P).
6. Murphy EA, Francis ME. The estimation of blood platelet survival. II. The multiple hit model. Thromb Diath Haemorrh. 1971;25(1):53–80.
7. Ballem PJ, Segal GM, Stratton JR, Gernsheimer T, Adamson JW, Slichter SJ. Mechanisms of thrombocytopenia in chronic autoimmune thrombocytopenic purpura. Evidence of both impaired platelet production and increased platelet clearance. J Clin Invest. 1987;80(1):33–40.
8. Hanson SR, Slichter SJ. Platelet kinetics in patients with bone marrow hypoplasia: evidence for a fixed platelet requirement. Blood. 1985;66(5):1105–9.
9. Tomer A, Hanson SR, Harker LA. Autologous platelet kinetics in patients with severe thrombocytopenia: discrimination between disorders of production and destruction. J Lab Clin Med. 1991;118(6):546–54.
10. Strom TS. A numerical analysis model for the interpretation of in vivo platelet consumption data. PLoS One. 2013;8(1), e55087.
11. Dowling MR, Josefsson EC, Henley KJ, Kile BT, Hodgkin PD. A model for studying the hemostatic consumption or destruction of platelets. PLoS One. 2013;8(3), e57783.
12. Roca M, Muniz-Diaz E, Mora J, Romero-Zayas I, Ramon O, Roig I, et al. The scintigraphic index spleen/liver at 30 minutes predicts the success of splenectomy in persistent and chronic primary immune thrombocytopenia. Am J Hematol. 2011;86(11):909–13.

13. von dem Borne AE, Helmerhorst FM, van Leeuwen EF, Pegels HG, von Riesz E, Engelfriet CP. Autoimmune thrombocytopenia: detection of platelet autoantibodies with the suspension immunofluorescence test. Br J Haematol. 1980;45(2):319–27.
14. Aster RH. Pooling of platelets in the spleen: role in the pathogenesis of "hypersplenic" thrombocytopenia. J Clin Invest. 1966;45(5):645–57.
15. AuBuchon JP, Herschel L, Roger J. Further evaluation of a new standard of efficacy for stored platelets. Transfusion. 2005;45(7):1143–50.
16. Holme S, Heaton A, Roodt J. Concurrent label method with 111In and 51Cr allows accurate evaluation of platelet viability of stored platelet concentrates. Br J Haematol. 1993;84(4):717–23.
17. Shao J, Wu CFJ. A general theory for jackknife variance estimation. The Annals of Statistics. 1989;17(3):1176–97.
18. Hoffmeister KM. The role of lectins and glycans in platelet clearance. J Thromb Haemost. 2011;9 Suppl 1:35–43.
19. Prislovsky A, Marathe B, Hosni A, Bolen AL, Nimmerjahn F, Jackson CW, et al. Rapid platelet turnover in WASP(−) mice correlates with increased ex vivo phagocytosis of opsonized WASP(−) platelets. Exp Hematol. 2008;36(5):609–23.
20. McMillan R, Wang L, Tomer A, Nichol J, Pistillo J. Suppression of in vitro megakaryocyte production by antiplatelet autoantibodies from adult patients with chronic ITP. Blood. 2004;103(4):1364–9.
21. Guo L, Yang L, Speck ER, Aslam R, Kim M, McKenzie CG, et al. Allogeneic platelet transfusions prevent murine T-cell-mediated immune thrombocytopenia. Blood. 2014;123(3):422–7.
22. Aledort LM, Hayward CP, Chen MG, Nichol JL, Bussel J. Prospective screening of 205 patients with ITP, including diagnosis, serological markers, and the relationship between platelet counts, endogenous thrombopoietin, and circulating antithrombopoietin antibodies. Am J Hematol. 2004;76(3):205–13.
23. Emmons RV, Reid DM, Cohen RL, Meng G, Young NS, Dunbar CE, et al. Human thrombopoietin levels are high when thrombocytopenia is due to megakaryocyte deficiency and low when due to increased platelet destruction. Blood. 1996;87(10):4068–71.
24. Kappers-Klunne MC, de Haan M, Struijk PC, van Vliet HH. Serum thrombopoietin levels in relation to disease status in patients with immune thrombocytopenic purpura. Br J Haematol. 2001;115(4):1004–6.
25. Makar RS, Zhukov OS, Sahud MA, Kuter DJ. Thrombopoietin levels in patients with disorders of platelet production: diagnostic potential and utility in predicting response to TPO receptor agonists. Am J Hematol. 2013;88(12):1041–4.

12

Emergency blood transfusion practices among anaemic children presenting to an urban emergency department of a tertiary hospital in Tanzania

Catherine R. Shari[1,2*], Hendry R. Sawe[1,2], Brittany L. Murray[1,2,3], Victor G. Mwafongo[1,2], Juma A. Mfinanga[1,2] and Michael S. Runyon[1,4]

Abstract

Background: Severe anaemia contributes significantly to mortality, especially in children under 5 years of age. Timely blood transfusion is known to improve outcomes. We investigated the magnitude of anaemia and emergency blood transfusion practices amongst children under 5 years presenting to the Emergency Department (ED) of Muhimbili National Hospital (MNH) in Tanzania.

Methods: This prospective observational study enrolled children under 5 years old with anaemia, over a 7-week period in August and September of 2015. Anaemia was defined as haemoglobin of <11 g/dL. Demographics, anaemia severity, indications for transfusion, receipt of blood, and door to transfusion time were abstracted from the charts using a standardized data entry form. Anaemia was categorized as severe (Hb <7 g/dL), moderate (Hb 7–9. 9 g/dL) or mild (Hb 10–10.9 g/dL).

Results: We screened 777 children, of whom 426 (55%) had haemoglobin testing. Test results were available for 388/426 (91%), 266 (69%) of whom had anaemia. Complete data were available for 257 anaemic children, including 42% (n = 108) with severe anaemia, 40% (n = 102) with moderate anaemia and 18% (n = 47) with mild anaemia. Forty-nine percent of children with anaemia (n = 125) had indications for blood transfusion, but only 23% (29/125) were transfused in the ED. Among the non-transfused, the provider did not identify anaemia in 42% (n = 40), blood was not ordered in 28% (n = 27), and blood was ordered, but not available in 30% (n = 29). The median time to transfusion was 7.8 (interquartile range: 1.9) hours. Mortality was higher for the children with severe anemia who were not transfused as compared with those with severe anaemia who were transfused (29% vs 10%, p = 0.03).

Conclusion: The burden of anaemia is high among children under 5 presenting to EMD-MNH. Less than a quarter of children with indications for transfusion receive it in the EMD, the median time to transfusion is nearly 8 h, and those not transfused have nearly a 3-fold higher mortality. Future quality improvement and research efforts should focus on eliminating barriers to timely blood transfusion.

Keywords: Anaemia, Emergency blood transfusion, Emergency medicine department, Paediatric, Tanzania

* Correspondence: catherinereuben50@yahoo.com
[1]Emergency Medicine Department Muhimbili University of Health and Allied Sciences, P.O Box 65001, Dar es Salaam, Tanzania
[2]Emergency Medicine Department, Muhimbili National Hospital, Dar Es Salaam, Tanzania
Full list of author information is available at the end of the article

Background

Anaemia is a significant contributor to mortality and morbidity globally, especially in children under 5 years old [1, 2]. It disproportionately affects children in Sub Saharan Africa [2]. In low income countries such as South East Asia and West Africa, anaemia has remained to be a significant health problem with even higher rates of mortality [3, 4]. In East Africa, anaemia is estimated to affect more than three quarters of children under 5 years [5, 6], and studies in Tanzania have shown even higher rates of anaemia [7–9].

Management of anaemia varies depending on the underlying etiology and severity, but in cases of severe and life threatening anaemia, blood transfusion has remained the most critical lifesaving intervention and is shown to improve outcomes [10, 11]. Studies have shown that blood transfusion is most beneficial when given early and that delayed transfusion leads to increased mortality [10, 12]. It has also been shown that with delay in treatment of severe anaemia, irreversible tissue damage can occur and patients may suffer morbidity that can persist for months after their initial treatment [13]. Therefore, early recognition and treatment of children with severe anaemia is vital to optimizing outcomes.

The WHO has produced guidelines for blood transfusion in severe anaemia; however, many children requiring transfusion under these guidelines do not receive blood. The availability of blood in emergencies is still a challenge in many developing countries [14]. The blood supply is not adequate to meet population demands in most of the low income countries such as Bangladesh, South East Asia, South and West Africa [3, 4, 15–18]. This lack of blood has been attributed to limited emergency and critical care services in these areas [19, 20]. In 2014, the National Blood and Transfusion Services (NBTS) in Tanzania estimated that the need for blood is about 450,000 units yearly, but only a third of that amount is collected [14]. Hence, the blood supply does not meet the population demand for blood transfusion [21]. In low income countries, adherence to WHO guidelines to transfusion is poor and most patients requiring blood do not get it in appropriate manner [12]. At Muhimbili National Hospital (MNH) in Dar es Salaam, Tanzania, emergency blood transfusion in the Emergency Department (ED) for those meeting the WHO guidelines is the expected standard of clinical practice. However, some patients who present with anaemia and indications for blood transfusion do not receive it in a timely manner. As a result, some patients die without being transfused. The emergency blood transfusion practices among anaemic children less than 5 years old presenting to the MNH-ED has not been previously studied. We aimed to assess the burden of anaemia in the children arriving at the MNH-ED, evaluate the emergency blood transfusion practices at our hospital, and report the outcomes of children with anaemia.

Methods

This was a prospective observational study of anaemic children who presented to the MNH-ED in August and September of 2015. MNH is located in Dar es Salaam, Tanzania and is the largest tertiary referral hospital and the main medical teaching hospital in the country. The MNH-ED was opened in 2010 and is the first and only 24-h/day full capacity ED in the country, attending to an average of 150 to 200 patients daily. Approximately 13% of the patients are children under the age of 5 years. The ED is staffed with seven medical doctors (registrars and residents) and 20 nurses who work under supervision of two emergency specialist and critical care nurses.

All children age 1 month to 5 years were consecutively screened for inclusion in the study. Laboratory testing was according to standard clinical care at the discretion of the treating doctor as part of standard care. Children found to be anaemic (laboratory confirmation of Hb < 11 g/dl) [22], were enrolled in the study. Signed, informed consent was obtained from the children's parent(s) or guardians. The study excluded children whose parent(s) or guardian(s) did not consent, children who were declared dead on arrival to the ED and those with incomplete or unavailable charts.

Patient screening and enrollment was performed by the principal investigator and one trained research assistant. Study data were recorded on a structured case report form. The indications for blood transfusion were as defined by WHO [22] and include:

1) Haemoglobin level less than 4 g/dl, or
2) Haemoglobin level of 4-7 g/dl with any of the following: shock, clinically detectable dehydration, impaired consciousness, respiratory acidosis revealed by deep labored breathing, heart failure, or more than 20% of red blood cells parasitized by malaria parasite.
3) Haemoglobin levels more than 4 g/dl with continuing bleeding

Our primary outcome was the proportion of anaemic children with WHO indications who received transfusion in the ED. Secondary outcomes included demographics, prevalence and severity of anaemia, variability in the indications for blood transfusion, time to blood transfusion, reasons for delays in transfusion, and in-hospital mortality. Age adjusted tachycardia was defined as heart rate > 180 beats/min in children less than 2 years and >140 beats/min in children aged 2–5 years, while age adjusted tachypnea was defined as respiratory rate > 34 breaths/min in children less than 2 years and >22 breaths/min in children 2–5 years.

Data are summarized with descriptive statistics, including the counts and percentages and medians and interquartile ranges (IQR). Categorical variables are presented as frequencies and percentages, and continuous variables are presented as medians and interquartile ranges (IQR). Ninety-five percent confidence intervals (CI) are presented where appropriate. The chi square test or Fisher's exact test were used to compare categorical variables and the Mann-Whitney U-test was used to compare continuous variables. Data were analysed using Microsoft Excel 2013 (Microsoft corporation, Redmond, WA, USA), Stata (version 13, StataCorp LP, Texas, USA), and StatsDirect (version 3.0.167, StatsDirect Ltd., Cheshire, UK).

Ethical clearance was obtained from the Research and Publications Committee of MUHAS and director of medical services of MNH.

Results

We screened 777 eligible children, representing 100% of children seen at the EMD during the study period. Of these, 426 (55%) had a haemoglobin level ordered, 388/426 (91%) had available results, and more than two thirds of all patients tested (68.6%, 95% CI: 63.7–73.1%) were found to be anaemic (Hb <11 g/dl) (Fig. 1).

Demographics and classification of anaemia

Of the 266 patients with anaemia, 257 (97%) had complete data for the primary outcome and were included in the analysis. The median age was 16 (IQR 8–31) months, 158 (61.5%) were male, and 108 (42%) had severe anaemia. There was no difference in the age or gender distribution among those children with and without transfusion indications. As expected, more children with severe anaemia had transfusion indications. Most patients (196; 76.3%) were referred from hospitals across Dar es Salaam and mainland Tanzania and those patients were more likely to have transfusion indications. (Table 1). The most common diagnoses were malaria (20.1%) and sickle cell disease (18.3%). Other diagnoses included sepsis (7.6%), pneumonia (7.3%), and malnutrition (5.4%). The most common chief complaints were fever (26%), vomiting (8.3%), cough (8.1%), general body malaise (7.6%), difficulty in breathing (6.5%), and diarrhea (5.7%).

Indications for blood transfusion and transfusion status

Overall, 125 (48.6%) children had WHO-defined indications for blood transfusion at the time of ED presentation. Of these children, 45 (36%) had Hb <4 g/dl, 76 (60.8%) had Hb between 4 g/dl and 7 g/dl with shock, and 4 (3.2%) had Hb > 4 g/dl with continuous bleeding.

Emergency physicians identified anaemia in 85 (68%) of the children with WHO-defined indications for blood transfusion, and ordered blood in 58 (68%). Blood was transfused in 29 (23.2%) of those with indications (Fig. 2).

Timing of blood processing and transfusion

The median 'door to transfusion' time (the time from arrival in the ED resuscitation room to the time transfusion started) was 468 min (IQR 410–525). The longest fraction of this time (190 min (IQR 180–280)

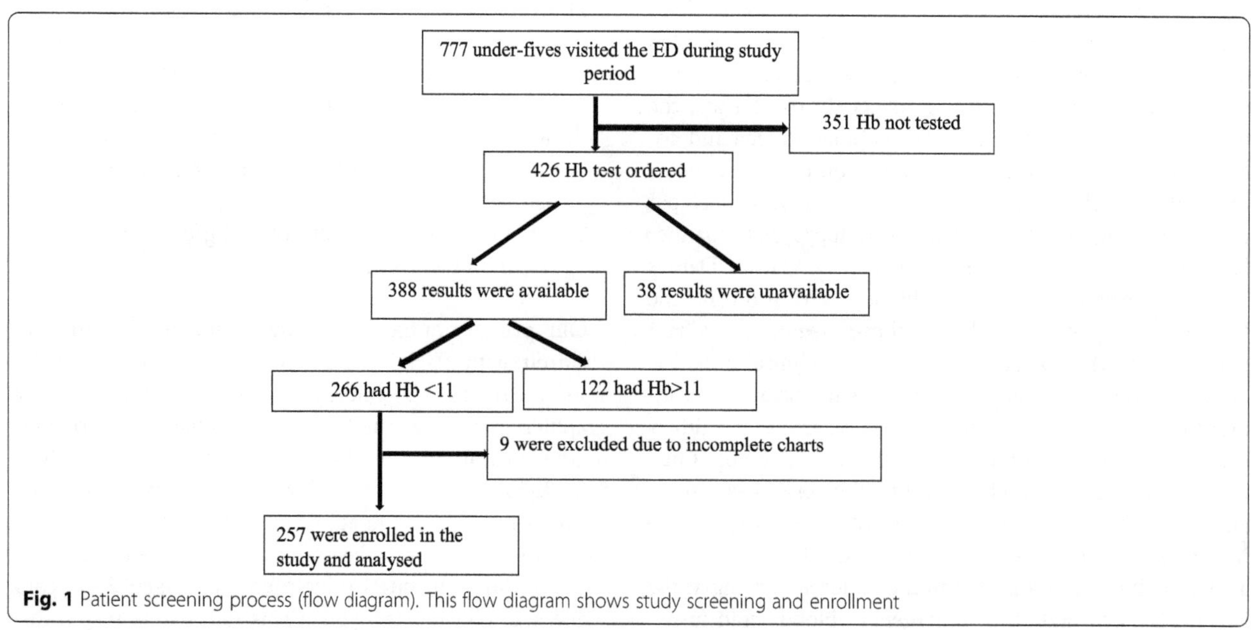

Fig. 1 Patient screening process (flow diagram). This flow diagram shows study screening and enrollment

Table 1 Demography and severity of anaemia[a]

Demographic characteristics	All (N = 257)	Indications (N = 125)	No indications (N = 132)	P-value
Gender				0.6
Male	158 (61.5%)	75 (60%)	83 (62.9%)	
Female	99 (38.5%)	50 (40%)	49 (37.1%)	
Age (months)	16 (8–31)	14 (6.5–26)	18 (9–34)	0.07
Referral				<0.0001
Patient presenting from home	61 (23.7%)	13 (10.4%)	48 (36.4%)	
Referral from another healthcare facility	196 (76.3%)	112 (89.6%)	84 (63.6%)	
Severity of anaemia				<0.0001
Mild	47 (18.3%)	0	47 (35.6%)	
Moderate	102 (39.7%)	24(19.2%)	78 (59.1%)	
Severe	108 (42.0%)	101 (80.8%)	7 (5.3%)	
Vitals				
Heart rate (beats/min)	147 (131–164)	151 (136–166)	143.5 (124–161.5)	0.02
Age-adjusted tachycardia[d]	58 (22.5%)	40 (32%)	29 (22%)	0.02
Respiratory rate (breath/min)	33 (29–38)	34 (30–49)	33 (28–36)	0.08
Age-adjusted tachypnea[b]	160 (64.3%)	59 (47.2%)	82 (62.1%)	0.01
SPO2% < 95%	23 (8.9%)	12 (9.6%)	11 (8.3%)	0.89
Temperature % < 36, > 38[c]	49 (20.2%)	29 (21.6%)	20 (15.2%)	0.21

[a]Data are summarized as counts (percentage) or median (interquartile range)
[b]Respiratory rate data were missing for 8 patients
[c]Temperature data were missing for 38 patients
[d]Age adjusted tachycardia was defined as heart rates >180 beats/min in children less than 2 years and >140 beats/min in children aged 2–5 years, while the age adjusted tachypnea was defined as respiratory rates >34 breaths/min in children less than 2 years and >22 breaths/min in children 2–5 years. (Cited from International paediatric sepsis consensus conference: definition for sepsis and organ dysfunction in paediatrics)
Table 1 shows overall patient demographics, severity of anaemia and comparison of these characteristics between those with indications for transfusion and those with no indications for transfusion

was the point from when the blood tubes for cross matching were sent to the laboratory until the patients received the transfusion, while the shortest fraction of time (30 min IQR 25–60) was from the doctor's order for crossmatch to the time that the samples was sent to the laboratory.

Anaemia recognition and plan for blood transfusion

Among the 125 patients with WHO-defined indications for blood transfusion, 96 (76.8%) did not receive transfusion while in the ED. In 40 (41.7%) of these patients, the physicians did not document the clinical features of anaemia, its severity, or blood transfusion indications. In

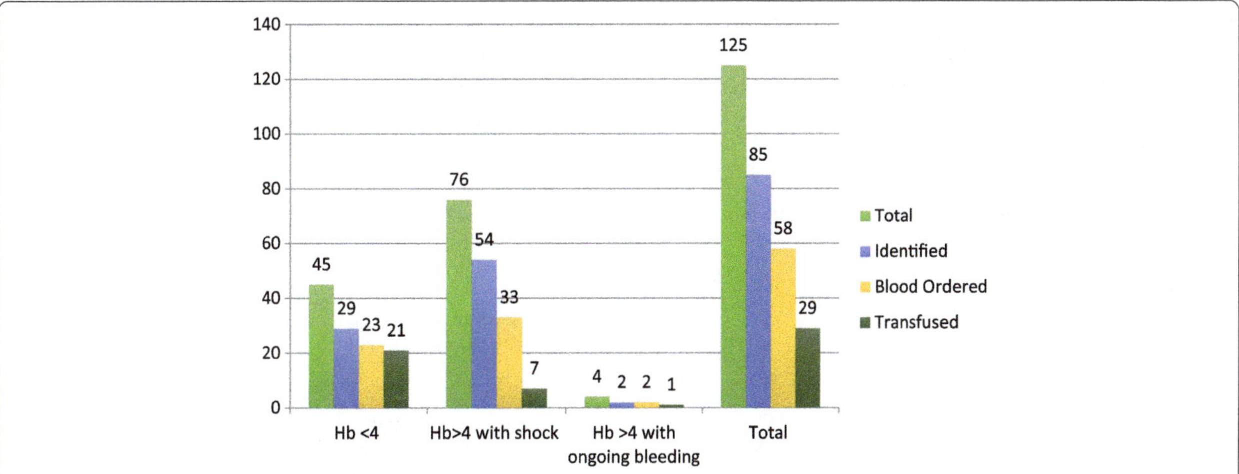

Fig. 2 Indications and transfusion status bar chart. Indicates number of children under 5 years old with indications for transfusion on the vertical axis and the horizontal axis indicates the transfusion indication categories as per WHO guidelines

27 (28.1%) of these patients anaemia was identified by the physician, but transfusion was not ordered, and in 29 (30.2%) of these patients, blood was ordered but it was unavailable.

ED outcome and patients disposition

Among the 257 children with anaemia, most (197; 76.7%) were admitted to the general pediatrics wards. Only 1.6% (4/257) were sent to the advanced paediatric care unit (APCU), 15.6% (40/257) were admitted to the pediatric surgery ward, 3.9% (10/257) were discharged to home from the ED, and 2.3% (6/257) died in the ED.

Overall patient outcomes and transfusion status

Among 241 Patients who were admitted to in-patient wards, 193 (80%) survived to discharge and 48 (20%) died while in the hospital.

Among 125 patients who had indications for blood transfusion at presentation to the ED, the overall mortality rates of those transfused and those not transfused at the ED were 10.3% and 29.2%, respectively (relative risk of 2.82, 95% CI 1.04–8.45). Table 2.

Inpatient transfusion practices

Among the 96 children with indications for blood transfusion who were not transfused in the ED, 59.4% (n = 57) did receive a blood transfusion in the wards before the time of their discharge or death.

Discussion

Our study has revealed a large burden of anaemia among children under the age of 5 years presenting to the MNH-ED. Since laboratory testing was at the discretion of the treating doctor, not all children were screened for anaemia. If we assume the unlikely scenario that anaemia was absent in all of the children who were not screened, we can conservatively estimate that at least one third (257/777) of children presenting to our ED are anaemic. We found that more than two thirds of all children tested in our ED have anaemia as compared to the estimated prevalence of anaemia globally (24.8%) [2], and that of developed countries [15, 16, 23, 24]. However, these findings were very similar to other low resource countries in South and Southeast Asia, and South and West Africa [3, 4, 16, 18]. The prevalence of anaemia in this study was lower compared to the study done in Ghana where more than a quarter of children admitted had anaemia, with as 71% of these children having severe anaemia which is higher compared to our study where children with severe anaemia comprised 42% of children with anaemia [4]. Our findings are also similar to the 2016 Tanzania Demographic and Health Survey (TDHS), which reported the prevalence of anaemia among children under 5 years-old to be 58% [25].

The proportion of anaemia found in our study is slightly lower than that previously reported among the MNH inpatient paediatric population, as documented by *Magesa* et al. who found a prevalence of 80.7% [8, 9]. Likewise, anaemia was found in 76% of children under 5 presenting to one of several hospitals in East Africa with severe infection [26]. The slightly lower rate of anemia in our cohort is likely due to the fact that we enrolled all children who underwent haemoglobin testing, regardless of their clinical condition or diagnosis. In fact, anemia was much more common in our cohort of children presenting to the ED than the 12% rate of anaemia reported in a study of 53,174 children admitted to one of 10 hospitals in Kenya [12].

The severity of anaemia in our study was striking. Although the proportion of anaemia in our study was similar to what is reported by TDHS [25], the distribution of severity of anaemia was very different. The proportion of anaemic under-fives with moderate to severe anaemia was higher (81.7%, 95% CI: 76.4–86.2%) in our population than the 32% rate of moderate or severe anaemia documented in the TDHS report [25]. This difference may reflect a different burden of disease that presents to MNH-ED. The patient population at MNH is largely referred from other hospitals, including 76.3% of our cohort, and these patients may be more likely to be anaemic and have transfusion indications than patients presenting to regional hospitals, either due to illness severity or simply because they were transferred to MNH specifically for blood transfusion due to lack of blood at the peripheral hospitals [2, 11]. The proportion of severe anaemia also raises the percentage of children meeting WHO transfusion criteria. Furthermore, the proportion of severe anaemia in our study is higher compared to

Table 2 Outcomes of anaemic under-fives with indications for BT (N = 125)

Outcome	Total n = 125 n (%) [95% CI]	Transfused in the ED n = 29 n (%) [95%CI]	Not Transfused in the ED n = 96 n (%) [95% CI]	P- value
ED mortality	6 (4.8%) (95%CI 1.05–8.55)	2 (6.9%) (95%CI −2.3-16.1)	4 (4.2%) (95% CI 0.19–8.21)	0.067
24 h mortality	19 (15.2%) (95% CI 8.91–21.49)	2 (6.9%) (95% CI −2.3-16.1)	17 (17.7%) (95% CI 10.1–25.3)	0.058
Overall mortality	31 (24.8%) (95% CI 17.23–32.37)	3 (10.3%) (95% CI −0.76-21.36)	28 (29.2%) (95% CI 20.01–38.19)	0.032

Table 2 shows the ED mortality, 24-h mortality, and overall mortality between the children with WHO indications for transfusion that received blood in the ED, and those that did not with their respective 95% confidence intervals other East African reports (12% in Kenya and 41% in Eastern Uganda) [26]. Despite the proportion of children with severe anaemia being high in our study (42%), it was lower compared to studies in Ghana where up to 71% present with severe anaemia [27]. The causes of anaemia in our study were found to be similar with a report from several Kenyan Hospitals where malaria was the leading cause of anaemia [12].

Our study showed that 48.6% of the anaemic under-fives presented at the ED with clear WHO defined indications for blood transfusion. Despite the high prevalence of anaemic under-fives with indications for transfusion in the MNH-ED, the transfusion rate was low (23.2%). This is quite low when compared to rates from EDs in the developed world [28]. We were unable to find data on transfusion rates in other ED settings in East Africa, but generally among paediatric inpatient populations in East Africa, transfusion rates have also been found to be low (20–45%), demonstrating poor adherence to WHO guidelines for transfusion [10, 26].

In our study, the low blood transfusion rate was associated with a number of different variables. The majority of patients who met transfusion criteria were not transfused because the physician either did not clearly diagnose anaemia or did not identify the indication for transfusion. This finding was in contrast to what was known in the past about physician gestalt. Although physicians in our ED have the ability to accurately diagnose anaemia based on clinical exam as reported by *Sawe* et al. [29], anaemia was not documented in many of the children in our study. There is a clear need for physicians to take time to properly examine children and look for signs of anaemia even when the primary chief complaint or referral diagnosis is not obviously related to anaemia or the need for blood transfusion. For example, in our setting some patients with complaints such as burn injuries and foreign bodies had severe anaemia with clear indications for blood transfusion. Moreover, when laboratory tests such as hemoglobin are often ordered, documentation of the results and their impact on clinical decision-making should be recorded in the physician documentation.

Physicians did not order blood transfusion in the ED for the majority of patients (67/125, 53.6%) who had indications according to the WHO guidelines. Even when transfusions were ordered in the ED, they were administered in only half of cases (29/58, 50%). This finding was similar to a study done in Kenya, where the majority of patients did not have an order for blood transfusion and 18% of those who did have an order did not receive the blood [12]. The reasons for these findings deserve further study. Possible reasons include both individual provider and system factors. For example, there may be a lack of clinical knowledge amongst providers regarding the criteria for ordering blood. Or, it could be due to the fact that blood and blood products continue to be a scarce resource at MNH and within Tanzania at large, as shown in previous NBTS reports [14]. According to the NBTS, only one third of the blood products that are needed in Tanzania each year are actually collected [14]. The scarcity of blood in Tanzania is not a novel finding. Blood has remained to be scarce in most developing countries and it significantly affect blood transfusion practices in most of these countries [4, 16, 18, 30]. Finally, some ED providers may find it inconvenient to order blood in the MNH-ED as it can increase the length of stay and contribute to overcrowding in the ED. This concern is illustrated in our study as the median time from door to transfusion is 7.8 (IQR 1.9) hours, which creates a backlog of patients in the resuscitation bay. It may have been hard for some physicians to accommodate these patients who needed to wait for blood for a very long time, especially during busy shifts and night shifts. Among those with indications for transfusion who did not receive it in the ED, only 60% were transfused after admission, further underscoring the importance of identifying and treating these children in the ED.

The median time interval to blood transfusion was very long in this study, nearly 8 h, with the blood processing at the laboratory taking the longest time interval. This may be explained by multiple possible factors including patients spending time on a queue to see a doctor, clearing registration/system issues, or in the laboratory for processing and preparation. This time interval is much longer than the guidelines from more mature healthcare systems, suggesting that uncross matched blood should ideally be available within 10 min, and group specific blood should be available within 30 min [31]. The specific cause of this delay in our department was not captured by our study methodology, but may include variables such as overcrowding in the ED, insufficient staff, a lack of blood products in the blood bank, or a lack of a systematic process to ensure availability of timely transfusion in the ED.

In this study, the overall mortality among patients with anaemia was 31/257 (12.1%, 95% CI: 8.6–16.6%), which is similar to prior reports from other locations in sub-Saharan Africa [32, 33]. The mortality rate among children who had indications for transfusion but were not transfused in the ED was almost three times higher than that of those who were transfused while in the ED (29.2% vs 10.3%, $p = 0.032$). Therefore, our study furthers the concept that early transfusion is associated with decreased mortality as found in other settings [13]. Our findings were similar to the study done by *Lackritz* et al. in Kenya among inpatient paediatric population, which showed a mortality benefit when blood was given early on the day of admission for those who presented with indications for blood transfusion as compared to those who received blood later [10]. However, the findings in our study did not take into account the other potential confounding factors that might contribute to the mortality difference.

The results from this study were disseminated internally to the practitioners at the MNH-ED and reasons for failure to identify anaemia and order indicated blood transfusions were explored. These included ED overcrowding necessitating a high patient turnover that did not allow time for physicians to wait for haemoglobin level results, impairing their ability to diagnose anaemia and make appropriate treatment decisions in a timely fashion. As a result of these findings, point of care haemoglobin testing was introduced to help physicians more rapidly diagnosis anaemia and initiate treatment. Furthermore, we provided targeted physician education on the clinical and laboratory assessment of anaemia, the WHO transfusion guidelines, and the importance of timely treatment in optimizing patients' outcomes.

Limitations

Our study limitations include that it was based at a single centre, which serves as the only full capacity ED in the country. This may limit the generalizability of our results. Another limitation is that we relied on physician documentation of anaemia and transfusion indications and this methodology may have underestimated recognition of these clinical diagnoses due to poor documentation. Despite this, our results are striking in that less than half of the patients with indications for transfusion had a transfusion order placed in the ED and only half of those for whom an order was placed were actually transfused. Finally, some paediatric patients presented to the ED during the study time period had no haemoglobin level measurements, which lead to their exclusion from the study; however, it is likely that some of those children were anaemic, resulting in an underestimation of the overall anaemia burden in our study population.

Conclusion

The burden of anaemia is high among children under 5 years-old presenting to EMD-MNH. Less than a quarter of children with indications for transfusion receive it in the EMD, mostly due to issues around low rates of anaemia diagnosis, transfusion orders, and blood availability. The median time to transfusion is nearly 8 h and among those who are not transfused in the ED have a nearly 3-fold higher mortality. Future quality improvement and research efforts should focus on larger scale studies in multiple centres aimed at eliminating barriers to timely blood transfusion.

Abbreviations

APCU: Acute Paediatric Care Unit; ED: Emergency Department; FBP: Full blood picture; Hb: Haemoglobin; MNH: Muhimbili National Hospital; MRN: Medical registration number; MUHAS: Muhimbili University of Health and Allied Sciences; NBTS: National Blood Transfusion Services; RBC: Red Blood Cell; TDHS: Tanzania Demographic and Health Surveys; US: United States of America; WHO: World Health Organization

Acknowledgements

We are deeply grateful to the Emergency Medicine Department at Muhimbili National Hospital for supporting this research, and the Ministry of Health Tanzania for providing financial support.

Funding

This study was accomplished using funds obtained from the Tanzania Ministry of Health, Community Development, Gender, Elderly and Children (MOHCDGEC) for Master of Medicine dissertation support to Dr. Catherine Reuben Shari.

Authors' contributions

CS conceived and designed the study, conducted the study, interpreted and analyzed the data, and developed the manuscript. HS provided guidance and review of the whole research, analysis, reporting and development of the manuscript. BM provided guidance and review in study design, data interpretation and analysis, assisted in development of the manuscript, and edited the manuscript for intellectual content and grammar. JM helped in shaping the ideas, methodology, material support and manuscript review. VM helped with data analysis and interpretation. MR assisted with the research idea development, data analysis and interpretation and edited the manuscript for important intellectual content and grammar. All listed authors have read and approved the manuscript for publication.

Competing interests

The authors declare that they have no competing interests.

Author details

[1]Emergency Medicine Department Muhimbili University of Health and Allied Sciences, P.O Box 65001, Dar es Salaam, Tanzania. [2]Emergency Medicine Department, Muhimbili National Hospital, Dar Es Salaam, Tanzania. [3]Division of Pediatric Emergency Medicine, Emory University School of Medicine, Emory University, Atlanta, GA, USA. [4]Department of Emergency Medicine, Carolinas Medical Center, Charlotte, NC, USA.

References

1. Chan M. Anaemia prevention and control [Internet]. WHO. 2014 [cited 2014 Dec 26]. Available from: http://www.who.int/medical_devices/initiatives/anaemia_control/en/.
2. McLean E, Cogswell M, Egli I, Wojdyla D, de Benoist B. Worldwide prevalence of anaemia, WHO vitamin and mineral nutrition information system, 1993-2005. Public Health Nutr. 2009;12(4):444–54.
3. Choudhury N. Blood transfusion in borderless South Asia. Asian J Transfus Sci. 2011;5(2):117–20.

4. Kubio C, Tierney G, Quaye T, Nabilisi JW, Ziemah C, Zagbeeb SM, et al. Blood transfusion practice in a rural hospital in northern Ghana, Damongo, west Gonja District. Transfusion (Paris). 2012;52(10):2161–6.
5. Murila FV, Macharia WM, Wafula EM. Iron deficiency anaemia in children of a peri-urban health facility. East Afr Med J. 1999;76(9):520–3.
6. Isanaka S, Spiegelman D, Aboud S, Manji KP, Msamanga GI, Willet WC, et al. Postnatal anemia and iron deficiency in HIV-infected women and the health and survival of their children. Matern Child Nutr. 2012;8(3):287–98.
7. Schellenberg D, Schellenberg JRMA, Mushi A, D de S, Mgalula L, Mbuya C, et al. The silent burden of anaemia in Tanzanian children: a community-based study. Bull World Health Organ. 2003;81(8):581–90.
8. Magesa AS, Magesa PM. Association between anaemia and infections (HIV, malaria and hookworm) among children admitted at Muhimbili National Hospital. East Afr J Public Health. 2012;9(3):96–100.
9. Magesa SA. A Profile of Acquired Causes of Childhood Anaemia in General Paediatric Wards at Muhimbili National Hospital Dar es Salaam, Tanzania [Internet] [masters]. Muhimbili University of Health and Allied Science; 2010 [cited 2016 Aug 8]. Available from: http://ihi.eprints.org/2120/.
10. Lackritz EM, Campbell CC, Ruebush TK, Hightower AW, Wakube W, Steketee RW, et al. Effect of blood transfusion on survival among children in a Kenyan hospital. Lancet. 1992;340(8818):524–8.
11. The clinical use of blood in general medicine,obstetrics, paediatrics,anaesthesia, surgery and burn [Internet]. [cited 2014 Dec 24]. Available from: http://www.who.int/bloodsafety/clinical_use/en/Manual_EN.pdf.
12. Thomas J, Ayieko P, Ogero M, Gachau S, Makone B, Nyachiro W, et al. Blood transfusion delay and outcome in county hospitals in Kenya. Am J Trop Med Hyg. 2017;96(2):511–7.
13. Phiri KS, Calis JCJ, Faragher B, Nkhoma E, Ng'oma K, Mangochi B, et al. Long term outcome of severe anaemia in Malawian children. PLoS One. 2008;3(8):e2903.
14. Tanzania national blood transfussion service policy guideline [Internet]. [cited 2014 Dec 30]. Available from: http://ihi.eprints.org/817/1/MoHSW.pdf_(46).pdf.
15. Islam MB. Blood transfusion services in Bangladesh. Asian J Transfus Sci. 2009;3(2):108–10.
16. Sharma R. South East Asia faces severe shortage of safe blood. BMJ. 2000; 320(7241):1026.
17. Lackritz EM, Ruebush TK, Zucker JR, Adungosi JE, Were JB, Campbell CC. Blood transfusion practices and blood-banking services in a Kenyan hospital. AIDS Lond Engl. 1993;7(7):995–9.
18. Salverda M, Ketharanathan N, van Dijk M, Beltchev E, Buys H, Numanoglu A, et al. A review of blood transfusions in a trauma unit for young children. SAMJ South Afr Med J. 2017;107(3):227–31.
19. Baker T, Lugazia E, Eriksen J, Mwafongo V, Irestedt L, Konrad D. Emergency and critical care services in Tanzania: a survey of ten hospitals. BMC Health Serv Res. 2013;13(1):140.
20. Reynolds TA, Mfinanga JA, Sawe HR, Runyon MS, Mwafongo V. Emergency care capacity in Africa: a clinical and educational initiative in Tanzania. J Public Health Policy. 2012;33(S1):S126–37.
21. Factsheet on Tanzania's blood Service: 2014 [Internet]. [cited 2015 Jan 1]. Available from: http://www.mamaye.org/sites/default/files/u214/TZ%20blood%20factsheet_2014_0.pdf.
22. World Health Organization. Pocket book of hospital care for children: guidelines for the management of common childhood illnesses. Second edition, 2013 edition. Geneva. Switzerland: World Health Organization; 2013. p. 412.
23. Dos Santos RF, Gonzalez ESC, de Albuquerque EC, de Arruda IKG, Diniz A da S, Figueroa JN, et al. Prevalence of anemia in under five-year-old children in a children's hospital in Recife, Brazil. Rev Bras Hematol E Hemoter. 2011; 33(2):100–4.
24. Quintero JP, Siqueira AM, Tobón A, Blair S, Moreno A, Arévalo-Herrera M, et al. Malaria-related anaemia: a Latin American perspective. Mem Inst Oswaldo Cruz. 2011;106(Suppl 1):91–104.
25. Tanzania Demographic and Health Survey 2010 [FR243] - FR243[24June2011].pdf [Internet]. [cited 2014 Dec 22]. Available from: http://dhsprogram.com/pubs/pdf/FR243/FR243%5B24June2011%5D.pdf.
26. Kiguli S, Maitland K, George EC, Olupot-Olupot P, Opoka RO, Engoru C, et al. Anaemia and blood transfusion in African children presenting to hospital with severe febrile illness. BMC Med. 2015;13:21.
27. Commey JO, Dekyem P. Childhood deaths from anaemia in Accra, Ghana. West Afr J Med. 1995;14(2):101–4.
28. Nunez TC, Dutton WD, May AK, Holcomb JB, Young PP, Cotton BA. Emergency department blood transfusion predicts early massive transfusion and early blood component requirement: RBC IN ED PREDICTS MASSIVE TRANSFUSION. Transfusion (Paris). 2010;50(9):1914–20.
29. Sawe HR, Mfinanga JA, Mwafongo V, Reynolds TA, Runyon MS. The test characteristics of physician clinical gestalt for determining the presence and severity of anaemia in patients seen at the emergency department of a tertiary referral hospital in Tanzania. Emerg Med J EMJ. 2016;33(5):338–44.
30. Vos J, Gumodoka B, van Asten HA, Berege ZA, Dolmans WM, Borgdorff MW. Changes in blood transfusion practices after the introduction of consensus guidelines in Mwanza region, Tanzania. AIDS Lond Engl. 1994;8(8):1135–40.
31. Calgary Laboratory Services. Emergency Transfusion [Internet]. [cited 2014 Dec 31]. Available from: http://www.calgarylabservices.com/lab-services-guide/transfusion-medicine/ordering-blood-components/emergency-transfusion.aspx.
32. Gumodoka B, Vos J, Kigadye FC, van Asten H, Dolmans WM, Borgdorff MW. Blood transfusion practices in Mwanza region, Tanzania. Bugando medical Centre. AIDS Lond Engl. 1993;7(3):387–92.
33. Muoneke VU, Ibekwe RC, Nebe-Agumadu HU, Ibe BC. Factors associated with mortality in under-five children with severe anemia in Ebonyi, Nigeria. Indian Pediatr. 2012;49(2):119–23.

13

KIR repertory in patients with hematopoietic diseases and healthy family members

Daniele Kazue Sugioka, Carlos Eduardo Ibaldo Gonçalves and Maria da Graça Bicalho*

Abstract

Background: Since the discovery of specific histocompatibility, literature has associated genes involved in the immune response, like the Human Leucocyte Antigen (HLA), with a better prognosis in transplantation. However, other non-HLA genes may also influence the immune process, such as the genes encoding the immunoglobulin-like receptors of natural killer cells (KIRs). The discovery that NK cell KIR receptors interact with conservative epitopes (C1, C2, Bw4) presented in HLA class I molecules that are genetically polymorphic, also observed in KIR genes, led to the investigation of the relevance of the KIR system to hematopoietic stem cell transplant. The cure of patients with leukemias and other hematological malignancies after bone marrow transplantation (BMT) has been attributed in part to the ability of the donor immune cells, present in the graft, to recognize and eliminate neoplastic cells of the patient. The cytotoxic activity of NK cells is mediated by the absence of HLA class I-specific ligands on the target cell surface to inhibitory KIR receptors (hypothesis of "missing-self").

Methods: We analyzed, by PCR typing-SSOP technique, the presence or absence of 16 KIR genes and haplotypes of 39 patients with hematopoietic disorders and 136 healthy individuals from Paraná State. The comparisons made between the patient and control group were performed using χ^2 test or Fisher exact test (bilateral *p*-value), as appropriated. Significance level was considered when *p*-value ≤ 0.05.

Results: Framework genes *KIR3DL3, KIR3DP1, KIR2DL4* and *KIR3DL2* were positive in all samples. The comparison between KIR repertoire of patients and healthy individuals revealed significant differences ($p < 0.05$) in inhibitors genes *KIR2DL2* ($p = 0.0005$) and *KIR2DL5* ($p = 0.0067$) and activating genes *KIR2DS1* ($p = 0.0013$), *KIR2DS2* ($p = 0.0038$), *KIR2DS3* ($p = 0.0153$) that are more frequent in controls than in patients. The *KIR2DS3* was significantly more frequent ($p = 0.0031$) in patients with acute myeloid leukemia (AML) when compared to patients with acute lymphoblastic leukemia (ALL). We observed a higher frequency of haplotype A (59 %) in the patients.

Conclusion: Our data suggests that susceptibility to leukemia can be influenced, at least, partly byKIR receptors.

Keywords: KIR, HLA, Leukemia

Background

Natural killer (NK) cells play a pivotal role in innate immunity providing immediate protection against infections as well as in the early steps of neoplastic cellular transformation [1]. The antileukemic role of Natural Killer (NK) cells has been brought into focus in recent years.

Killer cell immunoglobulin-like receptors (KIRs) interactions with their ligands regulate the cytotoxicity activity of NK cells. HLA-Cw is the primary ligand for a significant number of inhibitory KIRs. HLA-Cw allotypes are categorized into C1 and C2 groups based on a polymorphism at residue 80 in the HLA-Cw molecule. Inhibitory *KIR2DL2* and *KIR2DL3* are specific for the C1 ligand group, and inhibitory *KIR2DL1* is specific for the C2 ligand group. The inhibitory *KIR3DL1* receptor is specific for HLA molecules with the HLA-Bw4 epitope (HLA-B, HLA-A3 e HLA-A11) [2]. When inhibitory KIRs

* Correspondence: ligh@ufpr.br
Departamento de Genética, Laboratório de Imunogenética e Histocompatibilidade (LIGH), Universidade Federal do Paraná, R. Cel. Francisco H. dos Santos S/N, Centro Politécnico – Jardim das Américas, CEP 81.530.990, Curitiba, PR CP 19071, Brazil

encounter self-HLA class I ligands on target cells, they signal inhibition and establish tolerance.

KIR genotypes are organized into two main broad haplotypes termed A and B, according to KIR inhibitorys and activators genes content. Both A and B haplotype share four framework genes: *KIR2DL4, KIR3DL2, KIR3DL3* and *KIR3DP1*. Haplotype A gene organization includes up to eight genes, those of the framework content together with *KIR2DL1, KIR2DL3, KIR2DS4* and *KIR3DL1*. The activating *KIR* genes, *KIR2DS1, KIR2DS2, KIR2DS3, KIR2DS5,* and *KIR3DS1,* as well as the genes encoding inhibitory *KIRs, KIR2DL5A/B and KIR2DL2,* are the principal representants of the Group B haplotypes [3].

The "missing-self" concept presented by Kärre and colleagues in the 1980s, paved the way for the understanding of NK-derived allorecognition mechanism [1, 4]. In brief, NK cells, through the expressing of cognate inhibitory receptor learn to detect and kill cells with reduced or "missing" expression of "self" MHC class I ligands [5].

Since the early 70s hematopoietic progenitor cells transplantation from different sources, have been used as a therapeutic alternative for a broad spectrum of cancers and hematological diseases [6].

The past 10 years have witnessed dramatic progress in our understanding of possible exploitation of NK cells in cancer therapy. Haplo-Hematopoietic Stem Cell Transplantation (haplo-HSCT) outcoming showed a positive effect related to NK cells in adults with AML and also in children with high-risk ALL [7, 8]. The increased activity of NK cells after transplanting, even when the donor and recipient are HLA- identical, suggest that the cytotoxicity of these receptor cells from the donor can be an additional component previously unrecognized in the rejection process.

Several studies indicate an association with disease role in interactions between these KIRs and HLA loci and infectious diseases, autoimmune/inflammatory diseases, cancer and reproduction [9].

Only a few studies have investigated the association between the genetic diversity of activating and inhibitory KIR genes in humans and the susceptibility and resistance to leukemia [10]. Some results pointed out association between a group of activating and inhibitory KIR genes with relapse, overall survival and relative risk [11].

Some results pointed out the association between a group of activating and inhibitory KIR genes with relapse, overall survival and relative risk [11].

More studies on KIR allelic diversity are needed in order to clarify the role of NK cells in hematopoietic diseases. Among the three already well- known gene families which encode for NK cell receptors, we aimed to characterize the *KIR* genes repertoire in patients from Paraná State with hematopoietic disorders.

Methods

Samples

The sample consisted of 39 patients (as shown in Table 1) with HSCT indication from the Erasto Gaertner Hospital (Curitiba, Paraná State, Brazil) and 136 healthy family members from LIGH-UFPR (Laboratory of Immunogenetics and Histocompatibility, Federal University of Paraná) database, in the period of July 2007 to May 2008 to carry out pre-transplant histocompatibility testing. All participants signed an informed consent document. The study was approved by the Ethics Committee from UFPR-CEP-HC number 037ext.019/2001-07.

Table 1 General characteristics of patients ($N = 39$)

			Gender		Age		Ethnic group		
Disease	N	(%)	M	F	Average	Std. Dev.	White	Mulatto	Black
Bone Marrow Aplasia	1	0.03	0	1	30.0	0.00	1	0	0
Paroxysmal Nocturna Hemoglobinuria	2	0.05	2	0	31.5	2.10	2	0	0
NK Leukemia Cells	1	0.03	1	0	13.0	0.00	1	0	0
Non Hodgkin Lymphoma - Follicular	1	0.03	0	1	39.0	0.00	1	0	0
Acute Lymphoid Leukemia	13	0.33	7	6	15.2	16.70	11	2	0
Acute Myeloid Leukemia	11	0.28	7	4	35.7	17.80	3	0	0
Chronic Myeloid Leukemia	3	0.08	3	0	31.7	9.60	1	0	0
Myelodysplasia	1	0.03	1	0	23.0	0.00	2	0	0
Myelofibrosis	2	0.05	1	1	50.5	12.00	1	0	0
Multiple Myeloma	1	0.03	1	0	40.0	0.00	1	1	0
MyelodysplasticMyeloproliferativeSyndrome	2	0.05	1	1	42.0	1.40	10	1	0
Not Informed	1	0.03	1	0	NI	NI	1	0	0
Total	39	1	25	14			35	4	0

M male, *F* female, *Std. Dev.* standard deviation; IBGE ethnic classification

Extraction of genomic DNA

Two tubes with 10 milliliters (10 ml) of peripheral blood were collected from each individual by venous puncture into sterile tubes containing EDTA vacutainer type. These samples were centrifuged to obtain leucocyte layer from which the DNA was extracted by salting-out technique [12]. The DNA concentration of the samples was measured by reading optical density, using the spectrophotometer Gene Quantpro RNA/DNA calculator.

Typing of *KIR* genes

The *KIR* gene typing was performed by PCR-SSOP (Polymerase Chain Reaction - Sequence Specific Oligonucleotide Probes), amplifying the exons 3, 5 and 7–9, using the kit "Labtype*KIR* SSO Genotyping Test" (One Lambda Inc). The data analysis was performed using the HLA VISUAL version 2.0 software (One Lamda Inc.) that analyzes the combinations of probes in the microbeads detected by the instrument and consults an internal database that suggest what are the loci present.

Statistical analysis

Phenothypic frequencies regarding presence/absence of *KIR* genes for all samples (patient group and healthy control group) along with the haplotype frequencies were obtained by direct counting.

The frequencies of the 16 *KIR* genes obtained for ALL and AML patients group were compared using the χ^2 test, and the comparisons made between the patient and control group were performed using Fisher exact test (bilateral p-value), with the aid of BioEstat 5.0 software. When the sample size of the analyzed group was very small (less than 10), which can decrease the accuracy of the test χ^2, Yates correction was applied. The frequencies of haplotypes A and B were obtained by direct counting. The comparisons made between patient and controls were performed using χ^2test. Significance level was considered when p-value ≤ 0.05.

Results

The epidemiology of the 39 patients with HSCT indication was analyzed according to disease, gender, age and ethnic/racial group (Table 1). Age analysis of the patients ($N = 39$) indicated that 64 % of the patients were male (25) and 36 % were female (14). The average age of the patients was 28.50 + 17.74 years. According to the racial group suggested by the Brazilian Institute of Geography and Statistics (IBGE), 89 % of patients were classified as White and 11 % Mulattos (mixed-descendent of White *vs* Black).

The frequencies of the presence/absence of 16 KIR genes in the patients are presented in Table 2. These data were compared with 136 healthy family members and it was observed that the ***KIR2DL2*** ($p = 0.0005$); ***KIR2DL5*** ($p = 0.0067$); ***KIR2DS1*** ($p = 0.0013$); ***KIR2DS2*** ($p = 0.0038$) and ***KIR2DS3*** genes ($p = 0.0153$) were statistically more frequent in the healthy individuals than in the patients as can be seen in Table 3. The comparison between patients with acute lymphoid leukemia (ALL) and acute myeloid leukemia (AML) showed that the ***KIR2DS3*** gene ($p = 0.0013$) was more frequent in AML patients (Table 4).

We also observed a higher frequency of haplotype A in patients (59 % of haplotype A and 41 % of haplotype B).

Discussion

Fourteen KIR genes plus two pseudogenes are joined in the leukocyte receptor complex (LCR) on chromosome 19q13.4 and display a high degree of genetic diversity concerning gene content and allelic polymorphism [13]. This genomic structure drives to non-allelic homologous recombination events, which potentially generates considerable genetic diversity in KIR gene repertoire among individuals and populations [14].

HLA and *KIR* gene clusters are functionally linked but segregate independently creating a genetic diversity that could have a different impact on transplantation outcome. Hence, studies regarding KIR and HLA genes in different populations can provide valuable information to several scientific fields [15, 16].

In our study, we evaluated the repertoire of *KIR* genes in patients with hematopoietic disorders. Overall, the frequencies of the presence/absence of *KIR* genes were similar to the frequencies observed in European populations, which would be expected considering the predominance of White Euro-descendants in southern Brazil.

The framework genes *KIR3DL3, KIR3DP1, KIR2DL4* and *KIR3DL2* were observed in all samples, in accordance to their presence in all known KIR haplotypes. The remaining inhibitorys and activators *KIR* genes showed frequencies that varied between individuals. The distribution of *KIR* gene frequencies among patients showed low frequencies as follows: *KIR2DL2* (23 %), *KIR2DL5* (28 %), *KIR2DS1* (15 %), *KIR2DS3* (13 %), *KIR2DS5* (28 %) and *KIR3DS1* (26 %). Despite the small sample size, the results are in agreement with those observed for populations of Caucasian origin. The *KIR* genes that showed higher frequencies in the patient group were: *KIR2DL1* (90 %), *KIR2DL3* (92 %), *KIR2DP1* (95 %), *KIR2DS4* (92 %) and *KIR3DL1* (93 %).

A recent study of the association between polymorphisms in *KIR* and *HLA* genes and pediatric ALL in Hispanic and non-Hispanic children provided additional evidence about the contribution of genetic variation in ALL incidence. When the incidence and survival were evaluated between the two ethnic groups,

Table 2 Distribution of KIR genes frequenciesin patients ($N = 39$)

		KIR genes															
		2DL1	2DL2	2DL3	**2DL4**	2DL5	2DP1	2DS1	2DS2	2DS3	2DS4	2DS5	3DL1	**3DL2**	**3DL3**	**3DP1**	3DS1
Patients	absolutefrequency	35	9	36	39	11	37	6	12	5	36	11	37	39	39	39	10
$N = 39$	relativefrequency	0,90	0,23	0,92	1,00	0,28	0,95	0,15	0,31	0,13	0,92	0,28	0,95	1,00	1,00	1,00	0,26
	genefrequency	0,68	0,12	0,72	1,00	0,15	0,77	0,08	0,17	0,07	0,72	0,15	0,77	1,00	1,00	1,00	0,14
BoneMarrow Aplasia	absolutefrequency	1	0	1	1	1	1	1	0	0	1	1	0	1	1	1	1
$N = 1$	relativefrequency	1,00	0,00	1,00	1,00	1,00	1,00	1,00	0,00	0,00	1,00	1,00	0,00	1,00	1,00	1,00	1,00
	genefrequency	1,00	0,00	1,00	1,00	1,00	1,00	1,00	0,00	0,00	1,00	1,00	0,00	1,00	1,00	1,00	1,00
ParoxysmalNocturnaHemoglobinuria	absolutefrequency	2	0	2	2	0	2	0	1	0	2	0	2	2	2	2	0
$N = 2$	relativefrequency	1,00	0,00	1,00	1,00	0,00	1,00	0,00	0,50	0,00	1,00	0,00	1,00	1,00	1,00	1,00	0,00
	genefrequency	1,00	0,00	1,00	1,00	0,00	1,00	0,00	0,29	0,00	1,00	0,00	1,00	1,00	1,00	1,00	0,00
NK LeukemiaCells	absolutefrequency	1	0	1	1	0	1	0	0	0	1	0	1	1	1	1	0
$N = 1$	relativefrequency	1,00	0,00	1,00	1,00	0,00	1,00	0,00	0,00	0,00	1,00	0,00	1,00	1,00	1,00	1,00	0,00
	genefrequency	1,00	0,00	1,00	1,00	0,00	1,00	0,00	0,00	0,00	1,00	0,00	1,00	1,00	1,00	1,00	0,00
Non Hodgkin Lymphoma - Follicular	absolutefrequency	1	0	1	1	0	1	0	0	0	1	0	1	1	1	1	0
$N = 1$	relativefrequency	1,00	0,00	1,00	1,00	0,00	1,00	0,00	0,00	0,00	1,00	0,00	1,00	1,00	1,00	1,00	0,00
	genefrequency	1,00	0,00	1,00	1,00	0,00	1,00	0,00	0,00	0,00	1,00	0,00	1,00	1,00	1,00	1,00	0,00
AcuteLymphoidLeukemia	absolutefrequency	12	3	12	13	4	13	2	3	2	12	5	13	13	13	13	2
$N = 13$	relativefrequency	0,92	0,23	0,92	1,00	0,31	1,00	0,15	0,23	0,15	0,92	0,38	1,00	1,00	1,00	1,00	0,15
	genefrequency	0,72	0,12	0,72	1,00	0,17	1,00	0,08	0,12	0,08	0,72	0,22	1,00	1,00	1,00	1,00	0,08
AcuteMyeloidLeukemia	absolutefrequency	8	3	9	11	4	9	2	5	2	9	3	10	11	11	11	5
$N = 11$	relativefrequency	0,73	0,27	0,82	1,00	0,36	0,82	0,18	0,45	0,18	0,82	0,27	0,91	1,00	1,00	1,00	0,45
	genefrequency	0,48	0,15	0,57	1,00	0,20	0,57	0,10	0,26	0,10	0,57	0,15	0,70	1,00	1,00	1,00	0,26
ChronicMyeloidLeukemia	absolutefrequency	3	0	3	3	0	3	0	0	0	3	1	3	3	3	3	0
$N = 3$	relativefrequency	1,00	0,00	1,00	1,00	0,00	1,00	0,00	0,00	0,00	1,00	0,33	1,00	1,00	1,00	1,00	0,00
	genefrequency	1,00	0,00	1,00	1,00	0,00	1,00	0,00	0,00	0,00	1,00	0,18	1,00	1,00	1,00	1,00	0,00
Myelodysplasia	absolutefrequency	1	1	1	1	1	1	1	1	0	1	1	1	1	1	1	1
$N = 1$	relativefrequency	1,00	1,00	1,00	1,00	1,00	1,00	1,00	1,00	0,00	1,00	1,00	1,00	1,00	1,00	1,00	1,00
	genefrequency	1,00	1,00	1,00	1,00	1,00	1,00	1,00	1,00	0,00	1,00	1,00	1,00	1,00	1,00	1,00	1,00
Myelofibrosis	absolutefrequency	2	0	2	2	0	2	0	0	0	2	0	2	2	2	2	0
$N = 2$	relativefrequency	1,00	0,00	1,00	1,00	0,00	1,00	0,00	0,00	0,00	1,00	0,00	1,00	1,00	1,00	1,00	0,00
	genefrequency	1,00	0,00	1,00	1,00	0,00	1,00	0,00	0,00	0,00	1,00	0,00	1,00	1,00	1,00	1,00	0,00

Table 2 Distribution of KIR genes frequenciesin patients ($N = 39$) *(Continued)*

MultipleMyeloma	absolutefrequency	1	1	1	1	0	1	0	1	0	1	0	1	1	1	1	0
$N = 1$	relativefrequency	1,00	1,00	1,00	1,00	0,00	1,00	0,00	1,00	0,00	1,00	0,00	1,00	1,00	1,00	1,00	0,00
	genefrequency	1,00	1,00	1,00	1,00	0,00	1,00	0,00	1,00	0,00	1,00	0,00	1,00	1,00	1,00	1,00	0,00
MyelodysplasticMyeloproliferativeSyndrome	absolutefrequency	2	0	2	2	0	2	0	0	0	2	0	2	2	2	2	1
$N = 2$	relativefrequency	1,00	0,00	1,00	1,00	0,00	1,00	0,00	0,00	0,00	1,00	0,00	1,00	1,00	1,00	1,00	0,50
	genefrequency	1,00	0,00	1,00	1,00	0,00	1,00	0,00	0,00	0,00	1,00	0,00	1,00	1,00	1,00	1,00	0,29
NotInformed	absolutefrequency	1	1	1	1	1	1	0	1	1	1	0	1	1	1	1	0
$N = 1$	relativefrequency	1,00	1,00	1,00	1,00	1,00	1,00	0,00	1,00	1,00	1,00	0,00	1,00	1,00	1,00	1,00	0,00
	genefrequency	1,00	1,00	1,00	1,00	1,00	1,00	0,00	1,00	1,00	1,00	0,00	1,00	1,00	1,00	1,00	0,00

Genes in bold are those genes called "framewok genes

Table 3 Frequency of each KIR gene in patients ($N = 39$) and controls ($N = 136$)

	KIR gene	Patient ($n = 39$)	Control ($n = 136$)	*p*-value
Framework	*KIR2DL4*	39 (100 %)	136 (100 %)	1.0000
	KIR3DL2	39 (100 %)	136 (100 %)	1.0000
	KIR3DL3	39 (100 %)	136 (100 %)	1.0000
	KIR3DP1	39 (100 %)	136 (100 %)	1.0000
Haplotype A	*KIR2DS4*	36 (92 %)	129 (95 %)	0.6936
	KIR2DL1	35 (90 %)	130 (96 %)	0.2329
	KIR2DL3	36 (92 %)	118 (87 %)	0.4173
	KIR3DL1	37 (95 %)	129 (95 %)	1.0000
Haplotype B	***KIR2DS1***	6 (15 %)	59 (43 %)	**0.0013** ([a])
	KIR2DS2	12 (31 %)	78 (57 %)	**0.0038** ([a])
	KIR2DS3	5 (13 %)	45 (33 %)	**0.0153** ([a])
	KIR2DS5	11 (28 %)	45 (33 %)	0.6976
	KIR3DS1	10 (26 %)	53 (39 %)	0.1356
	KIR2DL2	9 (23 %)	75 (55 %)	**0.0005** ([a])
	KIR2DL5	11 (28 %)	72 (53 %)	**0.0067** ([a])
Haplotype A/B	*KIR2DP1*	37 (95 %)	131 (96 %)	0.6465

Genes in bold showed significance for the statistical test ([a])

a high incidence of ALL and a significantly worse survival was found in Hispanic children compared to non-Hispanic Whites. The genotypes diversity related to KIR and HLA ligands are very suggestive that these two loci may determine a different susceptibility effect depending on the ethnic groups. Such observed differences are probably multifactorial due to an interaction between KIR and environmental factors, e.g. patterns of infection, rather than merely allele frequencies differences between ethnic groups [14].

Table 4 Frequency of each KIR gene from patients with ALL ($N = 12$) and AML ($N = 11$)

	KIR GENE	All ($n = 12$)	AML ($n = 11$)	*p*-value
Framework	*KIR2DL4*	12 (100 %)	11 (100 %)	1.0000
	KIR3DL2	12 (100 %)	11 (100 %)	1.0000
	KIR3DL3	12 (100 %)	11 (100 %)	1.0000
	KIR3DP1	12 (100 %)	11 (100 %)	1.0000
Haplotype A	*KIR2DS4*	11 (92 %)	9 (82 %)	0.5921
	KIR2DL1	11 (92 %)	8 (73 %)	0.3168
	KIR2DL3	11 (92 %)	9 (82 %)	0.5901
	KIR3DL1	12 (100 %)	10 (91 %)	0.4783
Haplotype B	*KIR2DS1*	10 (83 %)	9 (82 %)	1.0000
	KIR2DS2	3 (25 %)	3 (27 %)	1.0000
	KIR2DS3	2 (17 %)	9 (82 %)	**0.0031** ([a])
	KIR2DS5	5 (42 %)	3 (27 %)	0.6668
	KIR3DS1	2 (17 %)	5 (45 %)	0.1930
	KIR2DL2	3 (25 %)	3 (27 %)	1.0000
	KIR2DL5	4 (33 %)	4 (36 %)	1.0000
Haplotype A/B	*KIR2DP1*	12 (100 %)	9 (82 %)	0.2174

Genes in bold showed significance for the statistical test ([a])

In a study carried out in Italian population Bontadini and colleagues reported the same general *KIR* gene patterns distribution observed in other Caucasian and non-Caucasian populations. Australian Aborigine, Chinese Han, and Japanese showed the most markedly different patterns, with significant differences from Italian population and other Caucasian populations, in particular for inhibitory gene *KIR2DL2* and non inhibitorys *KIR2DS1, KIR2DS2, KIR2DS3, KIR3DS1* [17–20]. The findings with respect to *KIR* gene diversity in different populations could provide relevant genomic diversity data for further studies on viral infection, autoimmune diseases, and reproductive fitness.

Inhibitorys genes *KIR2DL2* and *KIR2DL5B* were also found at lower frequencies in the Italian population, as well as the activating genes *KIR2DS3* and *KIR2DS4* [15]. Notably, as to *KIR2DS4* alleles, Han Chinese showed an inverse pattern compared to the Italian population [19].

The activating KIR2DS4 gene is unique in the haplotype A, whereas haplotype B contains up to five activating KIRs. Haplotypes A and B have been preserved in the human population (about 25 and 75 % in Caucasian), thus suggesting the occurrence of a balancing selection [13, 15].

Linkage disequilibrium or the non-random associations between alleles at two loci are also present in KIR genes repertoire. A high positive linkage disequilibrium between *KIR2DL1* and *KIR2DL3* has been observed in Caucasian and non-Caucasian populations [21]. Our data are consistent with this hypothesis since the frequencies of these two genes were the highest observed in both control and patient groups.

KIR repertoire comparisons between patients and healthy family members (Fig. 1) showed that the inhibitory genes *KIR2DL2* ($p = 0.0005$) and *KIR2DL5* ($p = 0.0067$), as well as the activating genes *KIR2DS1* ($p = 0.0013$), *KIR2DS2* ($p = 0.0038$), *KIR2DS3* ($p = 0.0153$) were more frequently found ($p < 0.05$) in healthy individuals than in patients.

HLA-KIR genotypes have been associated with susceptibility to a variety of diseases such as psoriatic arthritis, type I diabetes, infectious diseases, cancer, and reproduction. Just a few of these studies revealed an influence of HLA-KIR gene interactions on disease outcome [9]. Others studies have investigated the frequency of KIR genes in patients with hematologic malignancies [22]. Most of these investigations have been performed in patients with different diseases such as AML, CML and MDS [23–27].

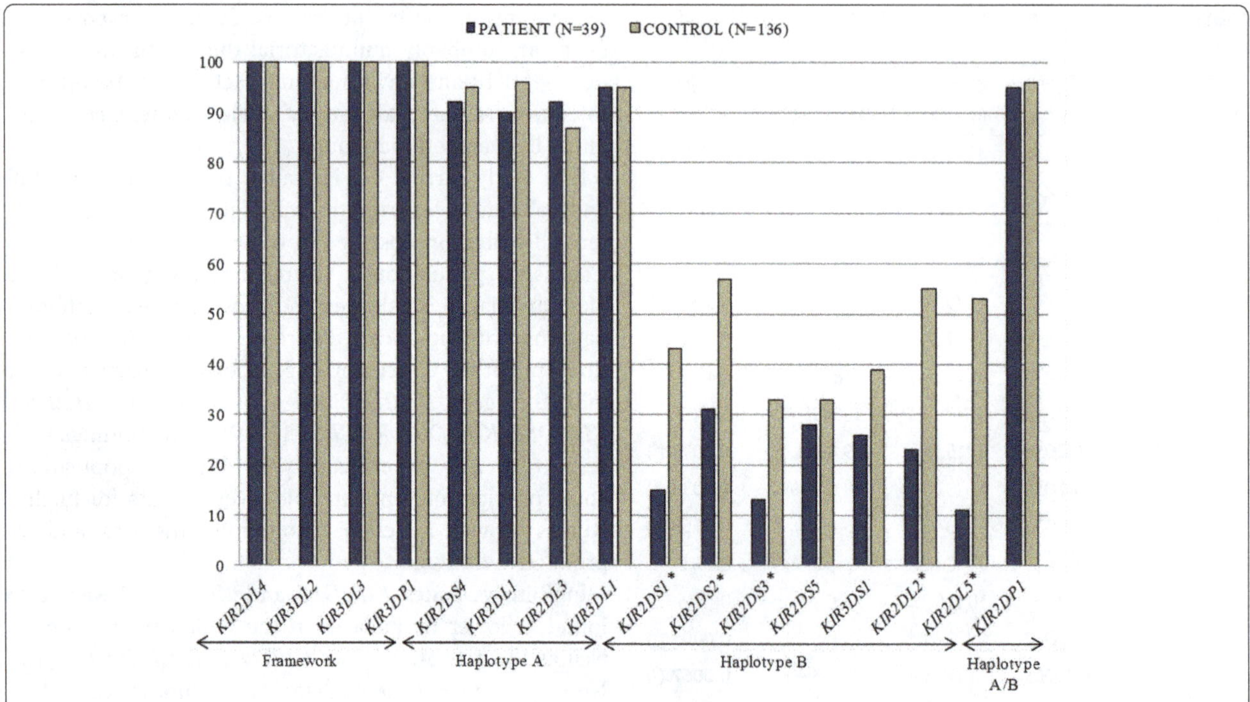

Fig. 1 Phenotypic frequency related to the presence/absence of *KIR* genes in patients ($N = 39$) and healthy controls ($N = 136$). Genes marked with (*) showed significance for the stastical test

There are several studies that investigate the association between *KIR* haplotypes distribution and diseases; it is observed that Haplogroups A and B vary considerably between ethnic groups [15, 28–30]. The association of *KIR* gene/haplotypes has been investigated in patients with indication for hematopoietic stem cell transplantation, highlighting the role of *KIR* genes in the transplant outcome [7].

The stratification of the patients according to AML *vs* ALL groups, revealed that the *KIR2DS3* gene presented higher frequencies ($p = 0.0031$) in AML when compared to ALL patients (Fig. 2). Although the sample size was relatively small, recent publications suggest important roles for specific KIR genes that may influence allogeneic hematopoietic stem cell transplantation (HSCT) outcome in HLA-compatible siblings, GvHD, relapse and other complications related to transplantation [31] in small and heterogeneous samples [32].

A study in China investigated KIR genotypes in 54 patients with hematopoietic malignancies, classified into two risk groups: standard and high. The frequency of activating *KIR* genes in standard-risk group was higher when compared to the high-risk group, specifically for *KIR2DS1*, *KIR2DS2* and *KIR3DS1*. A secondary analysis of this study, comparing standard-risk group *vs* high-risk group in AML patients, revealed higher frequencies of activating *KIR* genes in the standard-risk group, particularly for *KIR2DS1, KIR2DS2,* and *KIR2DS3* genes, the latter one in agreement with our findings in AML patients group [22].

In the same line of investigation, Kim and colleagues reported the influence of *KIR* genes in AML patients and HLA compatible donor siblings after HSCT. All the activating *KIR* genes in the donors showed an important role in transplant outcome and in the occurrence of acute graft-versus-host disease (GvHD) in HSCT in AML patients. Particularly, the *KIR2DS2* gene and the allele *KIR2DS4*003* were correlated with acute GvHD. This evidence suggests an immunogenic specificity in the Korean population compared to Caucasians since the frequency of *KIR2DL2* and *KIR2DS2* genes are comparatively lower in Koreans than in other countries. Long-term survival was noted even if the KIR2DS1 gene was only present in the donor and not in the recipient. The presence of both genes KIR2DS3-KIR2DS5 was more frequently found in a variety of complications related to transplant [31].

Mancusi and colleagues reported that donors, possessing KIR2DS1, KIR3DS1 or both activating genes, showed reduced infection rates and mortality, and a better event-free survival (EFS) [33].

Donor cells that express KIR haplotype B have been reported to contribute to relapse protection and improved survival after myeloablative allogeneic transplantation. Haplotype B/x donor cells have also been associated with a higher incidence of chronic GvHD. In

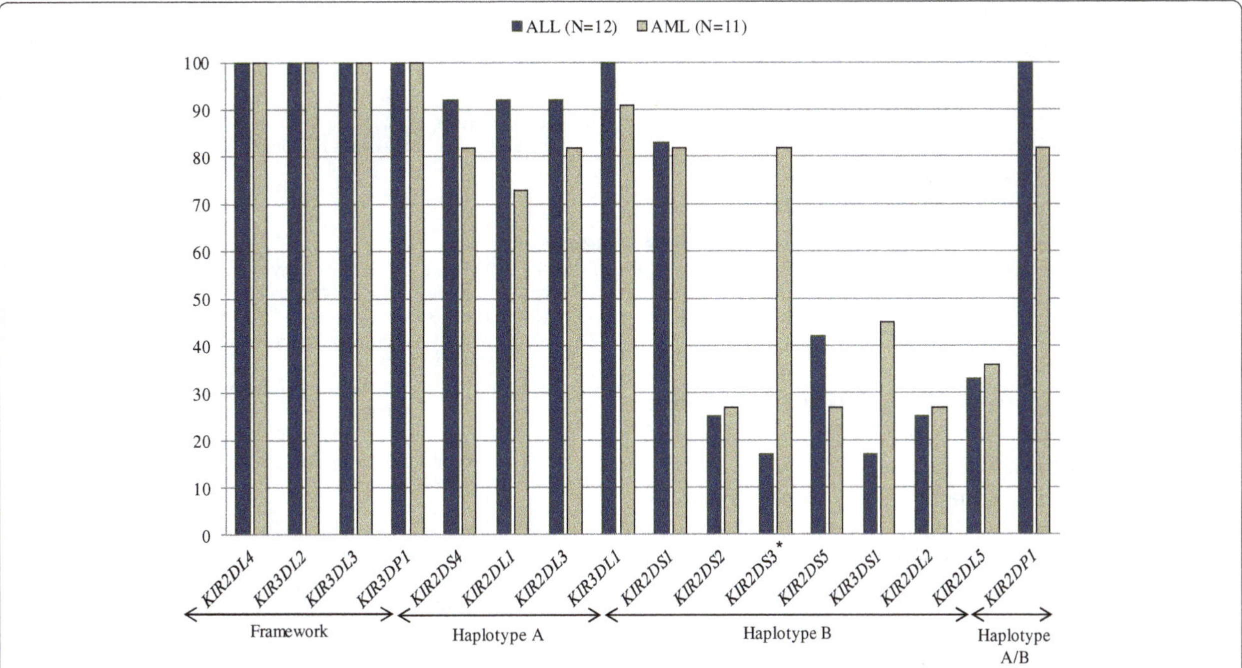

Fig. 2 Phenotypic frequency related to the presence/absence of *KIR* genes in ALL patients (*N* = 12) and AML patients (*N* = 11). Genes marked with (*) showed significance for the stastical test

HLA-haploidentical transplant setting, adonor *KIR* B haplotype has been associated with lower risk of relapse for patients with hematologic malignancies [2].

NK cells receptors of the family KIR may confer specific protector effect for different diseases. In a Turkish study carried out in a heterogeneous group of leukemia patients and controls, a protective effect was observed associated with KIR2DL2 and/or KIR2DS2 against CML [32].

From an evolutionary perspective, activating *KIRs* arose more recently from inhibitorys homologous genes [34]. A wide variation in *KIR* activators gene frequencies have been reported for different populational groups [35]. Nevertheless, the allelic diversity related to inhibitory receptors genes is limited when compared to activators genes [36]. The strong negative correlation observed between certain activating KIR and its ligands across populations, in contrast to weak positive correlations between several KIR inhibitory genes and their ligands, put forward a hypothesis that a pressure selection mechanism involving autoimmune disease is acting on the maintenance of lower frequencies of activator KIR receptor and their ligands [35].

KIR phenotypes analysis in Belgian leukemia patients indicated significantly higher frequencies of inhibitory *KIR2DL1, KIR2DL2,* and *KIR2DL3* genes, suggesting their contribution for the lack of antitumor responses of NK cells [10]. On another study, conducted in 35 patients with a lymphoproliferative NK cell disease, inhibitory genes *KIR2DL5A* and *KIR2DL5B* were more frequently found in patients compared to healthy controls [37].

Epstein-Barr virus has been associated to the development of Hodgkin's disease in some pathological conditions. An important review summarises current knowledge of the pathogenesis of Hodgkin's disease with particular emphasis on the association with EBV. Besson and colleagues identified in a family study a stronger protector effect related to *KIR2DS1/KIR3DS1* in patients with Hodgkin's lymphoma [38].

A total of 50 Han Chinese patients were studied to explore the correlation between *KIR* genes and susceptibility to leukemia. The comparison made between patient and control groups showed lower frequencies of *KIR3DL1* and *KIR2DL1* genes amongst patients. Additionally, the results highlighted a negative correlation between the pathogenesis of leukemia and *KIR3DL1, KIR3DS1, KIR2DL1,* and *KIR2DL5* genes [39], a very suggestive finding that *KIR* polymorphisms are associated with susceptibility to leukemia in Hans.

In the present study, patients had lower frequencies of *KIR3DS1* (26 % versus 39 %) and *KIR2DL5* (28 % versus 53 %) as compared to healthy family members group.

McQueen and collaborators analyzed *KIR* genes repertoire in donors, and found that *KIR2DS3* conferred a protective effect against chronic GvHD in transplantation with HLA-compatible unrelated donor [40] and with donors who have more than four activating KIR in haploidentical transplants.

NK cells were components previously not recognized in HSCT rejection process and GvHD. More recently, investigation of human health/disease effects associated with KIR receptors have been reported and the majority of the described associations have been with activators *KIR* genes. Our data suggest that susceptibility to leukemia can be influenced, at least, partly by KIR receptors and an increased sample can confirm these findings for further investigations.

Conclusion

Our study with KIR receptors in patients with hematologic diseases showed that inhibitory genes *KIR2DL2* and *KIR2DL5* and activating genes *KIR2DS1*, *KIR2DS2*, *KIR2DS3* were more frequently found in healthy family members than in patients. Also, the *KIR2DS3* was significantly more frequent in patients with AML when compared to patients with ALL. We observed a higher frequency of haplotype A in the patients group. All these data are crucial to understanding the mechanisms underlying the dysfunction of NK in leukemia. The characterization of the genetic profile of patients brings together relevant information to enable robust investigations of *KIR* genes and their influence on important diseases such as Acute Myeloid Leukemia, Acute Lymphoblastic Leukemia, and others.

Abbreviations

ALL: Acute lymphoblastic leukemia; AML: Acute myeloid leukemia; BMT: Bone marrow transplantation; CML: Chronic myeloid leucemia; DNTPs: Deoxynucleotide; EDTA: Ethylene tetraacetic acid; EFS: Event-free survival; GvHD: Graft-versus-host disease; HCT: Hematopoietic cell transplantation; HLA: Human leukocyte antigen; HSCT: Hematopoietic stem cell transplantation; IBGE: InstitutoBrasileiro de Geografia e Estatística; ILTs: Immunoglobulin-like transcript; *KIR*: Immunoglobulin-like receptors of natural killer; LCR: Leukocyte receptor complex; LIGH: Laboratório de imunogenética e histocompatibilidade; MDS: Myelodysplasia; MHC: Major histocompatibility complex; NK: Natural killer; PCR-SSOP: Polymerase chain reaction - sequence specific oligonucleotide probes

Acknowledgements

We are very grateful to the patients who generously accorded to provide samples for this study. We also thank the LIGH staff for technical support.

Funding

This study was supported by research funding from FUNPAR-LIGH and CAPES.

Authors' contributions

DKS: participated in the experimental design, performed DNA extraction and KIR typing, data collection, analysis and interpretation of data and writing of the manuscript. CEIG: participated in the writing of the manuscript, drawing up the tables and revision of the manuscript; MGB: participated in the experimental design and discussion of experiments, interpretation of data and writing of the manuscript. All authors read and approved the final manuscript.

Competing interests

The authors declare that they have no competing interests.

References

1. Lanier LL. NK cell recognition. Annu Rev Immunol. 2005;23:225–74.
2. Sobecks RM, Wang T, Askar M, Gallagher MM, Haagenson M, Spellman S, et al. Impact of KIR and HLA genotypes on outcomes after reduced-intensity conditioning hematopoietic cell transplantation. Biol Blood Marrow Transplant. 2015;21(9):1589–96.
3. Middleton D, Gonzelez F. The extensive polymorphism of KIR genes. Immunology. 2009;129:8–19.
4. Karre K, Ljunggren HG, Piontek G, Kiessling R. Selective rejection of H-2-deficient lymphoma variants suggests alternative immune defence strategy. Nature. 1986;319(6055):675–8.
5. Middleton D, Williams F, Halfpenny IA. KIR genes. Transpl Immunol. 2005; 14(3-4):135–42.
6. Holowiecki J. Indications for hematopoietic stem cell transplantation. Pol Arch Med Wewn. 2008;118(11):658–63.
7. Ruggeri L, Capanni M, Urbani E, Perruccio K, Hlomchik WD, Tosti A, et al. Effectiveness of donor natural killer cell alloreactivity in mismatched hematopoietic transplants. Science. 2002;295(5562):2097–100.
8. Marcenaro E, Carlomagn S, Pesce S, Chiesa MD, Moretta A, Sivor S. Role of alloreactive KIR2DS1(+) NK cells in haploidentical hematopoietic stem cell transplantation. J Leukoc Biol. 2011;90(4):661–7.
9. Kulkarni S, Martin MP, Carrington M. The Yin and Yang of *HLA* and *KIR* in human disease. Semin Immunol. 2008;20(6):343–52.
10. Verheyden S, Bernier M, Demanet C. Identification of natural killer cell receptor phenotypes associated with leukemia. Leukemia. 2004;18(12):2002–7.
11. Babor F, Fischer JC, Uhrberg M. The role of KIR genes and ligands in leukemia surveillance. Front Immunol. 2013;4:27.
12. John SW, Weitzner G, Rozen R, Scriver CR. A rapid procedure for extracting genomic DNA from leukocyte. Nucleic Acids Res. 1991;19(2):408.
13. Moretta L, Montaldo E, Vacca P, Zotto GD, Moretta F, Merli P, Locatelli F, Mingari MC. Human natural killer cells: origin, receptors, function, and clinical applications. Int Arch Allergy Immunol. 2014;164(4):253–64.
14. de Smith AJ, Walsh KM, Ladner MB, Zhang S, Xiao C, Cohen F, et al. The role of KIR genes and their cognate HLA class I ligands in childhood acute lymphoblastic leukemia. Blood. 2014;123(16):2497–503.
15. Uhrberg M, Parham P, Wernet P. Definition of content for nine commom group B haplotypes of the Caucasoid population: KIR haplotypes contain between seven and eleven KIR genes. Immunogenetics. 2002;54(4):221–9.
16. Toneva M, Lepage V, Lafay G, Dulphy N, Busson M, Lester S, et al. Genomic diversity of natural killer cell receptor genes in three populations. Tissue Antigens. 2001;57(4):358–62.
17. Bontadini A, Testi M, Cuccia MC, Martinetti M, Carcassi C, Chiesa A, et al. Distribution of killer cell immunoglobulin-like receptors genes in the Italian Caucasian population. J Transl Med. 2006;4:44.
18. Witt CS, Dewing C, Sayer DC, Uhrberg M, Parham P, Christiansen FT. Population frequencies and putative haplotypes of the killer cell immunoglobulin-like receptor sequences and evidence for recombination. Transplantation. 1999;68(11):1784–9.
19. Jiang K, Zhu FM, Lv QF, Yan LX. Distribution of killer cell immunoglobulin-like receptor genes in the Chinese Han population. Tissue Antigens. 2005; 65(6):556–63.
20. Yawata M, Yawata N, McQueen KL, Cheng NW, Guethlein LA, Rajalingam R, Shilling HG, Parham P. Predominance of group A KIR haplotypes in Japanese associated with diverse NK cell repertories of KIR expression. Immunogenetics. 2002;54(8):543–50.
21. Wilson MJ, Torkar M, Haude A, Milne S, Jones T, Sheer D, Beck S, Trowsdale J. Plasticity in the organization and sequences of human KIR/ILT gene families. Proc Natl Acad Sci U S A. 2000;97(9):4778–83.
22. Zhao XY, Chang YJ, Huang XJ. Differential expression levels of killer immunoglobin-like receptor genotype in patients with hematological malignancies between high-risk and standard-risk groups. Zhongguo Shi Yan Xue Ye Xue Za Zhi. 2008;16(4):746–9.

23. Ruggeri L, Capanni M, Casucci M, Volpi I, Tosti A, Perruccio K, Urbani E, Negrin RS, Martelli MF, Velardi A. Role of natural killer cells alloreactivity in HLA-mismatched hematopoietic stem cell transplantation. Blood. 1999;94(1):333–9.
24. Elmaagacli AH, Ottinger H, Koldehoff M, Peceny R, Steckel NK, Trenschel R, Biersack H, Grosse-Wilde H, Beelen DW. Reduced risk for molecular disease in patients with chronic myeloid leukemia after transplantation from a KIR-mismatched donor. Transplantation. 2005;79(12):1741–7.
25. Sconocchia G, Lau M, Provenzano M, Rezvani K, Wongsena W, Fujiwara H, Hensel N, Melenhorst J, Li J, Ferrone S, Barrett AJ. The antileukemia effect of HLA-matched NK and NK-T cells in chronic myelogenous leukemia involves NKG2D-target-cell interactions. Blood. 2005;106(10):3666–72.
26. Khakoo SI, Carrington M. KIR and disease: a model system or system of models? Immunol Rev. 2006;214:186–201.
27. Schellekens J, Rozemuller EH, Petersen EJ, Van Den Tweel JG, Verdonck LF, Tilanus MG. Activating KIRs exert a crucial role on relapse and overall survival after HLA-identical sibling transplantation. Mol Immunol. 2008;45(8):2255–61.
28. Shilling HG, Guethlein LA, Cheng NW, Gardiner CM, Rodriguez R, Tyan D, Parhan P. Allelic polymorphism synergizes with variable gene content to individualize human KIR genotype. J Immunol. 2002;168(5):2307–15.
29. Hsu KC, Chida S, Dupont B, Geragthy DE. The killer cell immunoglobulin-like receptor (KIR) genomic region: gene-order, haplotypes and allelic polimorphism. Immunol Rev. 2002;190:40–52.
30. Hsu KC, Liu XR, Selvakumar A, Mickelson E, O'Relly RJ, Dupont B. Killer Ig-like receptor haplotype analysis by gene content: evidence for genomic diversity with a minimum of six basic framework haplotypes, each with multiple subsets. J Immunol. 2002;169(9):5118–29.
31. Kim HJ, Choi Y, Min WS, Kim TG, Sho BS, Kim SY, Eom KS, Lee S, Min CK, Cho SG, Kim DW, Lee JW, Kim CC. The activating killer cell immunoglobulin-like receptors as important determinants of acute graft-versus host disease in hematopoietic stem cell transplantation for acute myelogenous leukemia. Transplantation. 2007;84(9):1082–91.
32. Middleton D, Diler AS, Meenagh A, Sleator C, Gourrau PA. Killer immunoglobulin-like receptors (*KIR2DL2* and/or *KIR2DS2*) in presence of their ligand (HLA-C1 group) protect against chronic myeloid leukaemia. Tissue Antigens. 2009;73(6):553–60.
33. Mancusi A, Ruggeri L, Urbani E, Pierini A, Massei MS, Carotti A, et al. Haploidentical hematopoietic transplantation from KIR ligand-mismatched donors with activating *KIRs* reduces nonrelapse mortality. Blood. 2015; 125(20):3173–82.
34. Abi-Rached L, Parham P. Natural selection drives recurrent formation of activating killer cell immunoglobulin-like receptor and Ly49 from inhibitory homologues. J Exp Med. 2005;201(8):1319–32.
35. Single RM, Martin MP, Gao X, Meyer D, Yeager M, Kidd JR, et al. Global diversity and evidence for coevolution of *KIR* and HLA. Nat Genet. 2007; 39(9):1114–9.
36. Hou L, Steiner NK, Chen M, Belle I, Kubit AL, et al. Limited allelic diversity of stimulatory two-domain killer cell immunoglobulin-like receptors. Hum Immunol. 2008;69(3):174–8.
37. Scquizzato E, Teramo A, Miorin M, Facco M, Piazza F, Noventa F, Trentin L, Agostini C, Zambello R, Semenzato G. Genotypic evaluation of killer immunoglobulin-like receptors in NK-type lymphoproliferative disease of granular lymphocytes. Leukemia. 2007;21(5):1060–9.
38. Besson C, Roetynck S, Williams F, Orsi L, Amiel C, Lependeven C, et al. Association of killer cell immunoglobulin-like receptor genes with Hodgkin's lymphoma in a familial study. PLoS One. 2007;2(5):e406.
39. Chen AM, Guo XM, Yan WY, Xie SM, Zhu N, Wang XD, Xu R, Liu QP. Polymorphism of killer cell immunoglobulin-like receptor gene and its correlation with leukemia. Zhongguo Shi Yan Xue Ye Xue Za Zhi. 2007;15(1):35–8.
40. McQueen KL, Dorighi KM, Guethlein LA, Wong R, Sanjanwala B, Parham P. Donor-recipient combinations of group A and B KIR haplotypes and HLA class I ligand affect the outcome of HLA-matched, sibling donor hematopoietic cell transplantation. Hum Immunol. 2007;68(5):309–23.

Drug-related problems and potential contributing factors in the management of deep vein thrombosis

Fekede Bekele Daba[1*], Fisihatsion Tadesse[2] and Ephrem Engidawork[3]

Abstract

Background: Patients receiving anticoagulant drugs must be carefully screened for drug-related problems, as such medications, including warfarin have narrow therapeutic ranges and a high potential for complications. Thus, this study was designed to assess drug-related problems in the management of patients with deep vein thrombosis at Tikur Anbessa Specialized Hospital.

Methods: A cross-sectional descriptive study involving retrospective chart review of adult patients with deep vein thrombosis was conducted from patients who visited the hospital from July 2012 to June 2013, using structured data collection format and this was complemented by key informant interview.

Results: The study included 91 patients with venous thromboembolism. Fifty three (58.2 %) were females. Mean age was 38.6 (±13.76) years and more than 2/3 were below the age of 44 years. About 54 % of them presented with concurrent medical conditions and most commonly with cancer. Adjustment of warfarin dose up or down was done in increments of 16 to 100 % for recent subtherapeutic International Normalized Ratios, 16 to 50 % for therapeutic and 11 to 66 % for overtherapeutic International Normalized Ratios, with the mean of 36.5 (±18.03) based on the cumulative weekly dose of warfarin. There was significant linear relationship between percentage of dose change and consequent International Normalized Ratio values ($R^2 = 0.419$; $p = 0.000$). Accordingly, more than 51 % of them presented with nontherapeutic International Normalized Ratio ranges following dose adjustment.

Conclusions: The most prevalent anticoagulation drug-related problems were subtherapeutic doses, overtherapeutic doses and potential drug interactions. Institutional validated decision support tools for dosing decisions during maintenance anticoagulation therapy should be developed and used accordingly in order to prevent recurrent and hemorrhagic complications and to improve clinical outcomes.

Keywords: Deep vein thrombosis, Drug-related problems, Warfarin, International Normalized Ratio, Tikur Anbessa Specialized Hospital

Background

A drug-related problem (DRP) is defined as an event or circumstance involving drug therapy that actually or potentially interferes with desired health outcomes. Categories of DRPs include unnecessary drug therapy, the needs for additional drug therapy, ineffective drug, dosage too low, dosage too high, adverse drug reaction (ADR) and patient noncompliance to the treatment [1].

DRPs are frequent and may result in reduced quality of life, and even morbidity and mortality. Despite excellent benefits and safety profile of most medications, DRPs pose a significant risk to patients, which adversely affect quality of life, increase hospitalization and overall health care cost. DRPs may arise at all stages of the medication process from prescription to follow-up of treatment [2].

Deep vein thrombosis (DVT) is the development of single or multiple blood clots within the deep veins of the extremities or pelvis, usually accompanied by inflammation of the vessel wall. The major clinical consequence is

* Correspondence: fekedeb2@gmail.com
[1]Department of Pharmacy, College of Health Sciences, Jimma University, P.O. Box 378, Jimma, Ethiopia
Full list of author information is available at the end of the article

embolization, usually to the lung [3]. Acquired risk factors for thrombosis include a prior thrombotic event, recent major surgery, presence of a central venous catheter, trauma, immobilization, malignancy, pregnancy, use of oral contraceptives, myeloproliferative disorders, and antiphospholipid syndrome.

It has long been known that hypercoagulability, stasis of blood flow, and venous endothelial injury, collectively known as the "Virchow's Triad" of pro-coagulant risk, are major factors in the pathophysiology of DVT. More recently, it has become apparent that susceptibility to venous disease is also governed by a complex interplay of gene expression, inflammation, lipid biology, and other processes. Because these processes remain incompletely characterized, standard treatment for DVT remains focused upon reducing recurrent events via the use of anticoagulant drugs.

Patients with venous thromboembolism (VTE) are generally managed with anticoagulant therapy with the aim of treating the acute event and preventing death due to pulmonary embolism (PE), in addition to minimizing the risk of postphlebitic symptoms and recurrent VTE. For most patient groups, initial therapy consists of administration of a parenteral anticoagulant drug with subsequent transition to long-term therapy with an oral vitamin K antagonist (VKA) such as warfarin for at least 3 months. Determination of the appropriate warfarin dose during initiation and maintenance therapy requires an understanding of patient factors that influence dose response: age, body weight, nutritional status, acute and chronic disease states, and changes in concomitant drug therapy and diet [4].

The goal with warfarin therapy is to maintain a balance between prevention of recurrence and excessive bleeding. This balance requires careful monitoring, typically by prothrombin time (PT)/International Normalized Ratio (INR). INR is only applicable for those taking warfarin and an INR range of 2.0 to 3.0 should be taken as therapeutic range with 2.5 as a target value for patients with DVT. INR is, therefore, used to adjust a patient's drug dosage to get the PT into the desired therapeutic range that is right for the patient and their condition. When INR is non-therapeutic, there are many options for dose adjustments. Patients whose INR is just outside the therapeutic range can be managed by either adjusting the dose up or down in increments of 5 to 20 % based on the cumulative weekly dose of warfarin or by more frequent monitoring, the latter with the expectation that the INR will return to therapeutic levels without a dosage change [5].

Patients receiving anticoagulant drugs such as DVT patients must be carefully screened for DRPs. While receiving anticoagulants, patients must be monitored closely to ensure effectiveness and to prevent side effects or overdosing. Hence, it has narrow therapeutic ranges and is associated with a high rate of DRPs thus failing to monitor warfarin therapy could increase the risk of recurrent thrombosis and hemorrhagic complications. Therefore, this study was initiated to address the possible DRPs that could occur in the management of patients with DVT in the study area.

Methods

The study was carried out at Tikur Anbessa Specialized Hospital (TASH), Ethiopia's largest general Public University Hospital. A cross-sectional descriptive study involving retrospective chart review of patients with objectively diagnosed VTE and key informant interview were carried out. Data of study population were abstracted from medical record charts of patients with objectively diagnosed VTE who visited the hospital from July 2012 to June 2013, using structured data collection format. Data abstracted included the following fields: patients' demographics, dosage schedule of the objective medications, type and number of concomitantly prescribed medications, number and types of concurrent medical conditions, series of patients' INR values and others related conditions. For the key informant interview, 3 physicians (2 hematologists and 1 consultant internist) who had long experience in the management of DVT and were working in the Hematology unit of TASH were interviewed. The data obtained from the interview included: the treatment guideline on which current DVT management depends in the study setting, factors need to be considered in deciding dose adjustments for a given nontherapeutic INR values; instructions regarding foods rich in vitamin K intake while patients are on anticoagulation therapy and other related factors.

Statistical analysis

Data entering and analysis were performed using SPSS software version 16.0. Descriptive statistics was calculated for demographic and clinical characteristics of patients. The percentage of warfarin dose change was calculated by dividing the difference of the total weekly dose before and after the time of adjustment by the total weekly dose before the time of adjustment and multiplying the quotient by 100 %. The association of the dosage change and the consequent change in INR value was done by simple linear regression analysis and the coefficient of determination (r^2 value) was taken to determine the relationship between the variables at 95 % CI and p-value < 0.05 was taken as statistically significant association. Cross-tabulation was performed for a 2x2 variables and Chi-square statistic (χ^2) was calculated to show the association between the variables at 95 % CI.

Ethical clearance

Prior to data collection, the study proposal was approved by the Ethical Review Board (ERB) of School of Pharmacy as well as Department of Internal Medicine of TASH, Addis Ababa University. During data collection, name of the patients was excluded and record card numbers were used. Data analysis was performed using a code number that had been given to each patient data collection instrument. Hence, confidentiality of all information obtained from the patient's medical record cards were kept and respected. Before conducting the interview, informed consent was obtained from the physicians.

Results

The study included 91 patients: 87.9 % with DVT, 4.4 % with PE, and 7.7 % with combined PE and DVT. Fifty three (58.2 %) were females. Mean age was 38.6 years (±13.76 years) and the age ranged from 16 to 70 years and more than 2/3 of the study population (69.2 %) was below age of 44 years. The most common concurrent medical condition was cancer. Thirty eight (41.8 %) patients were prescribed with warfarin and other medications concurrently that might potentially alter INR (Table 1).

Table 1 Demographic and clinical characteristics of patients with DVT ($n = 91$)

Patient characteristics		*n*	(%)
Sex	Female	53	(58.2)
	Male	38	(41.8)
Age (years)	16–22	4	(4.4)
	23–29	25	(27.5)
	30–36	23	(25.3)
	37–43	11	(12.1)
	44–50	7	(7.7)
	51–57	10	(11.0)
	58–64	3	(3.3)
	65–71	8	(8.8)
Co-morbidities	Cancer	14	(15.4)
	HIV/AIDS[a]	10	(11.0)
	Hypertension	7	(7.7)
	Anemia	6	(6.6)
	Others[c]	16	(17.6)
Number of prescribed drugs/patient	Less than 3	55	(60.4)
	Greater or equal to 3	36	(39.6)
Number of patients with concomitant drugs ($n = 38$)	Drugs that ↑INR[b]	21	(55.3)
	Drugs that ↓INR	13	(34.2)
	Drugs that ↑ or ↓INR	4	(10.5)

[a]HIV/AIDS: Human Immunodeficiency Virus/Acquired Immunodeficiency Syndrome
[b]INR: International normalized ratio
[c]Others include venous insufficiency, pulmonary tuberculosis, heart failure, diabetes mellitus, and dyslipidemia

Warfarin dose and INR

A total of 415 INRs were recorded over 12 months and "percent of measured INRs in range" was used to obtain the time in therapeutic range. Patients spent 49.2 %, 33.5 % & 17.3 % of time in subtherapeutic, therapeutic & supratherapeutic INR ranges, respectively (Fig. 1).

More than 66 % (276/415) of INR values were nontherapeutic and appropriate for warfarin dose adjustment, although clinical judgment might also be considered. Accordingly, the average daily dose of warfarin was increased, unchanged and decreased for 95 (46.6 %), 102 (50 %) and 7 (3.4 %) of subtherapeutic INR values, respectively. The average daily dose of warfarin was increased, unchanged and decreased for 3 (4.2 %), 25 (34.7 %) and 44 (61.1 %) for supratherapeutic INR ranges, respectively (Table 2).

The daily maintenance dose of warfarin before and after adjustment differed greatly between individuals; it was commonly between 1.25 mg/day and 12.5 mg/day during both periods. The average maintenance dose during the specified period was about 5.7 mg/day before and 5.4 mg/day after dose adjustment. The dose was lower in the elderly, which was 4.2 mg/day before and 2.5 mg/day after dosage change.

Effect of warfarin dose on the value of INR values was analyzed based on American College of Chest Physicians (ACCP) guideline [5]. Dose adjustment should be made based on the recent or current INR value and the previous cumulative weekly dose of warfarin. There had to be subsequently documented INR value at least for one week and within two months (56 days) following the dosage change to know the effect of dose. In this study, only 13.4 % (37/276) of nontherapeutic INRs were considered according to the above recommendation. Therefore, analysis of the effect of warfarin dose was performed for 41 patients. Among these, warfarin dosage was adjusted for more than 90 % of non-therapeutic and for about 10 % of therapeutic INRs (Fig. 2).

Association of warfarin dose and INR values

Adjustment of warfarin dose up or down was done in increments of 16 to 100 % for recent subtherapeutic INRs, 16 to 50 % for therapeutic and 11 to 66 % for overtherapeutic INRs with mean of 36.5 (±18.03) based on the cumulative weekly dose of warfarin. There was a moderate linear relationship between percentage of dosage adjusted and consequent INR values, which was statistically significant ($R^2 = 0.419$; $p = 0.000$). This analysis revealed that about 42 % of the variations in INR values were explained by changes in warfarin dosage. Accordingly, 21(51.2 %) of them had a non-therapeutic INR range following dosage adjustment (Table 3).

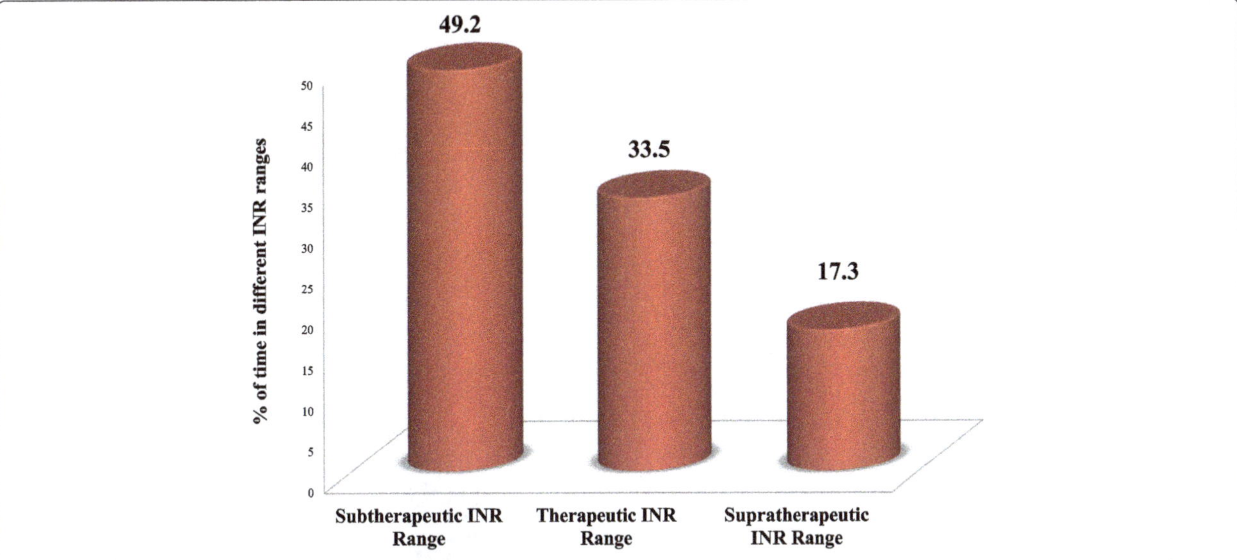

Fig. 1 Time spent in different International Normalized Ratio ranges in patients on warfarin therapy. A series of all recorded International Normalized Ratio (INR) values were collected over 12 months for each patient and calculated to determine whether they are in therapeutic range or not while on anticoagulation therapy

Warfarin interactions

Drug interaction with warfarin

More than 18 potentially interacting drugs were prescribed concomitantly with warfarin for 38 patients. Among these, 4 drugs were categorized as major interactions which are known to potentiate or inhibit warfarin effect by altering INR and 14 drugs as moderate interaction [6, 7] (Table 4). As a result, more than 55 % (21/38) and 34 % (13/38) of patients were prescribed with drugs that might increase and decrease INR when administered with warfarin, respectively (Table 1).

Among the patients whose warfarin dosage was adjusted, 46.3 % (19/41) of them were taking other medications during dosage adjustment that would have potential interaction with warfarin. This potential interaction appeared to contribute to fluctuation of INR values, as the values were out of range in a relatively higher proportion of (58 %) patients. Among the 22 patients that potential drug interaction was not a concern, INR was out of range in 45.5 % of the cases. Comparison was made between the two groups that had out-of-range INR to establish the relationship between drug-interaction and INR values. The analysis, however, did not produce any significant difference ($OR = 1.65$, $p = 0.43$), indicating the lack of association between the two factors (Fig. 3).

Table 2 Nontherapeutic INRs and warfarin dose adjustment

Nontherapeutic INRs	Decreased *n* (%)	Unchanged *n* (%)	Increased *n* (%)	Total *n* (%)
INR < 2	7 (3.4)	102 (50)	95 (46.6)	204 (100)
INR > 3	44 (61.1)	25 (34.7)	3 (4.2)	72 (100)

Food interaction with warfarin

Information about food interaction with warfarin was insufficiently documented except one instruction related to foods containing vitamin K. Thus, more than 12 %

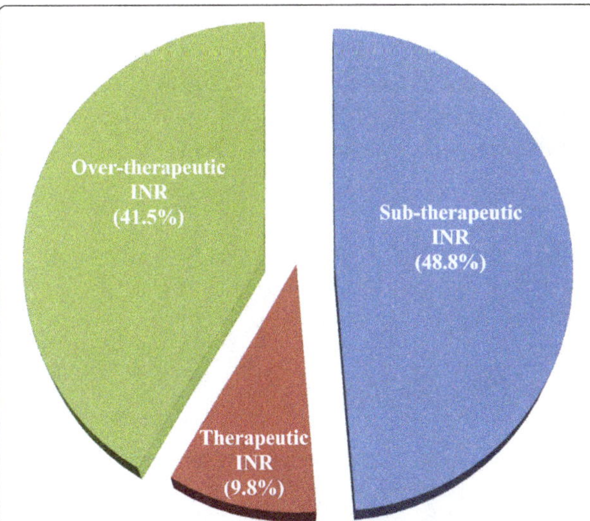

Fig. 2 Recent International normalized ratio for which warfarin dose was changed ($n = 41$). Effect of warfarin dose adjustment on the value of INR values was analyzed. Based on recommendations (ACCP 2008), analysis of the effect of warfarin dose was performed for 41 patients for those subsequently documented INR values at least for one week and within two months following the dosage change exists

Table 3 Percentage range of warfarin dose adjusted and its effect on the INR values ($n = 41$)

INR values for which warfarin dose was adjusted	n (%)	% weekly dose adjusted (mean)	INR after dose adjusted	n (%)
Less than 1.5	8 (19.5)	25–50 (37.5)↑	1.5–1.9	2 (25)
			2.0–3.0	5 (62.5)
			>4.0	1 (12.5)
1.5–1.9	12 (29.3)	16–100 (58)↑	1.5–1.9	1 (8.3)
			2.0–3.0	7 (58.3)
			3.1–4.0	2 (16.7)
			>4.0	2 (16.7)
2.0–3.0	4 (9.8)	16–50 (33) *(1 case = 16 %↑; 3 cases = 20-50 %↓)*	< 1.5	1 (25)
			1.5–1.9	2 (50)
			2.0–3.0	1 (25)
3.1–4.0	8 (19.5)	11–33 (22)↓	< 1.5	2 (25)
			1.5–1.9	2 (25)
			2.0–3.0	4 (50)
4.1–5.0	4 (9.8)	16–66 (41)↓	< 1.5	1 (25)
			1.5–1.9	1 (25)
			2.0–3.0	2 (50)
5.1–9.0	5 (12.2)	20–66 (43)↓	< 1.5	1 (20)
			1.5–1.9	3 (60)
			2.0–3.0	1 (20)

(11/91) of patients who were on anticoagulation medication were instructed to avoid green leafy vegetables (rich in vitamin K) during their anticoagulation treatment.

Adherence to warfarin treatment

Possible causes of non-adherence to anticoagulation treatment were documented in 6.6 % of the studied population and the most common was missing doses (4 of 6 possible causes) and the rest is related to availability of the product. Three of four patients with documented non-adherence had a nontherapeutic INR range.

Table 4 Types of drugs concurrently prescribed with warfarin known to have interaction and their potential effect on INR values ($n = 91$)

Drugs	Effect on INR	Severity
Norfloxacin, Metronidazole, Clarithromycin	Increase	Major
Rifampin	Decrease	Major
Isoniazid, Omeprazole, Tramadol, Ceftriaxone, Cimetidine, Allopurinol, Azithromycin	Increase	Moderate
Nevirapine, Neurobion, Mercaptopurine	Decrease	Moderate
Efavirenz, Hydrocortisone, Prednisolone	Increase/ Decrease	Moderate
Methotrexate, Vincristine, Furosemide, Simvastatin	Increase	Minor
Hydrochlorothiazide	Decrease	Minor

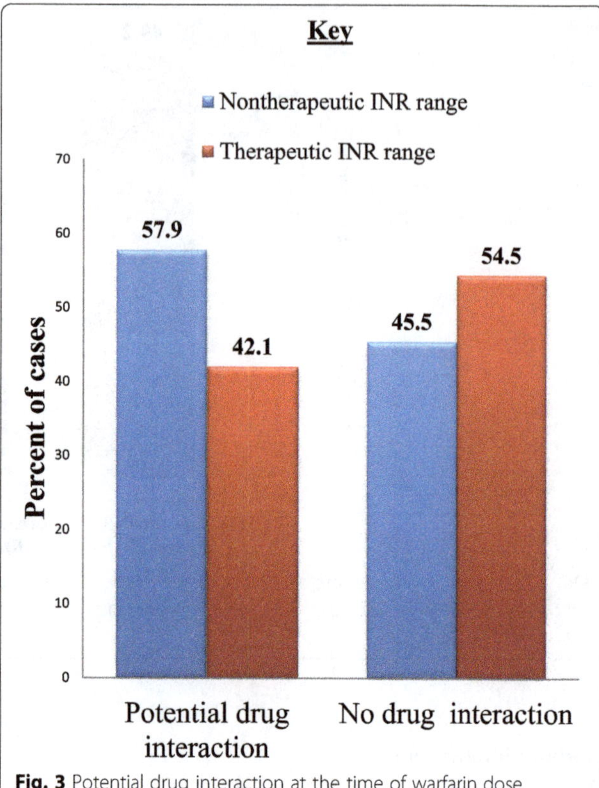

Fig. 3 Potential drug interaction at the time of warfarin dose adjustment and consequent INR value ($n = 41$)

ADR associated with warfarin therapy

About 9 % of patients who were on anticoagulation medication were documented to experience minor bleeding events (Fig. 4).

Discussions

Warfarin dose adjustment was performed for nontherapeutic INR values (more than 66 % of total INR values). Among these, warfarin dose was decreased in 3.4 % of subtherapeutic INRs and increased in 4.2 % of supratherapeutic INR ranges, although there was no clear reason documented for such paradox. In addition, the dose adjustments of only 13.4 % of nontherapeutic INRs were dependent on the recent INR values and cumulative weekly doses of warfarin, as recommended by ACCP guideline [5]. These imply that, most of anticoagulation management might have done by clinical evaluation of the patients' conditions. Although this approach have paramount importance, it would be much better if supported by available valid guidelines. Such practices might not allow someone to know the direct effect of changes in medication dose and might result in suboptimal quality

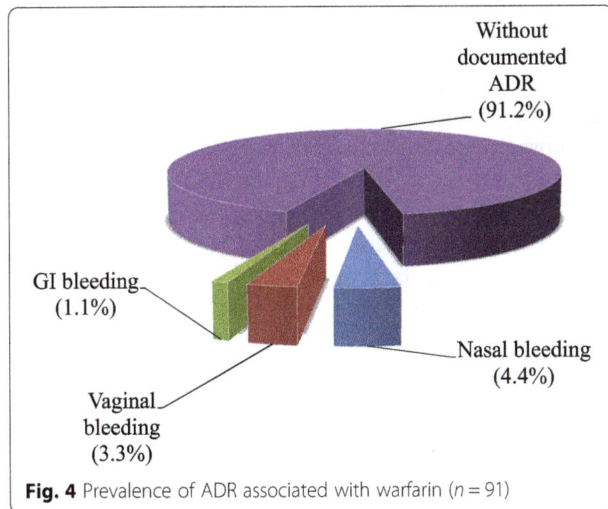

Fig. 4 Prevalence of ADR associated with warfarin ($n = 91$)

of anticoagulation management. This could be demonstrated by the low time patients stay in therapeutic INR range (33.5 %). Hence, the percentage of INRs in therapeutic range highly depends on the quality of dose management [5].

Among patients for which analysis of the effect of warfarin dose on the value of INR values was performed, nearly 10 % of INR values for which warfarin dosage had been adjusted were in the therapeutic range. The key informants stated that although dosage changes should be done based on the state of INR, patients' conditions were taken into account. For example, for patients with certain conditions such as peptic ulcer and other conditions of bleeding events, the risk-benefit ratio would be considered and dosage changes might be done accordingly, even if the INR values were within the therapeutic range. According to other studies, dosage change is not recommended for therapeutic INR values [8], for a single INR that is slightly out of range [9, 10]. ACCP guidelines also do not support dosage change for therapeutic INRs [5]. Therefore, it is important to consider the standard guidelines while deciding to modify/adjust the maintenance anticoagulant doses.

Warfarin weekly dose change ranged between 16 to 100 % for recent subtherapeutic INRs, 16 to 50 % for therapeutic and 11 to 66 % for overtherapeutic INRs. But, according to ACCP guidelines, patients whose INR is just outside the therapeutic range can be managed by either adjusting the dose up or down in increments of 5 to 20 % [5]. Other studies also recommended that dosage changes should be altered by the total weekly dose of 5 to 20 % [8, 9, 11, 12]. Variability in the amount or percentage of warfarin dosage change might be due to the absence of local dosing protocol or failure to adhere to the available international guideline. It is important to adhere to the international standard treatment guidelines where there are no local treatment protocols while deciding to modify/adjust the maintenance anticoagulant dosages for nontherapeutic INR values. Institutional protocols for dosing decisions during maintenance VKA therapy should be developed and used accordingly in order to minimize consequences of DRPs in patients with DVT.

In the present study, change in warfarin dose up or down showed significant linear relationship with consequent INR values ($p = 0.000$). Accordingly, about 42 % of the variations in INR values were accounted for by warfarin dosage change. As a result, percentage of weekly warfarin dosage reduction (up to 70 %) was related to the consequent nontherapeutic low INR values. Therefore, dose reductions might be one of the reasons for low INRs and dosage changes especially higher dose reductions could be major DRPs that might expose the patients to high risk of recurrent thrombosis complications. As evident from the current finding, more than 12 % were presented with significantly under-therapeutic INR range (INR less than 1.5) at weekly warfarin dose reduction of 21–70 %. This finding is in agreement with reports of different studies that, response to a previous change in warfarin dosage was the cause of under-anticoagulation [13] and low INR values [10, 14]. Therefore, high dosage changes greater than 20 % are not advisable and should be avoided in order to minimize complications such as recurrent thrombosis. But, there might be exceptions that need special considerations of higher doses including concurrent medications such as amiodarone and rifampin which need a total weekly dose reduction and increment of 50 %, respectively [15].

Five (12.2 %) patients presented with over-therapeutic INRs at weekly warfarin dosage increment ranging from 11 to 100 %. This might increase the risk of overanticoagulation and thus expose the patients to high risk of bleeding complications as supported by different studies [13, 16]. Dosage increment greater than 20 % should be avoided especially as the dosages become increased more than 40 % the risks might be more. There were 3 cases (7.3 %) in the current study that presented with an INR value greater than 4.0 at greater than 40 % dosage increment. It was not possible to say anything about these patients, as there were no documented adverse events except for some minor undesirable effects (9 %) such as nasal and vaginal bleeding, which were said to be not related to the above factor. But, INR values greater than 3.3 were recorded at the time of these bleeding events although there was no recent dose adjustment done that allows us to correlate with warfarin overdose. Nevertheless, the risk of bleeding should be an issue of utmost importance. Therefore, these trends should be guided by valid treatment guidelines in order to improve clinical outcomes and minimize unwanted complications due to anticoagulant drug overdose.

As the findings of this study showed, there had been potential interactions that could make INR to fall out of the therapeutic range. About 42 % of patients received warfarin concomitantly with 18 other medications that have potentially major or moderate interaction with warfarin. For more than 46 % (19/41) of patients, co-administration was made at the time of dosage adjustment. The fact that about 58 % of patients, in which drug-interaction was a concern, had non-therapeutic INR range suggests that whenever there is a need for dosage changes in patients with DVT the concurrent medications should be considered. It was stated that for most interactions a total weekly dose adjustment of either an increase or decrease of 30 % is needed except for certain drugs such as amiodarone and rifampin which need a total weekly dose reduction and increment of 50 %, respectively [15]. But, in the present study, both dose reductions and increments were done up to 50 % regardless of the type of concurrent medications and this might expose the patients to the risk of recurrent or hemorrhage complications.

Norfloxacin and metronidazole were prescribed for only one and two patients who were on warfarin, respectively. In both cases an increased INR value was showed but no apparent risk of bleeding since the increment was from low to therapeutic INR range. But one study reported that, metronidazole had shown an impact on bleeding risk when used with warfarin concomitantly [17]. In another study, all patients who received quinolone antibiotics concomitantly with warfarin had INR values above 3.5, suggesting drug-induced warfarin potentiation [18]. Rifampin was prescribed for 2 patients. Out of these, one patient's INR was dropped from 1.31 to 1.27 following warfarin increment of 33 % and the other patient's INR increased from 1.33 to 2.1 following warfarin increment of 50 %, suggesting major drug-drug interaction and need of large increment of warfarin dose. This is supported by a practice guideline [15], which stated that for rifampin interactions a cumulative weekly dose of warfarin increment of 50 % is needed. Whenever there is a need of anticoagulant dosage changes in patients with DVT, changes in concurrent medications especially those with major interactions with VKAs should be considered.

Tramadol was reported to increase the risk of bleeding [17]. In the present study, this drug was prescribed for 17 patients who were on warfarin therapy. Among these, INR values of 6 patients were increased to supratherapeutic ranges suggesting tramadol-induced warfarin potentiation but difficult to generalize since warfarin dose increment of 20–50 % was performed during this time. In addition, more than 41 % of tramadol prescriptions were written on a PRN (as required) basis without specified maximum daily doses. This might contribute to unintentional administration of over-dosage (more than 400 mg per day) and might also lead to increased effect of warfarin and its bleeding risk. Thus, it would be helpful to write full dosage schedule including the maximum daily dosage whenever medications are ordered especially when prescribed on the basis of PRN.

Vitamin K is known to reverse warfarin's pharmacologic activity, and many foods containing sufficient vitamin K reduce the anticoagulation effect of warfarin if a patient consumes them in large portions or repetitively within a short period of time. The present study showed that more than 12 % were instructed to avoid green leafy vegetables (rich in vitamin K) during their anticoagulation treatment. Responses from key informants regarding such practice were taken. Some of them suggested that unexplained changes in INR records might force to consider absolute avoidance of diets rich in vitamin K. This was not in agreement with other report that suggested considering abrupt changes rather than avoidance [19]. In the contrary, other informants said this was not the practice and strongly underlined to a consistent and moderate intake of such foods, as also supported by different studies [20, 21]. One study revealed that changes in dietary vitamin K intake were among the causes of INRs below 2.0 and above 4.0 [13]. Others also recommended that patients should be encouraged to maintain consistency in their vitamin K intake and should strive to meet the recommended dietary allowance for vitamin K [19, 21] because dietary content or extent of absorption of vitamin K might have effect on warfarin [16]. Patients should be given a list of vitamin K rich foods and encouraged to maintain consistency in their vitamin K intake rather than absolute avoidance and alternative sources of vitamin K, such as multivitamins and nutritional supplements should also be considered.

It is difficult to assess actual prevalence of patient non-adherence from medical charts. Regardless of this, some possible causes of non-adherence were documented in 6.6 % of studied population and the most common was missing doses. Although three of four patients with documented non-adherence had a nontherapeutic INR range, the low number of these cases compared to patients without non-adherence did not allow us to establish a sound association between non-adherence and INR values. But literature showed that, noncompliance was the cause of under-anticoagulation [13, 14]. Ensuring the patients' understanding about the benefits of adhering to the prescribed medications and the consequences of non-adherence to treatments is crucial in order to achieve the desired therapeutic goals. Hence patient compliance can influence the frequency of long-term INR monitoring [17].

Conclusion

In the present study, although young adults were among the commonly affected age groups, VTE is becoming the major cause of concern in all age groups. Managing patients with VTE is more complicated and prone to different DRPs for several reasons, including variable nature of anticoagulants such as warfarin, co morbidities, concurrent medications and other factors related to patients. In this study, different DRPs were identified and the most frequent were sub-therapeutic doses, over-therapeutic doses, and potential drug interactions, highlighting the importance of considering drugs as a possible cause of health problems and the need for their rational use. Warfarin dose adjustment can complicate the treatment course because it demands the knowledge of different factors. Thus, higher dosage changes were among the reasons for non-therapeutic INR values as one of the major DRPs that might expose patients to high risk of recurrent and hemorrhagic complications.

Abbreviations

ACCP: American College of Chest Physicians; ADR: adverse drug reaction; DRP: drug-related problem; DVT: deep vein thrombosis; FIP: International Pharmaceutical Federation; INR: International Normalized Ratio; OR: odds ratio; PT: prothrombin time; TASH: Tikur Anbessa Specialized Hospital; VKA: vitamin K antagonist; VTE: venous thromboembolism; WHO: World Health Organization.

Competing interests

The authors declare that they have no competing interests.

Authors' contributions

FBD was the principal investigator who conceived and designed the study; extracted, analyzed and interpreted the data and drafted the manuscript. EE supervised the whole research, guided the conception and design of the study and also assisted with manuscript preparation. FT has participated in the interpretation of the clinical data. All authors read and approved the final manuscript.

Acknowledgements

This study was supported by Jimma University and Addis Ababa University. We would like to acknowledge Nurse Getu Regassa for collecting the data and other nurses who were working in the hematology unit of TASH for their cooperation in facilitating the process of data collection.

Author details

[1]Department of Pharmacy, College of Health Sciences, Jimma University, P.O. Box 378, Jimma, Ethiopia. [2]Department of Internal Medicine, Tikur Anbessa specialized hospital, Addis Ababa University, Addis Ababa, Ethiopia. [3]Department of Pharmacology and Clinical Pharmacy, School of Pharmacy, College of Health Sciences, Addis Ababa University, P.O. Box 1176, Addis Ababa, Ethiopia.

References

1. WHO and FIP. Developing Pharmacy Practice: A focus on patient care-Handbook. Geneva: WHO; 2006. The Hague: FIP.
2. Nickerson A, MacKinnon J, Roberts N, Saulnier L. Drug-Therapy Problems, Inconsistencies and Omissions Identified During a Medication Reconciliation and Seamless Care Service. Healthc Q. 2005;8(Sp):65–72.
3. Domino FJ. The Five-Minute Clinical Consult 2011. 19th ed. Philadelphia: Lippincott Williams & Wilkins; 2010.
4. White PJ. Patient factors that influence warfarin dose response. J Pharm Pract. 2010;23(3):194–204.
5. Ansell J, Hirsh J, Hylek E, Jacobson A, Crowther M, Palareti G. Pharmacology and Management of the Vitamin K Antagonists: American College of Chest Physicians Evidence-Based Clinical Practice Guidelines, 8th Edition. Chest. 2008;133(Suppl):160S–98S.
6. Karen B. Stockley's Drug Interactions 2010 Pocket Companion. London: Pharmaceutical press; 2010.
7. Drug Interactions Checker [http://www.drugs.com/drug-interactions/warfarin.html]. Accessed 21 June 2013.
8. Van Spall HG, Wallentin L, Yusuf S, Eikelboom JW, Nieuwlaat R, Yang S, et al. Variation in warfarin dose adjustment practice is responsible for differences in the quality of anticoagulation control between centers and countries: an analysis of patients receiving warfarin in the randomized evaluation of long-term anticoagulation therapy (RE-LY) trial. Circulation. 2012;126(19):2309–16.
9. Gage BF, Fihn SD, White RH. Management and dosing of warfarin therapy. Am J Med. 2000;109(6):481–8.
10. Banet GA, Waterman AD, Milligan PE, Gatchel SK, Gage BF. Warfarin dose reduction vs. watchful waiting for mild elevations in the international normalized ratio. Chest. 2003;123(2):499–503.
11. BC Guideline warfarin therapy management [http://www2.gov.bc.ca/gov/content/health/practitioner-professional-resources/bc-guidelines/warfarin-therapy]. Accessed 17 July 2013.
12. American Society of Hematology. 2011 Clinical Practice Guide on Anticoagulant Dosing and Management of Anticoagulant-Associated Bleeding Complications in Adults [http://www.hematology.org/Clinicians/Guidelines-Quality/Quick-Ref/525.aspx]. Accessed 17 July 2013
13. Wittkowsky AK, Devine EB. Frequency and causes of over-anticoagulation and under-anticoagulation in patients treated with warfarin. Pharmacotherapy. 2004;24(10):1311–6.
14. Adam J, Ozonoff A, Grant RW, Lori E, Elaine M. Epidemiology of Subtherapeutic Anticoagulation in the United States. Circ Cardiovasc Qual Outcomes. 2009;2:591–7.
15. Warfarin Management - Adult - Ambulatory Clinical Practice Guideline [http://www.uwhealth.org/files/uwhealth/docs/pdf2/Ambulatory_Warfarin_Guideline.pdf]. Accessed 18 July 2013.
16. Alex S, Ross I, Beng H, Paul A. Consensus Guidelines for Warfarin Therapy. Med J Aust. 2000;172(12):600–5.
17. Holbrook A, Schulman S, Witt DM, Vandvik PO, Fish J, Kovacs MJ, et al. Evidence-Based Management of Anticoagulant Therapy: Antithrombotic Therapy and Prevention of Thrombosis, 9th ed: American College of Chest Physicians Evidence-Based Clinical Practice Guidelines. Chest. 2012;141(2_suppl):e152S–84S.
18. Njovane XW, Fasinu PS, Rosenkranz B. Comparative evaluation of warfarin utilization in two primary healthcare clinics in the Cape Town area. Cardiovasc J Afr. 2013;24(2):19–23.
19. Haines ST, Witt DM, Nutescu EA. Venous thromboembolism. In: Dipiro JT, Talbert RL, Yee GC, Matzke GR, Wells BG, Posey LM, editors. Pharmacotherapy: a pathophysiologic approach. 7th ed. New York: McGraw Hill Medical; 2008. p. 331–71.
20. Nutescu A, Shapiro L, Ibrahim S, West P. Warfarin and its interactions with foods, herbs and other dietary supplements. Expert Opin Drug Saf. 2006;5(3):433–51.
21. Hylek EM. Oral anticoagulants. Pharmacologic issues for use in the elderly. Clin Geriatr Med. 2001;17(1):1–13.

15

Comparative study of sickle cell anemia and hemoglobin SC disease: clinical characterization, laboratory biomarkers and genetic profiles

Milena Magalhães Aleluia[1,2], Teresa Cristina Cardoso Fonseca[3,4], Regiana Quinto Souza[3,4], Fábia Idalina Neves[3], Caroline Conceição da Guarda[1,2], Rayra Pereira Santiago[1,2], Bruna Laís Almeida Cunha[2], Camylla Villas Boas Figueiredo[1,2], Sânzio Silva Santana[1,2], Silvana Sousa da Paz[1], Júnia Raquel Dutra Ferreira[1,2], Bruno Antônio Veloso Cerqueira[5] and Marilda de Souza Gonçalves[1,2*]

Abstract

Background: In this study, we evaluate the association of different clinical profiles, laboratory and genetic biomarkers in patients with sickle cell anemia (SCA) and hemoglobin SC disease (HbSC) in attempt to characterize the sickle cell disease (SCD) genotypes.

Methods: We conducted a cross-sectional study from 2013 to 2014 in 200 SCD individuals (141 with SCA; 59 with HbSC) and analyzed demographic data to characterize the study population. In addition, we determined the association of hematological, biochemical and genetic markers including the β^S-globin gene haplotypes and the 3.7 Kb deletion of α-thalassemia ($-\alpha^{3.7Kb}$-thal), as well as the occurrence of clinical events in both SCD genotypes.

Results: Laboratory parameters showed a hemolytic profile associated with endothelial dysfunction in SCA individuals; however, the HbSC genotype was more associated with increased blood viscosity and inflammatory conditions. The BEN haplotype was the most frequently observed and was associated with elevated fetal hemoglobin (HbF) and low S hemoglobin (HbS). The $-\alpha^{3.7Kb}$-thal prevalence was 0.09 (9%), and it was associated with elevated hemoglobin and hematocrit concentrations. Clinical events were more frequent in SCA patients.

Conclusions: Our data emphasize the differences between SCA and HbSC patients based on laboratory parameters and the clinical and genetic profile of both genotypes.

Keywords: Sickle cell anemia, Hemoglobin SC disease, Biomarkers, Genetic profile

Background

Sickle cell disease (SCD) is a group of inherited diseases that includes sickle cell anemia (SCA), which is the homozygous state of the beta S (β^S) allele and the most severe SCD genotype. Likewise, the heterozygous state of the β^S allele is characterized by the presence of hemoglobin S (HbS) associated with changes in the structure or synthesis of the other globin chain and consists of a group of less severe SCD, including hemoglobin SC disease (HbSC). SCD has important implications for public health, as both worldwide incidence and prevalence are high, which reinforces it as a significant social problem in many countries [1, 2]. The clinical diversity of SCD includes hemolytic and vaso-occlusive episodes (VOE), infections, stroke, acute chest syndrome (ACS), pulmonary hypertension, multiple organ dysfunctions and other complications [3]. Several factors have been shown to modulate the clinical manifestations of SCD including hematological, biochemical, inflammatory and genetic

* Correspondence: mari@bahia.fiocruz.br
[1]Laboratório de Hematologia e Genética Computacional, Instituto Gonçalo Moniz - IGM, Fundação Oswaldo Cruz (Fiocruz), Rua Waldemar Falcão, 121, Candeal, Salvador, Bahia CEP 40296-710, Brazil
[2]Universidade Federal da Bahia (UFBA), Salvador, Bahia, Brazil
Full list of author information is available at the end of the article

markers, as well as environmental, sociodemographic, and socioeconomic characteristics [3, 4].

With respect to the genetic markers, SCA patients can also be carriers of one or more gene determinants such as the 3.7 Kb deletion of α-globin chain in α-thalassemia ($-\alpha^{3.7Kb}$-thal). In Afro-descendants, the heterozygous ($-\alpha/\alpha\alpha$) or homozygous ($-\alpha/-\alpha$) $-\alpha^{3.7Kb}$-thal genotype in SCA individuals is associated with a reduction in HbS concentration, which consequently lowers hemoglobin polymerization and cell damage and improves the hemolysis profile [5, 6]. In addition, this association promotes changes in hematological and biochemical parameters of SCA [5–7].

β^S globin gene haplotypes are constituted of polymorphisms in the β^S globin gene cluster, which are associated with specific levels of fetal hemoglobin (HbF), contributing to phenotypic diversity in SCA patients [8–10]. There are five main haplotypes, named Benin (BEN), Central African Republic (CAR), Senegal (SEN), Arab-Indian, and Cameroon (CAM), according to their geographical origin and ethnic groups [9, 11].

Considering the wide range of variability in the severity of SCA and HbSC individuals, laboratory biomarkers associated to hemolysis such as reticulocyte count and serum LDH, in addition to biomarkers of blood viscosity such as hemoglobin and hematocrit concentration, are important to perform a laboratorial characterization of the patients as well as to understand the disease physiopathology [12]. HbF levels, inflammatory response and endothelial dysfunction play a pivotal role in differentiating SCD sub-phenotypes [12, 13].

The severity of SCD arises from several clinical complications that influence each individual's immunity. Therefore, the use of medication, prophylactic vaccines and practicing healthy habits are recommended [14, 15]. However, another important point is the cost to the health care system and how much the government pays for each patient with SCD, including hospital admissions and readmissions, therapy and the spectrum of comorbidities that may require years of follow-up in different specialists [15, 16].

In this study, we investigated the association of different clinical manifestations, laboratory biomarkers and genetic profiles in patients with SCA and HbSC to establish parameters that highlight sub-phenotypes differences in these SCD genotypes.

Methods

Subjects

We conducted a cross-sectional study from 2013 to 2014 at the Itabuna Reference Center for Sickle Cell Disease in Itabuna, Bahia, Brazil, that develop the follow-up of 536 SCD patients from the south coast, extreme south and southwest regions of Bahia. Considering the cross-sectional nature of the study, the sample size calculation was performed on StatCalc, Epi Info, v.6.04 with a power of 95% and two-sided confidence level of 95%. Thus, we identify that a sample-size of 200 individuals with SCD would be a significant representation of the population, taking account a frequency of 1/650 children with SCD in Bahia state. Our sample size was 200 SCD patients (141 with SCA and 59 with HbSC) with a mean age of 16.06 ± 11.83 years and a median age of 13 years (range: 1–61 years). Clinical data were collected from the medical records. Each patient enrolled in the study was in a steady state, had not received a blood transfusion in the last six months and were not taking hydroxyurea (HU). Informed consent form was obtained from all adult participants as well as parents or guardians of the children also have assigned the informed consent form prior to the enrollment in the study. The study protocol was approved by the Ethics Research Board of the Gonçalo Moniz Institute of the Oswaldo Cruz Foundation (IGM-FIOCRUZ-BA) following the ethical principles of the Declaration of Helsinki of 1975 and its revision.

Hematological and biochemical parameters

Hematological analyses were carried out using Sysmex KX-21 N™ Automated Hematology Analyzer (Sysmex Corporation, Tokyo, Japan). Serum lipids and lipoproteins were analyzed using fully automated equipment (Cobas, Roche Diagnostics, Salt Lake City, Utah, USA). Hemoglobin profiles and HbF concentration were determined using High Performance Liquid Chromatography (HPLC, VARIANT I-Bio-Rad, CA, USA). Nitric oxide metabolites (NOm) were determined using the Griess reaction, as previously described [17].

Genetic analysis

Genomic DNA was extracted from leukocytes using a QIAamp® DNA Extraction Kit (Qiagen, Hilden, Germany) following the manufacturer's instructions. β^S globin gene cluster haplotypes were investigated using polymerase chain reaction (PCR) followed by restriction fragment length polymorphism (RFLP). The primers used detecting the β^S globin gene cluster haplotypes are: 5′γ^G gene 5′-AACTGTTGCTTTATAGGATTTT-3′ and 3′-AGGAG CTTATTGATAACTCAGAC-5′; γ^G /γ^A gene 5′-AAGTG TGGAGTGTGCACATGA-3′ and 3′-TGCTGCTAATGC TTCATTACAA-5′; γ^G /γ^A gene 5′- TGCTGCTAATG CTTCATTACAA-3′ and 3′-TAAATGAGGAGCATGCA CACAC-5′; Ψβ gene 5′-GAACAGAAGTTGAGATAGA GA-3′ and 3′-ACTCAGTGGTCTTGTGGGCT-5′; 3′Ψβ gene 5′-TCTGCATTTGACTCTGTTAGC-3′ and 3′-GG ACCCTAACTGATATAACTA-5′ [10, 18]. Allele-specific PCR was used to investigate the $-\alpha^{3.7Kb}$-thal deletion presence [19]. All analyses were performed in the Anemia Research Laboratory at the Federal University of Bahia and Laboratory of Hematology, Genetics and Computational Biology at the IGM-FIOCRUZ-BA.

Statistical analysis

Baseline values of selected variables were summarized as the mean and stratified according to percentile. Distribution of the quantitative variables was analyzed using Shapiro-Wilk test. Quantitative variables were compared between two groups using the t-test for data with a parametric distribution and the Mann-Whitney test for non-parametric data. The Chi-square test and Fisher exact test were used to analyze the qualitative or categorical variables. Statistical analyses were performed using the Statistical Package for the Social Sciences (SPSS) version 20.0 software (IBM, New York, NY, USA), and P values <0.05 were considered significant.

Results

In our study, we analyzed patients with SCA and HbSC and have identified that the majority of the SCD patients were female (52.0%; 104/200) and were aged either between 6 and 10 years (22.0%; 44/200) or 21 and 30 years (20.0%; 40/200). As recommended by the Brazilian Institute of Geography and Statistics the ethnicity was self-declared and the majority of patients were African derived people (89.0%; 178/200) (Table 1). With respect to patients' educational level, the frequency of uneducated or partially completed elementary school was 12.0% (24/200) in the age group of 11 to 15 years old, and 8.5% (17/200) in the age group older than 16 years old. In addition, in the age group older than 16 years old we also observed a frequency of 20.0% (40/200) of the patients only completed elementary school (Table 1). The age at first diagnosis of SCD was younger than 6 months of age in the majority of the patients (38.0%; 76/200), and 68 patients in this group were diagnosed through the newborn screening. In addition, 25.0% of the patients were diagnosed between the age of 7 months and 4 years (50/200) and 17.0% were diagnosed between the ages of 5 and 9 years (34/200) (Table 1). When we analyzed the number of patients who have any relatives with SCD, we found that 31.5% (63/200) had a sibling with the disease, and 28.5% (57/200) had four or more sibling with SCD (Table 1).

SCD patients were from several cities belonging to administrative regions, with 78.0% from the south coast of Bahia, 14.5% from the extreme south of Bahia, and 7.5% from the southwest of Bahia (Fig. 1). On the south coast, the city of Itabuna had the highest number of SCD patients, which represented 38.5% (77/200) of the study population, followed by Eunapólis, Ilhéus, Porto Seguro, and Camacan, which had 6.0% (12/200), 6.0% (12/200),

Table 1 Characterization of SCD patients followed by the Reference Center in the South of Bahia, Brazil

Age (years)	N (%)	Sex	N (%)	Ethnicity	N (%)	Region of Origin		N (%)
≤ 5	36 (18.0)	Female	104 (52.0)	Caucasian	13 (6.5)	South Coast		156 (78.0)
6 to 10	44 (22.0)	Male	96 (48.0)	African	178 (89.0)	Extreme South		29 (14.5)
11 to 15	37 (18.5)			Asian	9 (4.5)	Southwest		15 (7.5)
16 to 20	21 (10.5)							
21 to 30	40 (20.0)							
≥ 31	22 (11.0)							
Number of siblings with SCD	N (%)	Age at 1st Diagnosis	N (%)	Relatives with SCD	N (%)	Education (by age group)		N (%)
0	21 (10.5)	≤ 6 months	76 (38.0)	None	100 (50.0)	≤ 5	Uneducated or incomplete	36 (18.0)
1	47 (23.5)	7 months to 4 years	50 (25.0)	Father	4 (2.0)		elementary school	
2	42 (21.0)	5 to 9 years	34 (17.0)	Mother	3 (1.5)	6 to 10	Uneducated or incomplete	34 (17.0)
3	33 (16.5)	10 to 14 years	11 (5.5)	Brother	63 (31.5)		elementary school	
4 or More	57 (28.5)	15 to 17 years	15 (7.5)	Cousin	22 (11.0)		Elementary school	10 (5.0)
		≥ 17 years	14 (7.0)	Aunt and Uncle	1 (0.5)	11 to 15	Uneducated or incomplete	24 (12.0)
				Nephews	2 (1.0)		elementary school	
				Not heard	5 (2.5)		Elementary school	13 (6.5)
				Inform		≥ 16	Uneducated or incomplete	17 (8.5)
							elementary school	
							Elementary school	25 (12.5)
							High School	40 (20.0)
							University	1 (0.5)

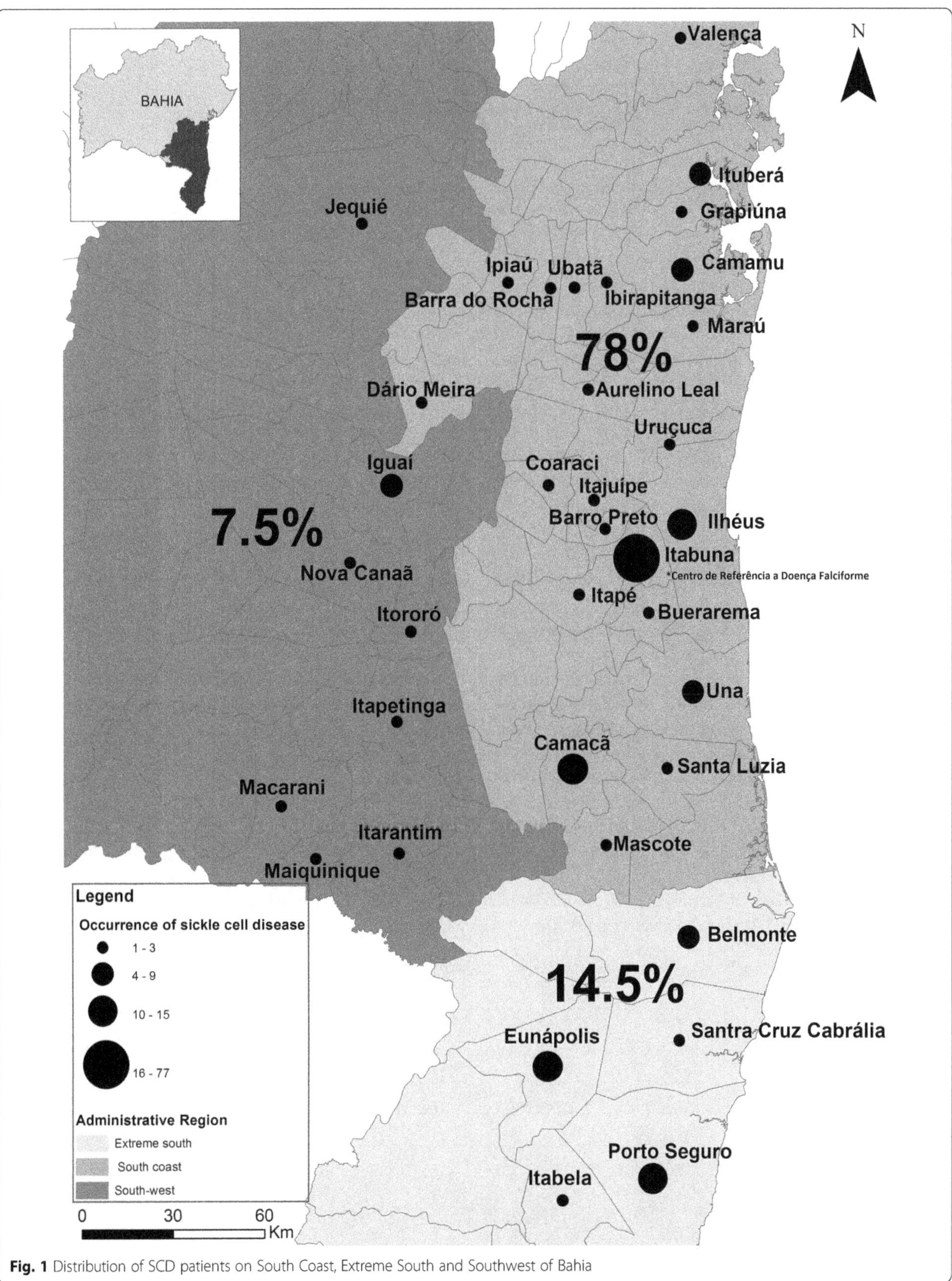

Fig. 1 Distribution of SCD patients on South Coast, Extreme South and Southwest of Bahia

5.5% (11/200), and 5.0% (10/200) of the SCD patients respectively.

We found that BEN haplotype (47.9%; 135/282) was the predominant haplotype in SCA patients, followed by CAR haplotype (45.0%; 127/282), and atypical haplotype (7.1%; 20/282). In the HbSC patients, 54.2% had BEN haplotype (32/59) and 45.8% had CAR haplotype (27/59). Regarding the genotype of the β^S globin gene cluster haplotypes among the SCA patients, 41.2% (58/141) had BEN/CAR genotype, followed by CAR/CAR genotype (22.7%; 32/141) and BEN/BEN genotype (24.8%; 35/141). Among the SCA patients, we found that 5.0% had BEN/Atypical genotype (7/141), 3.5% had CAR/Atypical genotype (5/141), and 2.8% the atypical genotype (4/141). When we analyzed the β^C globin gene cluster haplotypes associated to the HbSC, we found that 5.1% (3/59) had the BEN II genotype, 35.6% (21/59) had the CAR I genotype, 47.4% (28/59) had the BEN I genotype, 8.5% (5/59) had the CAR III genotype, 1.7% (1/59) had the CAR II genotype, and 1.7% (1/59) had the BEN III genotype (Table 2). The haplotypes are known to modulate HbF levels, thus, we analyzed 99 patients with SCA and 52 patients with HbSC who had no history of HU therapy and absence of the CAR haplotype lead to elevated HbF levels (Table 3).

We found that 168 patients had the wild type of the α-genotype and that 32 patients had the deletion ($-\alpha^{3.7Kb}$-thal). In this group, we observed 4 patients with the homozygous genotype (−α/−α) and 28 patients with the heterozygous genotype (−α/α) (Table 2). When we evaluated 98 patients with SCA and 52 patients with HbSC who had no history of HU therapy, we have found that hemoglobin and hematocrit concentrations were high and that mean cell volume (MCV) and mean corpuscular hemoglobin (MCH) were low in the presence of the $\alpha^{3.7Kb}$-thal in both SCD genotypes (Table 3).

Among the biomarkers of hemolysis, the red blood cell (RBC) count ($p < 0.001$), hemoglobin ($p < 0.001$) and hematocrit concentrations ($p < 0.001$) were low, and MCV ($p < 0.001$), MCH ($p < 0.001$) concentration and red blood cell distribution width (RDW) ($p < 0.001$) were high in SCA patients (Table 4). Additionally, in the same group, we found that the levels of total ($p < 0.001$), direct ($p < 0.001$) and indirect ($p < 0.001$) bilirubin, lactate dehydrogenase (LDH) ($p < 0.001$), NOm ($p = 0.047$) and reticulocyte count ($p < 0.001$) were high (Table 3). We also found that the total white blood cell (WBC) ($p < 0.001$), eosinophil ($p = 0.007$), lymphocyte ($p < 0.001$) and monocyte ($p = 0.003$) counts were high in SCA patients (Table 4). The platelet count was increased in SCA patients ($p < 0.001$). Conversely, we observed low levels of total cholesterol ($p = 0.012$) and high-density lipoprotein cholesterol (HDL-C) ($p < 0.001$) in these patients (Table 4).

We analyzed the distribution of clinical events in the different SCD genotypes (SCA and HbSC) with no history of HU therapy, and we found that hospitalization was strongly associated with the SCA genotype (91.8%; 90/98) ($p = 0.001$) (Table 5).

With regard to the use of prophylactic penicillin, we identified that 87.5% (70/80) of SCD pediatric patients received prophylactic penicillin therapy. Following the use of prophylactic penicillin therapy, 92.5% (185/200) of SCD patients in all age groups reported the use of folic acid everyday ($p = 0.046$). HU therapy was used by 25.0% (50/200) of SCD patients all older than 6 years and was more frequently used in patients aged 11 to 31 years ($p < 0.001$).

Discussion

The present study analyzed the laboratory, genetic, clinical and demographic characteristics of 200 SCD patients who were followed at the Reference Center living in the south of Bahia in the northeast of Brazil.

We observed low educational level in patients with SCD, which is in accordance with findings from studies

Table 2 Distribution of the genotypes and alleles of the β^S globin haplotype and $-\alpha^{3.7Kb}$-thalassemia in SCD

β^S globin Genotype				$-\alpha^{3.7Kb}$-Thalassemia Genotype			
HbSC	% (*N* = 59)	SCA	% (*N* = 141)	HbSC	% (N = 59)	SCA	% (N = 141)
BEN II	5.1 (3)	BEN/BEN	24.8 (35)	Absence	84.7 (50)	Absence	83.7 (118)
CAR I	35.6 (21)	BEN/CAR	41.2 (58)	Heterozygous	13.6 (8)	Heterozygous	14.2 (20)
BEN I	47.4 (28)	CAR/CAR	22.7 (32)	Homozygous	1.7 (1)	Homozygous	2.1 (3)
CAR III	8.5 (5)	BEN/Atypical	5.0 (7)				
CAR II	1.7 (1)	CAR/Atypical	3.5 (5)				
BEN III	1.7 (1)	Atypical	2.8 (4)				
β^S globin Haplotype in HbSC		β^S globin Haplotype in SCA		Frequency of $-\alpha^{3.7Kb}$-Thalassemia chromosome in SCD			
BEN	54.2 (32/59)	BEN	47.9 (135/282)	Presence 0.09 (36/400)			
CAR	45.8 (27/59)	CAR	45.0 (127/282)				
		Atypical	7.1 (20/282)				

Table 3 Distribution of the median (25th – 75th) hematological data among the β^S globin haplotypes and -α$^{3.7Kb}$-thalassemia

β^S globin Haplotype				-α$^{3.7Kb}$-Thalassemia			
HbSC (N = 52)		SCA (N = 99)		HbSC (N = 52)		SCA (N = 99)	
Median (25th – 75th)	Median (25th – 75th)	Median (25th – 75th)	Median (25th – 75th)	Median (25th – 75th)	Median (25th – 75th)	Median (25th – 75th)	Median (25th – 75th)
Absence CAR N = 26	Presence CAR N = 26	Absence CAR N = 29	Presence CAR N = 70	Absence -α$^{3.7Kb}$ N = 43	Presence -α$^{3.7Kb}$ N = 9	Absence -α$^{3.7Kb}$ N = 85	Presence -α$^{3.7Kb}$ N = 14
HbS		**HbS**		**Hb**		**Hb**	
50.0 (48.1–51.4)	50.6 (49.5–51.6)	83.0 (76.0–88.3)	88.3 (83.5–91.7)	10.8 (10.1–11.6)	10.9 (9.9–12.4)	7.6 (7.1–8.3)	8.2 (7.3–8.8)
$p = 0.301$		**$p = 0.004$**		$p = 0.735$		$p = 0.427$	
HbF		**HbF**		**Ht**		**Ht**	
1.9 (0.8–4.5)	1.3 (0.7–3.2)	12.9 (7.5–18.3)	7.7 (4.1–11.5)	30.7 (28.7–32.5)	31.7 (28.0–34.1)	21.7 (19.9–24.1)	23.8 (21.4–25.5)
$p = 0.181$		**$p = 0.005$**		$p = 0.961$		$p = 0.252$	
				MCV		**MCV**	
				76.1 (71.5–80.1)	71.6 (67.3–72.4)	88.0 (83.6–93.2)	80.3 (76.3–83.1)
				$p = 0.018$		**$p < 0.001$**	
				MCH		**MCH**	
				27.2 (24.6–28.8)	25.0 (23.4–26.5)	30.8 (28.8–32.7)	27.7 (25.7–29.0)
				$p = 0.071$		**$p < 0.001$**	

Hb hemoglobin, *Ht* hematocrit, *MCV* mean cell volume, *MCH* mean corpuscular hemoglobin. Bold values indicate significance at $p < 0.05$; p-value obtained using Mann-Whitney

in the United States and other Brazilian regions [20, 21]. Another study observed that sociodemographic characteristics had no influence on the development of SCD complications; however, age, low socioeconomic class and education level were associated with anemic crisis in SCD [22, 23].

Among our patients 38.0% were diagnosed younger than 6 months of age, and 25.0% were diagnosed between 7 months and 4 years old, which is consistent with a delayed diagnosis. Newborn screening for SCD started in 2001 in Brazil when the National Newborn Screening Program (PNTN)/Guthrie test was founded to test for hemoglobinopathies [24], establishing the important early diagnosis of SCD. Newborn screening for hemoglobinopathies resulted in a reduction of mortality and clinical complications in SCD patients in Brazil, due to the therapeutic and clinical monitoring of the child since the birth [24].

The evaluation of the geographic distribution of the SCD patients included in our study showed high occurrence of SCD patients on the south coast of Bahia, additionally, the majority of the patients were from the city of Itabuna. Itabuna was initially settled in 1867 by cowboys from Sergipe, when they started to immigrate to Vitória da Conquista [25]. Sergipean immigrants, from a state close to Bahia, initiated holdings on the Cachoeira River banks during the same period that the Jesuits provided a catechesis to the *Pataxó, Guerren* and *Camacã* natives on farms [25]. African derived people coming from the Sergipe and Bahia backlands in 1850 were attracted to the wealth of the region and the possibility of working on the cocoa farms [25]. In addition, slaves originated from different African tribes and African regions were brought from South Africa to the port of Ilhéus during the slave trade period.

Interestingly, some of the historical aspects suggest the possibility of greater dispersion of the β^S allele in Itabuna. The predominant haplotype in SCA patients was BEN/CAR, as well as in HbSC patients was the haplotype BEN I followed by CAR I. According to the literature, in 1678–1814, approximately 39 of the 1770 ships that exported tobacco from Bahia went to Congo and Angola, where they captured Africans for slave labor, which represents the genetic contribution from the central Atlantic region of Africa [26]. After 1815, Bahia was the only Brazilian state that restricted slave traffic through Ecuador, which explains the association between the genotypic frequencies in Bahia and Western Africa, principally the Benin region [27]. We found high levels of HbF and low levels of HbS in patients with the BEN haplotype. Most of the patients with the CAR haplotype had low HbF levels (below 5% of the total HbF), whereas carriers of the BEN haplotype had intermediate HbF levels (between 5 and 15%) and this is in agreement with a previous study [28].

In Brazil, the prevalence of -α$^{3.7Kb}$-thal is associated with different ethnic groups that constitute the population [29]. We observed a high prevalence of -α$^{3.7Kb}$-thal

Table 4 Comparison of the laboratory data between SCA and HbSC patients

Laboratory value	SCA (*N* = 98) Median (25th – 75th)	HbSC (N = 52) Median (25th – 75th)	p *value*
Hemolysis			
RBC, $\times 10^{12}$/L	2.60 (2.30–2.80)	4.15 (3.80–4.50)	**<0.001**
Hemoglobin, g/dL	7.60 (7.15–8.50)	10.90 (10.12–11.82)	**<0.001**
Hematocrit, %	21.80 (20.15–24.47)	30.80 (28.72–32.50)	**<0.001**
MCV, fL	86.05 (81.37–91.10)	74.40 (70.80–79.72)	**<0.001**
MCH, fL	30.15 (27.87–32.25)	26.60 (24.60–28.67)	**<0.001**
RDW, fL	24.80 (21.60–27.20)	18.65 (17.62–19.57)	**<0.001**
Total bilirubin, mg/dL	2.55 (1.67–3.72)	1.20 (0.80–1.67)	**<0.001**
Direct bilirubin, mg/dL	0.45 (0.30–0.60)	0.30 (0.20–0.40)	**<0.001**
Indirect bilirubin, mg/dL	2.20 (1.20–3.12)	0.90 (0.52–1.27)	**<0.001**
LDH, U/L	1094.00 (785.50–1684.50)	481.50 (381.75–567.25)	**<0.001**
Reticulocyte			
Reticulocyte count	5.40 (4.20–8.20)	3.65 (2.62–4.37)	**<0.001**
NO metabolites			
NOm, μM	35.62 (28.02–47.50)	31.34 (23.19–40.80)	**0.047**
Leukocytes			
WBC, $\times 10^9$/L	13.80 (11.17–16.10)	10.45 (7.22–12.90)	**<0.001**
Segment count, $\times 10^9$/L	5778.00 (4275.25–7203.50)	5182.00 (3498.50–6717.00)	0.080
Eosinophil count, $\times 10^9$/L	695.50 (281.50–1774.75)	421.50 (216.50–895.25)	**0.007**
Lymphocyte count, $\times 10^9$/L	5535.00 (4335.00–7156.50)	3356.50 (2492.00–4704.75)	**<0.001**
Monocyte count, $\times 10^9$/L	349.50 (219.00–670.75)	257.00 (144.50–402.75)	**0.003**
Platelets			
Platelet count, $\times 10^3$/mL	441.50 (365.25–547.00)	267.00 (189.50–389.00)	**<0.001**
MPV, fL	9.50 (8.80–10.40)	9.70 (9.30–10.40)	0.314
Lipid metabolism			
Total Cholesterol, mg/dL	122.00 (97.75–146.75)	133.50 (110.25–166.75)	**0.012**
HDL-C, mg/dL	32.00 (27.00–38.00)	37.00 (33.00–44.75)	**<0.001**
LDL-C, mg/dL	67.00 (41.75–88.25)	73.00 (57.00–109.75)	0.071
VLDL-C, mg/dL	22.00 (16.75–31.25)	21.00 (14.00–27.75)	0.178
Triglycerides, mg/dL	110.00 (82.75–156.50)	103.50 (68.50–138.50)	0.175

RBC red blood cells, *MCV* mean cell volume, *MCH* mean corpuscular hemoglobin, *RDW* red cell distribution width, *LDH* lactate dehydrogenase, *NOm*: nitric oxide metabolites, *WBC* white blood cell, *MPV* mean platelet volume, *HDL-C* high-density lipoprotein cholesterol, *LDL-C* low-density lipoprotein cholesterol, *VLDL-C* very low-density lipoprotein cholesterol; Bold values indicate significance at $p < 0.05$; *p*-value obtained using Mann-Whitney

deletion in the studied population. It is estimated that in Brazil, the overall frequency of the α-thalassemia trait is between 1% and 3% [30]. According to our results, the association with co-inheritance of $\alpha^{3.7Kb}$-thal deletion lead to increased hemoglobin levels, despite the microcytosis, hypochromia and increased hematocrit levels. The literature reports that the homozygous and heterozygous states of $-\alpha^{3.7Kb}$-thal, are characterized by mild anemia, hypochromia and microcytosis. However, increased hematocrit levels are observed, which contribute to enhance blood viscosity, increase vaso-occlusion and the occurrence of clinical events [7, 31].

Several studies have demonstrated the pathophysiological mechanisms underlying SCA and HbSC. We observed that SCA patients had a more prominent hemolytic pattern compared to HbSC patients who presented a lower RBC count and hemoglobin concentration, and increased LDH levels. This is in agreement with previous studies that described that in HbSC patients the HbC presence induces the HbS polymerization; however, it occur in a reduced degree when compared to SCA patients. Thus, HbSC patients exhibits a less severe hemolytic anemia [2, 32].

We identified increased reticulocytes count in SCA patients in response to hemolysis. This is related to anemic

Table 5 Clinical characterization of SCA and HbSC patients

Clinical characterization	SCA N = 98	HbSC N = 52	p value
Hospitalization	90/98 (91.8%)	36/52 (69.2%)	**0.001**
Pneumonia	38/98 (38.8%)	22/52 (42.3%)	0.728
Splenomegaly	40/98 (40.8%)	18/52 (34.6%)	0.486
Asthma	6/98 (6.1%)	3/52 (5.8%)	1.000
Pain crises	83/98 (84.7%)	41/52 (78.8%)	0.374
Infection	36/98 (36.7%)	18/52 (34.6%)	0.859
Priapism	10/50 (20.0%)	5/22 (22.7%)	0.764
Vaso-occlusion	89/98 (90.8%)	42/52 (80.8%)	0.119
Retinopathy	3/98 (3.0%)	4/52 (7.7%)	0.236
Cholelithiasis	17/98 (17.3%)	4/52 (7.7%)	0.139

Comparison of clinical events among the SCA and HbSC genotypes calculated using the Fisher's exact test. Bold values indicate significance at $p < 0.05$

stress that promotes the release of immature RBCs from the bone marrow, which consequently increases reticulocytes count on peripheral blood [33]. We observed a slight decrease in NOm in HbSC patients. The lysis of erythrocytes promotes the release of free Hb in the plasma, which promotes inflammatory and oxidative effects that contribute to endothelial dysfunction [12, 34]. Due to hemolysis, heme, reactive oxygen species (ROS) and arginase are released into the bloodstream, increasing oxidative stress and decreasing NOm levels [35, 36].

Patients with HbSC had lower leukocyte count than SCA patients. This result is consistent with previous findings that identify the same association [37]. Moreover, SCA patients had higher platelet counts; however, the mean platelet volume (MPV) was high in both the genotypes. An increase in platelet activation has been found in SCD patients during vaso occlusive events. Platelets regulate hemostasis, but they are also responsible for inducing inflammation [38].

The analysis of the lipid profile in SCD patients have shown lower HDL-C levels, as well as values below the reference value, which represents an important cardiovascular risk factor [39–41]. Hypertriglyceridemia and increased very low-density lipoprotein cholesterol (VLDL-C) were observed in SCA patients in this study, although these results were not statistically significant. According to previous reports, SCD individuals have decreased lipid plasma levels during hemolytic stress and compared with normal individuals [42].

Clinical manifestations are considered a limiting factor that may influence patient mortality; these include pain crisis, VOE and the coexistence of comorbidities, such as legs ulcers, infection, cholelithiasis, splenomegaly, retinopathy, vascular necrosis, and neurological disorders, which have a negative effect on the cognitive development of these patients [11, 16]. As demonstrated by our results, we found increased hospitalizations in SCA patients, once this is the most severe genotype of SCD characterized by a higher incidence of clinical complications and hospitalizations than HbSC [16].

We found that a high percentage of patients used oral prophylactic penicillin, including Benzathine, which was administered in patients prior to age 7 years. The prophylactic use of penicillin significantly reduces the risk of sepsis and death due to pneumococcal infection [43]. Another prescribed drug, folic acid, is used in cases of increased activity secondary to chronic hemolysis that results in high RBC destruction and leads to a deficit in folic acid [43, 44]. Our data showed daily high adherence to folic acid use in all age groups [45].

Conclusion

Our data highlight the differences between subphenotypes among SCA and HbSC patients, based on laboratory characterization, genetic profiles and clinical manifestations of both genotypes. The results of our analyses emphasize the need for specialized care services for SCA and HbSC patients, particularly because of their heterogeneous genetic, clinical and pathophysiological backgrounds, and indicate the need for public health policies that significantly improve the health of these patients.

Abbreviations

ACS: Acute chest syndrome; BEN: Benin; CAM: Arab-Indian, and Cameroon; CAR: Central African Republic; HbC: Hemoglobin C; HbF: Fetal hemoglobin; HbS: Hemoglobin S; HbSC: Hemoglobin SC disease; HDL-C: High-density lipoprotein cholesterol; HU: Hydroxyurea; LDH: Lactate dehydrogenase; MCH: Mean corpuscular hemoglobin; MCV: Mean cell volume; MPV: Mean platelet volume; NOm: Nitric oxide metabolites; PCR: Reaction polimerase chain; RBC: Red blood cell; RDW: Red blood cell distribution width; RFLP: Restriction fragment length polymorphism; ROS: Reactive oxygen species; SCA: Sickle cell anemia; SCD: Sickle cell disease; SEN: Senegal; VLDL-C: Very low-density lipoprotein cholesterol; VOE: Vaso occlusion events; WBC: White blood cell; -α$^{3.7Kb}$-thal: -α$^{3.7Kb}$-thalassemia

Acknowledgements

Not applicable.

Funding

No funding was received.

Authors' contributions

MMA, MSG and BAVC, performed conception and design of the study, acquisition of data, analysis and interpretation of data. RPS, CCG and JRDF drafting the article or revising it critically for important intellectual content. TCCF, FIN, RQS and BLAC assisted and performed the blood collection of the patients. CVBF and SSP helped perform the experiments, the hematological, biochemical and molecular analysis. SSS helped review the medical records and perform the statistical analyses. All authors read and approved the final manuscript.

Competing interests

The authors declare that they have no competing interests.

Author details
[1]Laboratório de Hematologia e Genética Computacional, Instituto Gonçalo Moniz - IGM, Fundação Oswaldo Cruz (Fiocruz), Rua Waldemar Falcão, 121, Candeal, Salvador, Bahia CEP 40296-710, Brazil. [2]Universidade Federal da Bahia (UFBA), Salvador, Bahia, Brazil. [3]Centro de Referência a Doença Falciforme, Itabuna, Bahia, Brazil. [4]Universidade Estadual de Santa Cruz (UESC), Ilhéus, Bahia, Brazil. [5]Universidade Estadual da Bahia (UNEB), Salvador, Bahia, Brazil.

References

1. WHO/AFRO. The health of the people: what works – the African Regional Health Report. Public health - organization and administration. 2014.
2. Grosse SD, Odame I, Atrash HK, Amendah DD, Piel FB, Williams TN. Sickle cell disease in Africa: a neglected cause of early childhood mortality. Am J Prev Med. 2011;41(6 Suppl 4):S398–405.
3. Steinberg MH. Genetic etiologies for phenotypic diversity in sickle cell anemia. ScientificWorldJournal. 2009;9:46–67.
4. Rees DC, Gibson JS. Biomarkers in sickle cell disease. Br J Haematol. 2012; 156(4):433–45.
5. Steinberg MH, Coleman MB, Adams JG, Rosenstock W. Interaction between HBS-beta-o-thalassemia and alpha-thalassemia. Am J Med Sci. 1984;288(5): 195–9.
6. Steinberg MH, Sebastiani P. Genetic modifiers of sickle cell disease. Am J Hematol. 2012;87(8):795–803.
7. Adorno EV, Couto FD, Moura Neto JP, Menezes JF, Rego M, Reis MG, et al. Hemoglobinopathies in newborns from Salvador, Bahia, Northeast Brazil. Cadernos de saude publica. 2005;21(1):292–8.
8. Charache S. Fetal hemoglobin, sickling, and sickle cell disease. Adv Pediatr. 1990;37:1–31.
9. Nagel RL, Fabry ME. Sickle cell anemia as a multigenetic disease: new insights into the mechanism of painful crisis. Prog Clin Biol Res. 1984;165: 93–102.
10. Goncalves MS, Bomfim GC, Maciel E, Cerqueira I, Lyra I, Zanette A, et al. BetaS-haplotypes in sickle cell anemia patients from Salvador, Bahia, Northeastern Brazil. Brazilian journal of medical and biological research = Revista brasileira de pesquisas medicas e biologicas / Sociedade Brasileira de Biofisica [et al]. 2003;36(10):1283–8.
11. Steinberg MH. Predicting clinical severity in sickle cell anaemia. Br J Haematol. 2005;129(4):465–81.
12. Kato GJ, Gladwin MT, Steinberg MH. Deconstructing sickle cell disease: reappraisal of the role of hemolysis in the development of clinical subphenotypes. Blood Rev. 2007;21(1):37–47.
13. Damanhouri GA, Jarullah J, Marouf S, Hindawi SI, Mushtaq G, Kamal MA. Clinical biomarkers in sickle cell disease. Saudi journal of biological sciences. 2015;22(1):24–31.
14. Steinberg MH, Barton F, Castro O, Pegelow CH, Ballas SK, Kutlar A, et al. Effect of hydroxyurea on mortality and morbidity in adult sickle cell anemia: risks and benefits up to 9 years of treatment. JAMA. 2003;289(13):1645–51.
15. Raphael JL, Dietrich CL, Whitmire D, Mahoney DH, Mueller BU, Giardino AP. Healthcare utilization and expenditures for low income children with sickle cell disease. Pediatr Blood Cancer. 2009;52(2):263–7.
16. Pizzo E, Laverty AA, Phekoo KJ, AlJuburi G, Green SA, Bell D, et al. A retrospective analysis of the cost of hospitalizations for sickle cell disease with crisis in England, 2010/11. J Public Health (Oxf). 2015;37(3):529–39.
17. Nims RW, Cook JC, Krishna MC, Christodoulou D, Poore CM, Miles AM, et al. Colorimetric assays for nitric oxide and nitrogen oxide species formed from nitric oxide stock solutions and donor compounds. Methods Enzymol. 1996; 268:93–105.
18. Sutton M, Bouhassira EE, Nagel RL. Polymerase chain reaction amplification applied to the determination of beta-like globin gene cluster haplotypes. Am J Hematol. 1989;32(1):66–9.
19. Chong SS, Boehm CD, Higgs DR, Cutting GR. Single-tube multiplex-PCR screen for common deletional determinants of alpha-thalassemia. Blood. 2000;95(1):360–2.
20. Carroll PC, Haywood C Jr, Hoot MR, Lanzkron S. A preliminary study of psychiatric, familial, and medical characteristics of high-utilizing sickle cell disease patients. Clin J Pain. 2013;29(4):317–23.
21. Loureiro MM, Rozenfeld S. Epidemiology of sickle cell disease hospital admissions in Brazil. Rev Saude Publica. 2005;39(6):943–9.
22. Adegoke SA, Adeodu OO, Adekile AD. Sickle cell disease clinical phenotypes in children from south-western. Nigeria Niger J Clin Pract. 2015;18(1):95–101.
23. Ballas SK, Kesen MR, Goldberg MF, Lutty GA, Dampier C, Osunkwo I, et al. Beyond the definitions of the phenotypic complications of sickle cell disease: an update on management. ScientificWorldJournal. 2012;2012:949535.
24. Serjeant GR. Screening for sickle-cell disease in Brazil. Lancet (London, England). 2000;356(9224):168–9.
25. Aleluia MM, Santiago RP, da Guarda CC, Fonseca TCC, Neves FI, Quinto RS, et al. Genetic Modulation of Fetal Hemoglobin in Hydroxyurea-Treated Sickle Cell Anemia. American journal of hematology. 2017:n/a-n/a.
26. Verger. Flux et Reflux de la Traite des Nègres Entre le Golfe de Benin et Bahia de Todos os Santos. Mouton Press, Paris, France. 1968.
27. Florentino M. Em Costas Negras. Companhia das Letras Press. 1997.
28. Powars DR. Beta s-gene-cluster haplotypes in sickle cell anemia. Clinical and hematologic features. Hematol Oncol Clin North Am. 1991;5(3):475–93.
29. Harteveld CL, Higgs DR. Alpha-thalassaemia. Orphanet journal of rare diseases. 2010;5:13.
30. Figueiredo MS, Kerbauy J, Goncalves MS, Arruda VR, Saad ST, Sonati MF, et al. Effect of alpha-thalassemia and beta-globin gene cluster haplotypes on the hematological and clinical features of sickle-cell anemia in Brazil. Am J Hematol. 1996;53(2):72–6.
31. Lyra IM, Goncalves MS, Braga JA, Gesteira Mde F, Carvalho MH, Saad ST, et al. Clinical, hematological, and molecular characterization of sickle cell anemia pediatric patients from two different cities in Brazil. Cadernos de saude publica. 2005;21(4):1287–90.
32. Kato GJ, Hebbel RP, Steinberg MH, Gladwin MT. Vasculopathy in sickle cell disease: biology, pathophysiology, genetics, translational medicine, and new research directions. Am J Hematol. 2009;84(9):618–25.
33. Discher DE, Ney PA. The reason sickle reticulocytes expose PS. Blood. 2015; 126(15):1737–8.
34. Belanger AM, Keggi C, Kanias T, Gladwin MT, Kim-Shapiro DB. Effects of nitric oxide and its congeners on sickle red blood cell deformability. Transfusion. 2015;55(10):2464–72.
35. Vilas-Boas W, Cerqueira BA, Zanette AM, Reis MG, Barral-Netto M, Goncalves MS. Arginase levels and their association with Th17-related cytokines, soluble adhesion molecules (sICAM-1 and sVCAM-1) and hemolysis markers among steady-state sickle cell anemia patients. Ann Hematol. 2010;89(9):877–82.
36. Dutra FF, Alves LS, Rodrigues D, Fernandez PL, de Oliveira RB, Golenbock DT, et al. Hemolysis-induced lethality involves inflammasome activation by heme. Proc Natl Acad Sci U S A. 2014;111(39):E4110–8.
37. Colella MP, de Paula EV, Machado-Neto JA, Conran N, Annichino-Bizzacchi JM, Costa FF, et al. Elevated hypercoagulability markers in hemoglobin SC disease. Haematologica. 2015;100(4):466–71.
38. Wun T, Paglieroni T, Tablin F, Welborn J, Nelson K, Cheung A. Platelet activation and platelet-erythrocyte aggregates in patients with sickle cell anemia. J Lab Clin Med. 1997;129(5):507–16.
39. Villagra J, Shiva S, Hunter LA, Machado RF, Gladwin MT, Kato GJ. Platelet activation in patients with sickle disease, hemolysis-associated pulmonary hypertension, and nitric oxide scavenging by cell-free hemoglobin. Blood. 2007;110(6):2166–72.
40. Executive Summary of The Third Report of The National Cholesterol Education Program (NCEP) Expert Panel on Detection, Evaluation, And Treatment of High Blood Cholesterol In Adults (Adult Treatment Panel III). Jama. 2001;285(19):2486–97.
41. Movva R, Rader DJ. Laboratory assessment of HDL heterogeneity and function. Clin Chem. 2008;54(5):788–800.
42. Gaston MH, Verter JI, Woods G, Pegelow C, Kelleher J, Presbury G, et al. Prophylaxis with oral penicillin in children with sickle cell anemia. A randomized trial. N Engl J Med. 1986;314(25):1593–9.
43. Dixit R, Nettem S, Madan SS, Soe HH, Abas AB, Vance LD, et al. Folate supplementation in people with sickle cell disease. Cochrane Database Syst Rev. 2016;2:Cd011130.
44. Martyres DJ, Vijenthira A, Barrowman N, Harris-Janz S, Chretien C, Klaassen RJ. Nutrient insufficiencies/deficiencies in children with sickle cell disease and its association with increased disease severity. Pediatr Blood Cancer. 2016;
45. Nwenyi E, Leafman J, Mathieson K, Ezeobah N. Differences in quality of life between pediatric sickle cell patients who used hydroxyurea and those who did not. Int J Health Care Qual Assur. 2014;27(6):468–81.

16

Prevalence of neutropenia in children by nationality

Srdjan Denic[1*], Hassib Narchi[2], Lolowa A. Al Mekaini[2], Suleiman Al-Hammadi[2], Omar N. Al Jabri[3] and Abdul-Kader Souid[2]

Abstract

Background: A high prevalence of neutropenia has been reported in several ethnic groups amongst whom many healthy individuals with low neutrophil counts undergo unnecessary investigations. This study aims to ascertain the prevalence of neutropenia (NP) in a large cohort of children from North African, Middle Eastern, and Asian countries residing in the United Arab Emirates.

Methods: Neutrophil counts of 26,542 children (one day to six years of age) from 86 countries were analyzed. The subjects were enrolled in the Well-Child-Care program of Ambulatory Health Services of Emirate of Abu Dhabi, United Arab Emirates. NP was defined as a neutrophil count $<1.5 \times 10^9$/L and severe NP $<0.5 \times 10^9$/L.

Results: The neutrophil counts reached a nadir in the fourth week of life and changed slightly from the age of six-months to six-years. The frequency of NP was (from West-to-East): North African Arabs 15.4 %, Green Crescent Arabs 9.8 %, Peninsular Arabs 10.9 %, Iranians 3.1 %, Afghanis 2.5 %, Pakistanis 5.6 %, Indians 10.2 %, and Filipinos 7.3 %. The frequency of severe NP in North African Arabs (Sudanese) was 2.8 %, Green Crescent and Peninsular Arabs ≤1 %, Indians 1.5 %, and Filipinos 1.8 %. In 12,703 Emirati children, the frequency of NP was 10.6 % similar to their adult counterparts.

Conclusion: The prevalence of childhood NP varied considerably by geoethnicity. Measures to prevent the inappropriate investigations of healthy children with benign neutropenia are proposed.

Keywords: Public health, Ethnicity, Monocyte count, Malaria hypothesis

Background

Neutropenia (NP) is common amongst several ethnic groups from Africa and Asia [1–8]. A NP frequency of up to 30 % from Africa has been reported [1]. Among African Americans, its prevalence is 4.4 % [3]. In United Arab Emirates (UAE), 10.7 % of the native population has absolute neutrophil counts less than 1.5×10^9/L [7]. The evidence suggests the inheritance of NP is autosomal dominant or co-dominant in people of Sudanese origin and among natives of Arabia [6, 7]. Molecular studies in some people of African ancestry, on the other hand, have shown a strong association between familial NP and the null Duffy genotype (Fy-/Fy-) and no association with the heterozygote (Fy-/Fy+) and wild-homozygote (Fy+/Fy+) genotypes, suggesting an autosomal recessive inheritance [9].

The benign nature of ethnic NP is based on reports of the absence of recurrent infections in such individuals [1–8]. However, many healthy individuals with low neutrophil counts often undergo unnecessary investigations to exclude pathologic NP. In addition, benign neutropenia often changes medical management such as delaying administration of myelosuppressants, premature stopping of drug therapy, postponing elective surgery and preventing recruitment into clinical trials [10–17]. This study ascertained the prevalence of NP in a large cohort of infants and children from North African, Middle Eastern and Asian countries who reside in UAE.

* Correspondence: s.denic@uaeu.ac.ae
[1]Department of Medicine, College of Medicine and Health Sciences, United Arab Emirates University, PO Box 17666, Al-Ain, United Arab of Emirates
Full list of author information is available at the end of the article

Methods

Study setting and population

This study was conducted in the Emirate of Abu Dhabi, UAE. The country's population is eight million, of which 15 % are Emiratis (ethnically Arab) and the remaining 85 % are temporary foreign workers from numerous countries including the Indian subcontinent, the Middle East and North Africa. The study cohort comprised 26,542 infants and children. Their ages ranged from 1 day to 6 years. These children were registered in the Well-Child Care Program at Ambulatory Health Services (AHS) funded by the Health Authority of Abu Dhabi. The blood samples were obtained at the treating physician's discretion between April 2008 and December 2013 at three hospitals (64 %), 26 outpatient AHS centers (19 %) or unidentified sites (17 %). Only one sample per child was used in the analysis. Written consent was not obtained as all blood counts were performed as part of the standard care.

Complete blood count

The blood samples were collected in BD Vacutainer® spray-coated K2EDTA tubes. The samples were mixed by inversion, transported at 2-8 °C, and tested as soon as they arrived at the laboratory. Blood cell counts were determined using the Cell-Dyne Ruby analyzers (Abbott Laboratories, Illinois, USA). The laboratories run daily internal quality controls before running patient samples and participate in External Quality Assurance program through the College of American Pathologists Proficiency Testing.

Definition of neutropenia and estimation of gene frequency

NP was considered mild, moderate and severe if the count was $<1.5 \times 10^9$/L, $<1.0 \times 10^9$/L and $<0.5 \times 10^9$/L, respectively. As the neutrophil count normally oscillates, some children with NP occasionally have $>1.5 \times 10^9$/L neutrophils. In a cross-sectional study, this fraction contributes to undetected (hidden) NP [7].

We hypothesized that severe NP in Emiratis was caused by a homozygote genotype and milder NP by a heterozygote genotype, i.e., inherited at a single locus with two alleles (q and $p = 1\text{-}q$). The native population of UAE is tribal, nearly half of the marriages are arranged between close cousins, and the mean coefficient of inbreeding in the population (F) is 0.022 [18–20]. Therefore, the frequency of the NP allele (q) in a large sample of Emiratis was determined using the Hardy-Weinberg equation adjusted for inbreeding. The frequency of homozygotes was $q^2(1\text{-}F) + qF$ and heterozygotes $2pq(1\text{-}F)$ [21].

Statistical analysis

As neutrophil counts did not follow a normal distribution (Shapiro-Wilk test $p < 0.001$), the non-parametric two-sample Wilcoxon rank-sum (Mann–Whitney) test was used to compare values between two categories, and Kruskal-Wallis rank test for three or more categories. The Spearman's correlation test was used to analyze the relation between neutrophil and monocyte counts. For all analyses, two-tailed p-value of < 0.05 defined statistical significance. Other standard descriptive and statistical methods were used. One subject was removed because of an impossible value.

Ethics approval

The study was approved by the Institutional Review Board of College of Medicine and Health Sciences – UAE University (#13/14).

Results

The enrolled children represented 86 nationalities, of which 25,435 (96 %) were from 32 countries in North Africa, the Middle East and Asia. The largest group (12,073) was that of Emirati nationals.

Figure 1 shows the neutrophil counts by age (26,542 children from 86 nationalities). The counts decreased during the first week of life, reached a nadir in the fourth week and changed slightly between six-months and six-years. In the first month, the median (±SD) count ($\times 10^9$/L) was lower ($p \leq 0.05$) in 2,856 males (6.4 ± 4.9) than in 3,551 females (7.3 ± 5.6), but later in life the differences were insignificant (Table 1). The median, 10th and 90th percentile neutrophil count for eight Arab population is shown in Additional file 1: Figure S1.

Figure 2 shows the prevalence of NP by nationality in six-month to six-year-old children. Analysis of the neutrophil counts by geoethnicity is shown in Table 2. NP was most common amongst African Arabs (14.7 to 20.2 %); in these populations, the 2.5th percentile count for 2-year-old children was 0.7×10^9/L and for 5 to 6 year-old children, 1.1×10^9/L. The frequency of NP in North Africans was 15.4 %, Peninsular Arabs 10.9 %, Indians 10.2 %, Green Crescent Arabs 9.8 %, Filipinos 7.3 %, Pakistanis 5.6 %, Iranians 3.1 %, and Afghanis 2.5 %. The prevalence of NP in Iranians and Afghanis was similar to that reported in Europeans [22–24]. The prevalence of severe NP in Sudanese was 2.8 %, Filipinos 1.8 %, Indians 1.5 %, and Middle Easterners ≤1 % (Fig. 2). The frequency of NP among eight Arab populations was not significantly different (see supplemental material).

We attempted to confirm the previously reported correlation between the monocyte and the neutrophil counts [7]. We found that the Spearman's correlation coefficients between neutrophil and monocyte counts in the four largest ethnic groups were as follows: Egyptians, 0.46; Sudanese, 0.51; Emiratis, 0.44; and Indians, 0.47.

In the 12,703 Emirati children (aged six-months to six-years), the prevalence of NP (Fig. 2) was 10.6 %, similar to

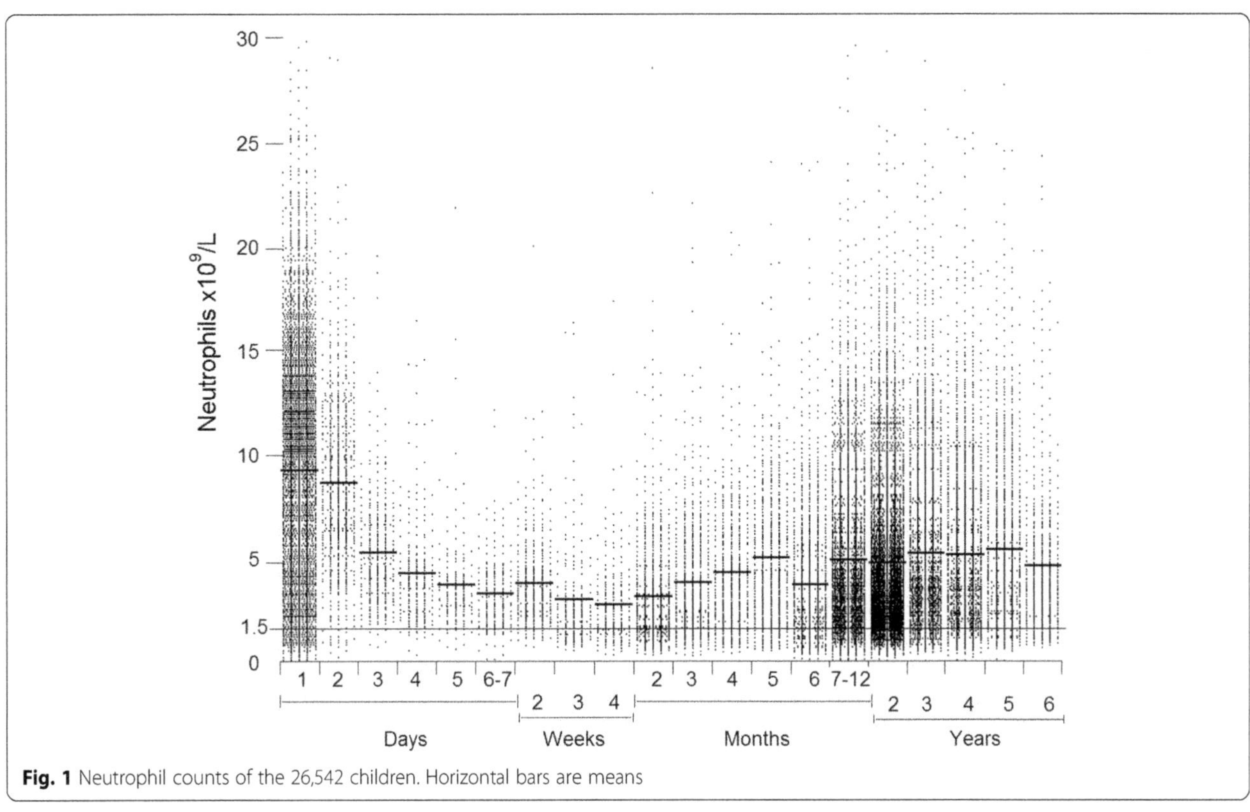

Fig. 1 Neutrophil counts of the 26,542 children. Horizontal bars are means

Table 1 Median and 2.5th percentile neutrophil counts of children from North Africa, Middle East and Asia

		Neutrophils × 10^9/L							
		Days		Weeks	Months	Years			
		1	2–7	2–4	2–12	2	3	4	5–6
All	Median	8.7	5.1	2.7	3.3	3.4	3.7	3.8	3.8
	2.5th	0.9	1.3	0.8	0.7	0.8	0.9	0.9	1.0
		(3,360)	(1,429)	(615)	(6,997)	(5,846)	(3,097)	(2,463)	(2,470)
Females	Median	9.7	5.6	3.1	3.3	3.4	3.9	3.8	3.8
	2.5th	1.1	1.4	0.8	0.7	0.9	0.9	1.0	0.9
		(1,511)	(647)	(274)	(3,109)	(2,748)	(1,454)	(1,172)	(1,207)
Males	Median	8.0	4.7	2.5	3.3	3.4	3.7	3.8	3.7
	2.5th	0.9	1.1	0.8	0.7	0.8	0.9	0.9	1.0
		(1,849)	(782)	(341)	(3,888)	(3,098)	(1,643)	(1,291)	(1,263)
Outpatient	Median	-	-	-	2.5	2.7	3.2	3.4	3.6
	2.5th				0.5	0.7	0.8	0.9	0.9
					(1,544)	(2,905)	(1,812)	(1,673)	(2,021)
Inpatient	Median	8.7	5.1	2.8	3.6	4.8	4.9	4.9	5.0
	2.5th	0.9	1.3	0.8	0.8	1.0	1.0	1.2	1.1
		(3,360)	(1,425)	(591)	(5,453)	(2,941)	(1,285)	(790)	(449)

Values in parenthesis are number of children (only for $n \geq 50$)

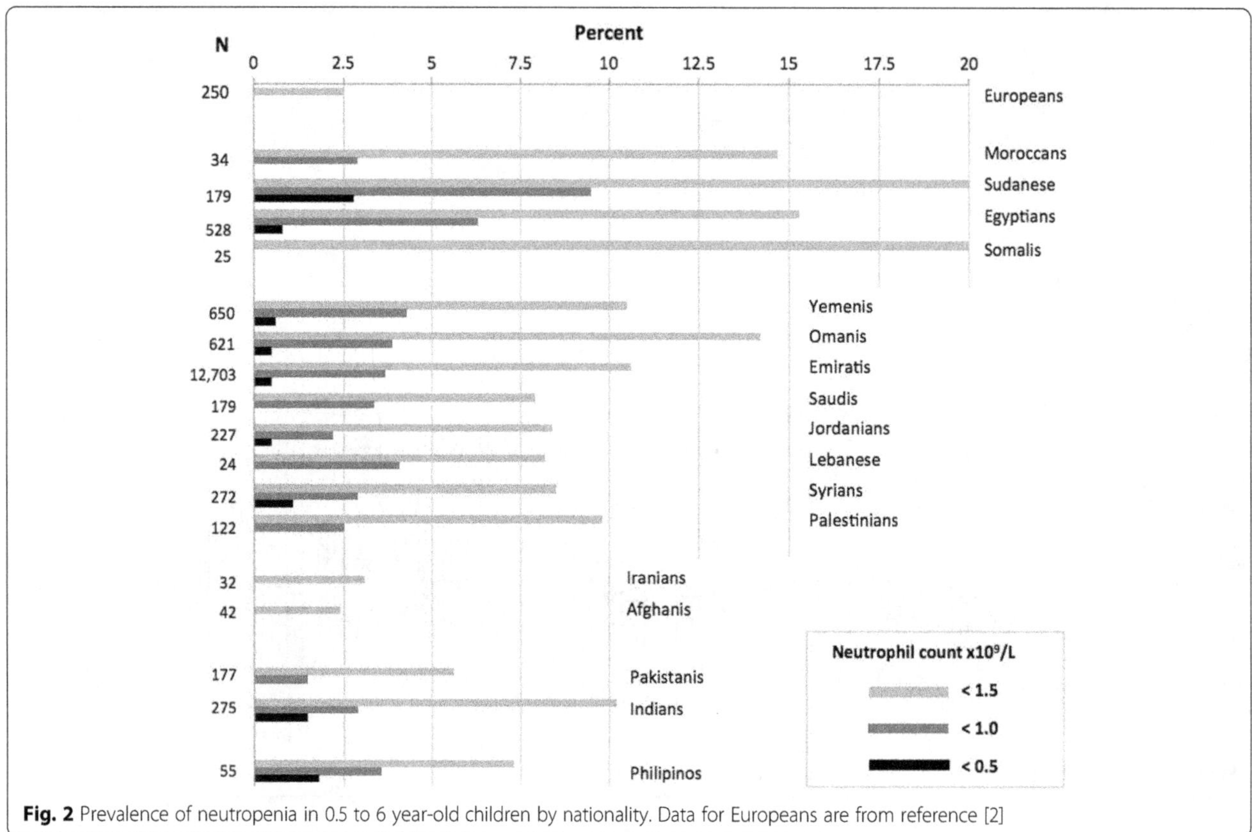

Fig. 2 Prevalence of neutropenia in 0.5 to 6 year-old children by nationality. Data for Europeans are from reference [2]

that of healthy adult Emiratis (10.7 %) [7]. The prevalence of severe NP of the children in this study was 0.53 %. For this sub-group we estimated frequency of NP allele which was 6.3 %, while the frequency of phenotype-derived heterozygosity was 11.6 %. The latter value was 1.51 % higher than the milder NP (10.7 % – 0.53 % = 10.07 %) observed in the studied population. This 1.51 % discrepancy in the frequency is explained by hidden NP.

Discussion

This study confirms that NP is common in people from North Africa, the Middle East and South Asia (Fig. 2 and Table 2). The neutrophil counts were highest at birth, decreased in the first seven days of life, and reached a nadir in the fourth week of life. Thereafter, the counts increased until 6 months of age and changed a little from six months to six years (Fig. 1). This pattern is similar to that in European children [22–24]. The median neutrophil count was lower in male neonates than female neonates (Table 1). In one study of adult Africans, males had lower neutrophil counts than females [16].

People from North African countries have the highest frequency of NP, ranging from 14.7 to 20.7 % (Fig. 2). Benign NP was first reported from Africa and from countries to which Africans have migrated [2, 3, 25]. A high prevalence of NP was found in the Sudanese who migrated to the Middle East, and amongst Yemenis and Ethiopian Jews who might have acquired the trait from neighboring African populations [6, 8]. This study shows that 10.5 % of Yemenis and 20 % children from the neighboring Somalia have NP. The frequency of NP in Peninsular Arabs ranged from 7.9 to 14.2 %, and Green Crescent Middle East residents from 8.2 to 9.8 % (Fig. 2). The Duffy negative blood group, strongly associated with benign NP in societies of African ancestry, is also common among Arab populations [26]. This finding is consistent with the historical mixing of Arabs with native African populations suggesting a common origin. In the geographically more distant Iranians and Afghanis, the frequency of NP is considerably lower (3.1 and 2.5 %, respectively) being similar to Europeans (<2.5 %) [23]. Furthermore, Iranians, Afghanis and Europeans share common pre-historic origins. In the Indian subcontinent, frequency of NP increased from 5.6 % in Pakistanis (closer to Afghanis) to 10.2 % in Indians.

This geoethnic distribution of frequencies raises a possibility that Afro-Arab and Indian NP have independent origins (involving the same or different genetic mutations). This hypothesis is supported by the absence of associations with the Duffy negative genotype (a biomarker for African NP) among Indians [9, 27]. High prevalence of NP is also found in Filipinos (Fig. 2); historically, this nation has received migrants from the Indian subcontinent and does not have the Duffy negative genotype [28].

Table 2 Median and 2.5th percentile neutrophil counts of children by geo-ethnicity

		Neutrophils × 10^9/L							
		Days		Weeks	Months	Years			
		1	2–7	2–4	2–12	2	3	4	5–6
North Africans	Median	5.8	4.6	-	2.7	2.6	3.0	3.1	3.8
	2.5th	0.9	0.9		0.5	0.7	0.7	0.6	0.9
		(171)	(84)		(252)	(363)	(132)	(104)	(108)
Peninsular Arabs	Median	9.0	5.3	2.7	3.4	3.6	3.8	3.8	3.5
	2.5th	1.0	1.3	0.8	0.7	0.8	1.0	1.0	1.0
		(2,585)	(969)	(529)	(5,929)	(4,782)	(2,187)	(1,399)	(776)
						2 - 6			
Green Crescent Arabs	Median	7.2	5.6	-	3.2	3.3			
	2.5th	0.7	1.4		0.9	1.0			
		(178)	(95)		(239)	(880)			
Iranians & Afghanis	Median	-	-	-	-	3.9			
	2.5th					1.4			
						(57)			
Indian Subcontinent	Median	7.5	5.1	-	3.2	3.2			
	2.5th	0.9	1.9		0.7	1.1			
		(180)	(98)		(211)	(510)			
Filipinos	Median	-	-	-	-	2.8			
	2.5th					1.4			
						(51)			

Values in parenthesis are number of children (only for $n \geq 50$)
North Africans (1,243): Egyptians (771), Sudanese (278), Moroccan (67), Somalis (44), Mauritanians (39), Tunisians (20), Ethiopians (10), Algerians (7), Eritreans (4), Libyans (2)
Peninsular Arabs (21,883): Emiratis (19,545), Yemenis (1,058), Omanis (952), Saudis (292), Qataris (18), Bahrainis (7), Bedouins (6), Kuwaitis (5)
Green Crescent Arabs (1,119): Syrians (448), Jordanians (365), Palestinians (222), Lebanese (51), Iraqis (33)
Indian Subcontinent (1,042): Indians (490), Pakistanis (448), Bangladeshis (82), Sri Lankans (16), Nepalese (6)

Considerable number of children have neutrophil counts <0.5 ×10^9/L (2.8 % of Sudanese, 1.8 % of Filipinos and 1.5 % of Egyptians and Indians). A different genetic mutation could account for this severe NP phenotype. On the other side, in pedigree analyses in earlier study, consanguineous parents of offspring with severe NP have milder phenotype, suggesting a co-dominant inheritance [7]. Severe NP, thus, could represent a homozygote genotype and milder NP (nearly always >0.8 ×10^9/L) a heterozygote genotype. This mode of inheritance is supported by our estimated frequency of presumed heterozygote ($2pq$, milder *plus* hidden phenotype) derived from frequency of severe NP (presumed homozygote, q^2) in 12,703 Emiratis. In over dozen kinship groups (data not shown), the frequency of both phenotypes correlates ($r = 0.468$), providing additional support that one mutation is a cause of benign NP. However, other genes and polymorphisms are known to impact neutrophil production and more than one gene could be involved in benign NP [29]. A possible effect of environmental factors that could affect gene expression could not be excluded.

In studied populations, two observations support the benign nature of NP. The prevalence of NP in 12,703 Emirati children (10.6 %) is similar to 10.7 % in 1,032 healthy adult Emiratis [7]. This unchanged frequency, over an estimated18-year-period, is an epidemiological evidence of its benign nature. The positive correlation between the monocyte and neutrophil counts in four large ethnic groups (Egyptians, Sudanese, Emiratis and Indians) supports benign rather than secondary NP, in which monocytosis is a more common finding [30–32]. In general, our findings agree with earlier reports of a high frequency of benign NP in children from Sudan and Jordan [4, 6].

The "malaria hypothesis" proposed as an explanation of high prevalence of benign NP is based on (i) a long history of endemic malaria in populations which have high prevalence of NP and (ii) its associated monocytopenia which is linked with a less intense phagocyte-mediated inflammation [7, 33–35]. The finding of low prevalence of NP among Iranians and Afghanis (whose ancestral population recently migrated from the north to this region) and a high prevalence among people from Indian subcontinent and Philippines (in whom NP has not been previously reported) supports the hypothesis (Fig. 2). In addition, the low monocyte count we found in four ethnic groups with NP (correlation coefficients, 0.44 to 0.51) supports the assertion of the benign nature of the observed NP and, indirectly, the "malaria hypothesis."

An important clinical implication of this study is that our suggested cutoff for NP (2.5th percentile) in African Arabs should be 0.9×10^9/L, in Middle Easterners 1.0×10^9/L, and in Indians 1.1×10^9/L (Table 2). In healthy adult Emiratis and adult Africans, this threshold should be 1.0×10^9/L and 0.9×10^9/L, respectively [7, 16]. These numbers are considerable lower than the commonly used NP cutoff of 1.5×10^9/L. Consequently, healthy individuals from these regions with neutrophil counts $<1.5 \times 10^9$/L often undergo unnecessary investigations and inappropriate treatment [15, 17]. This problem could be addressed in several ways: (i) issuing 'benign NP health cards' to identify subjects with NP; (ii) creating a national electronic registry for NP; (iii) the screening for NP by adding leucocyte differential count to the screening tests for hemoglobinopathies already performed in many countries, and (iv) developing ethnic/nation-specific neutrophil reference values. In addition, general guidelines for investigating apparently healthy neutropenic subjects could improve the quality of health care delivery and lower health care costs. In conclusion, at least 137 million of the consolidated 1.8 billion children and adults of the 16 countries represented in this study (Additional file 1: Table S1) could benefit from higher awareness of physicians about benign neutropenia, preventing investigation and management pitfalls in neutropenic patients.

Acknowledgment

Authors thank Mukesh M. Agarwal for the useful comments.

Authors' contributions

SD designed the study, performed research, interpreted data, and wrote the manuscript. HN performed research, interpreted data, and revised the manuscript. LAAM, SAH, OAJ, and AKS performed research and interpreted data. All authors read and approved the manuscript.

Competing interests

The authors declare that they have no competing interests.

Author details

[1]Department of Medicine, College of Medicine and Health Sciences, United Arab Emirates University, PO Box 17666, Al-Ain, United Arab of Emirates. [2]Department of Pediatrics, College of Medicine and Health Sciences, United Arab Emirates University, Al-Ain, United Arab of Emirates. [3]Ambulatory Healthcare Services, Abu Dhabi, United Arab of Emirates.

References

1. Haddy TB, Rana SR, Castro O. Benign ethnic neutropenia: What is a normal absolute neutrophil count? J Lab Clin Med. 1999;133:15–22.
2. Howells DP. Neutropenia in people of African origin. Lancet. 1971;2:1318–9.
3. Hsieh MM, Everhart JE, Byrd-Holt DD, Tisdale JF, Rodgers GP. Prevalence of neutropenia in the U.S. population: Age, sex, smoking status, and ethnic differences. Ann Intern Med. 2007;146:486–92.
4. Jumean HG, Sudah FI. Chronic benign idiopathic neutropenia in Jordanians. Acta haemat. 1983;69:59–60.
5. Kaab SA, Fadhli SA, Burhamah M, Al Jafar H, Khamis A. Lymphocyte subsets in healthy adult Kuwaiti Arabs with relative benign ethnic neutropenia. Immunology Letter. 2004;91:49–53.
6. Shoenfeld Y, Alkan ML, Asaly A, Carmell Y, Katz M. Benign familial leucopenia and neutropenia in different ethnic groups. Eur J Haematol. 1988;41:273–7.
7. Denic S, Showqi S, Klein C, Takala M, Nagelkerke N, Agarwal MM. Prevalence, phenotype and inheritance of benign neutropenia in Arabs. BMC Blood Disord. 2009;9:3.
8. Weingarten MA, Pottick-Schwartz EA, Brauner A. The epidemiology of benign leucopenia in Yemenite Jews. Isr J Med Sci. 1993;29:297–9.
9. Grann VR, Ziv E, Joseph CK, Neugut AI, Wei Y, Jacobson JS, et al. Duffy (Fy), DARC, and neutropenia among women from the United States, Europe and the Caribbean. Br J Haemat. 2008;143:288–93.
10. Kelly DL, Kreyenbuhl J, Dixon L, et al. Clozapine underutilization and discontinuation in African Americans due to leucopenia. Schizophr Bull. 2007;33:1221–4.
11. Kuno E, Rothbard AB. Racial disparities in antipsychotic prescription patterns for patients with schizophrenia. Am J Psychiatry. 2002;159:567–72.
12. Smith K, Wray L, Klein-Cabral M, Schuchter L, Fox K, Glick J, et al. Ethnic disparities in adjuvant chemotherapy for breast cancer are not caused by excess toxicity in black patients. Clin Breast Cancer. 2005;6:260–6.
13. Hershman D, Weinberg M, Rosner Z, et al. Ethnic neutropenia and treatment delay in African American women undergoing chemotherapy for early-stage breast cancer. J Natl Cancer Inst. 2003;15:1545–8.
14. Melia MT, Muir AJ, McCone J, Shiffman ML, King JW, Herrine SK, et al. Racial differences in hepatitis C treatment eligibility. Hepatology. 2011;54:70–8.
15. van Rooijen CR, Slieker WA, Simsek S. Benign ethnic neutropenia; an unrecognized cause of leukopenia in negroid patients. Ned Tijdschr Geneeskd. 2012;156:A4708.
16. Eller LA, Eller MA, Ouma B, Kataaha P, Kyabaggu D, Tumusiime R, et al. Reference intervals in healthy adult Ugandan blood donors and their impact on conducting international vaccine trials. Plos One. 2008;3:e3919.
17. Denic S, Nicholls MG. A call for screening for benign neutropenia in Arab populations. Saudi Medical Journal. 2011;32:738–9.
18. Heard-Bey F. The tribal society of the UAE and its traditional economy. In: Al Abed I, Hellyer P, editors. United Arab Emirates: A new perspective. London: Trident Press; 2001. p. 98–116.
19. Al-Gazali IL, Bener A, Abdulrazzaq MY, Micallef R, Al Khayat AI, Gaber T. Consanguineous marriages in the United Arab Emirates. J Biosoc Sci. 1997; 29:491–7.
20. Denic S. Aden B, Nagelkerke N, Al Essa A. Beta-thalassemia in Abu Dhabi: Consanguinity and tribal stratification are major factors explaining the high prevalence of disease. Hemoglobin. 2013. Early Online: 1–8.
21. Gillespie JH. Population Genetics: A Concise Guide Baltimore. Baltimore: The John Hopkins Univ Press; 1998.
22. Segel GB, Halterman JS. Neutropenia in pediatric practice. Pediatr Rev. 2008; 29(1):12–23.
23. Aldrimer M, Ridefelt P, Rödöö P, Niklasson F, Gustafsson J, Hellberg D. Population-based pediatric reference intervals for hematology, iron and transferrin. Scand J Clin Lab Invest. 2013;73:253–61.
24. Ahsan S, Noether J. Hematology, Chapter 14. In: The Harriet Lane. Philadelphia: Elsevier Mosby; 2011. p. 322–53.
25. Zezulka AV, Gill JS, Beevers DG. 'Neutropenia' in black west Indians. Postgrad Med J. 1987;63:257–61.
26. Sandler SG, Kravitz C, Sharon R, Hermoni D, Ezekiel E, Cohen T. The Duffy blood group system in Israeli Jews and Arabs. Vox Sanguinis. 1979;37:41–6.
27. Anita C, Sujata M, Yogesh Kumar J, Aparup D. Natural Selection Mediated Association of the Duffy (FY) Gene Polymorphisms with Plasmodium vivax Malaria in India. Plos One. 2012;7:e45219.
28. Peng CT, Tsai CH, Lee HH, Lin CL, Wang NM, Chang JG. Molecular analysis of Duffy, Yt and Colton blood groups in Taiwanese, Filipinos and Thais. Kaohsiung J Med Sci. 2000;16:63–7.

29. Reiner AP, Lettre G, Nalls MA, Ganesh SK, Mathias R, et al. Genome-Wide Association Study of White Blood Cell Count in 16,388 African Americans: the Continental Origins and Genetic Epidemiology Network (COGENT). PLoS Genet. 2011;7(6):e1002108.
30. Thobakgale FC, Ndung'u T. Neutrophil counts in persons of African origin. Curr Opin Hematol. 2014;21:50–7.
31. Bux J, Kissel K, Nowak K, Spengel U, Mueller-Eckhardt C. Autoimmune neutropenia: clinical and laboratory studies in 143 patients. Ann Hematol. 1991;63:249–52.
32. Coşkun O, Avci IY, Sener K, Yaman H, Ogur R, Bodur H, et al. Relative lymphopenia and monocytosis may be considered as a surrogate marker of pandemic influenza a (H1N1). J Clin Virol. 2010;47:388–9.
33. Chung BH, Chan GC, Lee T, Kwok JS, Chiang AK, Ho HK, et al. Chronic benign neutropenia among Chinese children. Hong Kong Med J. 2004;10:231–6.
34. Nathan C. Neutrophils and immunity: challenges and opportunities. Nature Rev Imm. 2006;6:173–82.
35. Nguyen PH, Day N, Pram TD, Ferguson DJ, White NJ. Intraleucocytic malaria pigment and prognosis in severe malaria. Trans R Soc Trop Med Hyg. 1995; 89:200–4.

17

Knowledge, attitude and practice of students towards blood donation in Arsi university and Adama science and technology university: a comparative cross sectional study

Habtom Woldeab Gebresilase[1], Robera Olana Fite[2*] and Sileshi Garoma Abeya[3]

Abstract

Background: Blood can save millions of lives. Even though people do not donate blood regularly, there is a constant effort to balance the supply and demand of blood. The aim of this study was, therefore, to determine the knowledge, attitude and practice of blood donation between university students.

Methods: The comparative cross sectional study design was used in Adama Science and Technology University and Arsi University from April 11–May 2, 2016.360 students were selected using stratified sampling. Frequencies and proportions were computed. Chi-Square and logistic regressions were carried out and associations were considered significant at $p<0.05$.

Result: The study revealed that there was a significant knowledge difference ($\chi 2 = 152.779$, $p<0.001$) and Attitude difference ($\chi 2 = 4.142$, $p = 0.042$) between Health Science students of Arsi University and Non-Health Science students of Adama Science and Technology University. The gender of the students (AOR = 3.150, 95% CI: 1.313, 7.554) was a significant predictor of the level of knowledge of Health Science students. The ethnicity of students (AOR = 2.085, 95% CI: 1.025, 4.243) was a significant predictor of the level of an attitude of Health Science students and gender of students (AOR = 0.343, 95% CI: 0.151, 0.779) was a significant predictor of the level of an attitude of Health Science students. Concerning Non-Health Science students, religion (AOR = 10.173, 95% CI: 1.191, 86.905) and original residence (AOR = 0.289, 95% CI: 0.094, 0.891) were a significant predictor of the level of knowledge of Non-Health Science students. Gender (AOR = 0.389, 95% CI: 0.152, 0.992) and Year of study (AOR = 0.389(0.164, 0.922) were significant predictor of level of attitude of Non-Health Science students. Year of study (AOR = 5.159, 95% CI: 1.611, 16.525) was a significant predictor of level of practice of Health Science students.

Conclusion: Significant knowledge difference and attitude difference were observed between students from Arsi University and Adama Science and Technology University.

Keywords: Knowledge, Practice, Attitude, Health science, Non-health science

* Correspondence: rolana2000@gmail.com
[2]Department of Nursing, College of Health Sciences and Medicine, Woliata Sodo University, PO-Box: 138, Woliata sodo, Ethiopia
Full list of author information is available at the end of the article

Background

The demand for the whole blood transfusion is rising in relation to increased life expectancy, accidents, severe anemia, cancer, chronic diseases, pregnancy-related complication and technological advancements in the healthcare delivery system demanding blood transfusion [1–3].

Among the different types of blood donors, the safest blood comes from voluntary blood donors. In different countries, the largest proportion of hospital obtained blood is replacement donation [4]. The World Health Organization (WHO) policy is to achieve 100% not-paid blood donation practice in 2020 [2].

There is a constant effort made to increase voluntary blood donation practice. Voluntary unpaid donors are the safest group who gives blood regularly [5]. Only 60% of the people in developing countries have adequate knowledge towards blood donation. The blood donation rate in low-income, middle-income, and high-income countries is 3.9, 36.8 and 11.7 per 1000 population, respectively [6, 7].

Willingness to donate blood without expecting financial reward is one major factor to influence blood donation practice. Donor eligibility, negative attitude and lack of education lead to blood shortage in various facilities [8]. Worldwide blood donation practices are increasing day by day, yet it is a big concern for many countries. Safe blood prevents blood borne infections from the donor to the recipient. Furthermore, it saves millions of lives each year. Blood donation is included as the main aspect of the preventive and therapeutic component of the health care delivery system [9]. Blood is a scarce product. There is an imbalance between the demand and supply [2]. In developing countries, the community accessed around 40% of the blood banks supply and from this, 60% are collected from paid blood donation [10]. This is associated with the hesitation to donate blood. People assume that they may develop complication from donating. This is a major misconception underlying the practice [11].

There is a need to establish a global and a nationwide organization in initiating and leading the practice of blood donation. Red Cross and Red Crescent society are institutions working in developing countries to address the blood donation for the mothers delivering, for patients undergoing surgery and for the patients who suffered from accidents [12].

Bleeding might be caused by accidents, medical procedures and giving birth.495,000 women die from bleeding associated with pregnancy and childbirth, which needs early medical interventions [13]. Worldwide people from all age groups require a blood donation to support continuity of life and improve the life quality [14]. This relates to the sophisticated medical surgical procedures requiring blood transfusion [15]. There is a growing need for blood. This is related to the advancement in the healthcare delivery [10]. WHO reported that 38% of voluntarily donated blood comes from those young people aged less than 25. There is a need to motivate young generations to meet 100% voluntary not-paid blood donation [16].

Young students are healthy, active, dynamic, resourceful and receptive; they constitute a greater proportion of the population so that those young students need encouragement and motivation to donate blood voluntarily. Absence of volunteer blood donation is a main challenge seen in our study area. Furthermore, no previous comparative study conducted in this area, this study tried to come up with the following major finding that fills the existing information gap on the level of knowledge, attitude and practice towards voluntary blood donation by comparing Health Science and Non-Health Science students of both universities.

Methods

Study area and period

The study was conducted in Adama Science and Technology University (ASTU) and Arsi university regular undergraduate Non-Health Science and Health Science students respectively. ASTU is found in Adama town East Shewa zone in Oromiya regional state. It is 100 km far from the capital city of Ethiopia, Addis Ababa. It has 9737 regular undergraduate students 7205 male & 2512 Female students among them 7448 are 3rd year and above. Arsi University is found in Oromiya regional state, Arsi zone, in Aselatown that is around 170 km far from Addis Ababa. There are around 1130 regular undergraduate Health Science students in this university.764 of them are male and 333 are female students. Among them, 538 are from 3rd year up to 5th year. The study was conducted from April 11–May 2, 2016.

Study design

An institution based comparative cross-sectional study design was used.

Population

The Source population was all undergraduate Health Science and Non-Health Science University students and the study population was sampled students who will fulfill the inclusion criteria.

Inclusion and exclusion criteria

ASTU Non-Health Science and Arsi university Health Science regular undergraduate at least 18 years old and those students who were from third-year up to the fifth-year were included. Those students who were critically ill during the data collection time, distance program students, weekend students, postgraduate students, students who had chronic disease and mentally challenged students were excluded.

Sample size and sampling procedure

Sample size determination

The sample size was calculated using Epi-Info version 21 by considering a 23.6% prevalence of blood donation practice from Ambo study [3], 95% confidence level, 80% power of the study, a risk ratio of 2, and one to one ratio (1:1)in comparison groups. After adding of 5% Non-response rate, the final sample size became 360(in each group it became 180).

Sampling procedure

First, the two universities were selected using a stratified sampling method, then the sample was equally distributed between both universities (half of the Health Science students and the other half of Non-Health Science students).Then the sample was proportional allocated using year of study. Finally, the simple random sampling method was used.

Operational definition

Knowledge A score of one was given for the correct response and zero for wrong response. Respondents who scored above the mean scored were considered as having good knowledge and others were considered as having poor knowledge.

Attitude A score of one was given for each correct response and zero for the wrong response. Respondents who scored above the mean scored were considered as having favorable attitude and others were considered as having unfavorable attitude.

Practice It was measured by asking about the history of blood donation.

Data collection tools

Structured questionnaire The structured questionnaire was adapted after a review of different literatures [3, 11, 13]. The questionnaire had four parts. The first part questions about the socio-demographic characteristics of the respondents. The second, third and fourth part questions about the knowledge, attitude and practice level of blood donation respectively.

Data collection procedure Four data collectors were recruited. One supervisor was used during the data collection period. Training was provided for the data collectors and the supervisor for two days by the principal investigator. The sessions of the training were the objective of the study, the meaning of each question and techniques of interview. In addition, the role of the data collector and the supervisor was covered.

Data quality assurance

Training was given to supervisors and data collectors. After completing the training, a pre-test did in rift valley University College Adama campus, accounting 5% of the total sample. During the data collection period, supervisors reviewed for the completeness, consistency, and accuracy of each questionnaire. Corrective measures were taken by discussing with the research team.

Data processing and analysis

Data checked manually for completeness and then coded and entered using EpiData version 3.1.The generated data were exported to SPSS version 20. The data were cleaned by visualizing, calculating frequencies and sorting. Frequencies and proportions were computed. The statistical association was done for categorical variables. Significance was determined by using crude and adjusted odds ratios with 95% confidence intervals. To assess the association between the dependent variables and independent variables, bivariable analysis was employed. Then multiple logistic regressions were employed to identify different predictor variables with considering *p*-value less than 0.05. Finally, the results were presented as tables, figures and sentence.

Result

Socio-demographic characteristics

In the study, 360 students participated in the study. The median age of Health Science students was 22 with a range of 21–23 and the Non-Health Science students were 23 with a range of 22–24. Among them, 294(81.7%) were males, 233(64.7%) were Orthodox religion followers, 139(38.6%) were Amhara and 199(55.3%) came from urban areas (Table 1).

Level of knowledge of blood donation

The majority of Health Science students 143(79.4%) of them has good knowledge regarding blood donation on the other hand only 25(13.9%) of Non-Health Science students shown to have good knowledge generally there is a significant knowledge difference was observed (Table 2).

Level of attitude on blood donation

Less than half 84(46.7%) and 64(35.6%) of Health and Non-Health Science students have favorable attitudes towards blood donation respectively. Generally, on chi-square test, a significant difference of attitude level observed, Health Science students shown to have a better level of attitude when compared to Non-Health Science (Table 3).

Table 1 Socio-demographic characteristics of Health Science students in Arsi University Health Science students and Adama science and Technology University Non-Health Science students, Ethiopia, April 11–May 2, 2016

Variables		Non-Health Science student		Health Science student		Total ($n = 360$)	
		N	(%)	N	(%)	N	%
Age	18–24	152	84.4	152	84.4	304	84.4
	25–30	28	15.6	28	15.6	56	15.6
Gender	Male	152	84.4	142	78.9	294	81.7
	Female	28	15.6	38	21.1	66	18.3
Religion	Orthodox	117	65	116	64.4	233	64.7
	Protestant	34	18.9	34	18.9	68	18.9
	Muslim	29	16.1	30	16.7	59	16.4
Ethnicity	Amhara	76	42.2	63	35	139	38.6
	Oromo	48	26.7	90	50	138	38.3
	Others	56	31.1	27	15	83	23.1
Original Residence	Rural	74	41.1	87	48.3	161	44.7
	Urban	106	58.9	93	51.7	199	55.3
year of study	Third year	90	50	72	40	162	45
	Fourth Year	50	27.8	65	36.1	115	31.9
	Fifth year	40	22.2	43	23.9	83	23.1

Level of practice of blood donation

Pertaining to blood donation practices 49 (27.2%) and 41 (22.8%) of Health and Non-Health Science students donate blood at least once in their lifetime respectively. A significant difference was observed regarding the level of blood donation practice between health and Non-Health Science students (Table 4).

Factors associated with the level of knowledge among health science students

Multivariable logistic regression was used to identify factors associated with the level of knowledge about blood donation. Consequently, coefficients were expressed as crude and adjusted OR relative to the referent category. The gender of the students was found as the significant predictor. Accordingly, female Health Science students were 3.2 times more likely to have a better knowledge than male Health Science students were (AOR = 3.150, 95% CI: 1.313, 7.554) (Table 5).

Factors associated with level of attitude among health science students

Multivariable logistic regression was used to identify factors associated with attitudes about blood donation. The ethnicity of the students was found as the significant predictor. Health Science students from the Oromo ethnic group were 2.1 times more likely to have a favorable attitude as compared to Health Science students from the Amhara ethnic group (AOR = 2.085, 95% CI: 1.025, 4.243) (Table 6).

Factors associated with level of practice among health science students

Multivariable logistic regression was used to identify factors associated with practice of blood donation. The gender of the students was found as the significant predictor. Accordingly, Female Health Science students were 65.7% less likely to donate blood than male Health Science students were (AOR = 0.343, 95% CI: 0.151, 0.779) (Table 7).

Table 2 Level of knowledge of blood donation among Health Science students in Arsi University and Non-Health Science students in Adama Science and Technology University, Ethiopia, April 11–May 2, 2016

Variables	Health Science students		Non-Health Science students		χ2	*P* value
	n	%	n	%		
Level of knowledge						
Good	143	79.4	25	13.9	152.779	<0.001[a]
Poor	37	20.6	155	86.1		

[a]Significant association

Table 3 Level of attitude on blood donation among Health Science students in Arsi University and Non-Health Science students in Adama Science and Technology University, Ethiopia, April 11–May 2, 2016

Variables	Health Science students		Non-Health Science students		χ2	P value
	n	%	n	%		
Level of Attitude						
Favorable	84	46.7	64	35.6	4.142	0.042[a]
Non-favorable	96	53.3	116	64.4		

[a]Significant association

Factors associated with level of knowledge among non-health science students

Multivariable logistic regression used to identify factors associated with the level of knowledge about blood donation. Before adjustment, Fifth-year Non-Health Science students were 66.7% less likely to have higher knowledge than third-year Non-Health Science (AOR = 0.333, 95% CI: 0.123, 0.900).However, it was not any more significant after adjustment.

After adjustment, Religion and residence of the students were significant predictors. Accordingly, Protestant religion follower Non-Health Science students were 10.2 times more likely to have a better knowledge than Orthodox religion follower Non- Health Science students (AOR = 10.173, 95% CI: 1.191,86.905). Urban living Non-Health Science students were 71.1% less likely to had good knowledge than rural living Non- Health Science students (AOR = 0.289, 95% CI: 0.094,0.891) (Table 8).

Factors associated with the level of attitude among non-health science students

Multivariable logistic regression used to identify factors associated with the level of attitude about blood donation. Before adjustment, other religion follower Non-Health Science students were 3.1 times more likely to have a favorable attitude than orthodox religion follower Non-Health Science students were(AOR = 3.110, 95% CI: 1.108,8.732). Nevertheless, it was not any more significant after adjustment. Gender and year of study of the students were the significant predictor.

Accordingly, Female Non-Health Science students were 61.1% less likely to have a favorable attitude than male Non-Health Science students were (AOR = 0.389, 95% CI: 0.152, 0.992). The fifth year Non-Health Science students were 61.1% less likely to had favorable attitude than third-year Non-Health Science (AOR = 0.389, 95% CI: 0.164, 0.922)(Table 9).

Factors associated with level of practice among non-health science students

Multivariable logistic regression used to identify factors associated with the level of knowledge. Accordingly, Fourth-year Non-Health Science students were 5.2 times more likely to donate blood than third-year Non- Health Science students (AOR = 5.159, 95% CI: 1.611, 16.525)(Table 10).

Discussion

Maintaining the required level of blood supply is the main concern of various organizations working on health. Therefore, identifying the level of knowledge, attitude and practice is very essential. An attempt was made to identify the knowledge, attitude, practice and factors associated factors with blood donation between Health Science students of Arsi University and Non-Health Science students of Adama Science and Technology University.

The study revealed that 79.4% of Health Science students shown to have good knowledge about blood donation. This is comparable to a study conducted in Addis Ababa university Health Science students, which was (83.6%) [17]; But this is higher when compared with the study conducted on Health Science students in Tamil Nadu, India in which around 35.6% of the respondents shown to have a good level of knowledge [18]. It is also higher than the study conducted on Health Science students of Manipur (9%) [19]. This difference might be related to the background of the students.

Table 4 Level of practice of blood donation among Health Science students in Arsi University and Non-Health Science students at Adama Science and Technology University, Ethiopia, April 11–May 2, 2016

Variables	Health Science students		Non-Health Science students		χ2	P value
	n	%	n	%		
Level of practice						
Yes	49	27.2	41	22.8	0.726	0.394
No	131	72.8	139	77.2		

Table 5 Factors associated with Level of knowledge on blood donation among Health Science students in Arsi University, Ethiopia, April 11–May 2, 2016

Variables		Knowledge level		COR(95% CI)	AOR(95% CI)
		Good	Poor		
Gender	Male[a]	118	24	1	1
	Female	25	13	2.557(1.148,5.696) [b]	3.150(1.313,7.554) [b]
Age	18-24[a]	118	34	1	1
	25–30	25	3	0.416(0.119,1.464)	0.391(0.100,1.528)
Religion	Orthodox[a]	91	25	1	1
	Protestant	27	7	0.944(0.368,2.420)	0.871(0.310,2.449)
	Others	25	5	0.728(0.253,2.096)	0.749(0.242,2.320)
Ethnicity	Amhara[a]	48	15	1	1
	Oromo	74	16	0.692(0.313,1.528)	0.823(0.347,1.951)
	Others	21	6	0.914(0.312,2.683)	0.896(0.270,2.974)
Year of study	Third year[a]	59	13	1	1
	Fourth year	47	18	1.738(0.773,3.906)	2.400(0.993,5.804)
	Fifth year	37	6	0.736(0.257,2.105)	0.890(0.286,2.774)
Residence	Rural[a]	69	18	1	1
	Urban	74	19	0.984(0.477,2.029)	1.027(0.465,2.266)

[a]Reference Category, [b]Significant association

Table 6 Factors associated with Level of attitude on blood donation among Health Science students in Arsi University, Ethiopia, April 11–May 2, 2016

Variables		Attitude level		COR(95% CI)	AOR(95% CI)
		Favorable	Unfavorable		
Gender	Male[a]	71	71	1	1
	Female	13	25	1.923(0.912,4.057)	1.972(0.884,4.399)
Age	18-24[a]	72	80	1	1
	25–30	12	16	1.200(0.532,2.707)	1.159(0.452,2.967)
Religion	Orthodox[a]	56	60	1	1
	Protestant	18	16	0.830(0.386,1.784)	0.649(0.283,1.493)
	Others	10	20	1.867(0.804,4.332)	1.475(0.607,3.588)
Ethnicity	Amhara[a]	36	27	1	1
	Oromo	36	54	2.000(1.041,3.844) [b]	2.085(1.025,4.243) [b]
	Others	12	15	1.667(0.672,4.134)	1.823(0.681,4.884)
Year of study	Third year[a]	32	40	1	1
	Fourth year	31	34	0.877(0.448,1.720)	0.913(0.442,1.886)
	Fifth year	21	22	0.838(0.393,1.787)	0.836(0.356,1.966)
Residence	Rural[a]	43	44	1	1
	Urban	41	52	1.239(0.689,2.229)	1.083(0.576,2.037)
Knowledge	Good[a]	69	74	1	1
	Poor	15	22	1.368(0.657,2.848)	1.346(0.613,2.952)

[a]Reference category, [b]Significant association

Table 7 Factors associated with Level of practice of blood donation among Health Science students in Arsi University, Ethiopia, April 11–May 2, 2016

Variables		Practice level		COR(95% CI)	AOR(95% CI)
		Yes	No		
Gender	Male[a]	32	110	1	1
	Female	17	21	0.359(0.170,0.761) [b]	0.343(0.151,0.779) [b]
Age	18-24[a]	39	113	1	1
	25–30	10	18	0.621(0.264,1.460)	0.820(0.307,2.188)
Religion	Orthodox[a]	34	82	1	1
	Protestant	8	26	1.348(0.555,3.273)	1.427(0.542,3.762)
	Others	7	23	1.362(0.534,3.473)	1.419(0.522,3.860)
Ethnicity	Amhara[a]	18	45	1	1
	Oromo	24	66	1.100(0.536,2.258)	0.896(0.405,1.982)
	Others	7	20	1.143(0.412,3.168)	1.046(0.338,3.237)
Year of study	Third year[a]	14	58	1	1
	Fourth year	20	45	0.543(0.247,1.192)	0.461(0.195,1.091)
	Fifth year	15	28	0.451(0.191,1.061)	0.466(0.177,1.229)
Residence	Rural[a]	21	66	1	1
	Urban	28	65	0.739(0.381,1.431)	0.792(0.385,1.629)
Knowledge	Good[a]	36	107	1	1
	Poor	13	24	0.621(0.287,1.346)	0.760(0.327,1.765)

[a]Reference category, [b]Significant association

Table 8 Factors associated with Level of knowledge on blood donation among Non-Health Science students in Adama Science and Technology University, Ethiopia, April 11–May 2, 2016

Variables		Knowledge		COR(95% CI)	AOR(95% CI)
		Good	Poor		
Gender	Male[a]	22	130	1	1
	Female	3	25	1.410(0.392,5.072)	1.846(0.444,7.674)
Age	18-24[a]	21	131	1	1
	25–30	4	24	0.962(0.303,3.051)	0.861(0.228,3.247)
Religion	Orthodox[a]	20	97	1	1
	Protestant	1	33	6.804(0.879,52.687)	10.173(1.191,86.905)[b]
	Others	4	25	1.289(0.404,4.111)	1.248(0.359,4.331)
Ethnicity	Amhara[a]	10	66	1	1
	Oromo	5	43	1.303(0.417,4.075)	1.171(0.345,3.973)
	Others	10	46	0.697(0.268,1.809)	0.501(0.175,1.435)
Year of study	Third year[a]	9	81	1	1
	Fourth year	6	44	0.815(0.272,2.439)	0.718(0.213,2.421)
	Fifth year	10	30	0.333(0.123,0.900) [b]	0.341(0.113,1.034)
Residence	Rural[a]	6	68	1	1
	Urban	19	87	0.404(0.153,1.067)	0.289(0.094,0.891) [b]

[a]Reference category, [b]Significant association

Table 9 Factors associated with Level of attitude on blood donation among Non-Health Science students in Adama Science and Technology University, Ethiopia, April 11–May 2, 2016

Variables		Attitude		COR(95% CI)	AOR(95% CI)
		Favorable	Unfavorable		
Gender	Male[a]	50	102	1	1
	Female	14	14	0.490(0.217,1.107)	0.389(0.152,0.992) [b]
Age	18-24[a]	53	99	1	1
	25–30	11	17	0.827(0.361,1.895)	0.842(0.319,2.225)
Religion	Orthodox[a]	46	71	1	1
	Protestant	13	21	1.047(0.477,2.294)	0.655(0.258,1.663)
	Others	5	24	3.110(1.108,8.732) [b]	2.778(0.934,8.263)
Ethnicity	Amhara[a]	28	48	1	1
	Oromo	18	30	0.972(0.460,2.053)	0.865(0.367,2.039)
	Others	18	38	1.231(0.594,2.553)	1.731(0.738,4.058)
Year of study	Third year[a]	28	62	1	1
	Fourth year	15	35	1.054(0.497,2.235)	1.036(0.447,2400)
	Fifth year	21	19	0.409(0.190,0.878) [b]	0.389(0.164,0.922) [b]
Residence	Rural[a]	25	49	1	1
	Urban	39	67	0.877(0.470,1.634)	0.914(0.448,1.868)
Knowledge level	Good[a]	12	13	1	1
	Poor	52	103	1.828(0.780,4.289	1.883(0.730,4.859)

[a]Reference category, [b]Significant association

Table 10 Factors associated with Level of practice of blood donation among Non-Health Science students in Adama Science and Technology University, Ethiopia, April 11–May 2, 2016

Variables		Practice level		COR(95% CI)	AOR(95% CI)
		Yes	No		
Gender	Male[a]	35	117	1	1
	Female	6	22	1.097(0.412,2.918)	1.830(0.619,5.411)
Age	18-24[a]	75	229	1	1
	25–30	15	41	1.428(0.506,4.026)	1.476(0.456,4.782)
Religion	Orthodox[a]	64	169	1	1
	Protestant	12	56	2.586(0.841,7.948)	2.093(0.592,7.397)
	Others	14	45	1.084(0.421,2.792)	1.184(0.422,3.326)
Ethnicity	Amhara[a]	38	101	1	1
	Oromo	32	106	1.786(0.715,4.458)	1.332(0.494,3.591)
	Others	20	63	1.181(0.529,2.638)	0.932(0.375,2.316)
Year of study	Third year[a]	41	121	1	1
	Fourth year	24	91	4.929(1.613,15.056) [b]	5.159(1.611,16.525) [b]
	Fifth year	25	58	1.286(0.552,2.996)	1.592(0.620,4.090)
Residence	Rural[a]	37	124	1	1
	Urban	53	146	0.894(0.438,1.822)	0.985(0.430,2.255)
Knowledge level	Good[a]	45	123	1	1
	Poor	45	147	2.162(0.875,5.342)	2.064(0.747,5.701)

[a]Reference category, [b]Significant association

The study also revealed that less than half (46.7%) of Health Science students had a favorable attitude. This finding is different from the finding of a study conducted in South Indian in which 87.3% of the respondents show favorable attitude [20]; it is also lower than the study conducted on Addis Ababa University health-science students of Ethiopia, in which 68% of the respondents had a favorable attitude [17]. This difference might occur due to sociocultural difference and educational attributes between the respondents. This suggests the need for more emphasis on blood donation in the Health Science curriculum.

A significant good level of knowledge difference observed between Health Science students (79.4%) and Non-Health Science students (13.9%). In addition, significant favorable attitude differences observed between Health Science students (46.7%) and Non-Health Science students (35.6%). This might be due to the effect of education delivered for Health Science students. In addition, direct exposure in the hospital environment might improve the knowledge and attitude of Health Science students.

Unlike previous reports year of study was not a significant association with knowledge towards blood donation among Health Science students [17, 21]. This might be due to the absence of special education related to blood donation delivered to senior students.

In the study, female Non-Health Science students were 61.1% less likely to have a favorable attitude than male Non-Health Science students did. This might be due to the less frequent mass-media exposure of females. This in turn might decrease access to information provided on blood donation. In addition, it might be due to the cultural taboo. This implies there is a need for health information delivery through campaigns and different sources of information.

Female Health Science students were 65.7% less likely to donate blood than male Health Science students were. This finding is consistent with similar studies [22–24]. This might be related to the limited opportunity and freedom of choice offered for females. This implies that females need to be advised more on the medical benefits of donating blood.

27.2% Health Science students have donated blood. This is contrary to a study conducted in South India in which 10.75% have donated blood [18], in Canada 43.8% have donated blood [25]. This might be due to the difference in the implementation of blood donation campaigns. In addition, the rate of blood donation in developing country is low [26]. This implies the health policy designed in those countries need to give due emphasis to blood donation practice. Furthermore, making Blood Banks available in different health institutions might strengthen the involvement of the institutions in promoting the practice.

Knowledge has no significant association with the level of practice among Health Science students. This is similar to different studies [27, 28]. This might be due to the lack of opportunity and have not asked for donating blood by donor recruitment programs. To increase the number of volunteer blood donors, students need to be constantly encouraged to donate blood through different blood campaigns.

The limitation of this study was the response might have been liable to social desirability bias. The study design cannot assess the cause and effect relationship. In addition, the factors expected to influence knowledge, attitude and practice may not be exhaustive. There could be other factors, which the study did not reveal. It has to be noted that the finding of this study mainly reflects the situation in Adama Science and Technology University and Arsi University. Therefore, the findings should be interpreted with caution.

The result signifies that the universities should establish or res-strengthen blood donation clubs. The students should receive training on voluntary blood donation. Furthermore, both universities need to work with various agencies to remove the misconceptions. Students also need to be motivated with recognitions. The national health policies need to focus on blood donation campaigns through the mobilization of students.

Conclusion

A significant level of knowledge difference and level of attitude difference observed between the Health Science of Arsi University and Non-Health Science students of Adama science and Technology University. There was no difference in the practice of blood donation between the two groups. The gender of the students was a significant predictor of the level of knowledge and level of practice of Health Science students. The ethnicity of the students was a significant predictor of the level of an attitude of Health Science students. Religion and residence of the students' was the significant predictor of the level of knowledge of Non-Health Science students. Gender and year of study of the students were significant predictors of the level of an attitude of Non-Health Science students. The year of a study of the students was a significant predictor of the level of practice of Non-Health Science students.

Abbreviations

AOR: Adjusted Odds Ration; ASTU: Adama Science and Technology University; CI: Confidence Interval; COR: Crude Odds Ration; WHO: World Health Organization

Acknowledgements

We would like to forward our deepest appreciation to the Adama General Hospital and Medical College for their cooperation on necessary materials and supports to undertake this study. Finally, our appreciation also goes to the data collectors, supervisors and students who participated in the study.

Funding
Adama Hospital and Medical College have covered the required funds for the research project. The funding body has no contribution in other activities of the research.

Authors' contributions
HWG conceptualized and designed the study. HWG, ROF and SGA analyzed, interpreted the data, drafted the manuscript and critically reviewed the manuscript. All the authors read and approved the manuscript.

Competing interests
The authors declare that they have no competing interests.

Author details
[1]Department of public Health, College of Health Sciences, Adama General Hospital and Medical College, Adama, Ethiopia. [2]Department of Nursing, College of Health Sciences and Medicine, Woliata Sodo University, PO-Box: 138, Woliata sodo, Ethiopia. [3]Department of Social and Population Health, Adama General Hospital and Medical College, Adama, Ethiopia.

References

1. Mohammed H, Osman T. Voluntary Blood Donation among Medical Students in a Resource-limited Country. JPHDC. 2016;2(3):257–67.
2. World Health Organization. Voluntary unpaid blood donations must increase rapidly to meet 2020 goal. http://www.who.int/campaigns/world-blood-donor-day/2016/event/en/. Accessed 17 Mar 2016.
3. Nigatu A, Demissie DB. Knowledge, Attitude and Practice on Voluntary Blood Donation and Associated Factors among Ambo University Regular Students, Ambo Town, Ethiopia. JCMHE. 2014;4(5). doi:10.4172/2161-0711.1000315.
4. Suchetha S, Muninarayana C, Venkatesha M, Anil NS. Blood donation awareness and beliefs among medical and nursing students. Int J Med Sci Public Health. 2015;4(10):1338–42.
5. Tapko JB, Toure B, Sambo LG. Status of blood safety in the WHO African region: report of the 2010 survey. Brazzaville: WHO Regional Office for Africa; 2014.
6. Riley W, Schwei M, McCullough J. The United States potential blood donor pool: estimating the prevalence of donor-exclusion factors on the pool of potential donors. Transfusion. 2007;47(7):1180–8.
7. World Health Organization. Blood safety and availability. WHO Fact Sheet. 2013(279). http://www.who.int/mediacentre/factsheets/fs279/en/. Accessed 17 Mar 2016.
8. Schreiber GB, Schlumpf KS, Glynn SA, Wright DJ, Tu Y, King MR, et al. Convenience, the bane of our existence, and other barriers to donating. Transfusion. 2006;46(4):545–53.
9. WHO, "Towards 100% voluntary blood donation a global framework for action,". Melbourne, 2010. http://www.who.int/bloodsafety/publications/9789241599696/en/. Accessed 17 Mar 2016.
10. Mitra K, Mandal PK, Nandy S, Roy R, Joaardar GKA. Study on awareness and perceptions regarding blood safety and blood donation among health care providers in a teaching hospital of Calcutta. Indian J Community Med. 2001;26(1):21–5.
11. Zubair H, Seema HS. Comparative Study on Knowledge Attitude and Practice regarding Blood Donation in Rural and Urban area of Bangalore. Int J Med Health Sci. 2015;4(3):309–14.
12. The International Federation of Red Cross and Red Crescent Societies. Voluntary blood donation towards safe and healthy living. http://www.ifrc.org/en/what-wedo/health/blood-services/global-actiontowards-100-per-cent-voluntary-nonremunerated-blood-donation/. Accessed 20 June 2016.
13. Hosain GM, Anisuzzaman M, Begum A. Knowledge, Attitude and practice on blood donation among Dhaka university students in Bangladesh. East Afr Med J. 1997;74(9):549–53.
14. Damesyn MA, Glynn SA, Schreiber GB, Ownby HE, Bethel J, Fridey J, et al. Behavioral and infectious disease risks in young blood donors: implications for recruitment. Transfusion. 2003;43(11):1596–603.
15. Lives S. Universal access to safe blood transfusion: scaling up the implementation of the WHO strategy for blood safety and availability for improving patient health and saving lives. Geneva: World health Organization; 2015.
16. Van Hulst M, SmitSibinga CT, Postma MJ. Health economics of blood transfusion safety–focus on sub-Saharan Africa. Biologicals. 2010;38(1):53–8.
17. Misganaw C, Tenkir M, Deresa A, Tesfaye M, Tessema TT, Taye H. The level and associated factors of knowledge, attitude and practice of blood donation among health science students of Addis Ababa university. IJMHSR. 2014;1(10):105–18.
18. Manikandan S, Srikumar R, Ruvanthika PN. A study on knowledge, attitude and practice on blood donation among health professional students in Chennai, Tamil Nadu, South India. IJRSP. 2013;3(3):1–4.
19. Syiemlieh AJ, Akoijam BS, Kumar S. Assessment of Knowledge, Perception & Practice of Voluntary Blood Donation among Health Professional Students in RIMS, Imphal, Manipur. IOSR-JDMS. 2016;15(10):26–30.
20. Karakkamandapam S, Raghavan V, Sabu KM. Knowledge, attitude and practice on blood donation among health science students in a university campus. South India OJHAS. 2011;10(2):1–3.
21. Singh S, Muninarayana C, Venkatesha M, Anil NS. Blood donation awareness and beliefs among medical and nursing students. Int J Med Sci Public Health. 2015;4(10):1338–42.
22. Mamatya A, Prajapati R, Yadav R. Knowledge and practice of blood donation: a comparison between medical and non-medical Nepalese students. Nepal Med Coll J. 2012;14(4):283–6.
23. Safizadeh H, Pourdamghan N, Mohamadi B. University students Awarness and Attitude towards Blood Donation in Kerman City. IJBC. 2009;1(3):107–10.
24. Alethea Z, Silveira MF, Dumith SC. Blood donation prevalence and associated factors in Pelotas,Southern Brazil. Rev Saude Publica. 2010;44(1):112–20.
25. Lemmens KPH, Abrham C, Ruiter RAC, Veldhuizen IJT, Bos AER, Schaalma HP. Identifying blood donors willing to help with recruitment. Vox Sang. 2008;95(3):211–7.
26. World Health organization. Global status report on road safety: time for action 2009. http://www.who.int/violence_injury_prevention/road_safety_status/2009/en/. Accessed 5 June 2017.
27. Sabu KM, Remya A, Binu VS, Vivek R. Knowledge, Attitude and Practice on Blood Donation among Health Science students in a university campus, South India. Online J Health Allied SCS. 2011;10(2):6.
28. Bharatwaj RS, Vijaya K, Rajaram P. A Descriptive Study of Knowledge, Attitude and Practice with regard to Voluntary Blood Donation among Medical Undergraduate Students in Pondicherry, India. J Clin Diagnos Res. 2012;6(4):602–4.

Biochemical and hematological changes among anemic and non-anemic pregnant women attending antenatal clinic at the Bolgatanga regional hospital, Ghana

Benjamin Ahenkorah[1,4,5*], Kwabena Nsiah[2], Peter Baffoe[3] and Enoch Odame Anto[5,6,7]

Abstract

Background: Anemia in pregnancy may not only be associated with maternal morbidity and mortality but can also be detrimental to the fetus. A definitive diagnosis of anemia is a pre-requisite to unravelling possible cause(s), to allow appropriate treatment intervention. It is hypothesised that measured hemoglobin (HGB), complemented by biochemical and other hematological parameters would enhance anemia diagnosis.

Methods: This was a cross-sectional study among 400 pregnant women comprising 253 anemic and 147 non-anemic pregnant women, attending an antenatal clinic at Bolgatanga Regional Hospital, Ghana. Venous blood was collected and hemoglobin genotype, complete blood count and biochemical parameters [ferritin, iron, total iron binding capacity (TIBC), transferrin saturation (TfS), C-reactive protein (CRP) and bilirubin] were determined. Thick blood films were prepared for malaria parasitemia, while early morning stool and midstream urine samples were examined for enteric and urogenital parasites, respectively.

Results: There were significantly reduced levels of HGB ($p < 0.0001$), HCT ($p < 0.0001$), MCV ($p < 0.0001$), iron (0.0273), ferritin ($p = 0.018$) and transferrin saturation (0.0391) and increased WBC ($p = 0.006$), RDW ($p = 0.0480$), TIBC ($p = 0.0438$) and positivity of CRP in anemic, compared to non-anemic pregnant women. Anemic women were associated with increased proportion of hemoglobinopathies (AS, SS and SC), *Plasmodium falciparum, Schistosoma hematobium* and intestinal parasite infections.

Conclusion: Anemic pregnant women are associated with a significant derangement in hematological and iron indices that implicate iron deficiency. This was influenced by hemoglobinopathies and parasitic infections.

Keywords: Anemia, Pregnant women, Hematological, Biochemical, Iron deficiency

Background

Anemia is the most prevalent nutritional deficiency problem during pregnancy. Iron deficiency anemia is the leading cause of anemia in most developing countries [1]. Anemia and iron deficiency anemia are often used interchangeably and the prevalence of anemia taken to be the same as that of iron deficiency [1]. It has been reported that 56% of pregnant women in low income countries are affected [2], in contrast to 18% in high income countries [3].

In Ghana, anemia has been attributed to poor bioavailability of iron in the diet, which is due to the low intake of foods that enhance absorption of iron [4–6]. During pregnancy, there is disproportionate increase in the plasma volume, relative erythrocyte number, leading to a fall in hemoglobin concentration [7]. Moreover, the iron requirement generally exceeds the amount provided in the diet [8]. Intestinal iron absorption increases during pregnancy but becomes poor in cases of associated parasitic infectious diseases, such as hookworm and roundworm infestations [9].

* Correspondence: benahenkorah.cos@gmail.com; bennahie@yahoo.com
[1]Biochemistry and Hematology Units, Bolgatanga Regional Hospital, P.O. Box 26, Bolgatanga-Upper East Region, Ghana
[4]Department of Biochemistry and Molecular Medicine, School of Medical and Health Science, University for Development Studies, Tamale, Ghana
Full list of author information is available at the end of the article

Anemia during pregnancy is associated with a number of maternal and fetal disorders including the risks of preterm births, low birth weight babies, perinatal mortality and intrauterine growth retardation [10, 11]. Formation of fetal hemoglobin and myoglobin requires iron. Fetal iron is obtained from maternal stores, which progressively leads to depletion of iron in the mother. Therefore, adequate iron is required for a successful pregnancy and fetal outcomes [12].

A number of hematological [13, 14] and iron-related indices [15] have been used in the diagnosis of anemia in pregnancy. Although serum ferritin concentration of less than 12 μg/L is usually used as an indicator of iron deficiency [16], in tropical countries, a cut-off of 30 μg/L has been recommended as being the best indicator of deficient iron stores [17]. Elevated ferritin level, serum transferrin, transferrin receptor (TfR), TIBC, erythrocyte sedimentation rate, and C-reactive protein concentrations, and reduced serum iron concentrations and transferrin saturation are usually associated with anemia of chronic disease [18].

The routine assessment of anemia has been based on hemoglobin levels of < 11 g/dl. However, other red cell indices such as MCV, MCH, MCHC and RDW have been widely employed in anemia diagnosis [18]. A reduced Hb, MCV below the lower reference limit for normal and an increased RDW above the upper reference limit for normal have been associated with microcytic anemia in pregnancy [19].

Although the anemic condition is progressive throughout pregnancy and is known to alter the red cell indices and iron status, few studies have studied both factors in pregnancy. Some studies, apart from measuring these factors independently, did not simultaneously consider the effect of Plasmodium parasite, intestinal parasites and *Schistosoma hematobium* infestation. It is against this background that we determined the changes in iron status and red cell indices, along with the presence of sickle cell and parasitic infections, among anemic and non-anemic pregnant women, visiting an antenatal clinic at the Bolgatanga Regional Hospital, Ghana.

Methods

Study design and setting

This hospital-based cross-sectional case-control study was conducted in the Obstetrics and Gynecology Department of the Regional Hospital Bolgatanga (RHB), Ghana, West Africa from May, 2013 to May, 2014.

Study population and participant recruitment

A total of 400 pregnant women, comprising 253 anemic pregnant women with hemoglobin concentration < 11 g/dl using WHO criteria [20], were considered as cases and 147 non-anemic pregnant women of hemoglobin concentration > 11 g/dl, were purposively recruited as control.

Inclusion and exclusion criteria

The study included all pregnant women attending their first antenatal care, of ages ranging from 15 to 48 years. Pregnant women in need of emergency care or having an at-risk pregnancy such as gestational diabetes, pre-eclampsia and eclampsia, were excluded. Antenatal pregnant women reporting for repeat visits during the study period and subjects who had been confirmed to be HIV positive were also excluded from the study.

Specimen collection and processing

Five (5) milliliters (mls) of participants' venous blood samples were drawn for hematological and biochemical analysis, between the hours of 8:00 am and 9:00 am. About 2mls were collected into BD vacutainers, containing EDTA for determination of hematological parameters and 3mls into BD Vacutainers with SST II Advance semi-separator gel, for determination of biochemical parameters. Samples in SST were centrifuged at 3000 rpm for 10 min and serum samples were aliquoted into cryotubes and stored at -80° C until assay. Also, about 2 drops (6 μl) of blood were collected on a slide for the preparation of thick blood film to detect the presence of malaria parasites, according to the protocol described by Ahenkorah et al. [21].

About two grams (2 g) of early morning stool and 10 mls midstream early morning urine samples were also collected into sterile containers. The urine was used for the determination of *Schistosoma hematobium* ova/cyst and the stool for the determination of intestinal parasites. The collected samples were transferred in a cold box to the Biochemistry and Hematology Laboratory of RHB, for the required investigations.

Hematological assay

Full blood count was performed using the Sysmex KX-21 N Automated Hematology Analyzer (Sysmex Corporation Kobe, Japan) Whole Blood Mode. The parameters for the full blood count determination were; WBC, HGB, HCT, RDW, MCHC and MCV. Routine quality control checks were run on control specimen within specified limits per the manufacturer's instructions. Hematology analyzer was calibrated per the instructions of the manufacturer when there was a change of reagent. The presence of Hb variants was detected on a hemolysate prepared from EDTA sample on cellulose acetate paper at pH 8.5, using an electrophoresis set-up (Beijing Liuyi Instrument Factory, China).

Biochemical assay

Serum ferritin was measured, using the AXSYM, MEIA quantitative technique. Serum iron and UIBC were assayed by the modified method of Henry (1984), using the BT3000 Plus Chemistry Analyser (Biotecnica Instruments, Rome, Italy). Transferrin saturation index was calculated by dividing serum iron by TIBC and expressing the result as a percentage. Bilirubin determination was based on the modification of Tietz's method (1994). Daily quality control checks were run on control specimen within specified limits per the manufacturer's instructions. Clinical chemistry analyzer was calibrated per the instructions of the manufacturer when there was a change of reagent.

The CRP Latex test was used to determine the level of inflammation. It is a rapid slide agglutination test for the qualitative and semi-quantitative detection of C-reactive protein in serum. The reagent, containing particles coated with specific anti-human C-reactive protein antibodies, agglutinates in the presence of CRP in the patient's serum.

Malaria parasite screening

Parasitemia was determined using both the parasite density and plus (+) system. All the thick blood smears were stained with 10% Giemsa and examined under the × 100 oil immersion objective lens of a light microscope. For parasite density determination, the number of asexual parasites was counted against 200 leucocytes, where an average leucocytes count of 8000/μL was assumed. The blood smear was considered negative when 200 high power fields had been examined without visible parasite [22].

For the plus (+) system counting of parasite, the results were categorised as follows:

1–9 parasites per 100 microscopic fields (+); 10–99 parasites per 100 microscopic fields (++); 1–9 parasites per microscopic field (+++); more than 10 parasites per microscopic field (++++). The examination of the blood film for malaria parasites was done by two certified microscopists independently who were blinded to each other's results [23].

Stool and urine analysis

The formol-ether concentration method was used in the preparation of stool samples for microscopy and detection of intestinal parasite.

The urine sedimentation technique was used to detect the presence of *S. hematobium* ova. About 10 mls of urine was filtered using paper filters and the egg/ova count was recorded per 10 mls of urine.

Statistical analysis

Data were entered into Microsoft Excel worksheet. Results were presented as mean ± standard deviation (SD) and frequency (percentage) and geometric mean (95% CI), where necessary. The Fischer's exact test or Chi-square (X^2) was used to assess the statistical significance of categorical variables. Unpaired sample t-test was used to compare between two means of continuous variables for normally distributed data and Mann-Whitney U test was used to compare between two medians of continuous variable for non-parametric variables. *P*-value less than 0.05 was considered statistically significant. Analysis was performed using GraphPad Prism 5 Project software (GraphPad software, San Diego California USA, www.graphpad.com).

Results

Table 1 shows the biochemical profiles of study participants. There was no statistically significant difference between the mean ages of anemic pregnant women (27.53 ± 5.31 years), compared to non-anemic pregnant women (28.02 ± 4.97 years) ($p = 0.309$). Anemic pregnant women had a significantly lower mean HGB, HCT, MCV, MCHC than their non-anemic counterparts ($p < 0.0001$). Conversely, there was a significantly higher mean WBC and RDW amongst anemic pregnant women ($p < 0.05$). There were statistically significant increased levels of TIBC in anemic pregnant women, compared to the non-anemic pregnant women. The anemic pregnant women also had significantly lower median levels of serum ferritin ($p = 0.0180$), iron ($p = 0.0273$) and %TfR saturation ($p = 0.0391$). Bilirubin (total, direct and indirect) levels were lower in the anemic than the non-anemic pregnant women ($p > 0.05$). A higher proportion of anemic pregnant women had MCV < 80 fl (16.9% vs 5.4%; $p = 0.0115$), RDW > 15.0% (15.0% vs. 3.4%; $p = 0.0052$), serum iron < 40 μg/dl (18.6% vs. 6.1%; $p = 0.0092$), ferritin < 12 ng/ml (16.2% vs. 6.1%; $p = 0.0400$) and TIBC> 500 μg/dl (15.4% vs. 3.4%; $p = 0.0015$), compared to non-anemic pregnant women.

Table 2 shows the association between anemia and parasitemia. Higher proportion of women with anemia had malaria parasitemia, and intestinal parasitic infections. There was a statistically significant association between anemia and malarial parasitemia ($p = 0.0111$), as well as intestinal parasite ($p = 0.0152$). The proportion of + 1 (20.6% vs. 9.5%) and 2++ (4.0% vs. 0.7%) malaria parasite was significantly higher in anemic, compared to non-anemic. There was a significantly increased geometric mean of ring trophozoite of *Plasmodium falciparum* among anemic pregnant women (2159 pa/μl blood), compared to their non-anemic counterparts (809.4 pa/μl blood) ($p = 0.0487$). The proportion of intestinal parasite 1+ among anemic women (27.7%) was significantly higher, compared to non-anemic (18.4%) counterparts ($p = 0.0152$). All schistosomiasis infections were found in anemic participants, giving a proportion

Table 1 Hematological and biochemical profile stratified according to anemic and non-anemic pregnant women

Parameters	Anemic	Non-anemic	*p*-value
	(*n* = 253)	(*n* = 147)	
Maternal age (years)	27.53 ± 5.31	28.02 ± 4.97	0.309
Hematological profile			
HGB (g/dl)	9.31 ± 1.34	11.89 ± 0.80	< 0.0001
WBC (/μL)	10.26 ± 1.68	6.13 ± 1.39	0.0006
HCT (%)	29.08 ± 3.34	35.43 ± 4.76	< 0.0001
MCHC (g/dl)	31.88 ± 2.02	33.43 ± 1.58	< 0.0001
MCV (fl)	78.72 ± 9.02	85.94 ± 8.32	< 0.0001
RDW (%)	16.87 ± 5.95	14.79 ± 3.55	0.048
Biochemical profile			
Serum ferritin (ng/ml)[a]	19.7 (15.2–94.0)	29.3 (21.4–106)	0.0180
Serum iron (μg/dl)[a]	88.3 (73.9–182)	152.7 (81.0–201)	0.0273
TIBC (μg/dl)[a]	369 (118.0–532.0)	302 (93–379)	0.0438
TfS (%)[a]	20.7 (6.6–26.4)	24.6 (8.1–27.5)	0.0391
Total Bilirubin (μmol/l)	18.09 ± 6.63	18.64 ± 6.33	0.564
Direct Bilirubin (μmol/l)	5.45 ± 2.13	5.82 ± 2.37	0.249
Indirect Bilirubin (μmol/l)	12.79 ± 6.08	13.26 ± 6.06	0.593
MCV (< 80 fL)[b]	43 (16.9%)	8 (5.4%)	0.0115
RDW (> 15%)[b]	38 (15.0%)	5 (3.4%)	0.0052
Serum iron(< 40 μg/dl)[b]	47 (18.6%)	9 (6.1%)	0.0092
Ferritin (< 12 ng/ml)[b]	41 (16.2%)	9 (6.1%)	0.0400
TIBC(> 500 μg/dl)	39 (15.4%)	5 (3.4%)	0.0015

TIBC Total iron binding capacity, *TfS* Transferrin saturation, *HGB* hemoglobin, *WBC* White blood cells, *HCT* Hematocrit, *MCHC* Mean corpuscular hemoglobin concentration, *MCV* Mean corpuscular volume, *RDW* Red cell distribution width. $p < 0.05$ was considered statistically significant different
Values are presented as mean ± standard deviation, [a]median (interquartile range). [b]frequency (percentages)

Table 2 Association between anemia and malaria infection, intestinal parasite and Schistosomiasis among pregnant women

Characteristics	Anemic (*n* = 253)	Non-anemic (*n* = 147)	Statistics X^2 value, df	*p*-value
Plasmodium falciparum			6.455, 1	0.0111
Not seen	186 (73.5%)	132 (89.8%)		
1+	52 (20.6%)	14 (9.5%)		
2++	10 (4.0%)	1 (0.7%)		
Parasite density(pa/ul)#	2159 (926.2–7205.3)	809.4 (479.3–941.5)		0.0487
Intestinal parasite			8.371, 2	0.0152
Not seen	183 (72.3%)	120 (81.6%)		
1+	70 (27.7%)	27 (18.4%)		
Schistosomiasis			–	–
Not seen	251 (99.2)	147 (100.0%)		
S. haematobium (++)	1 (0.4%)	–		
S. mansoni (++)	1 (0.4%)	–		

Values are presented as frequency (percentage); #: geometric mean (confidence interval). X^2: Chi-square value; df: degree of freedom of 0.4% (1/253) each of S. *hematobium* (1+) and *S. mansoni* (1+) infection.

Also, from Table 3, the proportions of AA and CC genotypes between the anemic and non-anemic pregnant women were not statistically significantly different ($p > 0.05$). A significantly higher percentage of the non-anemic (21.8%) had AC genotype, compared to the anemic (9.4%) ($p = 0.0327$). On the other hand, a significantly higher percentage of AS genotype was found among the anemic (16.2%), compared to non-anemic (4.1%) pregnant women ($p = 0.0081$). Additionally, SC 4.7% (12/253) and SS genotypes 0.4% (1/253) were found in only the anemic pregnant women.

Subjects who had anemia had a more positive response to C-reactive protein 52.2% (48/92) than the non-anemic pregnant women 28.8% (19/66) (Fig. 1).

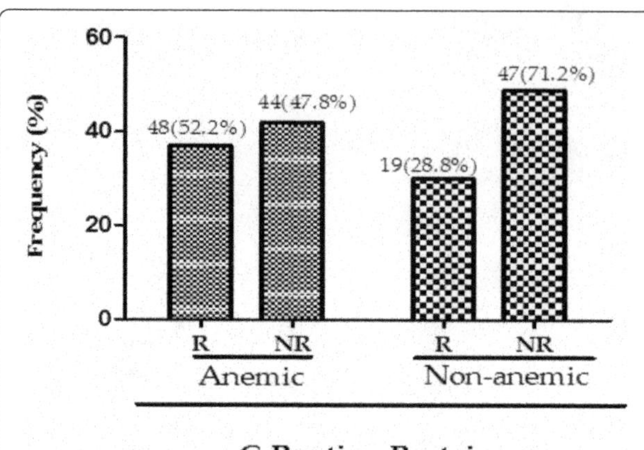

Fig. 1 C - reactive protein of study participants. R: Reactive; NR: Non-reactive. Values in parentheses represent proportions of the responses between the two groups of women

Discussion

This study determined the hematological and biochemical changes, along with the occurrence of sickle cell and parasitic infections among anemic and non-anemic pregnant women.

In this study, hematological indices such as Hb, HCT, MCHC and MCV levels were lower in anemic pregnant women, compared to their non-anemic counterparts. This is consistent with several studies [24–26] among anemic pregnant women. The mean Hb level of 9.31 g/dl observed among the anemic pregnant women fell within the moderate anemia ($7.0 < \text{Hb} < 9.9$ g/dl) category, as per WHO classification criteria for anemia [20]. The reduced HCT can be attributed to the reduced Hb concentration [27]. Additionally, a reduced HCT may arise from increase in plasma volume and hormonal changes during pregnancy, which cause hemodilution and fluid retention [28].

This study also observed a significantly low mean MCV level among anemic pregnant women, as 16.9% of them had MCV < 80 fL. A reduced MCV below the lower reference limit, suggests microcytic anemia or iron deficiency anemia [25]. Our finding that MCV levels were reduced in anemic pregnant women is consistent with that of Erhabor et al. who had a similar study [29] among anemic pregnant women in Sokoto, Nigeria. Erhabor and colleagues linked their findings to microcytic hypochromic anemia. The low MCV in our study is further supported by a significant rise in RDW level in the anemic pregnant women, which was above the cut-off point of 15%. The significantly higher proportion of anemic pregnant women who had RDW > 15% is consistent with the observation made by Tasneem et al. [13].

Table 3 Hemoglobin genotypes of the pregnant women with and without anemia

Hb Genotype	Anemic $n = 253$	Non-Anemic $n = 147$	*p*-value
AA	166 (65.6%)	105 (71.4%)	0.5428
AC	24 (9.5%)	32 (21.8%)	0.0327
AS	41 (16.2%)	6 (4.1%)	0.0081
CC	9 (3.6%)	4 (2.7%)	0.4448
SC	12 (4.7%)	–	–
SS	1 (0.4%)	–	–

Values are presented as *n* (%). Comparisons between proportions of anemic and non-anemic groups were performed using Fischer's exact test. $p < 0.05$ was considered statistically significant different

The significantly lower serum iron, ferritin and transferrin saturation among anemic pregnant women supports the finding by Nuzhat et al. [30]. Low levels of iron, ferritin and transferrin are suggestive of iron deficiency anemia. Our study observed that the proportion of anemic pregnant women with low iron (< 40μg/dl) and ferritin (< 12 ng/ml), were significantly higher among anemic pregnant women; this is another evidence of iron deficiency anemia [15]. We also observed a significantly higher TIBC in the anemic pregnant women. A higher than normal TIBC is an indication of iron-deficiency anemia. Our result corroborates that of Bleyere et al. [31], in a study among pregnant women in Cote d'lvoire. The probable explanation to the high TIBC levels among anemic pregnant women could be the reduced iron and % transferrin saturation [32].

The present study shows non-significantly lower levels of bilirubin among anemic pregnant women. The low bilirubin levels among the anemic pregnant women probably rules out hemolysis of the red cells.

Increased WBC could be as a result of increased inflammation and/or defensive immune response to infection [33]. This study observed a non-significantly increased levels of total WBC count among anemic pregnant women, compared to non-anemic women. Luppi [34] observed an increasing level of total lymphocyte count throughout pregnancy, which could be due to maternal body's attempt to build up immunity. Our present study observed that majority of anemic pregnant women had parasitic infections like malaria and schistosomiasis; hence the elevated WBC is more likely to be attributed to these infections [33]. Although the mean WBC of anemic pregnant women in this study was elevated, it was within the reference range.

In the present study, the positive response of anemic pregnant women to C-reactive protein was 52.2% while non-anemic pregnant women showed 28.8%. A study by Mburu et al. [35] indicated that C-reactive protein levels > 6 ng/ml is indicative of increased inflammatory response, due to parasitic infections and or hemoglobinopathies.

From this study, Hb genotypes AS, SC and SS may have contributed to the higher number of anemic pregnant women due to the increased proportion of sickle cell trait and disease in the participants. Anemia is a major feature of sickle cell disease due to defective haemoglobin structure [36]. Anemia in pregnancy complicated by sickle cell disease or trait had been reported by Desai et al. [37]

In our previous study, an increased proportion of *Plasmodium falciparum* malaria and intestinal helminthes infections were observed among anemic pregnant women, compared to non-anemic pregnant women. Our current study supports our previous study [21] that anemic pregnant women reported with an increased proportion of *Plasmodium falciparum, Schistosoma hematobium* and intestinal parasites. This confirms the explanation that malaria and intestinal parasite infections coexist with micronutrient deficiencies, culminating in anemia [38].

The main strength of this study is the fact that despite working from a less resourced setting, we have been able to combine the measurement of biochemical and hematological parameters, unlike many other studies, where the two types of tests had been done independently. These measurements were done concurrently on same subjects, whereas in other studies, different subjects were used.

Despite these strengths, there were some limitations of our study. The use of single slide for parasite detection, cross-sectional nature of the study, inability to analyse all samples for CRP and the general lack of reference intervals specific to the local condition in Bolgatanga, which necessitated the comparison of the results of this study with data from countries whose socio-demographic variables vary from our local setting. Other micronutrients such as vitamin A, folate, cyanocobalamin, and zinc were not assessed in this study. Their influence on the burden of anemia in this setting can therefore become a subject for further scientific investigation.

Conclusion

Anemic pregnant women are associated with some changes in hematological and iron indices including significantly reduced Hb, HCT, MCV, iron, ferritin and transferrin saturation and increased WBC, RDW, TIBC and positivity of CRP. These changes could have been influenced by a higher proportion of hemoglobinopathies, *Plasmodium falciparum, Schistosoma hematobium* and intestinal parasite.

Abbreviations

CHRPE-KNUST/KATH: Committee on Human Research, Publication and Ethics of Kwame Nkrumah University of Science and Technology and Komfo Anokye Teaching Hospital; CRP: C-reactive protein; EDTA: Ethylenediaminetetraacetic acid; HCT: Hematocrit; HGB/Hb: Hemoglobin; IRB-NHRC: Institutional Review Board of the Navrongo Health Research Centre; MCH: Mean Corpuscular Hemoglobin; MCHC: Mean Corpuscular Hemoglobin Concentration; MCV: Mean Corpuscular Volume; MEIA: Microparticle Enzyme Immunoassay; PCV: Packed Cell Volume; RBC: Red Blood Cell; RDW: Red Cell Distribution Width; RHB-ANC: Regional Hospital Bolgatanga Antenatal Clinic; SST: Serum Separator Tube; TfS: Transferrin Saturation; TIBC: Total Iron Binding Capacity; UIBC: Unbound Iron Binding Capacity; WBC: White Blood Cell

Acknowledgements

We are grateful to the Committee on Human Research, Publication and Ethics of Kwame Nkrumah University of Science and Technology and Komfo Anokye Teaching Hospital (CHRPE-KNUST/KATH) and the Institutional Review Board of the Navrongo Health Research Centre (IRB-NHRC), for approving this study. The authors of this paper are also grateful to all the participating women, the midwives and administrative staff of Bolgatanga Regional Hospital. Our special thanks go to all staff of the Bolgatanga Regional Hospital Laboratory department for their immense technical support in the assay of our specimens.

Funding

This was self-funded by the corresponding author.

Authors' contributions

BA, KN and PB designed the study and BA carried out the clinical and laboratory work, BA and KN drafted the paper and KN revised the paper. BA provided reagents and consumables for the study. EOA interpreted and analysed the data. All authors read and approved the final manuscript and they are guarantors of the paper.

Competing interests

The authors declare that they have no competing interests.

Author details

[1]Biochemistry and Hematology Units, Bolgatanga Regional Hospital, P.O. Box 26, Bolgatanga-Upper East Region, Ghana. [2]Department of Biochemistry and Biotechnology, Kwame Nkrumah University of Science and Technology, Kumasi, Ghana. [3]Obstetrics and Gynecology Unit, Bolgatanga Regional Hospital, P.O. Box 26, Bolgatanga-Upper East Region, Ghana. [4]Department of Biochemistry and Molecular Medicine, School of Medical and Health Science, University for Development Studies, Tamale, Ghana. [5]Department of Molecular Medicine, School of Medical Science, Kwame Nkrumah University of Science and Technology, Kumasi, Ghana. [6]Department of Medical Laboratory Technology, Royal Ann College of Health, Atwima-Manhyia, Kumasi, Ghana. [7]School of Medical and Health Science, Edith Cowan University, Perth, WA, Australia.

References

1. Nguyen V, Wuebbolt D, Thomas H, Murphy K, D'souza R. Iron deficiency Anemia in pregnancy and treatment options: a patient-preference study [1L]. Obstet Gynecol. 2017;129:122S.
2. Balarajan Y, Ramakrishnan U, Özaltin E, Shankar AH, Subramanian S. Anaemia in low-income and middle-income countries. Lancet. 2011; 378(9809):2123–35.
3. Mwangi MN, Prentice AM, Verhoef H. Safety and benefits of antenatal oral iron supplementation in low-income countries: a review. Br J Haematol. 2017;177(6):884–95.
4. Tay SCK, Nani EA, Walana W. Parasitic infections and maternal anaemia among expectant mothers in the Dangme East District of Ghana. BMC Res Notes. 2017;10(1):3.
5. Gernand AD, Aguree S, Pobee R, Murray-Kolb LE. Micronutrient deficiencies in Ghanaian women before pregnancy. FASEB J. 2017;31(1 Supplement) 786.720–786.720
6. Anlaakuu P, Anto F. Anaemia in pregnancy and associated factors: a cross sectional study of antenatal attendants at the Sunyani municipal hospital, Ghana. BMC Res Notes. 2017;10(1):402.
7. Otto JM, Plumb JO, Clissold E, Kumar S, Wakeham DJ, Schmidt W, Grocott MP, Richards T, Montgomery H. Hemoglobin concentration, total hemoglobin mass and plasma volume in patients: implications for anemia. Haematologica. 2017; 2017.169680
8. Arimond M, Vitta BS, Martin-Prével Y, Moursi M, Dewey KG. Local foods can meet micronutrient needs for women in urban Burkina Faso, but only if rarely consumed micronutrient-dense foods are included in daily diets: a linear programming exercise. Matern Child Nutr. 2017;
9. Percy L, Mansour D, Fraser I. Iron deficiency and iron deficiency anaemia in women. Best Prac Res Clin Obstet Gynaecol. 2017;40:55–67.
10. Orlandini C, Torricelli M, Spirito N, Alaimo L, Di Tommaso M, Severi FM, Ragusa A, Petraglia F: Maternal anemia effects during pregnancy on male and female fetuses: are there any differences? J Matern Fetal Neonatal Med 2017, 30(14):1704–1708.
11. Yildiz Y, Özgü E, Unlu SB, Salman B, Eyi EGY. The relationship between third trimester maternal hemoglobin and birth weight/length; results from the tertiary center in Turkey. J Matern Fetal Neonatal Med. 2014;27(7):729–32.
12. Darnton-Hill I, Mkparu UC. Micronutrients in pregnancy in low-and middle-income countries. Nutrients. 2015;7(3):1744–68.
13. Tasneem S, Sultana N, Snover A, Alam K. Clinical utility of red blood cell count, red cell distribution width: will it provide more accurate differentiation of Beta thalassemia trait and iron deficiency anemia in pregnancy? Rawal Med J. 2016;41(4):424–7.
14. Rayis DA, Ahmed MA, Abdel-Moneim H, Adam I, Lutfi MF. Trimester pattern of change and reference ranges of hematological profile among Sudanese women with normal pregnancy. Clin Prac. 2017;7(1):888.
15. Lopez A, Cacoub P, Macdougall IC, Peyrin-Biroulet L. Iron deficiency anaemia. Lancet. 2016;387(10021):907–16.
16. World Health Organization. Iron deficiency anaemia: assessment, prevention, and control. In: A guide for programme managers. Geneva: WHO; 2001. *NHD Publicação* 2015(01.3).
17. Daru J, Allotey J, Peña-Rosas JP, Khan KS. Serum ferritin thresholds for the diagnosis of iron deficiency in pregnancy: a systematic review. Transfus Med. 2017;27(3):167–74.
18. Abdelgader EA, Diab TA, Kordofani AA, Abdalla SE. Haemoglobnin level, RBCs indices, and iron status in pregnant females in Sudan. Basic Res J Med Clin Sci. 2014;3(2):8–13.
19. Tunkyi K, Moodley J. Anemia and pregnancy outcomes: a longitudinal study. J Matern Fetal Neonatal Med. 2017:1–5.
20. World Health Organization: Worldwide prevalence of anaemia 1993-2005: WHO global database on anaemia 2008.
21. Ahenkorah B, Nsiah K, Baffoe P. Sociodemographic and obstetric characteristics of Anaemic pregnant women attending antenatal clinic in Bolgatanga regional hospital. Scientifica. 2016;2016:1–8.
22. Haggaz AD, Elbashir LM, Adam GK, Rayis DA, Adam I. Estimating malaria parasite density among pregnant women at Central Sudan using actual and assumed white blood cell count. Malar J. 2014;13(1):6.
23. WHO. Basic Malaria Microscopy – Part I: Learner's guide. Second edition www.who.int/malaria/publications/atoz/9241547820/en/; 2010.
24. Karaoglu L, Pehlivan E, Egri M, Deprem C, Gunes G, Genc MF, Temel I. The prevalence of nutritional anemia in pregnancy in an east Anatolian province, Turkey. BMC Public Health. 2010;10(1):329.
25. Getahun W, Belachew T, Wolide AD. Burden and associated factors of anemia among pregnant women attending antenatal care in southern Ethiopia: cross sectional study. BMC Res Notes. 2017;10(1):276.
26. Susanti AI, Sahiratmadja E, Winarno G, Sugianli AK, Susanto H, Panigoro R. Low hemoglobin among pregnant women in midwives practice of primary health care, Jatinangor, Indonesia: Iron deficiency Anemia or β-thalassemia trait? Anemia. 2017:5. Article ID 6935648.
27. James TR, Reid HL, Mullings AM. Are published standards for haematological indices in pregnancy applicable across populations: an evaluation in healthy pregnant Jamaican women. BMC pregnancy and childbirth. 2008;8(1):8.
28. Stevens GA, Finucane MM, De-Regil LM, Paciorek CJ, Flaxman SR, Branca F, Peña-Rosas JP, Bhutta ZA, Ezzati M, Group NIMS. Global, regional, and national trends in haemoglobin concentration and prevalence of total and severe anaemia in children and pregnant and non-pregnant women for 1995–2011: a systematic analysis of population-representative data. Lancet Glob Health. 2013;1(1):e16–25.
29. Erhabor O, Isaac I, Isah A, Udomah F. Iron deficiency anaemia among antenatal women in Sokoto, Nigeria. Br J Med Health Sci. 2013;1(4):47–57.
30. Raza N, Sarwar I, Munazza B, Ayub M, Suleman M. Assessment of iron deficiency in pregnant women by determining iron status. J Ayub Med Coll Abbottabad. 2011;23(2):36–40.
31. Bleyere MN, Bi ASN, Kone M, Sawadogo D, Yapo PA: Iron status and red cell parameters in pregnant and non-pregnant adolescents in Côte d'Ivoire (West Africa). 2014.
32. Villers M, Grimsley A, James A, Heine RP, Cooper A, Swamy G. 512: collaboration of care improves outcomes among pregnant women with iron deficiency anemia. American Journal of Obstetrics & Gynecology. 2016; 214(1):S278.
33. Adikwu P, Amuta E, Obande G, Adulugba A, Abba E. Studies on malaria parasite and Haemoglobin level among pregnant women attending antenatal at Benue state general hospital, Otukpo, Nigeria. Am J Med Med Sci. 2017;7(6):265–70.
34. Luppi P. How immune mechanisms are affected by pregnancy. Vaccine. 2003;21(24):3352–7.
35. Mburu AS, Thurnham DI, Mwaniki DL, Muniu EM, Alumasa F, De Wagt A: The influence and benefits of controlling for inflammation on plasma ferritin and hemoglobin responses following a multi-micronutrient supplement in apparently healthy, HIV+ Kenyan adults. J Nutr 2008, 138(3):613–619.
36. Yu C, Stasiowska E, Stephens A, Awogbade M, Davies A. Outcome of pregnancy in sickle cell disease patients attending a combined obstetric and haematology clinic. J Obstet Gynaecol. 2009;29(6):512–6.
37. Desai G, Anand A, Shah P, Shah S, Dave K, Bhatt H, Desai S, Modi D. Sickle cell disease and pregnancy outcomes: a study of the community-based hospital in a tribal block of Gujarat, India. J Health Popul Nutr. 2017;36(1):3.
38. Anchang-Kimbi JK, Elad DM, Sotoing GT, Achidi EA. Coinfection with Schistosoma haematobium and Plasmodium falciparum and Anaemia severity among pregnant women in Munyenge, Mount Cameroon area: A cross-sectional study. J Parasitol Res. 2017:12. Article ID 6173465.

19

Prevalence of anemia before and after initiation of antiretroviral therapy among HIV infected patients at Black Lion Specialized Hospital, Addis Ababa, Ethiopia: a cross sectional study

Gashaw Garedew Woldeamanuel[1*] and Diresibachew Haile Wondimu[2]

Abstract

Background: Anemia is the most common hematological abnormality in Human immunodeficiency virus (HIV) positive patients and a significant predictor of its progression to AIDS or death. This study was aimed to assess the prevalence of anemia before and after initiation of antiretroviral therapy (ART) among HIV positive patients attending Black Lion Specialized Hospital, Addis Ababa, Ethiopia.

Methods: A cross sectional study was conducted from January to April, 2017 in Black Lion Specialized Hospital, Addis Ababa, Ethiopia. A total of 255 patients on ART were selected using simple random sampling techniques. Socio-demographic and clinical characteristics of the study subjects were collected using structured questionnaire. Measurements of complete blood cell counts and CD4 + T cell counts were made using Sysmex XT 2000i hematology analyzer and BD FACS Count CD4 analyzer, respectively. Statistical analysis of the data (Chi-square, paired T-test, logistic regression) was done using SPSS version 20. A *p*-value < 0.05 was considered as significant.

Results: Prevalence of anemia before and after ART initiation was 41.9 and 11.4% respectively. There are a significance differences in CD4 + T cell count, RBC count, hemoglobin values and RBC indices in HIV patients before and after ART initiation (*p*-value < 0.05). WHO clinical stages and CD4+ T cell counts were found to be associated with the prevalence of anemia before ART initiation. Among the total number of anemic cases, normocytic normochromic anemia was present in 71% of the cases before ART and in 58.6% of the cases after ART. The prevalence of macrocytic normochromic anemia before and after ART initiation was 4.7 and 27.6% respectively.

Conclusions: It is evident from this study that there is a remarkable reduction in the prevalence of anemia after ART initiation. However, a significant proportion of HIV patients remained anemic after 6 months of ART initiation suggesting the need for routine screening and proper treatment of anemia to mitigate its adverse effects.

Keywords: HIV, ART, Anemia, Ethiopia

* Correspondence: gashawgaredew05@gmail.com
[1]Department of Medicine, College of Medicine and Health Sciences, Wolkite University, P.O. Box 07, Wolkite, Ethiopia
Full list of author information is available at the end of the article

Background

Hematologic abnormalities are among the most common manifestations of advanced human immunodeficiency virus (HIV) infection and acquired immunodeficiency syndrome (AIDS) [1]. Low blood cell counts, are the most common of these disorders [2]. The frequency and severity of these hematological manifestations increased with the decline in CD4 counts [3] with anemia being the most common hematologic abnormality in HIV patients and is associated with disease progression and decreased survival [4]. However, the prevalence of anemia in HIV patients varies considerably, ranging from 1.3 to 95%. Several factors including stage of HIV, age, sex and the definition of anemia used are said to account for the variations in HIV prevalence [5].

Anemia is multifactorial. HIV infection itself causes anemia, probably as a consequence of HIV infection of stromal cells. Other common causes of anemia in AIDS are anemia of chronic disease, bone marrow suppression by ART, and hemolytic anemia induced by oxidant drugs [6, 7]. Cytokines such as interleukin 1, tumor necrosis factor and the interferon play a role in impairing erythropoietin response by reducing concentration of marrow progenitors and erythroid colonies. As ART generally diminishes these cytokines, anemia is less common than in the pre ART era. But commonly used myelosuppressive drugs in the HIV setting may contribute to anemia and even in the era of ART, anemia continues to contribute to morbidity and diminished quality of life [8].

Overall, the treatment of HIV infection with ART reduces the incidence of anemia and increases hemoglobin levels over time [9]. However, zidovudine (AZT) has also been clearly demonstrated to cause anemia [10]. Marrow erythroid hypoplasia, aplasia, and megaloblastic maturation have developed as a result of AZT therapy [8]. The effect of AZT is modest when taken as ART than administered as a single dose [11].

Different studies were conducted to assess the prevalence of anemia in HIV infected individuals. But there are only few published reports in Ethiopia on the assessment of anemia among HIV positive patients. Therefore, this study gave information about the prevalence of anemia before and after initiation of antiretroviral therapy among HIV patients who attended at ART clinic of Black Lion Specialized Hospital, Addis Ababa, Ethiopia.

Methods

Study setting and study population

Cross sectional study design was conducted at ART clinic of Black Lion Specialized Hospital, Addis Ababa, Ethiopia. This hospital is selected based on the availability of patients from all parts of the country as it is referral and specialized teaching hospital in Ethiopia. This study was conducted from January to April, 2017. During the study period, 2675 HIV infected adults were on ART. Among those on ART, a total of 255 HIV infected patients taking ART for at least 6 months were selected randomly and included in this study. Sample size was estimated using a single population proportion formula, taking $p = 20.9\%$ (expected prevalence rate of anemia) [11], 5% level of precision (d) with 95% confidence interval. The inclusion criteria for this study includes; HIV positive adults greater than 18 years old at the time of ART initiation, those who were on ART for at least 6 months, patients having complete hematological values at the baseline and those who were volunteered to participate in the study. Patients transferred from other health institutions, those who were on medication, pregnant, diagnosed as having hematological diseases and other medical conditions by medical experts were excluded from the study.

Data collection

The data was collected using a structured questionnaire by five nurses working in the ART clinic. The collected information includes socio-demographics, clinical characteristics, and immunohematological profile of patients at baseline and after 6 months of ART initiation. Data on socio-demographic, clinical characteristics and baseline information of the study participants were collected by interview and review of medical records. Anthropometric measurements were carried out according to the WHO recommendations. Then, the study participants were sent to the laboratory for determination of blood cell counts. Hemoglobin concentration, RBC count and RBC indices were determined using Sysmex XT 2000i hematology analyzer whereas CD4+ T cells were assayed using the BD FACS Count system. The instruments and the procedures used for analysis of blood cell counts were the same during the two time points.

To ensure good quality data, training of data collectors, pre-testing of data collection instrument and continuous supervision of the data collection process were carried out.

Definition of outcome variable and statistical analysis

The data were cleaned, edited, checked for completeness and entered into SPSS version 20 for analysis. Anemia was defined as Hgb concentration less than 13 g/dl for adult males and less than 12 g/dl for adult females. It was further classified into mild (11–11.9 g/dl for women and 11–12.9 g/dl for men), moderate (8–10.9 g/dl) and severe (< 8 g/dl) for both sexes [12]. Microcytosis was defined as MCV < 80 fl, macrocytosis as MCV > 100 fl and hypochromia was defined as MCHC value < 31 g/dl [13].

Descriptive statistics was used to get a clear picture of dependent and independent variables. After checking the normality of the data, paired T-test was used and also chi square was computed to determine association between dependent and independent variables. Multivariable logistic regression analysis was performed to obtain the adjusted effect of different risk factors on the odds of being anemic at baseline and after 6 months of ART initiation. A p-value < 0.05 was considered as statistically significant.

Results

General characteristics of study participants

A total of 255 HIV positive patients, of which 148 (58%) women and 107 (42%) men were involved in this study. The overall mean age was 40.6 ± 9.4 years, within the range of 20–70 years old. The majority of patients were within 40–49 years of age. About 95 (37.3%) participants were under WHO clinical stage III and the most widely used ART regimen (62.7%) in this study was 1e (TDF-3TC-EFV). At the time of study, 61.6% of them were taking cotrimoxazole prophylaxis therapy (Table 1).

Table 1 Sociodemographic and clinical characteristics of HIV positive patients taking ART at Black Lion Specialized Hospital, Addis Ababa, Ethiopia, 2017

Variables	Frequency (n = 255)	Percentage (%)
Age (in years)		
20–29	33	12.9
30–39	86	33.7
40–49	96	37.6
50–59	30	11.8
60–69	9	3.5
70–79	1	4
Sex		
Male	107	42
Female	148	58
Marital Status		
Single	67	26.3
Divorced	43	16.9
Married	106	41.5
Widowed	39	15.3
Educational status		
illiterate	27	10.6
Primary school	101	39.6
High school	91	35.7
Certificate and above	36	14.1
Employment status		
Employed in public organization	26	10.2
Employed in private organization	23	9
Self employed	57	22.4
Unemployed	149	58.4
WHO clinical stages at baseline		
Stage I	41	16.1
Stage II	56	22
Stage III	95	37.3
Stage IV	63	24.6
Types of ART regimens		
1c	40	15.7
1d	30	11.8
1e	160	62.7
1f	25	9.8
Cotrimoxazole prophylaxis		
Yes	157	61.6
No	98	38.4

1c = AZT-3TC-NVP, 1d = AZT-3TC-EFV, 1e = TDF-3TC-EFV, 1f = TDF-3TC-NV

Red blood cell parameters and CD4$^+$ T cell counts of HIV positive patients before and after initiation of ART

There were statistically significant differences in the mean values of RBC count (4.41 ± 0.71 × 10^6/μl vs. 4.28 ± 0.59 × 10^6/μl), hemoglobin (12.8 ± 1.99 g/dl vs. 14.34 ± 1.89 g/dl), MCV (86.34 ± 6.42 fl vs. 96.33 ± 8.80 fl), MCH (29.1 ± 2.69 pg vs. 32.78 ± 4.09 pg), MCHC (33.52 ± 1.75 g/dl vs 34.18 ± 1.86 g/dl), RDW (14.91 ± 2.66% vs. 13.66 ± 1.58%) and CD4+ T cell counts (162.5 ± 108.6 cells/μl vs. 347 ± 183.17cells/μl) before and after ART initiation respectively. Patients after ART initiation have high hemoglobin level, MCV, MCH, MCHC and CD4+ T cell counts when compared to ART naïve patients (p < 0.001) (Table 2).

Prevalence of anemia among HIV positive patients before and after initiation of ART

The prevalence of anemia in HIV patients was 41.9% (107/255) before ART initiation and 11.4% (29/255) after ART initiation. About 90 (84.1%) had mild anemia and 17 (15.9%) had moderate anemia before ART initiation.

From anemic patients after ART initiation, about 22 (75.9%) had mild anemia and 7 (24.1%) had moderate anemia. Severe anemia was not found in this study. The prevalence of anemia after ART initiation was significantly decreased by 30.5%.

Risk factors of anemia in HIV infected patients before and after ART initiation

From anemic patients before ART initiation, about 43.9% (47/107) were males and 40.5% (60/148) were females. Similarly 42.5% (48/113) of patients were within the age of 30 to 40 years and 49.4% of patients with CD4 cell count < 200 cells/μl developed anemia. There were

Table 2 Red blood cell parameters and CD4$^+$ T cell counts of HIV positive adult patients at baseline and after 6 months of ART at Black Lion Specialized Hospital, Addis Ababa, Ethiopia, 2017

Parameters	Before initiation of ART ($n = 255$) Mean ± SD	After 6 months of ART initiation ($n = 255$) Mean ± SD	*P*-value
RBC (×10^6/μl)	4.41 ± 0.71	4.28 ± 0.59	0.009
Hgb (g/dl)	12.8 ± 1.99	14.34 ± 1.89	< 0.001
MCV (fl)	86.34 ± 6.42	96.33 ± 8.80	< 0.001
MCH (pg)	29.1 ± 2.69	32.78 ± 4.09	< 0.001
MCHC (g/dl)	33.52 ± 1.75	34.18 ± 1.86	< 0.001
RDW (%)	14.91 ± 2.66	13.66 ± 1.58	< 0.001
CD4 (Cells/μl)	162.5 ± 108.6	347 ± 183.17	< 0.001

significant associations between anemia with CD4 cell count and WHO clinical stage before ART initiation. HIV patients with CD4 cell count < 200 cells/μl before ART initiation had higher prevalence of anemia (49.4%, $p < 0.001$). Similarly about 48.4% ($p < 0.05$) patients with WHO clinical stage III/IV had anemia before ART initiation. However, there was no significant association of anemia with sex and age (Table 3).

Multiple logistic regression analysis was performed to obtain the adjusted effect of different risk factors on the odds of being anemic before initiation of ART. Table 3 summarizes the result of the final regression model. The variables; age, sex, WHO clinical stages and CD4 counts were included in the analysis. After adjusting for these factors in a multiple logistic regression analysis; clinical stage III/IV and CD4 count < 200 cells/mm^3 were significantly associated with increased odds of being anemic.

From anemic patients after ART initiation, about 9.3% (10/107) were males and 12.8% (19/148) were females. Similarly 21.2% of patients with the age of < 30 years and 16.2% of patients with CD4 cell count < 200 cells/μl developed anemia. Although, HIV patients with CD4 cell count < 200 cells/μl had higher prevalence of anemia (16.2%) after ART initiation, there was no significant association between anemia and CD4 cell counts ($p = 0.27$). Similarly sex, age and ART regimen types had no significant association with anemia after ART initiation (Table 4). In multivariable logistic regression analysis, increased risk of anemia after 6 months of ART was observed among participants with age less than 30 years and CD4 count < 200 cells/mm^3 whereas the odds of being anemic was lower among individuals with TDF based ART regimen, BMI 18.5–24.9 kg/m^2 and male participants.

Types of anemia among HIV positive patients before and after ART initiation

From the total anemic HIV infected patients at the baseline, 71% had normocytic-normochromic anemia followed by microcytic-normochromic anemia 14.9%. After 6 months of ART initiation, normocytic-normochromic anemia was present in 58.6% of the cases followed by macrocytic-normochromic anemia in 27.6% of the cases (Fig. 1).

Table 3 Anemia and its associated factors before ART initiation in HIV positive patients attending Black Lion Specialized Hospital, Addis Ababa, Ethiopia, 2017

Variables	Anemic	Non anemic	X^2	*P* value	AOR (95% CI)
Age(in years)					
<30	13 (39.4%)	20 (60.6%)	0.10	0.95	1.13 (0.49–2.63)
30–40	48 (42.5%)	65 (57.5%)			1.02 (0.58–1.78)
>40	46 (42.2%)	63 (57.8%)			1.00
Sex					
Male	47 (43.9%)	60 (56.1%)	0.21	0.65	1.09 (0.64–1.86)
Female	60 (40.5%)	88 (59.5%)			1.00
WHO clinical stages					
Stage I/II	32 (32%)	68 (68%)	6.70	**0.01**	1.00
Stage III/IV	75 (48.4%)	80 (51.6%)			1.83 (1.06–3.15)
CD4 count (cells/mm^3)					
<200	89 (49.4%)	91 (50.6%)	14.07	< **0.001**	2.91 (1.57–5.39)
≥200	18 (24%)	57 (76%)			1.00

Numerical data in bold indicates the level of significance ($p < 0.05$), *AOR* Adjusted odds ratio, *CI* Confidence interval, 1.00 = reference group

Table 4 Anemia and its associated factors after ART initiation in HIV positive patients attending Black Lion Specialized Hospital, Addis Ababa, Ethiopia, 2017

Variables	Anemia	Non anemic	X^2	*P* value	AOR (95% CI)
Age(in years)					
<30	7 (21.2%)	26 (78.8%)	6.23	0.05	4.01 (1.24–13.02)
30–40	15 (13.3%)	98 (86.7%)			2.25 (0.84–5.98)
>40	7 (6.4%)	102 (93.6%)			1.00
Sex					
Male	10 (9.3%)	97 (90.7%)	1.19	0.28	0.79 (0.34–1.85)
Female	19 (12.8%)	129 (87.2%)			1.00
ART regimen					
TDF based	21 (11.4%)	164 (88.6%)	0.000	0.99	0.99 (0.40–2.46)
AZT based	8 (11.4%)	62 (88.6%)			1.00
Cotrimoxazole					
NO	9 (8.9%)	92 (91.1)	1.01	0.32	0.74 (0.29–1.86)
Yes	20 (13%)	134 (87)			1.00
CD4 count (cells/mm^3)					
<200	10 (16.2%)	52 (83.9%)	2.62	0.27	2.04 (0.70–5.96)
200–349	10 (12.2%)	72 (87.8%)			1.44 (0.52–3.99)
≥350	9 (8.1%)	102 (91.9%)			1.00
BMI(Kg/m^2)					
<18.5	4 (12.9%)	27 (87.1%)	0.08	0.96	0.81 (0.21–3.17
18.5–24.9	18 (11.2%)	143 (88.8%)			0.76 (0.29–2.01)
≥25	7 (11.1%)	56 (88.9%)			1.00

AOR Adjusted odds ratio, *BMI* Body mass index, *CI* Confidence interval, 1.00 = reference group

Discussion

Anemia is the most common hematological abnormality and it has been associated with an increased HIV disease progression among HIV infected patients [13]. As recovery from anemia led to improvements in patient survival, screening for anemia among HIV infected patients should be performed to decrease the risk of death and to enhance the individual's functional status [4]. All subjects in this study were under first line of antiretroviral therapy.

The present study revealed that the prevalence of anemia at the baseline was 41.9% with 84.1% mild and 15.9% moderate anemia. After 6 months of ART, the prevalence of anemia was reduced to 11.4%. This finding is in agreement with a study done in Addis Ababa, Ethiopia reported that the prevalence of anemia at the

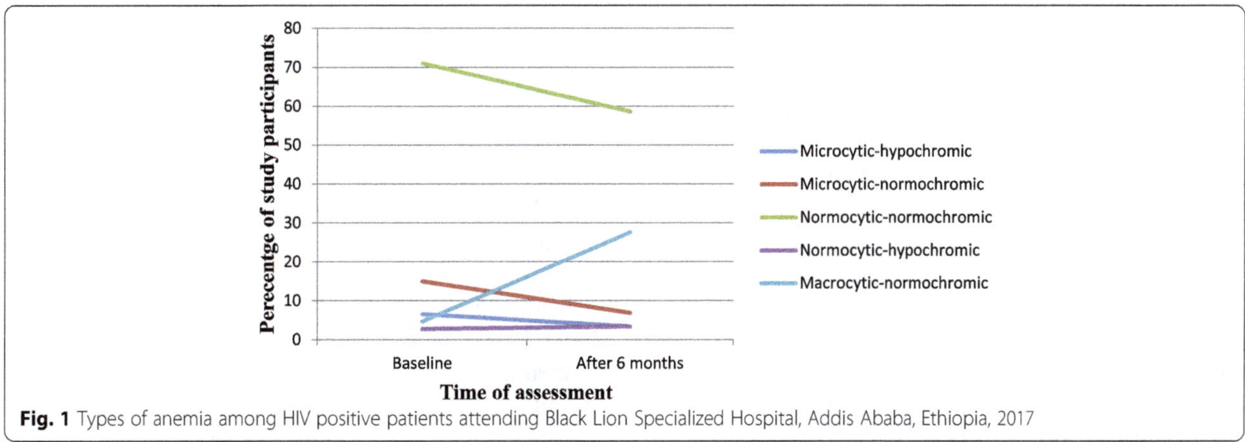

Fig. 1 Types of anemia among HIV positive patients attending Black Lion Specialized Hospital, Addis Ababa, Ethiopia, 2017

baseline was 42.9% with 79, 15.6 and 5.3% mild, moderate and severe anemia respectively. The study also added that at 12 months of ART initiation the prevalence of anemia was reduced to 14.3% [11]. In a separate study at Arba Minch, Ethiopia the prevalence of anemia at baseline was 52.3% with 28.1, 22.9 and 1.3% mild, moderate and severe anemia respectively [4]. Other studies also found different prevalence rates of anemia. A study from Hawassa, Ethiopia reported the prevalence of anemia as 23.4% before ART and 12.0% after ART [14]. A study from Jimma, Ethiopia reported the prevalence as 29.9% before ART and 16.2% after ART [13]. The baseline prevalence of anemia reported from Hawassa and Jimma is lower than the present study. On the other hand, a study from North eastern Nigeria stated a prevalence rate of anemia in ART-naive patients was 57.7% and it was reduced to 24.3% in ART-experienced patients [15]. The reasons for the observed differences might be due to the difference in the study population, sample size, study design and variability in the definition of anemia.

The decrease in the prevalence of anemia after ART initiation is attributed to the positive effect of ART on the differentiation and survival of erythrocytes. HIV infection of marrow stromal cells, decrease in serum erythropoietin levels, auto-antibodies to erythropoietin, or marrow suppression by opportunistic infections, may contribute to the anemia commonly observed in HIV-infected patients. ART may ameliorate many of these effects in an indirect manner simply by decreasing the HIV viral burden [15].

In this study, the prevalence of anemia observed across sex groups was higher in men than in women before ART initiation (43.9% vs 40.5%), and lower after ART initiation (9.3% vs. 12.8%). In agreement with this finding, a report from Benin city, Nigeria showed that among ART naive HIV patients, men had higher prevalence of anemia than their women counterparts (76.42% vs 63.43%), and lower in those patients on ART (44.19% vs 55.73%) [16]. The findings in this study differ from the findings of a study in Hawassa, Ethiopia [14] and Addis Ababa, Ethiopia [17]. Female gender has been reported as a risk factor for anemia among HIV patients [8]. In the present study, the same finding was obtained among HIV patients who were receiving ART. Although statistically insignificant, the prevalence of anemia post ART initiation was dropped from 43.9 to 9.3% in men and from 40.5 to 12.8% in women.

We found that, the prevalence of anemia was increased with decreasing CD4 count both before and after ART initiation with a high prevalence among patients with CD4 count < 200 cells/mm^3. In agreement with this finding, various studies reported that anemia was more prevalent among HIV patients with CD4 count < 200 cells/mm^3 [3, 4, 11, 18]. In general, in the advanced stage of the disease, the blood cell counts were lower than the early stage of the diseases. This might be due to the increasing trend in the frequency of bone marrow abnormalities with progressive immunologic deterioration and advanced disease due to HIV [19, 20].

The types of anemia were also assessed in this study. Among the total number of anemic cases, normocytic normochromic anemia was present in 71 and 58.6% of the cases before and after ART initiation respectively. A study conducted in Gondar, Ethiopia reported that the prevalence of normocytic normochromic anemia in ART naive patients was 48.9%, which reduced to 29.4% in those patients on ART [21]. This difference might be due to a difference in the definition of the types of anemia.

In the present study the relatively higher risk of developing microcytic hypochromic anemia was found in HIV positive patients before ART as compared to those on ART. Another cross sectional study in Ghana showed that, the likelihood of developing microcytic hypochromic anemia in ART-naive patients was five times more compared to those on ART [22]. This may reflect the overall nutritional deficiencies (malnutrition and malabsorption) associated with HIV patients.

This study also found that macrocytic normochromic anemia was present in 4.7% of anemic subjects at the baseline which was increased to 27.6% after ART initiation. This showed that the average MCV for patients on ART were significantly higher compared to their ART naïve patients and the degree of macrocytosis is more to the group receiving zidovudine. In agreement with the current findings, studies conducted in Ghana [22] and Ethiopia [21] reported that macrocytic normochromic anemia was more common after ART than before ART initiation. This is probably due to the effect of ART particularly AZT which is responsible for the development of macrocytosis.

This study assesses the prevalence of anemia before and after initiation of ART. However, this study had limitations such as lack of age and sex matched healthy control group. Also the study does not address viral load and albumin levels because of lack of resources. In addition, this study did not include baseline data on BMI. Nevertheless, this study provides valuable information about the burden of anemia among HIV positive patients before and after ART.

Conclusions

There was a remarkable reduction in the prevalence of anemia after ART initiation. WHO clinical stages and CD4 + T cell counts were associated with the prevalence of anemia before ART initiation. Normocytic normochromic anemia was the commonest type of anemia before and after ART initiation. Based on the present findings, a significant proportion of HIV patients remained anemic after 6 months of ART initiation suggesting the need for routine screening and proper treatment of anemia to mitigate its adverse effects.

Abbreviations

3TC: Lamivudin; AIDS: Acquired immunodeficiency syndrome; ART: Antiretroviral treatment; AZT/ZDV: Azidothymidine/Zidovudine; BMI: Body mass index; CD4: Cluster of differentiation 4; EVF: Efavirenz; Hgb: Hemoglobin; HIV: Human immunodeficiency virus; MCH: Mean cell hemoglobin; MCHC: Mean cell hemoglobin concentration; MCV: Mean cell volume; NVP: Nevirapine; RBC: Red blood cell; RDW: Red cell distribution width; TDF: Tenofovir

Acknowledgments

The authors would like to extend their deepest appreciation to staff member of ART clinic of Black Lion Specialized Hospital for their cooperation, who providing the necessary information for this study. We also would like to thank all study participants for their cooperation. We are grateful to thank Addis Ababa University for sponsoring this research project.

Funding

This study was funded by Addis Ababa University. The funders had no role in study design, data collection and analysis, decision to publish, or preparation of the manuscript.

Authors' contributions

GGW: Develop proposal and data collection sheet, collected data, analyzed it and wrote the draft of the manuscript. DHW: Conceived the study, supervised the data collection and reviewed the draft of the manuscript. Both authors read and approved the final draft of the manuscript.

Competing interests

The authors declare that they have no competing interests.

Author details

[1]Department of Medicine, College of Medicine and Health Sciences, Wolkite University, P.O. Box 07, Wolkite, Ethiopia. [2]Department of Medical Physiology, School of Medicine, College of Health Sciences, Addis Ababa University, Addis Ababa, Ethiopia.

References

1. Erhabor O, Ejele OA, Nwauche CA, Buseri FI. Some haematological parameters in human immunodeficiency virus (HIV) infected Africans: the Nigerian perspective. Niger J Med. 2005;14(1):33–8.
2. Kyeyune R, Saathoff E, Ezeamama AE, Loscher T, Fawzi W, Guwatudde D. Prevalence and correlates of cytopenias in HIV-infected adults initiating highly active antiretroviral therapy in Uganda. BMC Infect Dis. 2014;14:496.
3. Dikshit B, Wanchu A, Sachdeva RK, Sharma A, Das R. Profile of hematological abnormalities of Indian HIV infected individuals. BMC Blood Disord. 2009;9:5.
4. Alamdo AG, Fiseha T, Tesfay A, Deber MK, Tirfe ZM, Tilahun T. Anemia and its associated risk factors at the time of antiretroviral therapy initiation in public health facilities of Arba Minch town, Southern Ethiopia. Health. 2015; 7(12):1657–64.
5. Belperio PS, Rhew DC. Prevalence and outcomes of anemia in individuals with human immunodeficiency virus: a systematic review of the literature. Am J Med. 2004;116(Suppl 7A):27S–43S.
6. Bain BJ. Pathogenesis and pathophysiology of anemia in HIV infection. Curr Opin Hematol. 1999;6(2):89–93.
7. Volberding P. The impact of anemia on quality of life in human immunodeficiency virus–infected patients. J Infect Dis. 2002;185:110–4.
8. Moyle G. Anemia in persons with HIV infection: prognostic marker and contributor to morbidity. AIDS Rev. 2002;4(1):13–20.
9. Moore RD, Forney D. Anemia in HIV-infected patients receiving highly active antiretroviral therapy. J Acquir Immune Defic Syndr. 2002;29:54–7.
10. Curkendall SM, Richardson JT, Emons MF, Fisher AE, Everhard F. Incidence of anaemia among HIV-infected patients treated with highly active antiretroviral therapy. HIV Med. 2007;8(8):483–90.
11. Assefa M, Abegaz WE, Shewamare A, Medhin G, Belay M. Prevalence and correlates of anemia among HIV infected patients on highly active anti-retroviral therapy at Zewditu Memorial Hospital, Ethiopia. BMC Hematol. 2015;15:6.
12. WHO. Hemoglobin concentrations for the diagnosis of anemia and assessment of severity. Vitamin and mineral nutrition information system. Geneva: World Health Organization; 2011.
13. Gedefaw L, Yemane T, Sahlemariam Z, Yilma D. Anemia and risk factors in HAART naive and HAART experienced HIV positive persons in south West Ethiopia: a comparative study. PLoS One. 2013;8(8):e72202.
14. Daka D, Lelissa D, Amsalu A. Prevalence of anemia before and after the initiation of antiretroviral therapy at ART center of Hawassa University Referral Hospital, Hawassa, South Ethiopia. Sch J Med. 2013;3(1):1–6.
15. Denu BA, Kida IM, Hammagabdo A, Dayar A, Sahabi MA. Prevalence of anemia and immunological markers in HIV-infected patients on highly active antiretroviral therapy in Northeastern Nigeria. Infect Dis. 2013;6:25–33.
16. Omoregie R, Omokaro EU, Palmer O, Ogefere HO, Egbeobauwaye A, Adeghe JE, Osakue SI, Ihemeje V. Prevalence of anaemia among HIV-infected patients in Benin City, Nigeria. Tanzan J of Health Res. 2009; 11(1):1–4.
17. Adane A, Desta K, Bezabih A, Gashaye A, Kassa D. HIV-associated anemia before and after initiation of antiretroviral therapy at ART Centre of Minilik II Hospital, Addis Ababa, Ethiopia. Ethiop Med J. 2012;50(1):13–21.
18. Tesfaye Z, Enawgaw B. Prevalence of anemia before and after initiation of highly active antiretroviral therapy among HIV positive patients in Northwest Ethiopia: a retrospective study. BMC Res Notes. 2014;7(1):1–5.
19. Santiago-Rodríguez EJ, Mayor AM, Fernández-Santos DM, Hunter-Mellado RF. Profile of HIV-Infected Hispanics with Pancytopenia. Int J Environ Res Public Health. 2015;13(1):38–45.
20. Dhurve SA, Dhurve AS. Bone marrow abnormalities in HIV disease. Mediterr J Hematol Infect Dis. 2013;5(1):e2013033.
21. Enawgaw B, Alem M, Addis Z, Melku M. Determination of hematological and immunological parameters among HIV positive patients taking HAART and treatment naïve in the antiretroviral therapy clinic of Gondar University Hospital, Gondar, Northwest Ethiopia: a comparative cross-sectional study. BMC Hematol. 2014;14:8.
22. Owiredu WK, Quaye L, Amidu N, Addai-Mensah O. Prevalence of anemia and immunological markers among Ghanaian HAART-naive HIV-patients and those on HAART. Afri Health Sci. 2011;11(1):2–15.

20

Useful clinical features and hematological parameters for the diagnosis of dengue infection in patients with acute febrile illness: a retrospective study

Juthatip Chaloemwong, Adisak Tantiworawit*, Thanawat Rattanathammethee, Sasinee Hantrakool, Chatree Chai-Adisaksopha, Ekarat Rattarittamrong and Lalita Norasetthada

Abstract

Background: Dengue infection patients are presented with acute febrile illness. Clinical presentations may mimic other infections. The serology for definite diagnosis is costly and inaccessible in many hospitals. We sought to identify the clinical features and hematologic parameters from a complete blood count (CBC) which distinguish dengue infection from other causes.

Methods: This was a retrospective single center study from Chiang Mai University Hospital. All patients who presented with acute fever between September 2013 and July 2015 were included. The diagnosis of dengue infection must be confirmed by serology. The control groups were patients who presented with acute febrile illness without localizing signs. Clinical data and CBC results were reviewed and compared. The Chi-square test was used to compare categorical variables. The CBC parameters were analyzed using the linear mixed model.

Results: One hundred and fifty-four dengue and 146 control patients were included. Headache, nausea, loss of appetite and bleeding diathesis were significantly symptoms in dengue patients ($p < 0.05$). There was some diversity in the the CBC in the dengue patients compared to the control group. Moreover, this study also identified the day of fever which these parameters were statistically significant. The dengue group had higher hemoglobin and hematocrit from day 3 to day 10 ($p < 0.001$), lower white blood cell count from day 1 to day 10 ($p < 0.001$), lower platelet count from day 3 to day 10 ($p < 0.001$), higher monocyte on day 1–4 ($p < 0.001$), higher atypical lymphocyte percentage on day 5–9 ($p < 0.001$) and higher eosinophil percentage on day 9–10 ($p = 0.001$). Furthermore, the neutrophil to lymphocyte percentage ratio of dengue group was > 1 on the first 5 days then reversed on day 6 to Day 9 but in non-dengue group, the ratio was always > 1.

Conclusion: We identified important clinical features and CBC parameters to differentiate dengue patients from other patients who had acute febrile illness from other causes. This identification could be done in local hospitals to give an accurate diagnosis, enabling further investigation to be tailored and treatment commenced earlier.

Keywords: Dengue infection, Diagnosis of dengue, Acute febrile illness, Complete blood count, Hematological parameters

* Correspondence: adisak.tan@cmu.ac.th; atantiwo@yahoo.com
Division of Hematology, Department of Internal Medicine, Faculty of Medicine, Chiang Mai University, 110 Intravaroros road, A. Muang, Chiang Mai 50200, Thailand

Background

Dengue is an infection caused by Dengue virus which transmitted by the bite of an infected mosquito. The disease is found in approximately 50 million people worldwide annually and 2.5 billion in dengue endemic countries [1]. The data from the population of Thailand from 1 January 2016 to 20 November 2016 shows a total of 34,677 cases, a morbidity rate of 0.01/100,000 population [2].

Dengue infection severity varies from mild illness to dengue shock syndrome. The clinical presentation of dengue patients is acute febrile illness with no localizing signs and symptoms which may mimic other infections. Therefore the laboratory tests such as a complete blood count (CBC), serological test or blood culture need to be used to differential and confirm the diagnosis.

The CBC in dengue patients change by the day of the fever, specifically on days 3 to 8, starting with progressive leukopenia followed by thrombocytopenia and hemoconcentration due to plasma leakage [3, 4]. The data from Brazil demonstrated mean white blood cell count (WBC) of dengue infected patients was 4.6×10^9/L with the lowest count of 0.7×10^9/L and the mean platelet count was 26.4×10^9/L with the lowest count registered was less than 1×10^9/L [5].

Currently, the serological test is used to confirm the diagnosis of dengue infection such as the detection of the dengue NS1 antigen (sensitivity 76% and specificity 98%) or the dengue IgM antibody by the ELISA method (sensitivity 90% and specificity 93%) [6]. Nevertheless, these serological tests may be inaccessible in underdeveloped countries or in some small local hospitals, so the clinical clues from the history taking, physical examination and the routine laboratory tests are still important. There was a study in Puerto Rico in 2011 which revealed that the dengue patients had enhanced leukopenia at 87% and a positive tourniquet test in 52% of patients. Hence patients with acute febrile illness with leukopenia and a positive tourniquet test were more likely to be infected with dengue than influenza, leptospirosis and enteroviruses [7].

The CBC parameters such as hemoglobin (Hb), hematocrit (Hct), WBC count, differential percentages of the WBCs and platelet count alter each day of the fever in patients infected with dengue. Little evidence exists to date to identify these daily changes ensuring dengue infection is distinguished from the other causes of acute febrile illness without localizing signs. Our aim was to find the most useful clinical features and CBC parameters which enable dengue to be distinguished from other infections in cases of acute febrile illness patients.

Methods

We retrospectively reviewed medical records of patients age 15 years or older who presented at Chiang Mai University Hospital for both inpatient and outpatient between September 2013 and July 2015. The inclusion criteria were patients with acute febrile illness (less than 7 days) without any identified source of infection. Patients must have had serology test or blood culture to confirm the diagnosis to be included in the study. Dengue infected patients were identified by a positive result of either the dengue NS1 antigen or dengue IgM antibody. The control group consisted of patients who also presented with fever without localzing signs and symptom including rickettsial infection (scrub typhus IgM or murine typhus IgM positive titer more than 1:400), primary bacteremia (positive blood culture without other primary source of infection), leptospirosis (positive leptospirosis IgM) and malarial infection (identified of *Plasmodium* spp. on thick or thin film). This study excluded patients with previously documented anemia (Hb less than 13 g/dl in men, 12 g/dl in women or mean corpuscular volume (MCV) value outside the range 80–100 fl), WBC count less than 5000 per cu.mm., platelet count less than 140,000 or more than 400,000 per.cu.mm, other hematologic diseases, chronic liver disease, chronic kidney disease, immunodeficiency patients, patients with malignancy during chemotherapy, and patients who were receiving any immunosuppressive drugs. We excluded the acute febrile illness patients with uncertain diagnosis. The dengue infected patients with evidence of co-infection were also excluded. The sample size was calculated using the formula $N = p \times (100 - P) \times z2/d2$ in which P was the anticipated prevalence, d was the desired precision and z was the appropriate value from the normal distribution for the desired confidence. We estimated an anticipated prevalence of 20% with 95% confidence ($Z = 1.96$) of achieving a precision of 10%. The calculated sample size was 300 patients, divided in to 2 groups; the dengue group and control group. The data concerning the control group was limited due to the lack of serological confirmed diagnosis of any one particular disease. To achieve the sample size, the control group needed to include patients with varying diseases; specifically rickettsia disease, leptospirosis, malaria, and primary bacteremia.

Clinical data was collected from medical records and compared between the dengue and control groups included demographic data, clinical presentations and all parameters from the CBC. Leukopenia was defined as a total WBC count of less than 4000 per cu.mm.; thrombocytopenia was defined as a total platelet count of less than 100,000 per.cu.mm; monocytosis was defined as a monocyte level of more than 10%; eosinophilia was defined as having an eosinophil level of more than 3%, and basophilia was defined as a basophil level of more than 2% of the total WBC. The CBC parameters were collected every time the blood test was performed related to days of fever until disease recovery at tenth day or when the blood component was transfused since post transfused CBC would not be analyzed. The frequency of blood test was depend on physician decision as individual case. Complete blood counts were performed using automated hematology analyzers, Siemens ADVIA® 2120 which are calibrated for standardization of results every 6 months.

The data was analyzed using SPSS statistical software version 17.0. Demographic data and laboratory data were presented as descriptive statistics including frequency, percentage, mean and range. The Chi-square test was used to compare categorical variables. The CBC parameters were analyzed using the linear mixed model as there were repeated measurements which were unbalanced and there were missing observations within the data for some subjects. A p-value of less than 0.05 was considered as statistically significant.

Results

A total of 154 patients were enrolled onto the dengue group, the dengue being serologically confirmed and 146 patients in the control group were enrolled. The serologic result for dengue group was positive for NS1 antigen in 57.79% (89/154), dengue IgM antibody in 27.92% (43/154) and both in 14.29% (22/154). There were 46 of 154 (29.8%) dengue infected patients classified in severe dengue infection. The control group included 103 (70.5%) patients with rickettsial disease, 30 (20.5%) with primary bacteremia, 8 (5.5%) with malaria and 5 (3.4%) with leptospirosis.

Table 1 demonstrates the baseline characteristics of the dengue and control groups. The sex and mean ages were slightly different between groups. The dengue group had a lower proportion of male patients (49.4% vs. 62.3%; $p = 0.024$) and a lower mean age (27 vs. 45 years; $p = 0.05$).

When compared to the control group, the dengue group had significant presentations of headache (47.4% vs. 34.2%, $p = 0.021$), loss of appetite (34.4% vs.15.8%, $p < 0.001$), nausea (33.8% vs.15.1%, $p < 0.001$) and bleeding diathesis (5.8% vs. 0%, $p = 0.003$). Chill symptoms were found more frequently in the control group (0.6% vs. 22.6%, $p < 0.001$). The others symptoms including myalgia, arthralgia, abdominal pain, rash, sore throat and diarrhea were not statistically different when the groups were compared (Table 2).

There were several hematologic parameters from the CBC which were diverse in the dengue patients. Also this study identified the days of fever when these parameters were statistically significantly different between the two groups. The dengue group had significantly higher hematocrit and also higher hemoglobin levels than the control group from day 3 to day 10 (Fig. 1). The highest was on day 7 of the fever: hemoglobin level [14.3 g/dl (13.98–14.55) vs. 12.9 g/dl (12.59–13.38)] and hematocrit [43.3% (42.29–43.89) vs. 39.2% (38.42–40.67)], respectively ($p < 0.001$).

As shown in Fig. 2, the dengue group had a lower total WBC count than the control group. The lowest mean WBC count was on day 4 of the fever; [3333 (2706 – 4136) vs. 8561 (8091 - 10,107) per cu.mm, $p < 0.001$]. Leukopenia was found from day 2 of fever (30.8%) and the incidence increased on successive days of the fever until day 5 (78.8%) and then there was a gradual recovery (Table 3).

The differential WBC count between the dengue and controls group by day of the fever are demonstrated in Fig. 3. The dengue group had a higher monocyte percentage than the control group on day 1 to 4 with the highest being on day 2 [11.7 vs. 5.4% ($p < 0.001$)]. Monocytosis was found in 62.5, 71.8, 50.8 and 44.9% of patients on days 1 to 4 of the fever respectively. The neutrophil percentage of the dengue group gradually decreased in a negative correlation with the increase in the percentage of lymphocytes in successive days of the fever. Dengue patients had higher neutrophil percentage predominately in the first 5 days of the fever then this was reversed and the

Table 1 Baseline characteristics of dengue and control group

	Dengue group (N = 154)	Control group (N = 146)	p-value
	N (%)	N (%)	
Sex			0.024
• Male	76(49.4)	91(62.3)	
• Female	78(50.6)	55 (37.7)	
Mean Age (year)	27(15–67)	45 (15–83)	< 0.001
Underlying disease	4 (2.6)	11(7.5)	0.050

Table 2 Comparison of the clinical presentations in dengue and control patients

	Dengue (N = 154)		Control (N = 146)		p-value
	N	Percent	N	Percent	
Fever	154	100	146	100.0	
Chills	1	0.6	33	22.6	< 0.001
Headache	73	47.4	50	34.2	0.021
Myalgia	75	48.7	63	43.2	0.335
Rash	10	6.5	8	5.5	0.712
Arthralgia	2	1.3	5	3.4	0.223
Abdominal pain	9	5.8	7	4.8	0.686
Nausea	52	33.8	22	15.1	< 0.001
Bleeding	9	5.8	0	0	0.003
Loss of appetite	53	34.4	23	15.8	< 0.001
Sore throat	14	9.1	12	8.2	0.789
Diarrhea	8	5.2	15	10.3	0.098

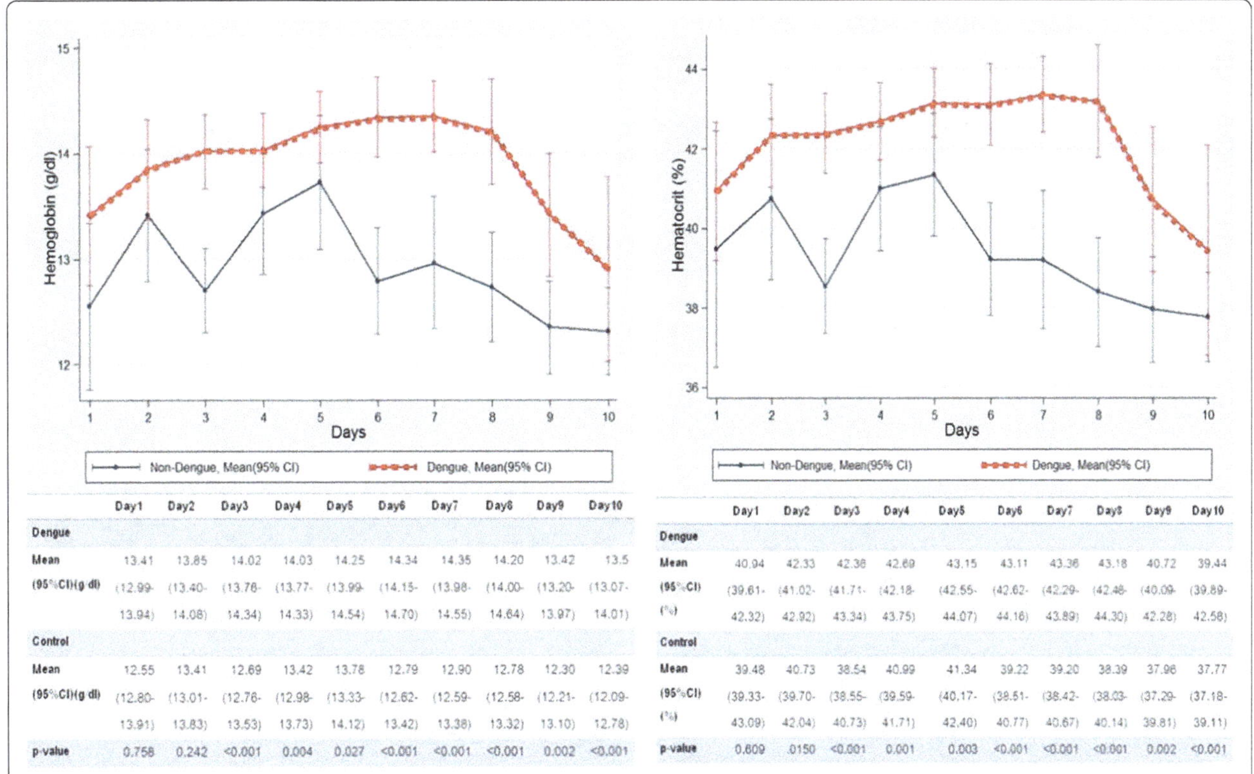

	Day1	Day2	Day3	Day4	Day5	Day6	Day7	Day8	Day9	Day10
Dengue										
Mean	13.41	13.85	14.02	14.03	14.25	14.34	14.35	14.20	13.42	13.5
(95%CI)(g/dl)	(12.99-13.94)	(13.40-14.08)	(13.76-14.34)	(13.77-14.33)	(13.99-14.54)	(14.15-14.70)	(13.98-14.55)	(14.00-14.64)	(13.20-13.97)	(13.07-14.01)
Control										
Mean	12.55	13.41	12.69	13.42	13.78	12.79	12.90	12.78	12.30	12.39
(95%CI)(g/dl)	(12.80-13.91)	(13.01-13.83)	(12.76-13.53)	(12.98-13.73)	(13.33-14.12)	(12.62-13.42)	(12.59-13.38)	(12.58-13.32)	(12.21-13.10)	(12.09-12.78)
p-value	0.758	0.242	<0.001	0.004	0.027	<0.001	<0.001	<0.001	0.002	<0.001

	Day1	Day2	Day3	Day4	Day5	Day6	Day7	Day8	Day9	Day10
Dengue										
Mean	40.94	42.33	42.38	42.69	43.15	43.11	43.36	43.18	40.72	39.44
(95%CI) (%)	(39.61-42.32)	(41.02-42.92)	(41.71-43.34)	(42.18-43.75)	(42.55-44.07)	(42.62-44.16)	(42.29-43.89)	(42.48-44.30)	(40.09-42.28)	(39.89-42.58)
Control										
Mean	39.48	40.73	38.54	40.99	41.34	39.22	39.20	38.39	37.96	37.77
(95%CI) (%)	(39.33-43.09)	(39.70-42.04)	(38.55-40.73)	(39.59-41.71)	(40.17-42.40)	(38.51-40.77)	(38.42-40.67)	(38.03-40.14)	(37.29-39.81)	(37.18-39.11)
p-value	0.609	.0150	<0.001	0.001	0.003	<0.001	<0.001	<0.001	0.002	<0.001

Fig. 1 Comparison of hemoglobin and hematocrit between dengue and control group by day of fever. Shows that the dengue group had higher hemoglobin and hematocrit significantly on day 3 to day 10 (highest on day7)

percentage of lymphocytes increased. Reversed neutrophil to lymphocyte ratios occurred on day 6 to 9 of fever (69.3, 89.4, 83.3 and 80% respectively). On the other hand, the neutrophil percentage in the control group predominated from the first day of the fever until recovery (Fig. 4). The dengue group had significantly higher percentage of atypical lymphocytes on day 5 to 9 of the fever than did the control group [4.25 vs. 0%; $p = 0.004$, 9.29 vs.0%; $p < 0.001$, 13 vs. 0.48%; $p < 0.001$, 10.85 vs. 0.13%; $p < 0.001$ and 6.56 vs. 0%; $p = 0.001$ respectively] with the highest being on day 7. The mean eosinophil percentage was higher in cases of dengue infection on day 9 and 10 (2.2 vs. 0.7% and 1.88 vs. 1.14%, $p < 0.001$). Eosinophilia was found in 28% and 20% of dengue patients on day 9 and 10 respectively. Basophil percentages were no different between the groups.

The mean platelet count was lower in the dengue than the control group on day 3 to 10 with the lowest on day 6 (68,910 vs. 196,137 per cu.mm., $p < 0.001$) as shown in Fig. 5. The thrombocytopenia occurred in more than 50% of patients on day 4 and reached the highest level of 80% on day 6.

Discussion

Dengue infected patients present with acute febrile illness without localized signs and symptoms and the clinical presentations may resemble other infections hence making a differential diagnosis difficult in distinguishing it from other infections such as tropical infection (rickettsial disease, leptospirosis or malaria), other viral infection and primary bacteremia. Our study identified the significant differences of clinical features and CBC parameters to facilitate the distinguishing of dengue infection from the other causes.

The clinical presentations in dengue infection are fever, headache, loss of appetite, nausea, bleeding diathesis, myalgia, abdominal pain, sore throat and diarrhea [5, 8, 9]. These symptoms are not specific and can be found in other infections. From our study, we found that headache, nausea, loss of appetite and bleeding diathesis were commonly found in dengue patients but chills presented significantly more frequently in the control group. Therefore, these clinical presentations may be helpful in distinguishing dengue infection from the other infections at presentation.

The demographic data between dengue and the control group in our study were different as regards gender, mean age and preexisting underlying diseases. The mean age of the dengue group was 27 years. They showed a strong correlation with the epidemiology of known dengue infection in Thailand, namely that the highest proportion of cases by age group is 15–24 years [2]. The

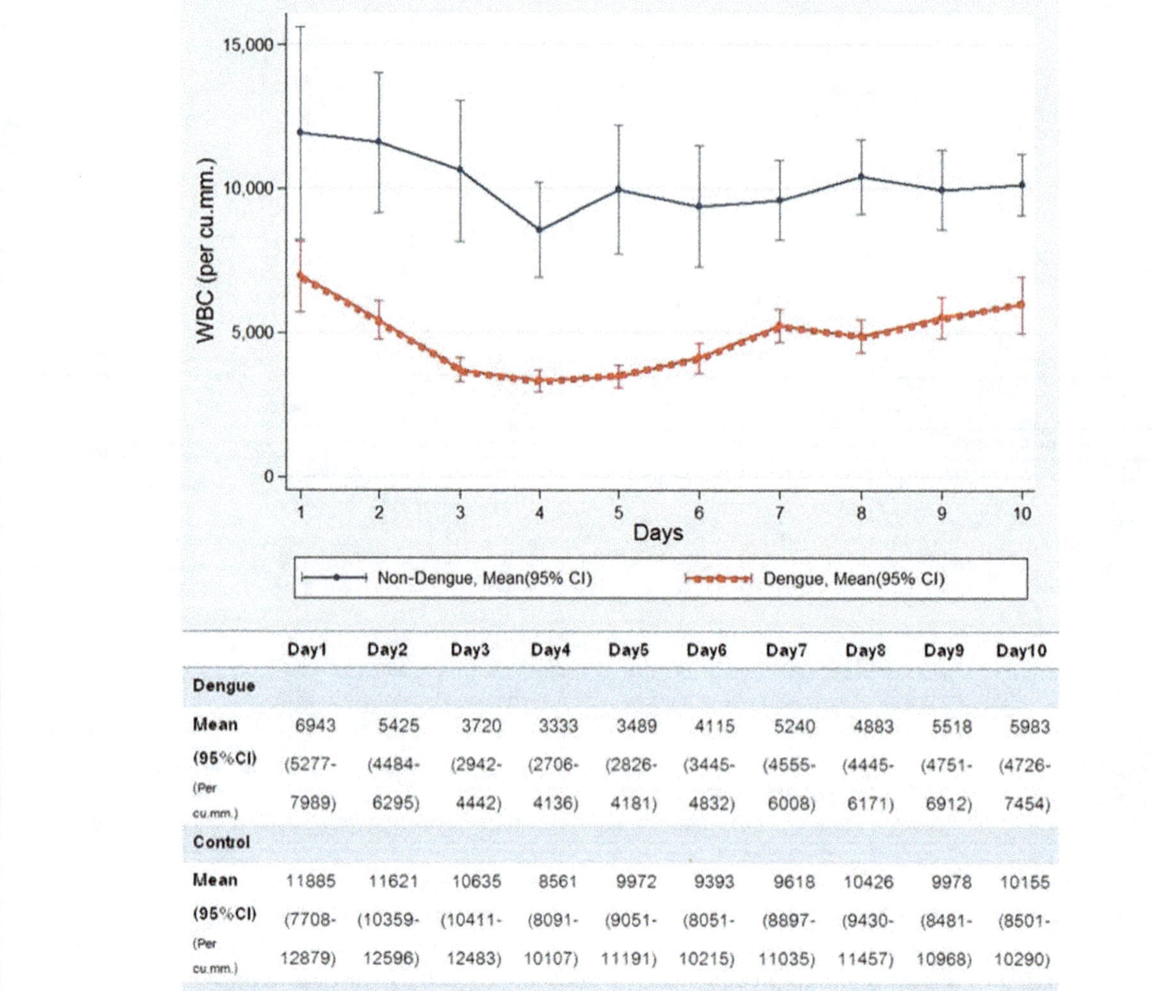

	Day1	Day2	Day3	Day4	Day5	Day6	Day7	Day8	Day9	Day10
Dengue										
Mean	6943	5425	3720	3333	3489	4115	5240	4883	5518	5983
(95%CI) (Per cu.mm.)	(5277-7989)	(4484-6295)	(2942-4442)	(2706-4136)	(2826-4181)	(3445-4832)	(4555-6008)	(4445-6171)	(4751-6912)	(4726-7454)
Control										
Mean	11885	11621	10635	8561	9972	9393	9618	10426	9978	10155
(95%CI) (Per cu.mm.)	(7708-12879)	(10359-12596)	(10411-12483)	(8091-10107)	(9051-11191)	(8051-10215)	(8897-11035)	(9430-11457)	(8481-10968)	(8501-10290)
p-value	<0.001	<0.001	<0.001	<0.001	<0.001	<0.001	<0.001	<0.001	<0.001	<0.001

Fig. 2 Comparison of WBC between dengue and control group by day of fever. Shows that the dengue group had lower white blood cell (WBC) count significantly from day 1 to day 10 (lowest on day 4)

Table 3 CBC parameters of dengue and control groups by day of fever

Day of fever	Avaliable CBC data		Leukopenia		Monocytosis		Neutrophil < 50%		Eosinophilia		Thrombocytopenia	
	Dengue ($N = 154$)	Control ($N = 146$)	Dengue N(%)	Control N(%)	Dengue N(%)	Control N(%)	Dengue N(%)	Control N(%)	Dengue N(%)	Control N(%)	Dengue N(%)	Control N(%)
1	16	12	0(0)	0(0)	10(62.5)	1(8.3)	0(0)	0(0)	2(12.5)	1(8.3)	0(0)	1(8.3)
2	39	27	12(30.8)	2(7.4)	28(71.8)	3(11.1)	3(1.9)	0(0)	1(2.6)	2(7.4)	3(7.7)	4(14.8)
3	61	32	40(65.6)	0(0)	31(50.8)	9(28.1)	10(16.4)	0(0)	2(3.3)	8(25)	18(29.5)	6(18.8)
4	69	33	53(76.8)	2(6.1)	31(44.9)	6(18.2)	18(26.1)	4(12.1)	4(5.8)	3(9.1)	36(52.2)	2(6.1)
5	80	29	63(78.8)	3(10.3)	33(41.3)	6(20.7)	30(37.5)	3(10.3)	5(6.3)	4(13.8)	46(57.5)	5(17.2)
6	75	29	44(58.7)	0(0)	36(48)	9(31)	52(69.3)	4(13.8)	16(21.3)	3(10.3)	60(80)	4(13.8)
7	66	30	20(30.3)	1(3.3)	26(39.4)	5(16.7)	59(89.4)	4(13.3)	9(13.6)	4(13.3)	50(75.8)	11(36.7)
8	42	32	12(28.6)	1(3.1)	13(31)	6(18.8)	35(83.3)	3(9.4)	7(16.7)	5(15.6)	29(69)	11(34.4)
9	25	20	4(16)	0(0)	9(36)	9(45)	20(80)	7(35)	7(28)	0(0)	9(36)	6(30)
10	15	45	3(20)	0(0)	11(73.1)	14(31.1)	11(73.3)	11(24.4)	3(20)	3(6.7)	4(26.7)	3(6.7)

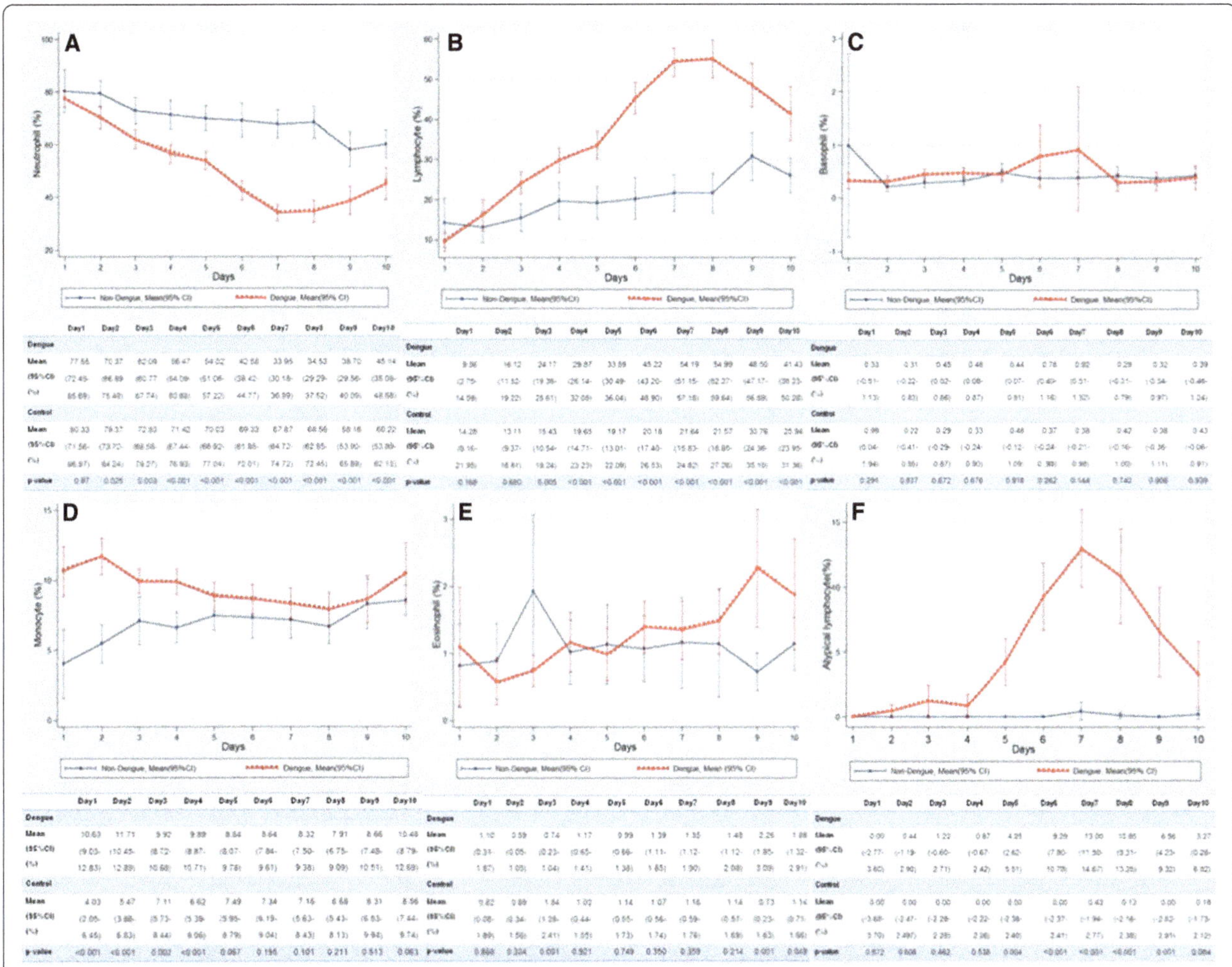

Fig. 3 Comparison of differential WBC count between dengue and control group by day of fever. Shows that the dengue group had lower neutrophil on day 4–10 (**a**), higher lymphocyte on day 3–10 (**b**), basophils not different (**c**), higher monocytes on day 1–4 (**d**), higher eosinophils on day 9–10(**e**) and higher atypical lymphocytes on day 5–9 (**f**)

control group was older (mean age of 45 years old) which may be explained by the higher level of preexisting underlying diseases in this group compared to the dengue group.

In addition to the clinical features, there were several hematologic parameters that were useful in distinguishing dengue infection from other infections using the CBC which is an accessible laboratory test in almost all hospitals.

In summary, the dengue group had higher hemoglobin levels and a higher hematocrit from day 3 to day 10 (highest on day 7), lower white blood cell (WBC) count from day 2 to day 10 (lowest on day 4) and lower platelet count from day 3 to day 10 (lowest on day 6). The details of the differential WBC percentage were that the samples from the patients with dengue showed higher monocyte on day 1–4 (highest on day 2), higher atypical lymphocytes day 5–9 (highest on day 7) and higher eosinophils on day 9–10 (highest on day 9) than control group. Furthermore, the neutrophil to lymphocyte ratio in the dengue group was >1 on the first 5 days then reversed on day 6 to day 9.

The dengue group had higher hemoglobin levels and a higher hematocrit as a result of the plasma leakage. An in vitro study revealed a cross-reaction of proinflammatory mediators such as tumor necrosis factor (TNF)--alpha and anti-NS1 antibodies with surface proteins on endothelial cells causing apoptosis of these cells and subsequently plasma leakage [10].

The total white blood cell count was significantly lower in the dengue group than the control group. Leukopenia occurred from day 2 and was lowest on day 5 of the fever in the dengue group. A hypothesis regarding the occurrence of the leukopenia in the cases of dengue infection was that it was caused by the destruction or inhibition of myeloid progenitor cells as the bone marrow examination showed mild hypocellularity in the first seven days of fever then normal cellularity in the convalescent phase [11].

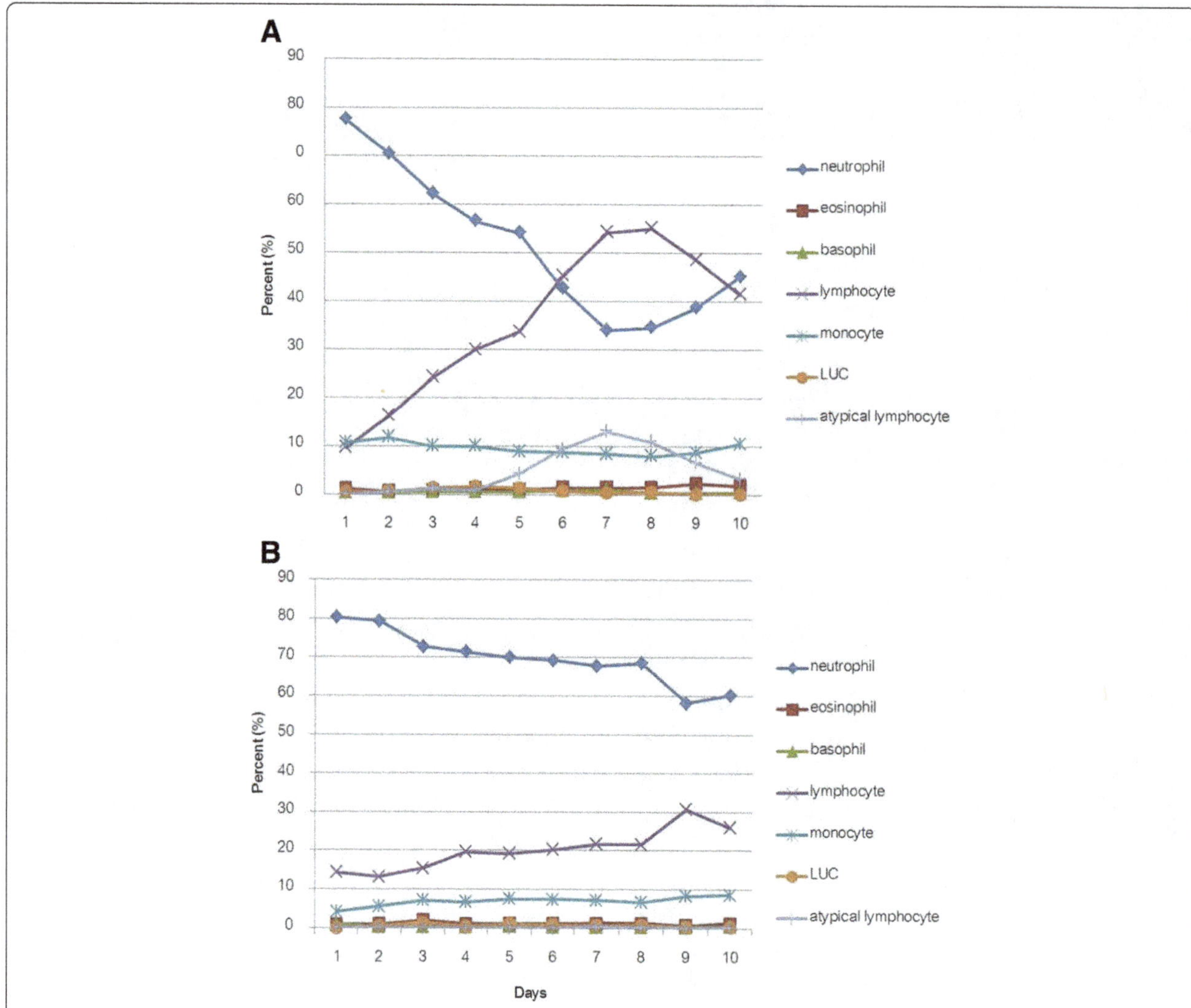

Fig. 4 The change in differential WBC count of dengue and control group by day of fever. Shows differential white blood cell count of dengue group (**a**) and control group (**b**). The neutrophil to lymphocyte ratio of dengue group was > 1 on the first 5 days then reversed on day 6 to Day 9 but in control group, the ratio was always > 1

Monocytosis occurred in 60–70% of patients in our study which was similar to previous study which found it in 84.6% of patients [12]. Another study showed that monocytosis was found in cases of dengue hemorrhagic fever more often than dengue fever [8]. Thus, monocytosis might be a parameter which can be used to predict the severity of dengue infection. A hypothesis as to why there is an increase in monocytes in the first few day of the fever is that monocytes and macrophages are the part of the primary immune which carry out phagocytosis of microorganisms and present the resulting carried antigen to the T helper cells. However, there were several conditions associated with monocytosis, for example other viral infections, enteric fever, malaria, tuberculosis, HIV, malignancy or pyrexia of unknown origin [13], so the monocytosis was not specific to dengue infection.

The neutrophils percentage was predominant in the first 5 days of the fever, a condition which was reversed, lymphocytes then predominating. This result was in agreement with a previous study which showed that lymphocytes predominated on day 10 of the fever [14].

A study from Brazil and Pakistan had similar results to this study in terms of eosinophilia, the study showing that around 20% of patients had a higher eosinophil count on day 10 of the fever [5, 9]. In cases of dengue infection, eosinophil levels were low in the acute phase due to the response to the inflammatory process, the levels then returning to baseline and increasing in the convalescence phase [15].

Atypical lymphocytes increased on days 5–9 in the dengue group. The higher atypical lymphocyte percentage was found in cases of dengue hemorrhagic fever more than dengue fever [12]. Therefore the percentage of atypical

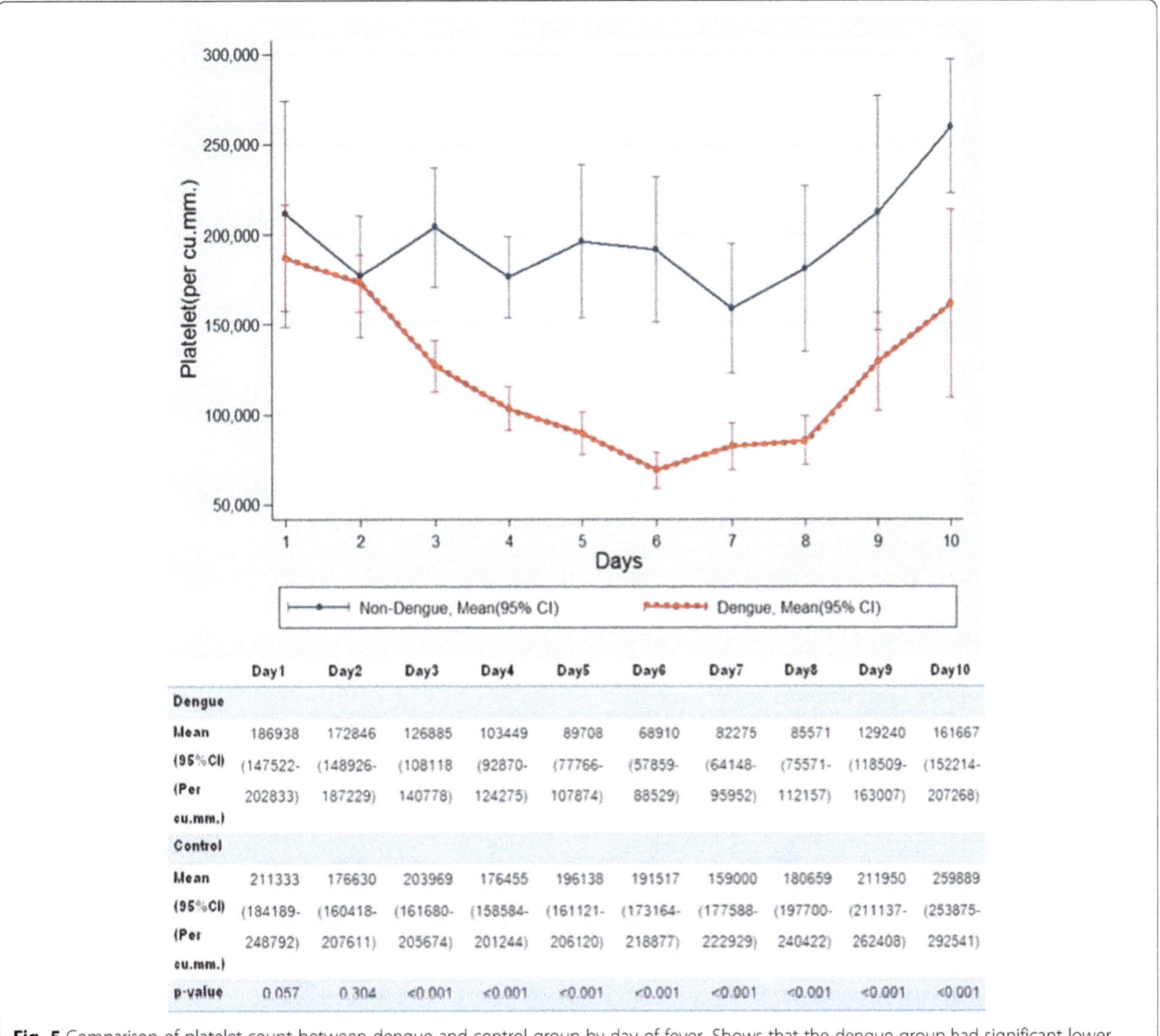

	Day1	Day2	Day3	Day4	Day5	Day6	Day7	Day8	Day9	Day10
Dengue										
Mean (95%CI) (Per cu.mm.)	186938 (147522- 202833)	172846 (148926- 187229)	126885 (108118 140778)	103449 (92870- 124275)	89708 (77766- 107874)	68910 (57859- 88529)	82275 (64148- 95952)	85571 (75571- 112157)	129240 (118509- 163007)	161667 (152214- 207268)
Control										
Mean (95%CI) (Per cu.mm.)	211333 (184189- 248792)	176630 (160418- 207611)	203969 (161680- 205674)	176455 (158584- 201244)	196138 (161121- 206120)	191517 (173164- 218877)	159000 (177588- 222929)	180659 (197700- 240422)	211950 (211137- 262408)	259889 (253875- 292541)
p-value	0.057	0.304	<0.001	<0.001	<0.001	<0.001	<0.001	<0.001	<0.001	<0.001

Fig. 5 Comparison of platelet count between dengue and control group by day of fever. Shows that the dengue group had significant lower platelet count from day 3 to day 10 (lowest on day 6)

lymphocytes may be another parameter useful in the prediction of the severity of dengue infection in addition to monocytosis.The study from India showed basophilia (basophil > 2%) in 52.9% of dengue patients [12]. On the contrary to this result, the basophils were not elevated in our study. The cause of basophilia may be due to recovery from the bone marrow suppression in the convalescence phase [16].

Half of the patients had thrombocytopenia on day 4 and increased up to approximately 80% of cases on day 6. Although almost patients had thrombocytopenia, but most of them were non-severe form of dengue infection so the bleeding diathesis of our study was low(5.8%). There are several hypotheses to explain this such as an infected megakaryocyte by the virus, peripheral destruction and cross-reaction of antibodies against platelets [17]. The platelets of dengue infected patients had mitochondrial dysfunction which activated the apoptosis cascade and led to cell death [18]. Prolonged thrombocytopenia was found in dengue hemorrhagic fever more frequently than in cases of dengue fever [12], so the duration of thrombocytopenia is considered to be the predictor of the severity of dengue infection. Currently, the new parameter to reflect the rate of thrombopoiesis is the immature platelet fraction (IPF) which can be used to predict platelet recovery in dengue patients [19]. Cytopenia is the major parameter from the CBC which can distinguish dengue infection from the others. A review of a bone marrow study in dengue patients showed the transient suppression of hematopoiesis within 3–4 days of infection then the host inflammatory response which occurred to eliminate infected cells. Therefore, the cytopenia is probably a protective mechanism to limit injury to the marrow stem cells during the subsequent process of the eradication of infected cells [16]. In addition, the dengue-infected endothelial cells are potentially bound to white blood cells, neutrophils, lymphocytes, platelets, and large lymphocytes in vitro but the monocytes, basophils, and eosinophils had no interaction. The increased binding of neutrophils and platelets to infected endothelial cells may explain neutropenia and thrombocytopenia in dengue patients [20].

In addition to a previous study, our study included the changes in all CBC parameters on each successive day of the fever. The first parameter was monocytosis, followed by leukopenia, thrombocytopenia, a raised hematocrit, increased atypical lymphocytes and a reversed neutrophil to lymphocyte ratio respectively. The recovery phase started with the increase of white blood cell, hematocrit and platelet. We also found eosinophilia at this phase.

A study in Indonesia identified the possible use of new parameters to enable the differentiation of dengue from leptospirosis and enteric fever using flow cytometry to quantitate the atypical lymphocyte area, high-fluorescent lymphocyte counts, immature granulocytes and IPF [21]. These investigations may give high accuracy for diagnosis but are inaccessible in all hospitals. Furthermore, there were other parameters which would probably be useful for diagnosis of dengue infection, such as prolonged activated partial thromboplastin time, prothrombin time, thrombin time and elevated liver enzymes [22], but these data in our cohort were limited. Many laboratory parameters are not only useful for diagnosis but also enable the prediction of severity such as monocytosis, duration of thrombocytopenia, high atypical lymphocyte percentage, high serum lactate and lactate dehydrogenase levels [23, 24]. The last enzyme test was not performed routinely in our study.

The limitation of this study was that it was a retrospective study. Much information which may be useful for comparison and the diagnosis of dengue infection was not available from the database and as it was retrospective could not be addressed. The control group was made up of patients with many diseases which make the data inhomogeneous when comparing it with the dengue group especially malaria or leptospirosis which were few cases in that group so some data may be masked. Hence, other CBC parameters and further work needs to be done using a specific disease group to compare to the dengue group. Another limitation, the CBC result was done on physician decision as individual case. This limitation might influence the results obtained in our study as the CBC was not done on the daily basis. The enrollment in the study was done from diagnosis and reviewed for history of fever which was matched the inclusion criteria. This may effect the selection bias of case and quality of the study. Prospective study in this topic can be done in the future to correct the limitation of our study.

Conclusions

We identified important clinical presentations and useful CBC parameters to enable the differentiation of dengue patients from other patients with other causes of acute febrile illness. These findings can be applied to local hospital situations as the data can be amassed from a CBC. An accurate diagnosis using these data will enable further investigation to be tailored and early treatment for the patient.

Abbreviations

CBC: Complete blood count; Hb: Hemoglobin; Hct: Hematocrit; IPF: Immature platelet fraction; MCV: Mean corpuscular volume; TNF: Tumor necrosis factor; WBC: White blood cell count

Acknowledgements

I would like to sincerely thank Ms. Antika Wongthani, Head of Analytical & Statistical data unit, Research Institute for Health Sciences, Chiang Mai University for suggestion in statistics of this study.

Funding

This study was supported by a research grant from the Faculty of Medicine, Chiang Mai University.

Authors' contributions

J.C. collected, summarized, analyzed clinical data and wrote the paper; A.T. designed the research, obtained researched grant, analyzed data, wrote the paper and corresponding author; T.R., S.H., E.R.,C.C., L.N. wrote, revised the manuscript and gave critical comment. "All authors read and approved the final manuscript".

Competing interests

All of the authors declare no competing interests.

References

1. WHO Guidelines Approved by the Guidelines Review Committee. Dengue: guidelines for diagnosis, treatment, prevention and control: new edition. Geneva: World Health Organization World Health Organization; 2009.
2. Bureau of Epidemiology DoDC. Ministry of Public Health Dengue fever. Thailand: Bureau of National disease surveillance (Report 506) Epidemiology MoPH; 2015.
3. Oliveira EC, Pontes ER, Cunha RV, Froes IB, Nascimento D. Hematological abnormalities in patients with dengue. Rev Soc Bras Med Trop. 2009;42(6):682–5.
4. Ali N, Usman M, Syed N, Khurshid M. Haemorrhagic manifestations and utility of haematological parameters in dengue fever: a tertiary care Centre experience at Karachi. Scand J Infect Dis. 2007;39(11–12):1025–8.
5. Denys Eiti Fujimotoa SK. Clinical and laboratory characteristics of patients with dengue hemorrhagic fever manifestations and their transfusion profile. Brazilian Journal of Hematology and Hemotherapy. 2014;36(2):115–20.
6. Prevention CfDCa. Laboratory guidance and diagnostic testing of dengue infection September 27, 2012.
7. Gregory CJ, Lorenzi OD, Colon L, Garcia AS, Santiago LM, Rivera RC, et al. Utility of the tourniquet test and the white blood cell count to differentiate dengue among acute febrile illnesses in the emergency room. PLoS Negl Trop Dis. 2011;5(12):e1400.

8. Khan E, Kisat M, Khan N, Nasir A, Ayub S, Hasan R. Demographic and clinical features of dengue fever in Pakistan from 2003-2007: a retrospective cross-sectional study. PLoS One. 2010;5(9):e12505.
9. Riaz MM, Mumtaz K, Khan MS, Patel J, Tariq M, Hilal H, et al. Outbreak of dengue fever in Karachi 2006: a clinical perspective. JPMA The Journal of the Pakistan Medical Association. 2009;59(6):339–44.
10. Martina BE, Koraka P, Osterhaus AD. Dengue virus pathogenesis: an integrated view. Clin Microbiol Rev. 2009;22(4):564–81.
11. Lin SF, Liu HW, Chang CS, Yen JH, Chen TP. Hematological aspects of dengue fever. Gaoxiong yi xue ke xue za zhi = The Kaohsiung journal of medical sciences. 1989;5(1):12–6.
12. Malathesha AHN MK. Hematological Manifestations in Dengue Fever – An Observational Study. J Evol Med Dent Sci. 2014;3(09):2245–50.
13. ShweSina* LL, Aunga TY, TheingiMaungMaungb, KhaingSwea K. Approach to the Patients with Monocytosis IOSR. Journal of Dental and Medical Sciences. 2015;14(5):81–6.
14. Jameel T, Mehmood K, Mujtaba G, Choudhry N, Afzal N, Paul RF. Changing haematological parameters in dengue viral infections. Journal of Ayub Medical College, Abbottabad : JAMC. 2012;24(1):3–6.
15. Beeson P, Bass DA. The eosinophil. In: Smith LH, editor. Major problems in internal medicine, vol. 14; 1977. p. 215–34.
16. La Russa VF, Innis BL. Mechanisms of dengue virus-induced bone marrow suppression. Baillieres Clin Haematol. 1995;8(1):249–70.
17. Mendez A, Gonzalez G. Abnormal clinical manifestations of dengue hemorrhagic fever in children. Biomedica : revista del Instituto Nacional de Salud. 2006;26(1):61–70.
18. Hottz ED, Medeiros-de-Moraes IM, Vieira-de-Abreu A, de Assis EF, Vals-de-Souza R, Castro-Faria-Neto HC, et al. Platelet activation and apoptosis modulate monocyte inflammatory responses in dengue. J Immunol. 2014; 193(4):1864–72.
19. Dadu T, Sehgal K, Joshi M, Khodaiji S. Evaluation of the immature platelet fraction as an indicator of platelet recovery in dengue patients. Int J Lab Hematol. 2014;36(5):499–504.
20. Butthep P, Bunyaratvej A, Bhamarapravati N. Dengue virus and endothelial cell: a related phenomenon to thrombocytopenia and granulocytopenia in dengue hemorrhagic fever. The Southeast Asian journal of tropical medicine and public health. 1993;24(Suppl 1):246–9.
21. Oehadian A, Michels M, de Mast Q, Prihatni D, Puspita M, Hartantri Y, et al. New parameters available on Sysmex XE-5000 hematology analyzers contribute to differentiating dengue from leptospirosis and enteric fever. Int J Lab Hematol. 2015;37(6):861–8.
22. Wahid SF, Sanusi S, Zawawi MM, Ali RA. A comparison of the pattern of liver involvement in dengue hemorrhagic fever with classic dengue fever. The Southeast Asian journal of tropical medicine and public health. 2000;31(2):259–63.
23. Sirikutt P, Kalayanarooj S. Serum lactate and lactate dehydrogenase as parameters for the prediction of dengue severity. Journal of the Medical Association of Thailand = Chotmaihet thangphaet. 2014;97(Suppl 6):S220–31.
24. Thanachartwet V, Oer-Areemitr N, Chamnanchanunt S, Sahassananda D, Jittmittraphap A, Suwannakudt P, et al. Identification of clinical factors associated with severe dengue among Thai adults: a prospective study. BMC Infect Dis. 2015;15:420.

21

Albumin, copper, manganese and cobalt levels in children suffering from sickle cell anemia at Kasumbalesa, in Democratic Republic of Congo

Olivier Mukuku[1*†], Joseph K. Sungu[2†], Augustin Mulangu Mutombo[2], Paul Makan Mawaw[3], Michel Ntetani Aloni[4], Stanislas Okitotsho Wembonyama[2] and Oscar Numbi Luboya[1,2,3]

Abstract

Background: Sickle Cell Anemia (SCA) is characterized by high levels of oxidative stress markers and low levels of antioxidant capacity. Antioxidant defence mechanisms against the harmful effects of ROS requires cellular and extracellular enzymes. These enzymes requires micronutrient for complete activity. Information on micronutrients such as manganese, cobalt and copper in SCA population was poorly documented in the literature.

Methods: Plasma copper, manganese, cobalt and albumin concentrations determined by atomic absorption spectrophotometry were compared between two groups of children: 76 with SCA (Hb-SS) and 76 without SCA (controls). This study was conducted in the Muhona Hospital of Kasumbalesa, which is situated in a rural and low in resources.

Results: The mean age was 10.0 years (SD = 5.4) in SCA children and 9.2 years (SD = 4.7) in the control group. The levels of cobalt, manganese, copper and albumin were not different between the two groups ($p > 0.05$).

Conclusion: In our study, albumin, manganese, cobalt and copper values did not differ between SCA children in steady state and Hb-AA children. The lack of differences in plasma elemental concentrations between the two groups in context of increased demands in the SCA group, may represent adequate compensatory intake or elemental dyshomeostasis in the SCA group.

Keywords: Sickle cell Anemia, Children, Trace elements, Africa

Background

Sickle cell anaemia (SCA) remains the most common genetic diseases and major problem in public health in the world. The incidence is estimated to range from 30,000 to 40,000 neonates per year in a recent report [1].

The disease is characterized by chronic hemolysis, chronic inflammation, immune deficiency, a heterogeneous clinical phenotype and organ damage [2–7]. Pathogenic mechanism in sickle cell disease is mainly due to chronic inflammation with oxidative stress. This situation leads to high levels of oxidative stress markers and low levels of antioxidant capacity in SCA patients. Antioxidant defence mechanisms against the harmful effects of reactive oxygen species (ROS) requires cellular and extracellular enzymes such as peroxidase, glutathione reductase, catalase and superoxide dismutase (SOD). These enzymes require micronutrients for complete activity.

SCA is associated with increased risks of multiple micronutrient deficiencies but no significant differences found in the levels of copper and albumin in SCA adults compared to Hb-AA adults [8]. These nutriments have a major role in the protection of the red cell membrane against stress free radical mediated by oxidation in SCA [9–11]. Children suffering from SCA have significantly lower serum levels of zinc, magnesium and selenium

* Correspondence: oliviermukuku@yahoo.fr
†Olivier Mukuku and Joseph K. Sungu contributed equally to this work.
[1]Department of Research, High Institute of Techniques Medicales, Lubumbashi, Democratic Republic of Congo
Full list of author information is available at the end of the article

[12]. SOD is a copper and zinc-containing enzyme that converts superoxide radicals to hydrogen peroxides. Copper is essential for this enzyme's catalytic activity and antioxidant functions; it plays an important role in the functions of cytochrome c oxidase [13]. A recent study shows a correlation between the oxidant/antioxidant imbalance and alteration in the serum copper level in patients suffering from SCA [14]. A copper excess may contribute to free radical production and oxidative damage [2].

This study is part of a project to evaluate micronutrients in sickle-cell anemia in the African environment. A first study showed that zinc, selenium and magnesium values were significantly lower in SCA children compared to children with normal hemoglobin (Hb-AA) [12]. The objective of this second study was to determine the cobalt, copper, manganese and albumin serum levels among SCA children in steady state. The findings could be a starting point for future research in the understanding of the disease in a context of tropical, malnutrition and in highly resource-scarce settings environment such as the Democratic Republic of Congo (DRC).

Methods

This study was conducted from January 2014 to June 2014 in the Muhona Hospital of Kasumbalesa, which is situated in the southeastern part of the DRC. This hospital receives all SCA children from the health area of Kasumbalesa which is a rural and low in resources.

We consecutively recruited SCA children (Hb-SS) between the age of 2 years and 15 years after written informed consent provided by their legal guardians. All SCA children were in steady state, free of pain for at one month and had not been hospitalized or transfused for at least 100 days before the study [6]. We excluded subjects (i) under iron therapy (ii) under chronic transfusion program. For each case, one control patient (Hb-AA) matched for age, sex and place of residence were recruited into the study, and 76 SCA children were compared to 76 Hb-AA children.

Data collection procedure and blood analysis

Five ml of venous blood sample was drawn from each study participant into an EDTA tube, used to determine laboratory parameters.

Five ml of venous blood sample was drawn from each study participant into an EDTA tube, used to determine hemoglobin electrophoresis. Sickle cell screening was performed using isoelectric focusing method.

Cobalt, manganese and copper levels were estimated in blood samples using a Perkin Elmer Model 2380 Atomic absorption Spectrophotometer (Norwak, Connecticut, USA). Albumin was measured in blood samples by the bromocresol green dye binding method. Trace elements were performed at Mineralogy Laboratory of the Société de Développement Industriel et Minier du Congo (SODIMICO) at Kasumbalesa, in DRC.

Ethics statement

The approval to conduct the study and authorizations were obtained from the Medical Ethic Committee of the University of Lubumbashi (UNILU/CEM/048/2015). Data was used with high confidentiality and no names were recorded.

Data management and analysis

Results were analyzed using the Epi Info 7.1 (CDC Atlanta, USA) and they were exported on STATA 12 for further analysis. Data are represented as means ± standard deviation (SD) when the distribution was normal and median with range when the distribution was not normal. The analysis of Student's t-test was used for comparisons of means. Chi square test was also used to compare the difference between groups regarding age groups and gender. Statistical significance level was set at $p < 0.05$.

Results

A total of 152 children, 76 SCA children and 76 no-SCA children were recruited into the study over the 6 months. The mean age of the Hb-SS group was 10.0 (SD = 5.4) years while that of the Hb-AA group was 9.2 (SD = 4.7) years. The sex-ratio male to female in the SCA group and control group was respectively 1:1.8 and 1:1.1 (Table 1).

The Fig. 1 shows that the mean albumin level in Hb-SS group tended to be lower than in Hb-AA group. However, there was no statistically difference between the two groups (43.71 ± 1.10 g/L vs 48.46 ± 2.78 mg/L; $p = 0.50$).

In the Hb-SS group, the mean value of manganese was similar to that of the Hb-AA group (0.12 ± 0.04 μg/L vs 0.03 ± 0.01 μg/L; $p = 0.057$) as shown in the Fig. 1.

In the Hb-SS group, the mean cobalt level tended to be higher than in the Hb-AA group (0.81 ± 0.13 μg/L vs 0.48 ± 0.10 μg/L; $p = 0.065$). However, there was no statistical difference between the two groups (Fig. 1).

Table 1 Demographics characteristics of the two study groups

Variable	Hb-SS group ($n = 76$)	Hb-AA group (n = 76)	p
Age			
< 5 years	15 (19.7%)	17 (22.4%)	0.7195
5–9 years	21 (27.6%)	24 (31.6%)	
≥ 10 years	40 (52.6%)	35 (46.0%)	
Mean ± SD	10.0 ± 5.4	9.2 ± 4.7	0.3324
Sex			
Female	49 (64.5%)	40 (52.6%)	0.1877
Male	27 (35.5%)	36 (47.4%)	

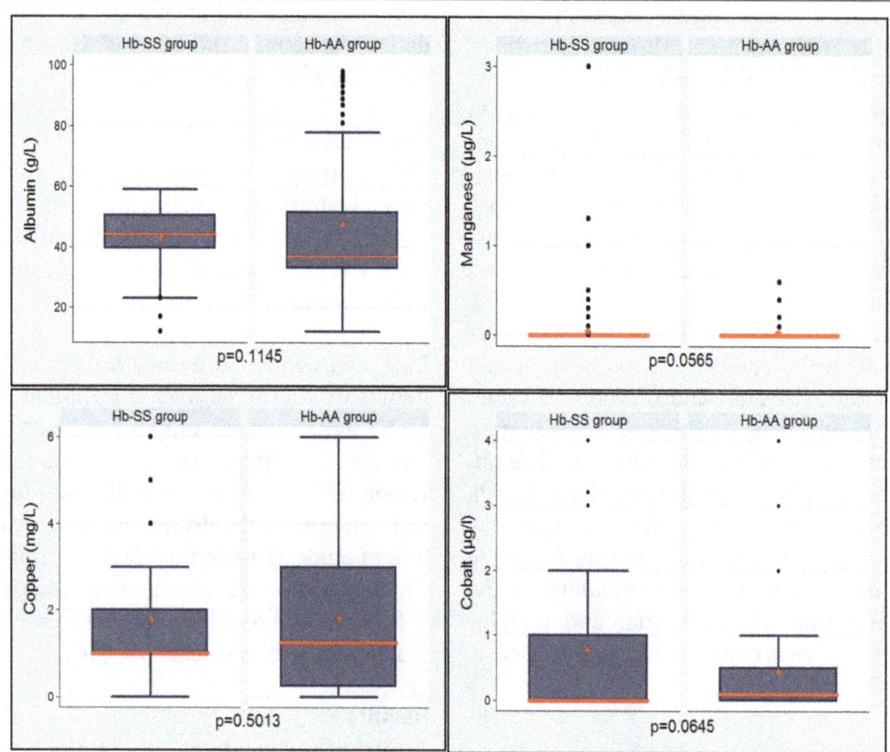

Fig. 1 Albumin, manganese, copper and cobalt levels according hemoglobin status. Red line: median; Red cross: means; Line at the furthest lower of the box: first quartile (25%); Line at the furthest upper of the box: third quartile (75%); Dot: outlier; Line at the furthest lower: lowest value (minimum) excluding outliers; Line at the furthest upper: highest value (maximum) excluding outliers. Student's t-test was used to compare the two groups.

The Fig. 1 shows that the mean copper level did not vary significantly between the two groups (1.72 ± 0.15 mg/L vs 1.89 ± 0.20 mg/L; $p = 0.50$).

Discussion

Our study is the first to look at albumin, manganese, cobalt and copper values in SCA children living in the Central Africa. Albumin exerts its anti-oxidant effect in the body by binding copper ions and heme tightly and iron ions weakly. It thus plays a role in preventing copper and iron from participating in lipid peroxidation. In our series, there was no significant difference in the levels of albumin in the SCA patients compared to controls. Our findings are in consonance with previous reports from Nigeria and Sudan [4].

Manganese is a trace element that is required as a cofactor for many antioxidant enzymes such as glutathione peroxidase and superoxide dismutase [5–7]. Thus, this trace element plays a key role in oxidative damage without deleterious side effects of Fenton chemistry. In the SCA group, the mean values of manganese were similar to those of the control group. In his study, Kehinde et al. in Nigeria reported similar findings [15]. By contrast, in their Nigerian series, Digban et al. found that manganese level was significantly decreased in sickle cell patients when compared with apparent controls [16]. On the other hand, Kehinde et al. reported that manganese values were higher in the SCA patients in crisis [15]. We postulate that the metabolism of manganese and are not influenced by the presence of sickle cell anemia in steady state.

In the SCA group, the mean values of cobalt were similar to those of the control group. There is still a lack of information on cobalt in SCA children in the medical literature. Cobalt is an essential element, but at high concentrations, possesses the ability to produce reactive radicals such as superoxide anion radical and nitric oxide in biological systems. This oxidative stress contributes to cell toxicity and death [9, 10]. Cobalt is integral part of vitamin B_{12}, its alone function known in human physiology. In the SCA group, the median values of cobalt were similar between sickle cell patients and children with Hb-AA. By contrast, in their Nigerian series, Digban et al. found that cobalt level was significantly decreased in sickle cell patients when compared with apparently controls [16]. There is still a lack of information on cobalt in SCA children in the medical literature. We postulate that the metabolism of cobalt are not influenced by the presence of sickle cell anemia or may be due to normal dietary intake of vitamin, in our series. In addition, we speculate that environment and genetic factors may explain this difference between these two studies.

In this study, the mean copper level did not vary significantly between the two groups, which is similar to the findings reported by Alayash et al. in Saudi Arabia, and by Kehinde et al. in Nigeria [11, 15]. However, our results are different with the previous worldwide reports in which they found a significantly higher serum copper in sickle cell patients compared with controls [2, 14, 17–19]. We therefore speculate that environment and genetic factors may explain this difference between these studies. In addition, rates of child malnutrition remain very high in the DRC in general and particularly in the health zone of Kasumbalesa, which is a rural and low in resources [20].

Conclusion

The first literature on the subject of albumin, manganese, cobalt and copper values in SCA is briefly reported in Africa. In our study, albumin and these trace elements did not differ between SCA children in a steady state and Hb-AA children. The lack of differences in plasma elemental concentrations between the two groups in context of increased demands in the SCA group, may represent adequate compensatory intake or elemental dyshomeostasis in the SCA group. Further investigations will focus on data on these trace elements in SCA children in crisis compared to those in steady state.

Abbreviations

DRC: Democratic Republic of Congo; Hb-AA: Hemoglobin AA; Hb-SS: Hemoglobin SS; ROS: Reactive oxygen species; SCA: Sickle Cell Anemia; SD: Standard deviation; SOD: Superoxide dismutase

Acknowledgements

The authors gratefully thank the staff of the laboratories of SODIMICO and Muhona Hospital. Warm thanks to Doctor Gloria Bundutidi and the Nurse Team of Saint-Crispin Medical Center as well as all the patients for their invaluable contribution to the present study.

Authors' contributions

OM, JKS, AMM, PMM and ONL conceived, designed, deployed and directed the study at the Muhona Hospital and at the Faculty of Medicine of University of Lubumbashi. JKS, PMM and OM carried out patient recruitment and follow-up, sample collection, storage and transport. OM and MNA wrote the manuscript. MNA brought some precious corrections. OM, JS, AMM, PMM, MNA, SOW and ONL analysed data. OM and MNA edited the English and made corrections. All authors read and approved the final manuscript.

Competing interests

The authors declare that they have no competing interests.

Author details

[1]Department of Research, High Institute of Techniques Medicales, Lubumbashi, Democratic Republic of Congo. [2]Department of Pediatrics, University Hospital of Lubumbashi University of Lubumbashi, Lubumbashi, Democratic Republic of Congo. [3]School of Public Health, University of Lubumbashi, Lubumbashi, Democratic Republic of Congo. [4]Division of Hemato-oncology and Nephrology, Department of Paediatrics, University Hospital of Kinshasa, School of Medicine, University of Kinshasa,, Kinshasa, Democratic Republic of Congo.

References

1. Piel FB, Hay SI, Gupta S, Weatherall DJ, Williams TN. Global burden of sickle cell anaemia in children under five, 2010-2050: modelling based on demographics, excess mortality, and interventions. PLoS Med. 2013;10(7): e1001484. https://doi.org/10.1371/journal.pmed.1001484.
2. Hasanato RM. Zinc and antioxidant vitamin deficiency in patients with severe sickle cell anemia. Ann Saudi Med. 2006;26(1):17–21.
3. Ballas SK. More definitions in sickle cell disease: steady state v base line data. Am J Hematol. 2012;87:338. https://doi.org/10.1002/ajh.22259.
4. Yahaya IA. Biochemical features of hepatic dysfunction in Nigerians with sickle cell anaemia. Niger Postgrad Med J. 2012 Dec;19(4):204–7.
5. Parmalee NL, Aschner M. Manganese and aging. Neurotoxicology. 2016 Sep; 56:262–8. https://doi.org/10.1016/j.neuro.2016.06.006.
6. Takada Y, Hachiya M, Park SH, Osawa Y, Ozawa T, Akashi M. Role of reactive oxygen species in cells overexpressing manganese superoxide dismutase: mechanism for induction of radioresistance. Mol Cancer Res. 2002 Dec;1(2):137–46.
7. Aguirre JD, Culotta VC. Battles with iron: manganese in oxidative stress protection. J Biol Chem. 2012 Apr 20;287(17):13541–8. https://doi.org/10.1074/jbc.R111.312181.
8. Arinola OG, Olaniyi JA, Akiibinu MO. Evaluation of antioxidant levels and trace element status in Nigerian sickle cell disease patients with Plasmodium parasitaemia. Pak J Nutr. 2008;7:766–9.
9. Battaglia V, Compagnone A, Bandino A, Bragadin M, Rossi CA, Zanetti F, Colombatto S, Grillo MA, Toninello A. Cobalt induces oxidative stress in isolated liver mitochondria responsible for permeability transition and intrinsic apoptosis in hepatocyte primary cultures. Int J Biochem Cell Biol. 2009 Mar;41(3):586–94. https://doi.org/10.1016/j.biocel.2008.07.012.
10. Jomova K, Valko M. Advances in metal-induced oxidative stress and human disease. Toxicology. 2011 May 10;283(2–3):65–87. https://doi.org/10.1016/j.tox.2011.03.001.
11. Alayash AI, Dafallah A, Al-Quorain A, et al. Zinc and copper status in patients with sickle cell anemia. Acta Haematol. 1987;77:87–9.
12. Sungu JK, Mukuku O, Mutombo AM, Mawaw P, Aloni MN, Luboya ON. Trace elements in children suffering from sickle cell anemia: a case-control study. J Clin Lab Anal. 2017 Feb 15; https://doi.org/10.1002/jcla.22160.
13. Osredkar J, Sustar N. Copper and zinc, biological role and significance of copper/zinc imbalance. J Clinic Toxicol. 2011;S3:001. https://doi.org/10.4172/2161-0495.S3-001.
14. Al-Naama LM, Hassan MK, Mehdi JK. Association of erythrocytes antioxidant enzymes and their cofactors with markers of oxidative stress in patients with sickle cell anemia. Qatar Med J. 2016 Jan 20;2015(2):14. https://doi.org/10.5339/qmj.2015.14.
15. Kehinde MO, Jaja SI, Adewumi OM, Adeniyi IM, Nezianya MO, Ayinla EO. Liver enzymes and trace elements in the acute phase of sickle cell anaemia. West Afr J Med. 2010 Jul-Aug;29(4):244–8.
16. Digban AK, Okogun GRA, Adu M, Jemikalajah JD. Evaluation of some micronutrients in sickle cell disease. International Journal of Innovative Research and Development. 2016;5:309–13.
17. Akenami FO, Aken'Ova YA, Osifo BO. Serum zinc, copper and magnesium in sickle cell disease at Ibadan. South western Nigeria Afr J Med Sci. 1999;28:137–9.

18. Pellegrini Braga JA, Kerbauy J, Fisberg M. Zinc, copper and iron and their interrelations in the growth of sickle cell patients. Arch Latinoam Nutr. 1995;45:198–203.
19. Bashir NA. Serum zinc and copper levels in sickle cell anaemia and beta-thalassaemia in North Jordan. Ann Trop Paediatr. 1995;15:291–3.
20. Kandala NB, Madungu TP, Emina JB, Nzita KP, Cappuccio FP. Malnutrition among children under the age of five in the Democratic Republic of Congo (DRC): does geographic location matter? BMC Public Health. 2011 Apr 25;11:261.

Factor V Leiden G1691A and prothrombin G20210A mutations among Palestinian patients with sickle cell disease

Fekri Samarah[1*] and Mahmoud A. Srour[2,3]

Abstract

Background: Vascular thrombosis is an important pathophysiological aspect of sickle cell disease (SCD). This study aimed to investigate the prevalence and clinical impact of factor V Leiden G1691A (FVL) and prothrombin G20210A mutations among Palestinian sickle cell disease (SCD) patients.

Methods: A total of 117 SCD patients, including 59 patients with sickle cell anemia (SS), 33 patients with sickle β-thalassemia and 25 individuals with sickle cell trait (AS) were studied. The control group consisted of 118 healthy individuals. FVL and prothrombin G20210A mutations were determined by RFLP PCR.

Results: Analysis of the clinical history of SCD patients revealed that seven patients have had vascular complications such as ischemic stroke or deep vein thrombosis. In SCD patients, the inheritance of the FVL mutation showed a significantly higher incidence of pain in joints, chest and abdomen as well as regular dependence on blood transfusion compared to SCD with the wild type. Age- and sex-adjusted logistic regression analysis revealed a significant association between FVL and sickle cell anemia with an odds ratio (OR) of 5.6 (95% confidence intervals [CI] of 1.91–39.4, $P = 0.039$) in SS patients. However, increased prevalence of the FVL in AS subjects and sickle β-thalassemia patients was not statistically significant compared to controls (OR 3.97, 95% CI 0.51–28.6, $P = 0.17$ and OR 3.59, 95% CI 0.35–41.6, $P = 0.26$, respectively). The distribution of prothrombin G20210A mutation among SCD patients compared to controls was not significantly different, thus our findings do not support an association of this mutation with SCD.

Conclusions: FVL was more prevalent among SS patients compared to controls and it was associated with higher incidence of disease complications among SCD patients.

Keywords: Factor V Leiden, Prothrombin G20210A, Sickle cell disease, Palestine

Background

Sickle cell disease (SCD) is an inherited disorder of β-globin gene and HbS was one of the first structural variants of hemoglobin to be discovered. HbS results from the substitution of valine for glutamic acid at the sixth codon of β-globin gene. SCD is a term used to describe not only homozygous HbSS but also includes cases of compound heterozygotes with other β-globin gene disorders such as β-thalassemia (β^0 or β^+) [1]. Although sickle hemoglobin is the product of one mutated gene, the disease phenotype is multigenetic, and gene polymorphisms dictate the different variations seen in SCD patients [2]. The contribution of inherited thrombophilia to the pathophysiology of SCD has been tackled by many reports. The mortality rate of SCD patients has been shown to increase with the presence of acute chest syndromes, as well as occlusive strokes [3]. In addition, a hypercoagulable state in SCD patients has been established that is attributed to several factors including the interaction of sickle cells with the endothelium. The adherence of sickle cells to endothelium is attributed to the increased levels of circulating interleukins as well as platelet and monocyte activation [4].

The coinheritance of genetic thrombophilia thus may exacerbate the hypercoagulable state in SCD patients. The identification of SCD patients with risk factors for developing thrombosis should be valuable in the

* Correspondence: fekri.samarah@aauj.edu
[1]Department of Medical Technology, Faculty of Allied Health Sciences, Arab American University in Jenin, Jenin, Palestine
Full list of author information is available at the end of the article

management and prevention of vasoocclusive crisis through pharmacological intervention using antithrombotic medications [5].

A well-established genetic predisposition to venous thrombosis that occurs in approximately 5% of Caucasian populations is a single-point mutation in the gene encoding coagulation factor V (G1691A) or Factor V Leiden (FVL). FVL is associated with a 7-fold increased risk of venous thrombosis in heterozygote individuals and a 50-fold to 100-fold increased risk of venous thrombosis in homozygote individuals [6]. The second most common risk factor for venous thrombosis is the prothrombin G20210A mutation which is also specific for Caucasian populations (2%) [7]. The prothrombin G20210A mutation is associated with a higher plasma prothrombin levels and a three-fold greater risk of venous thrombosis.

In this study, the prevalence of FVL G1691A and prothrombin G20210A mutation was assessed in 117 SCD individuals and 118 healthy controls from the West Bank of Palestine.

Methods

Study design and subjects

A cross-sectional study was conducted with the objective to investigate the prevalence and clinical impact of factor V Leiden G1691A (FVL) and prothrombin G20210A mutations among Palestinian (of Caucasian race) sickle cell disease (SCD) patients. Sickle cell and sickle β-thalassemia patients were all recruited from Al-Watani Hospital in Nablus. This Hospital is the referral center for these disorders in Northern Governorate of Palestine. And the majority of Sickle cell anemia cases in Palestine are registered in the Northern Governorates of Palestine. For selection of the patients, the medical files of patients registered as Sickle cell anemia or Sickle β-thalassemia (S/βthal) at Al-Watani Hospital were reviewed and patients that fulfilled the inclusion criteria were contacted and asked to participate. Information about the health status or clinical complications was collected from medical files. In addition, all patients who accepted to participate in the study were asked to to state their age, sex and confirm their diagnosis using an interview-based questionnaire. The inclusion criteria were: confirmed diagnosis of Sickle cell anemia, Sickle cell trait, or S/βthal, did not experience vascular crisis or chest syndrome at time of sampling, did not show thrombotic events or have family history of thrombosis, and were not transfused during the last 4 weeks prior to sample collection. Patients comprised 117 individuals with SCD, of whom 59 were SS (30 males and 29 females) aged 16 ± 9.9 years (mean ± SD), 25 were AS (14 males and 11 females) aged 21.2 ± 9.1 years (mean ± SD), and 33 were S/β thalassemia (18 males and 15 females) aged 15.1 ± 5.1 years (mean ± SD). The control group included 118 apparently healthy individuals (77 males and 41 females) aged 20.6 ± 5.5 years (mean ± SD). The inclusion criteria for controls were: individuals did not experience any past or current thrombotic events or had a family history of venous or arterial thrombosis (including stroke, deep venous thrombosis or pulmonary embolism), and were recruited either from blood donors, or medical staff. Blood samples were collected after a written informed consent was obtained from each patient or their guardians/parents before entry to the study.

Main outcome measures

The primary outcome measure was the frequency of FVL and Prothrombin G20210A mutations among SCD compared to controls. Secondary outcomes included type and frequency of clinical complications among SCD positive for FVL or/and Prothrombin G20210A mutations compared to those with wild type genotype.

Laboratory methods

Hematological data including complete blood counts and red cell indices were measured using a cell counter Sysmex Kx21 (Kobe, Japan) for all study patients and controls.

The sickle cell phenotype was diagnosed by conventional electrophoresis methods (cellulose acetate at alkaline and acid pH) [8]. In addition, hemoglobin electrophoresis was performed for controls to ascertain absence of β-thalassemia trait. DNA was isolated from peripheral blood leukocytes with the QIAamp Blood kit (QIAGEN, Heldin/Germany) according to manufacturer's recommendations and kept at −20 °C until analyzed. DNA analysis was used to confirm the diagnosis of sickle cell anemia, sickle cell trait and sickle β-Thalassemia. Homozygosity or heterozygosity for the β^S mutation was ascertained by polymerase chain reaction (PCR) followed by digestion with the restriction enzyme DdeI [9]. The β^S haplotype was determined by RFLP PCR as described earlier [10]. The Benin β^S haplotype was the most predominant haplotype among our patients corresponding to about 88% of all haplotypes. The β-thalassemia alleles in S/βthal patients were screened by PCR reverse dot blot (PCR-RDB) technique [11].

Detection of factor V Leiden mutation

The FVL G1691A mutation was identified as described earlier [6]. Briefly, a 267-bp fragment of exon 10 of coagulation factor V gene was amplified using the following primer pair: forward primer 5'-TGC CCA GTG CTT AAC AAG ACC A-3′; reverse primer 5′-TGT TAT CAC ACT GGT GCT AA-3′. The PCR product was digested with MnlI restriction enzyme and analyzed on a 3% agarose gel. The normal G allele was confirmed by the presence of three fragments (163, 67, and 37 bp), while the mutant A allele was confirmed by the presence of two fragments (200 and 67 bp).

Detection of prothrombin G20210A mutation

The prothrombin G20210A mutation was identified as described earlier [7]. Briefly, a 345-bp fragment spanning the 3′ sequence of exon 14 and 5′ sequence of 3′-untranslated region of the prothrombin gene was amplified using the primer pair: forward 5'-TCT AGA AAC AGT TGC CTG GC-3′ and reverse 5′-ATA GCA CTG GGA GCA TTG AAG C-3′. The PCR product was digested with HindIII restriction enzyme and analyzed on a 3% agarose gel. The presence of intact 345 bp fragment on the agarose gel indicates the presence of normal G allele, while the presence of two fragments (322 and 23 bp) indicates the presence of mutant A allele.

Statistics

Allele frequency was calculated using the gene counting method. The observed genotype frequencies for FVL and prothrombin G20210A mutations among patients and healthy individuals were compared and tested for Hardy–Weinberg equilibrium using the Chi-Square test. The significance of the difference of observed alleles and genotypes between the groups was tested using the Chi-Square analysis after grouping individuals as normal and heterozygous/homozygous carriers of the FVL and prothrombin G20210A mutations. Odds ratio (OR), both unadjusted and age- and sex-adjusted as well as their 95% confidence intervals (CI) were calculated using SPSS logistic regression to estimate the relative risk for the disease. A P-value < 0.05 was considered statistically significant. The SPSS software package version 15.0 was used for the statistical analysis.

Results

Clinical characteristics

The general and hematological characteristics of study patients are summarized in Table 1. The type of β-thalassemia mutation was determined in 26 out of 33 sickle/β-thalassemia patients. Seven different mutations were determined: IVS-I-1 (G → A), IVS-II-1 (G → A), Codon 39 (C → T), Fs8 (–AA), Codon 30 (AGG → ACG), IVS-I-110 (G → A), and Codon 37 (G → A). Around 80% of the later mutations were associated with β^0-thalassemia. Relevant clinical information was recorded in all SCD patients. Vascular occlusive cerebral disease (stroke) was diagnosed in four patients based on computerized tomography and focal neurologic defect. One patient out of four was with Sickle/β^0-thalassemia with IVS-II-1 (G → A) mutation, the remaining three patients were with sickle cell anemia (SS). In addition, three patients were diagnosed with venous thrombosis. The later three patients developed a thrombosis associated with central vein catheter; the diagnosis was based on clinical data. For chronic complications leg ulcers were present in nine patients (6 males, 3 females), all were with sickle cell anemia (SS). X-ray documented avascular bone necrosis (AVN) in seven patients (4 females, 3 males), two of them were with Sickle/β^0-thalassemia with IVS-II-1 (G → A) and Codon 39 (C → T) mutations. Priapism occurred at the post-pubertal

Table 1 Charecteristics of SS, AS, S/β^{Thal} patients and controls. Data are presented as mean ± SD for the age and hematological data and frequency for sex and clinical complications

	AS ($n = 25$)	SS ($n = 59$)	S/βThal ($n = 33$)	Controls ($n = 118$)
Sex, F/M	11/14	29/30	15/18	41/77
Age, years	21.2 ± 9.1	16 ± 9.9	15.1 ± 5.1	20.6 ± 5.5
Hematological data				
Hb (mg/dL)	12.9 ± 1.67	8.4 ± 1.09	8.32 ± 1.33	14.1 ± 1.58
MCV (fL)	81.4 ± 7.39	87.4 ± 8.0	69.16 ± 7.91	85.2 ± 4.08
MCH (pg)	26.78 ± 2.91	28.7 ± 2.88	23.34 ± 3.41	31.1 ± 2.76
HbF (%)	1.1 ± 0.63	5.14 ± 3.3	7.98 ± 3.43	0.9 ± 0.23
HbS (%)	36.3 ± 6.1	86.6 ± 7.4	69.8 ± 10.56	0
Hb A2 (%)	2.61 ± 0.41	2.1 ± 0.52	4.46 ± 0.74	2.4 ± 0.52
Clinical complications				
DVT	0	0	3	0
Stroke	0	3	1	0
Priapism	0	2	0	0
Leg ulcers	0	9	0	0
AVN	0	5	2	0

Hb hemoglobin, *MCV* mean corpuscular volume, *MCH* mean corpuscular hemoglobin, *HbF* hemoglobin F, *HbS* hemoglobin S, *HbA2* hemoglobin A2. *AS* Sickle cell trait, *SS* Sickle cell anemia, *S/βThal* Sickle β-thalassemia, *DVT* deep vein thrombosis, *AVN* avascular bone necrosis age in two males presenting with sickle cell anemia (SS) (Table 1).

Analysis of factor V Leiden G1691A mutation

The frequency of FVL mutation in the study population and its association with SCD is summarized in Table 2. The FVL mutation in its homozygous and heterozygous forms was found in 20 out of 117 patients for an overall prevalence of 17%. Analysis of the SS patients for the FVL mutation revealed that 11 of 59 (18.64%) SS patients were heterozygotes (frequency of A allele 9.32%), while none of the SS patients were homozygote for this mutation. Among the AS patients, one patient was heterozygote and one patient was homozygote for the FVL mutation with a prevalence of 8% and the frequency of A allele was 6%. Analysis of the S/βthal patients revealed that 4 patients were heterozygotes and three were homozygotes for the FVL mutation with a prevalence of 21.21% and the frequency of A allele was 30.3%. Among the control group, 18 individuals were heterozygotes and two were homozygotes for the FVL mutation (16.94%) and the frequency of A allele was 9.32%. Frequency of FVL genotypes in SS, AS and S/βthal patients and controls revealed no statistically significant difference when compared with the predicted genotypes from the Hardy–Weinberg equilibrium (*P* values 0.92, 0.90, 0.89, and 0.72, respectively). Analysis of the association of gender with FVL mutation showed that among the SS patients, four males and seven females were heterozygotes of FVL mutation. While among the controls two males were homozygotes and 18 females were heterozygotes for FVL mutation. In the AS group, one male was heterozygote and another one was homozygote for the FVL mutation. While in S/βthal patients, 2 females and 2 males were heterozygotes and 1 female and 2 males were homozygote for the FVL mutation. Taking the results of FVL mutation altogether, a significantly high prevalence of FVL was observed in Palestinian SS patients compared to controls.

Logistic regression analysis of age- and sex-adjusted data revealed a significant association between FVL mutation and sickle cell anemia (OR = 5.6; 95% CI = 1.91–39.4, $P = 0.039$) in SS patients (Table 2). However, elevated prevalence of FVL in AS subjects and S/βthal patients was not statistically significant when compared to controls (OR = 3.97, 95% CI = 0.51–28.6, $P = 0.17$ and OR = 3.59, 95% CI = 0.35–41.6, $P = 0.26$, respectively).

Heterozygous FVL mutation was reported in one patient out of seven (14%) with AVN documented by X-ray, and the remaining 6 patients with AVN were normal for this mutation. The later differences were not statistically significant.

Analysis of the prothrombin G20210A mutation

The frequency of prothrombin G20210A mutation among the study population and its association with SCD is summarized in Table 3. None of the SCD patients were homozygous for prothrombin G20210A mutation, but 8 of the 117 patients were heterozygous for the mutation for an overall prevalence of 6.83%. Heterozygous prothrombin G20210A mutation was found in 3 of 59 (5.08%) SS patients (allele A frequency 2.54%), one of 25 (4%) AS subjects (allele A frequency 2%), 4 of 33 (12.12%) S/βthal patients (allele A frequency 6.06%) and 6 of 118 (5.08%) controls (allele A frequency 2.54%). The frequency of prothrombin G20210A genotypes in SS, AS, and S/βthal patients and controls revealed no significant difference when compared to the predicted genotypes from the Hardy–Weinberg equilibrium (*P* values 0.95, 0.92, 0.91, and 0.83, respectively). In SS patients, 3 males were carriers of prothrombin G20210A mutation while in 118 controls, 2 females possessed this mutation. In AS subjects one male carried the prothrombin G20210A mutation. While in S/βthal patients the mutation was found in 2 females and 2 males.

Logistic regression analysis of age- and sex-adjusted data showed that the prevalence of the prothrombin G20210A in SS, AS individuals and S/βthal patients, was not statistically significant compared to controls (OR 6.3, 95% CI 1.17–33.9, $P = 0.12$, OR 3.71, 95% CI 0.46–26.1, $P = 0.18$ and OR 3.39, 95% CI 0.33–43.4, $P = 0.21$, respectively) (Table 3).

Heterozygous prothrombin G20210A mutation was found in one of the 4 patients (25%) with stroke, and the remaining 3 patients with stroke were normal for this mutation. But, the later differences were not statistically significant.

Table 2 Prevalence of factor V Leiden mutation and its association with SCD in Palestinian patients

Patient (*n*)	FV Leiden			Crude		Adjusted	
	G/G	G/A	A/A	OR (95% CI)	*P* value	OR (95% CI)	*P* value
SS (59)	48	11	0	9.31(2.1–61.9)	0.027	5.6 (1.91–39.4)	0.039
AS (25)	23	1	1	8.4 (1.12–64.7)	0.038	3.97 (0.51–28.6)	0.17
S/βThal (33)	26	4	3	7.2 (0.63–75.4)	0.19	3.59 (0.35–41.6)	0.26
Controls	98	18	2	1	–	1	–

Table 3 Prevalence of prothrombin G20210A mutation and its association with SCD in Palestinian patients

Patient (*n*)	Prothrombin G20210A			Crude		Adjusted	
	G/G	G/A	A/A	OR (95% CI)	*P* value	OR (95% CI)	*P* value
SS (59)	56	3	0	8.4(1.8–56.4)	0.16	6.3(1.17–33.9)	0.12
AS (25)	24	1	0	5.5(1.1–66.2)	0.13	3.71(0.46–26.1)	0.18
S/Thal (33)	29	4	0	9.4(1.9–54.4)	0.09	3.39(0.33–43.4)	0.21
Controls	112	6	0	1	–	1	–

Clinical symptoms of SCD patients and thrombophilic mutations

The clinical symptoms of SCD patients enrolled in this study are shown in Table 4. The association between clinical manifestation of SCD patients and the co-inheritance of either the FVL or mutant allele of prothrombin G20210A was explored by chi-square analysis (Table 4). SCD patients having the FVL mutation showed a significantly higher incidence of pain in joints, chest and abdomen, as well as regular dependence on blood transfusion compared to SCD patients with the wild-type genotype. However, SCD patients having the mutant allele for prothrombin G20210A mutation showed no significant association with the clinical manifestations investigated in this study, except for blood transfusion, when compared to SCD patients with the wild-type genotype.

Discussion

Thrombosis is a common complication in patients with sickle cell disease, where coagulation and fibrinolytic abnormalities lead to the development of a hypercoagulability state in such patients [12]. Acute chest syndrome and occlusive strokes have been evidenced in patients with SCD as major causes of death, which results from previous thromboembolism events [3].

FVL and prothrombin G20210A are the major inherited risk factors for venous thrombosis and their presence increases the risk of thrombosis 5–10-folds among patients with deep venous thrombosis [13].

Nowadays, there is no single clinical or laboratory test that can predict which patients are at high risk for developing thrombotic complications of SCD. Inherited predisposition factors to thrombosis could coexist with other endothelial, erythrocyte, and coagulation abnormalities and leads to an increased risk of thrombotic complications [14]. However, the role of inherited thrombophilia in the pathogenesis of SCD has been tackled by few studies but the findings were not conclusive or even controversial. For example, a low prevalence of FVL and prothrombin G20210A was reported in SCD patients from Saudi Arabia representing Saudi nationals [15], Brazilians with African descent [16] or African Americans in the United States [17]. In contrast, a high prevalence of FVL but not prothrombin G20210A was reported among Indian [18] and Iranian SCD patients [19]. In the present study, a significantly higher prevalence of FVL was observed among SS patients compared to controls while the frequency of prothrombin G20210A mutation was not significantly different among SCD patients compared to controls. Our findings were consistent with previous reports concerning FVL and prothrombin G20210A [18, 19] but in contrast to other studies [15–17]. The different findings concerning prevalence of FVL and prothrombin G20210A among SCD patients may be partially due to the different

Table 4 Clinical symptoms observed among SCD patients with the FVL G1691A and prothrombin G20210A mutations versus SCD patients without these mutations. Results are expressed as frequency and percentages

	FVL mutant (*N* = 20)	FVL wild (*N* = 97)	*P*-value	Prothrombin mutant (*N* = 8)	Prothrombin wild (*N* = 109)	*P* value
Joints pain	16 (80%)	41 (42.2%)	0.0132	4 (50%)	55 (50.4%)	NS[a]
Chest pain	18 (90%)	52 (53.6%)	0.006	4 (50%)	57 (52.2%)	NS
Abdominal pain	14 (70%)	48 (49.5%)	0.0311	4 (50%)	61 (55.9%)	NS
Splenomegaly	18 (90%)	53 (54.6%)	0.0071	3 (37.5%)	49 (44.9%)	NS
Frequency of Blood transfusion (no./year)						
0–2	2 (10%)	21 (21.6%)	NS	1 (12.5%)	29 (26.6%)	NS
3–5	3 (15%)	7 (7.2%)	0.047	2 (25%)	45 (41.3%)	NS
6–9	11 (55%)	4 (4.1%)	0.018	4 (50%)	23 (21.1%)	0.003
≥ 10	1 (5%)	0 (0%)	NS	———	———	———

[a]*NS* not significant

genetic background of the different ethnicities of study patients as well as the limited sample size in some studies.

In the present study, we also examined the role of inherited mutations FVL and prothrombin G20210A in the thrombotic complications of Palestinian SCD patients. Inherited risk factors for vascular disease, including venous as well as arterial thrombosis, have been described in the world population [20, 21]. However, the risk factor resulting from the prothrombin gene variant was distributed similarly among patients of Caucasian descent as well as patients of African descent [22].

In this study, the development of thrombosis and occlusive stroke were compared and no distinct prevalence of the risk factors was found. This is in agreement with the lack of correlation between FVL mutation and cerebral ischemia among patients with SCD [17], as well as in the general population. Also, the presence of chronic complications was not related to the presence of risk factors studied. In addition, our results indicated a higher incidence of pain and increased dependence on blood transfusion among SCD patients with FVL. While SCD patients with prothrombin G20210A mutation showed a significant association with increased dependence on blood transfusion but no significant association with pain in chest and joints and splenomegaly.

The high prevalence rate of FVL among healthy subjects from Palestine was interestingly matched with similarly high rates from neighboring Jordan [23], Israeli Arabs [24] and Lebanon [25]. This suggested that FVL mutation must have originated as a single mutational event outside of Europe, then spreading by migration of mutation-carrying individuals [26].

Prothrombin G20210A mutation was also present among healthy controls from Palestine, but at a lower frequency than FVL. Our results (2.54%) were comparable to that reported for communities of Caucasian descent, including Turkey (2.7%) [27] and Italy (3.2%) [28].

Conclusions

This study is the first report that shows the prevalence and clinical impact of FVL and prothrombin G20210A mutations among Palestinian SCD patients. FVL was more prevalent among SS patients compared to normal subjects (control group). SCD patients with FVL showed a significantly higher incidence of pain in chest, abdomen and bone joints making these SCD patients dependent on regular blood transfusion to modify the vasoocclusive crises. The high frequency of FVL and its significant correlation with sickle cell anemia from Palestine could be an important risk factor for developing occlusive crisis. Studies that include a larger number of patients and controls are necessary to define specific guidelines. It is still possible that other inherited thrombophilic mutations may contribute to thrombotic complications in SCD. Mutations and polymorphisms in the fibrinogen gene, C677T mutation in the methylenetetrahydrofolate reductase (MTHFR) gene, C1565T mutation in the platelet glycoprotein IIIa (GPIIIa) gene, and factor VII gene and others should be analyzed to determine the contribution of inherited thrombophilic mutations to thrombotic complications in patients with SCD.

Abbreviations

AS: Sickle cell trait; AVN: Avascular bone necrosis; CI: Confidence interval; FVL: Factor V Leiden; GPIIIa: Platelet glycoprotein IIIa gene; MTHFR: Methylene tetrahydrofolate reductase; OR: Odds ratio; RDB-PCR: Reverse dot blot polymerase chain reaction; RFLP PCR: Restriction fragment length polymorphism – polymerase chain reaction; SCD: Sickle cell disease; SS: Homozygote sickle cell anemia; β^S: Hemoglobin S

Acknowledgments

The authors are grateful to the staff of the Thalassemia and Hematology departments at Al-Watani hospital/Nablus and the Palestinian Ministry of Health for their help in patient's recruitment and sample collection.

Funding

None.

Authors' contributions

FS conducted experimental design, sample collection and analysis, data interpretation and manuscript writing. MAS conducted experimental design, interpretation of data and was a major contributor to manuscript writing. Both authors read and approved the final manuscript.

Authors' information

FS is an assistant professor of Hematology at the Department of Medical Technology, Faculty of Allied Health Sciences, Arab American University, Jenin, Palestine.
E-mail: fekri.samarah@aauj.edu.
MAS is an assistant professor at the Department of Medical Laboratory Sciences, Faculty of Health professions, Al-Quds University, Jerusalem, Palestine.E-mail: msrour@yahoo.com. Present address: Department of Biology & Biochemistry, Faculty of Science, Birzeit University, Birzeit, Palestine.

Competing interests

The authors declare that they have no competing interests.

Author details

[1]Department of Medical Technology, Faculty of Allied Health Sciences, Arab American University in Jenin, Jenin, Palestine. [2]Department of Medical Laboratory Sciences, Faculty of Health professions, Al-Quds University, Jerusalem, Palestine. [3]Present address: Department of Biology & Biochemistry, Faculty of Science, Birzeit University, Birzeit, Palestine.

References

1. Stuart MJ, Nagel RL. Sickle-cell disease. Lancet. 2004;346:1343–60.
2. Kutlar A, Kutlar F, Turker I, Tural C. The methylene tetrahydrofolate reductase (C667T) mutation as a potential risk factor for avascular necrosis in sickle cell disease. Hemoglobin. 2001;25:213–7.
3. Manci EA, Culberson DE, Yang YM, Gardner TM, Powell R, Haynes J Jr, et al. Investigators of the cooperative study of sickle cell disease. Causes of death in sickle cell disease: an autopsy study. Br J Haematol. 2003;123:359–65.
4. Montes RA, Eckman JR, Hsu LL, Wick TM. Sickle erythrocyte adherence to endothelium at low shear: role of shear stress in propagation of vaso-occlusion. Am J Hematol. 2002;70:216–27.
5. Andrade FL, Annichino-Bizzacchi JM, Saad STO, Costa FF, Arruda VR. Prothrombin mutant, factor V Leiden, and thermolabile variant of methylenetetrahydrofolate reductase among patients with sickle cell disease in Brazil. Am J Hematol. 1998;59:46–50.
6. Weingarz L, Schindewolf M, Schwonberg J, Hecking C, Wolf Z, Erbe M. Thrombophilia and risk of VTE recurrence according to the age at the time of first VTE manifestation. Vasa. 2015;44(4):313–23.
7. Poort SR, Rosendaal FR, Reitsma PH, Bertina RM. A common genetic variation in the `3-untranslated region of the prothrombin gene is associated with elevated plasma prothrombin levels and an increase in venous thrombosis. Blood. 1996;88(10):3698–703.
8. Wild BJ, Bain BJ. Investigation of abnormal hemoglobins and thalassemia. In: Bain BJ, Bates I, Laffan MA, Lewis SM, editors. Dacie and Lewis practical Haematology. 11th ed. London: Elsevier Churchill Livingstone; 2011. p. 301–32.
9. Kulozik AE, Lyons J, Kohne E, Bartram CR, Kleihaur E. Rapid and non radioactive prenatal diagnosis of β-thalassemia and sickle cell disease: application of the polymerase chain reaction (PCR). Br J Haematol. 1988;70(1):455–8.
10. Samarah F, Ayesh S, Athanasiou M, Christakis J, Vavatsi N. Beta(S)-Globin gene cluster haplotypes in the West Bank of Palestine. Hemoglobin. 2009;33(2):143–9.
11. Bhardwaj U, Zhang YH, Lorey F, McCabe LL, McCabe ER. Molecular genetic confirmatory testing from newborn screening samples for the common African-American, Asian Indian, southeast Asian, and Chinese beta-thalassemia mutations. Am J Hematol. 2005;78(4):249–55.
12. Kenneth IA, Eugene PO. Hypercoagulability in sickle cell disease: a curious paradox. Am J Med. 2003;115:721–8.
13. Klaassen IL, van Ommen CH, Middeldorp S. Manifestations and clinical impact of pediatric inherited thrombophilia. Blood. 2015;25(7):1073–7.
14. Pandey SK, Meena A, Kishor K, Mishra RM, Pandey S, Saxena R. Prevalence of factor V Leiden G1691A, MTHFR C677T, and prothrombin G20210A among Asian Indian sickle cell patients. Thromb Hemost. 2012;18(3):320–3.
15. Fawaz NA, Bashawery L, Al-Sheikh I, Qatari A, Al-Othman SS, Almawi WY. Factor V-Leiden, prothrombin G20210A, and MTHFR C677T mutations among patients with sickle cell disease in eastern Saudi Arabia. Am J Hematol. 2004;76:307–9.
16. Neto FM, Lourenco DM, Noguti MAE, Morelli VM, Gil ICP, Beltrao ACS, Figueiredo MS. The clinical impact of MTHFR polymorphism on the vascular complications of sickle cell disease. Braz J Med Biol Res. 2006;39:1291–5.
17. Mj K, Scher C, Rozans M, Michaels RK, Leissinger C, Krause J. Factor V Leiden is not responsible for stroke in patients with sickling disorders and is uncommon in African Americans with sickle cell disease. Am J Hematol. 1997;54:12–5.
18. Nishank SS, Singh MPSS, Yadav R. Clinical impact of factor V Leiden, prothrombin G20210A and MTHFR C677T mutations among sickle cell disease patients of central India. Eur J Haematol. 2013;91:462–6.
19. Rahimi Z, Raygani AV, Nagel RL, Muniz A. Thrombophilic mutations among southern Iranian patients with sickle cell disease: high prevalence of factor V Leiden. J Throm Thrombolys. 2008;25:288–92.
20. De Stefano V, Finazzi G, Mannucci PM. Inherited thrombophilia: pathogenesis, clinical syndromes and management. Blood. 1996;87(9):3531–344.
21. Lane DA, Mannucci PM, Bauer KA, Bertina RM, Bochkov NP, Boulyjenkov V, et al. Inherited thrombophilia: part 1. Thromb Haemost. 1996;76(5):651–62.
22. Arruda VR, Annichino-Bizzachi JM, Goncalves MS, Costa FF. Prevalence of the prothrombin gene variant (20210A) in venous thrombosis and arterial disease. Thromb Haemost. 1997;78(6):1430–3.
23. Eid SS, Rihani G. Prevalence of factor V Leiden, prothrombin G20210A, and MTHFR C677T mutations in 200 healthy Jordanians. Clin Lab Sci. 2004;17(4):200–2.
24. Rosen E, Renbaum P, Heyd J, Levy-Lahad E. High frequency of factor V Leiden in a population of Israeli Arabs. Thromb Haemost. 1999;82(6):1768.
25. Almawi WY, Keleshian SH, Borgi L, Fawaz AN, Abboud N, Mitraoui N, et al. Varied prevalence of factor V G1691A (Leiden) and Prothrombin G20210A single nucleotide polymorphisms among Arabs. J Thromb Thrombolys. 2005;20(3):163–8.
26. Zivelin A, Griffin JH, Xu X, Pabinger I, Samama M, Conard J, et al. A single genetic origin for a common Caucasian risk factor for venous thrombosis. Blood. 1997;89:397–402.
27. Batioglu F, Atmaca LS, Karabulut HG, Beyza Sayin D, Factor V. Leiden and prothrombin gene G20210A mutations in ocular Behcet disease. Acta Ophthalmol Scand. 2003;81:283–5.
28. Atherosclerosis, Thrombosis, and Vascular Biology Italian Study Group. No evidence of association between prothrombotic gene polymorphisms and the development of acute myocardial infarction at a young age. Circulation. 2003;107:1117–22.

23

The clinical presentation, utilization, and outcome of individuals with sickle cell anaemia presenting to urban emergency department of a tertiary hospital in Tanzania

Hendry R. Sawe[1,2*], Teri A. Reynolds[1,3], Juma A. Mfinanga[1,2], Michael S. Runyon[1,4], Brittany L. Murray[1,5], Lee A. Wallis[6] and Julie Makani[7,8]

Abstract

Background: Sickle cell anaemia (SCA) is prevalent in sub-Saharan Africa, with high risk of complications requiring emergency care. There is limited information about presentation of patients with SCA to hospitals for emergency care. We describe the clinical presentation, resource utilization, and outcomes of SCA patients presenting to the emergency department (ED) at Muhimbili National Hospital (MNH) in Dar es Salaam, Tanzania.

Methods: This was a prospective cohort study of consecutive patients with SCA presenting to ED between December 2014 and July 2015. Informed consent was obtained from all patients or patients' proxies prior to being enrolled in the study. A standardized case report form was used to record study information, including demographics, relevant clinical characteristics and overall patients outcomes. Categorical variables were compared with chi-square test or Fisher's exact test; continuous variables were compared with two-sample t-test or Mann-Whitney U-test.

Results: We enrolled 752 (2.7%) people with SCA from 28,322 patients who presented to the MNH-ED. The median age was 14 years (Interquartile range [IQR]: 6–23 years), and 395 (52.8%) were female. Pain 614 (81.6%), fever 289 (38. 4%) were the most frequent presenting complaint. Patients with fever, hypoxia, altered mental status and bradycardia had statistically significant relative risk of mortality of 10.4, 153, 50 and 12.1 ($p < 0.0001$) respectively, compared to patients with normal vitals. Overall, 656 (87.2%) patients received Complete Blood Cell counts test, of these 342 (52.1%) had severe anaemia (haemoglobin < 7 g/dl), and a 30.3 ($p = 0.02$) relative risk of relative risk of mortality compare to patients with higher haemoglobin. Patients who had malaria, elevated renal function test and hypoglycemia, had relative risk of mortality of 22.9, 10.4 and 45.2 ($p < 0.0001$) respectively, compared to patient with normal values. Most 534 (71.0%) patients were hospitalized for in patients care, and the overall morality rate was 16 (2.1%).

Conclusions: We described the clinical presentation, management, and outcomes of patients with SCA presenting to the largest public ED in Tanzania, as well as information on resource utilization. This information can inform development of treatment guidelines, clinical staff education, and clinical research aimed at optimizing care for SCA patients.

Keywords: Sickle cell anaemia, Emergency department, Anaemia, Sub-Saharan Africa

* Correspondence: hendry_sawe@yahoo.com
[1]Emergency Medicine Department, Muhimbili University of Health and Allied Sciences, P.O. Box 54235, Dar es salaam, Tanzania
[2]Emergency Medicine Department, Muhimbili National Hospital, Dar es salaam, Tanzania
Full list of author information is available at the end of the article

Background

Sickle cell disease (SCD) is one of the most common genetic diseases in the world, with the highest prevalence in sub-Saharan Africa, the Caribbean, the Middle East and India [1]. The morbidity and mortality from Sickle Cell Anaemia (SCA) in developed countries has improved significantly over the last five decades, with studies showing median survival rates beyond the fifth decade of life [2]. In developing countries, however, SCA still causes significant morbidity and mortality with the greatest burden of the disease in sub-Saharan Africa. The World Health Organization (WHO) estimates over half of children born with SCA in sub-Saharan Africa will die before they reach adulthood [3]. Infectious diseases, such as malaria and pneumococcal disease (meningitis, pneumonia, and septicaemia) are thought to be the major cause of morbidity and mortality [4, 5].

Tanzania ranks fifth in the world for number of SCD births with an estimated prevalence of 6 [interquartile range (IQR) 1–13] per 1000 births, equivalent to 11,000 SCD births per year [4, 6]. A study conducted at a university teaching hospital in Tanzania reported a SCA mortality rate of 1.9 per 100 person years of observation (PYO), with the highest incidence of death occurring in the first five years of life [7]. Overall median survival in this study was 33 years. Of note, life expectancy of Tanzanian residents is 52 years. Similar to other developing countries, morbidity and mortality due to SCA in Tanzania is highly influenced by comorbid conditions, such as infections (particularly malaria), anaemia, and poor nutrition [4].

Emergency department (ED) presentations of SCA complications are well characterized in developed countries, with the majority of these patients presenting with pain crisis [8–12]. Most of these patients are treated with aggressive pain management and fluid therapy and discharged home, with less than one-third admitted to the hospital. In 2010, Muhimbili National Hospital (MNH), which is the main University Teaching Hospital, opened the first full capacity, high-volume ED in Tanzania. This ED has provided an opportunity for early stabilization and resuscitation of acutely ill patients, including those with SCA. The study on mortality in SCA in Africa published in 2011 was conducted at the same hospital, at that time had no full capacity ED [7]. This is critical as little is known about the acute or emergent manifestations, management, and outcomes of SCA complications in Tanzania. The primary aim of this investigation is to describe the clinical presentation, ED management, and hospital outcomes of individuals known or suspected to have sickle cell disease and presenting to the MNH ED.

Methods

Study design and setting

This was a prospective observational study of consecutive patients presenting to the MNH ED in Dar es Salaam, Tanzania, from 1 December 2014 to 31 July 2015. MNH has a bed capacity of 1500 and serves as the top referral hospital in Tanzania. The ED was established in 2010 via a partnership between the Ministry of Health and Social Welfare, and Abbott Fund Tanzania. The ED is the first full capacity public ED in Tanzania, and the training site for the only emergency medicine (EM) residency program in the country. The department is staffed 24 h, seven days a week by locally trained specialist emergency physicians, who oversee the care of patients and training of interns, registrars, and EM residents. The ED sees an average of 45,000 patients annually, with an admission rate of around 65%. The top disease categories in all age groups are trauma, infectious disease, and mental health [13]. MNH is one of the largest SCD treatment and research centre in Tanzania. The diagnosis of SCA at MNH is normally confirmed by the haemoglobin electrophoresis, after initial sickling test or clinical suspicion at most of the referring hospitals. Patients confirmed to have SCA are enrolled into a Sickle Cell clinic, provided with dedicated medical record number and special follow up card. In this study, all patients with confirmed evidence of SCA presenting with acute illness at the ED were eligible for enrolment.

Study protocol

Screening and enrolment was completed by a research assistant and the study investigator (HS). A structured data sheet was used to record study information, including demographics, pre-referral information, chief complaints, initial vital signs, history and physical examination findings, laboratory results, treatment delivered, and final ED diagnoses and disposition. All diagnostic, treatment, and disposition decisions were made at the discretion of the treating physician. The research assistant followed up on all enrolled patients throughout the duration of their hospital study and recorded lengths of stay in hospital and intensive care unit (ICU) or high acuity ward, as well as final hospital diagnosis and clinical outcome (discharge or death) for each patient.

Data analysis

Information collected from the handwritten data sheets were transferred into an Excel spreadsheet (Microsoft Corporation, Redmond, WA, USA), verified, and checked for any errors and outliers. Data were subsequently imported into StatsDirect (version 3.0.167, StatsDirect Ltd., Cheshire, UK) for analysis. Categorical variables were summarized as frequencies and percentages, and continuous variables as means and standard deviations (SD) or medians and interquartile ranges (IQR), depending on data distribution. Normality was assessed using the Shapiro-Wilk test. Ninety-five percent confidence intervals (CI) are presented where appropriate, and were calculated by the Clopper-Pearson (exact) method. Categorical variables were compared with chi-square test or Fisher's exact test; continuous variables were compared with two-sample t-test or Mann-Whitney U-test. Two-tailed *p*-values of < 0.05 were considered statistically significant.

Results

We enrolled 752 (2.7%) people with SCA from 28,322 patients who presented to the MNH ED from 1 December 2014 to 31 July 2015. The median age of enrolled patients was 14 years (Interquartile range (IQR) of 6–23 years), with 19.7% younger than age 5, and 52.9% were female. A total of 299 (40.2%) patients were referred from peripheral hospitals, the median length of admission at these peripheral facilities prior to referral was 2 days (IQR 1.3 days) Table 1.

Patients' baseline variables and presenting complaints

Tachypnea 336 (44.7%) was the most frequent abnormal vital sign among enrolled patients, while bradycardia 14 (1.9%) was the least frequent abnormal sign. All the abnormality are based on age-appropriate vital signs [14]. Patients who presented fever 289 (17.4%), hypoxia 67 (8.9%), altered mental status 59 (7.8%) and bradycardia 14 (1.9%) had a statistically significant higher relative risk of death compared with those without bradycardia. Pain 614 (81.6%) and urinary symptoms 6 (0.8%) were most and least frequent presenting complaints respectively Table 2.

Investigations ordered in the ED

Nearly all patients 744 (99%) had at least one laboratory test done while receiving ED care. Complete blood cell counts were ordered for 656 (87.2%) patients. Of these 346 (52.7%) had elevated white blood counts (> 11 K/uL)

Table 1 Patient demographics

Demographics	Number	Percentage (%)
Sex	$N = 747$	
Female	395	52.9
Male	352	47.1
Age Group	$N = 741$	
1 month–< 5 years	146	19.7
5 years–< 18 years	304	41.0
≥ 18 years	291	39.3
Referral Status	$N = 744$	
Self referral	445	59.8
Referred	299	40.2

and 342 (52.1%) had severe anaemia (Hb < 7 g/dL) of which 166 (25.3%) had (Hb < 5 g/dL). Of the 415 patients tested for malaria, 48 (11.6%) were positive. The relative risk of death among those with severe anaemia, malaria test positive, elevated renal function test and hypoglycaemia was 30.3, 22.9,10.4 and 45.2 respectively. X-ray of the chest was ordered in 85 (11.3%) of patients, and the relative risk of death among those with an abnormal chest x-ray was 4.0 (Table 3).

Final ED diagnosis

The top three ED diagnoses were painful crisis ($n = 472$; 62.8%), malaria ($n = 176$; 23.4%), and severe anaemia ($n = 117$; 15.6%) (Table 4).

ED treatment and interventions

In the ED, intravenous fluid bolus and intravenous dextrose were given to 370 (49.2%) and 129 (17.2%) of enrolled patients, respectively. A total of 489 patients (65.0%) received analgesics for pain, with 350 (71.6%) receiving opioid analgesics. Antimalarial were administered in the ED to 123 (16.4%) patients, while 220 (29.3%) received antibiotics, the majority of whom (89.2%) received intravenous ceftriaxone. Seventy-two patients (9.6%) received blood products (fresh whole blood, packed red cells, or fresh frozen plasma), with the majority (91.2%) receiving fresh whole blood.

Patients' disposition and hospital outcomes

Of the 752 SCA patients seen in the ED, 534 (71%) were hospitalized for inpatient care, while five patients (0.7%) died in the ED. The median length of stay in hospital was 3 days (Interquartile range (IQR): 1–5) days. The overall morality (ED plus inpatient) was 16 (2.1%). Overall, 8 (50%) of deaths' occurred within 24 h of ED presentation (Table 5).

Discussion

The opening of a full capacity ED at MNH provided a unique opportunity for rapid assessment and early stabilization of acutely ill individuals, including those with SCA. Our study reports on the clinical profile and management of acutely ill individuals with SCA presenting to an urban ED in Tanzania. This information on ED access and resource utilization can be useful in developing local and countrywide strategies to improve access, treatment guidelines, and health outcomes among individuals with SCA.

In our study, the prevalence of SCA among acutely ill patients presenting ED was found to be 2.7%, and most of the patients were self-referral, highlighting the role of ED as a major mode of healthcare utilization in this patient population in Tanzania. Most of our patients were children below eighteen years, an observation

Table 2 Patients' baseline variables and presenting complaints

Clinical characteristics	Overall $N = 752$ n (%)	Died $N = 16$ n (%)	Survived $N = 736$ n (%)	Relative risk RR (95%CI)	*P*-value
Tachypnea [b]	336 (44.7)	10 (62.5)	326 (44.3)	2.1 (0.8–5.7)	0.16
Tachycardia[b]	186 (24.7)	5 (31.3)	181 (24.6)	1.4 (0.5–3.9)	0.5
Febrile ($T > 37.5$ °C)[c]	131 (17.4)	11 (68.8)	120 (16.3)	10.4 (3.7–29.5)	< 0.0001
SpO_2[a] < 95%	67 (8.9)	15 (93.8)	52 (7.1)	153 (20–1143)	< 0.0001
Altered mental status	59 (7.8)	13 (81.3)	46 (6.3)	50 (15–174)	< 0.0001
Bradycardia[b]	14 (1.9)	3 (18.8)	11 (1.5)	12.1 (3.9–38.0)	< 0.0001
Pain	614 (81.6)	12 (75.0)	602 (81.8)	0.7 (0.2–2.1)	0.5
Fever	289 (38.4)	10 (62.5)	279 (37.9)	2.7 (1.0–7.3)	0.06
Abdominal Symptoms	159 (21.1)	2 (12.5)	157 (21.3)	0.5 (0.1–2.3)	0.4
Respiratory Symptoms	156 (20.7)	11 (68.8)	145 (19.7)	8.4 (3.0–23.8)	0.0001
Cardiovascular Symptoms	83 (11.0)	2 (12.5)	81 (11.0)	1.2 (0.3–5.0)	0.9
Jaundice	80 (10.6)	1 (6.3)	79 (10.7)	0.6 (0.1–4.2)	0.6
Body Swelling	54 (7.2)	2 (12.5)	52 (7.1)	1.9 (0.4–7.9)	0.4
Neurological Symptoms	45 (6.0)	6 (37.5)	39 (5.3)	9.4 (3.6–24.8)	< 0.0001
Long Lasting Erection	20 (2.7)	1 (6.3)	19 (2.6)	2.4 (0.3–17.6)	0.4
Urinary Symptoms	6 (0.8)	1 (6.3)	5 (0.7)	8.3 (1.3–53.1)	0.03

[a]*SpO_2* Saturation of oxygen in peripheral capillary [b]Age-adjusted variables [c] Measurements were all axillary

consistent with previously published literature in the same settings [7].

Pain was the most common presenting complaints among patients presenting to ED. Vaso-occlusive painful crisis phenomena is a well documented reason for ED visit among sickle cell patients in different settings [7, 8], and it has been shown to be a potential marker of serious illness, which may be associated with increased morbidity and mortality [7, 15]. Respiratory compromise, denoted by tachypnea and hypoxia (oxygen saturation < 95%), was the most common physical examination finding at presentation. In this population, the most common reason for respiratory compromise was chest infection (pneumonia), followed by acute chest syndrome. Infection is the leading cause of preventable morbidity and mortality in patients with SCA, and

Table 3 Investigations ordered in the ED

	Overall n/N (%)	Died n/N (%)	Survived n/N (%)	Relative risk RR (95%CI)	*P*-value
Laboratory Tests					
WBC [Ω] (> 11 K/uL)	346/656 (52.7)	11/16 (68.8)	335/640 (52.3)	2.0 (0.7–5.6)	0.2
Haemoglobin (< 7 g/dL)	342/656 (52.1)	16/16 (100)	326/640 (50.9)	30.3 (1.8–503)	0.02
Abnormal urine results [δ]	11/63 (17.5)	1/16 (6.3)	10/47 (21.3)	0.3 (0.04–2.11)	0.2
Malaria test positive	48/415 (11.6)	12/16 (75)	36/399 (9.0)	22.9 (7.7–68)	< 0.0001
Elevated RFT[β]	24/219 (11.0)	9/16 (56.3)	15/203 (7.4)	10.4 (4.2–25.5)	< 0.0001
Low RBG[ɳ] (< 3 mmol/L)	39/627 (6.2)	12/16 (75)	27/611 (4.4)	45.2 (15.3–133.8)	< 0.0001
Imaging Tests					
Abnormal chest x-ray [α]	30/85 (35.3)	11/16 (68.8)	19/69 (27.5)	4.0 (1.5–10.5)	0.004
Abnormal brain CT scan [ρ]	7/26 (26.9)	5/16 (31.3)	2/10 (20)	1.2 (0.67–2.2)	0.5

[Ω] WBC-White Blood Cell

[δ] Presence of blood in urine, leukocytes, nitrites, albumin, or glucose

[α] Signs of infection or stroke

[β] RFT-Renal function test

[ɳ] RBG-Random Blood Glucose

[α] Pneumonic changes

[ρ] Signs of stroke

Table 4 Final ED diagnosis

Final ED Diagnosis	$N = 752$	% (95% CI)
Painful crisis	472	62.8 (59.3–66.2)
Malaria	176	23.4 (20.5–26.6)
Severe anaemia	117	15.6 (13.2–18.3)
Pneumonia	105	14.0 (11.7–16.6)
Acute chest syndrome	49	6.5 (5.0–8.5)
Hypoglycaemia	42	5.6 (4.2–7.5)
Urinary tract infection	41	5.5 (4.0–7.3)
Acute kidney injury	27	3.6 (2.5–5.2)
Priapism	18	2.4 (1.5–3.8)
Cerebral vascular accident	16	2.1 (1.3–3.4)

previous studies reported mortality as high as 38% in the USA, in absence of aggressive treatment [16, 17]. Standardized treatment and prevention (i.e. prophylactic penicillin and vaccination against pneumococcal infections) have significantly improved the outcome and quality of life [18]; however, these interventions are not routinely available to our patient population as they are not part of standard care [19]. When present, bradycardia, altered mental status, and hypoxia were each associated with a relative risk of death of greater than 10 in our study population compared to when these features were absent.

In addition to physical examinations, most of these patients received laboratory and imaging tests. More than three-quarters of patients had a complete blood cell count as part of their ED care, more than half of who had severe anaemia. All patients who died had severe anaemia at presentation. Severe anaemia was associated with a significantly higher relative risk of death when compared with higher haemoglobin levels. These findings are similar to previous literature in similar settings, which have shown low haemoglobin to be an independent predictor of mortality in patients with SCA [16, 20]. Severe anaemia is reported to negatively impact outcome and quality of life in SCA patients [20]. In our patient cohort, only 21% of patients with severe anaemia received blood transfusion in the ED. The current local guideline for management of severe anaemia in patients with SCA recommends blood transfusion to all SCA patients with haemoglobin (Hb) less than 5 g/dL, regardless of presenting complaint, and to those with Hb < 7 g/dL if symptomatic [21]. In this study population, 25.3% of patients had haemoglobin less than 5 g/dL, but overall more than half of patients who should receive blood products as part of their ED care did not receive it. Several factors may impact availability, access, and transfusion practices in our ED, including lack of enough eligible donors, lack of testing and storage equipment, lack of recognition and late presentation [22, 23]. We are unable to determine the exact reasons for the low rate of transfusion in our study. Thus, we recommend further study to address what appears to be a significant opportunity for improvement in emergency care of acute SCA cases. The findings of hypoglycaemia, positive malaria test, abnormal renal function tests and abnormal chest x-ray findings were all associated with a significantly higher relative risk of death compared to patients with normal results. All of these abnormal findings are easily manageable at MNH, and at most of the basic facilities within Tanzania, hence further studies should focus on addressing the challenges associated with care and factors associated with mortality within these conditions so as to ensure death from these conditions are prevented.

Painful crisis, malaria and severe anaemia were the top three ED providers' diagnosis. Malaria was diagnosed in 176 patients by ED providers, while only 48 of patients tested positive, this might indicate an over diagnosis by ED providers, however we were unable to detect whether the providers used syndrome approach to treatment of malaria which calls for use of antimalarial for suspicious cases regardless of the malaria test results [24].

Over two-thirds of patients were admitted for inpatient care after initial stabilization in the ED. This is a much higher admission rate than reported in many developed countries [8, 10, 12], but similar to the overall ED disposition patterns in our setting [13]. The overall mortality in our study population was 2.1%, with 50% of the deaths occurring within the first 24 h of presentation to the ED. Our results show that severe anaemia, infection (malaria and bacterial infection), and hypoxia are associated with increase in mortality in our study population. These contributors should receive focused attention in the design of ED care protocols for SCA and further studies.

Table 5 Patients' disposition and hospital outcomes

Disposition	$N = 752$	% (95% CI)
Admitted	534	71.0 (67.6–74.2)
Discharged from ED	213	28.3 (25.1–31.7)
Died in ED	5	0.7 (0.3–1.5)
Death within 24-h of ED presentation ϖ	8	1.1 (0.5–2.1)
Inpatient mortality φ	11	2.1 (1.2–3.7)
Overall mortality	16	2.1 (1.3–3.4)
	Median	IQR
Median length of hospital stay	3 days	1–5 days

ϖ Includes ED and inpatient deaths
φ Includes only in patients' deaths (denominator: $N = 534$) those who were admitted

Limitations

The generalizability of our results may be limited due to the single-centre nature of our study. The ED at MNH is the entry point to the largest tertiary referral hospital in Tanzania, and receives acutely ill patients from all over the country. Therefore, the sample seen at the MNH ED might be different than that seen at the district hospitals and health centres. The exclusion of undiagnosed SCD in our study might have under-estimated the overall proportion of SCD in our study population. In addition, the assessment of factors associated with mortality was limited by the number of deaths in our study population.

Conclusions

We have provided a description of the clinical presentation, management, and outcomes of patients with SCA presenting to the largest public emergency department in a tertiary referral hospital in Tanzania. These data will inform development of strategies to provide education for clinical staff, treatment guidelines, and clinical research aimed at optimizing care of the SCA patient population.

Abbreviations

CBC: Complete Blood Count; CRF: Case Report Form; ED: Emergency Department; MNH: Muhimbili National Hospital; MUHAS: Muhimbili University of Health and Allied Sciences; WHO: World Health Organization

Acknowledgements

The authors thank the patients and staff of Muhimbili National Hospital, Muhimbili University of Health and Allied Sciences, and the Emergency Medicine Department.

Funding

This project was supported by a National Institutes of Health (NIH) Research Training Grant #R25 TW009343 funded by the Fogarty International Center and the National Heart, Lung, and Blood Institute, as well as the University of California Global Health Institute (UCGHI). The content is solely the responsibility of the authors and does not necessarily represent the official views of the NIH or UCGHI. NIH or UCGH did not have any role in designing, collection, analysis, interpretation or writing of this manuscript.

Authors' contributions

HS contributed to the conception and design of the study; acquired, analysed, and interpreted the data; and drafted and revised the manuscript. JAM contributed to the design of the study, data acquisition and entry, and also revised the manuscript. BLM each contributed to the conception of the study; assisted in initial design of the study; and revised the manuscript. JM, LW, and TR contributed to the conception and assisted in the initial design of the study, data interpretation, and critically revised the manuscript. MSR contributed to the conception and assisted in the initial design of the study; analysed and interpreted the data; and revised the manuscript. All authors read and approved the final manuscript.

Competing interests

The authors declare no conflicts of interest.

Author details

[1]Emergency Medicine Department, Muhimbili University of Health and Allied Sciences, P.O. Box 54235, Dar es salaam, Tanzania. [2]Emergency Medicine Department, Muhimbili National Hospital, Dar es salaam, Tanzania. [3]Department of Emergency Medicine, University of California San Francisco, San Francisco, CA, USA. [4]Department of Emergency Medicine, Carolinas Medical Center, Charlotte, NC, USA. [5]Division of Pediatric Emergency Medicine, Emory University School of Medicine/Children's Hospital of Atlanta, Atlanta, GA, USA. [6]Division of Emergency Medicine, University of Cape Town, Cape Town City, South Africa. [7]Nuffield Department of Medicine, University of Oxford, Oxford, UK. [8]Department of Haematology and blood transfusion, Muhimbili University of Health and Allied Sciences, Dar es Salaam, Tanzania.

References

1. CDC - Sickle Cell Disease, Data and Statistics - NCBDDD [Internet]. [cited 2013 Mar 13]. Available from: http://www.cdc.gov/ncbddd/sicklecell/data.html.
2. Platt OS, Brambilla DJ, Rosse WF, Milner PF, Castro O, Steinberg MH, et al. Mortality in sickle cell disease – life expectancy and risk factors for early death. N Engl J Med. 1994;330(23):1639–44.
3. Weatherall DJ. The inherited diseases of hemoglobin are an emerging global health burden. Blood. 2010;115(22):4331–6.
4. Fleming AF. The presentation, management and prevention of crisis in sickle cell disease in Africa. Blood Rev. 1989;3(1):18–28.
5. Oniyangi O, Omari AA. Malaria chemoprophylaxis in sickle cell disease. In: Cochrane Database of Systematic Reviews [Internet]. John Wiley & Sons, Ltd; 1996 [cited 2013 Mar 15]. Available from: https://www.ncbi.nlm.nih.gov/pubmed/17054173.
6. Piel FB, Patil AP, Howes RE, Nyangiri OA, Gething PW, Dewi M, et al. Global epidemiology of sickle haemoglobin in neonates: a contemporary geostatistical model-based map and population estimates. Lancet. 2013; 381(9861):142–51.
7. Makani J, Cox SE, Soka D, Komba AN, Oruo J, Mwamtemi H, et al. Mortality in sickle cell anemia in Africa: a prospective cohort study in Tanzania. PLoS One. 2011;6(2):e14699.
8. Tanabe P, Myers R, Zosel A, Brice J, Ansari AH, Evans J, et al. Emergency department management of acute pain episodes in sickle cell disease. Acad Emerg Med. 2007;14(5):419–25.
9. Tanabe P, Hafner JW, Martinovich Z, Artz N. Adult emergency department patients with sickle cell pain crisis: results from a quality improvement learning collaborative model to improve analgesic management. Acad Emerg Med. 2012;19(4):430–8.
10. Yusuf HR, Atrash HK, Grosse SD, Parker CS, Grant AM. Emergency department visits made by patients with sickle cell disease: a descriptive study, 1999-2007. Am J Prev Med. 2010;38(4 Suppl):S536–41.
11. Gray A, Anionwu EN, Davies SC, Brozovic M. Patterns of mortality in sickle cell disease in the United Kingdom. J Clin Pathol. 1991;44(6):459–63.
12. Reddin CDRC, Cerrentano E, Tanabe P. Sickle cell disease management in the emergency department: what every emergency nurse should know. J Emerg Nurs. 2011;37(4):341–5 quiz 426.
13. Reynolds T, Sawe HR, Lobue N, Mwafongo V. Most frequent adult and pediatric diagnoses among 60,000 patients seen in a new urban emergency Department in Dar Es Salaam, Tanzania. Ann Emerg Med. 2012;60(4):S39.
14. Fleming S, Thompson M, Stevens R, Heneghan C, Plüddemann A, Maconochie I, et al. Normal ranges of heart rate and respiratory rate in children from birth to 18 years: a systematic review of observational studies. Lancet. 2011;377(9770):1011–8.

15. Heimlich JB, Chipoka G, Kamthunzi P, Krysiak R, Majawa Y, Mafunga P, et al. Establishing sickle cell diagnostics and characterizing a paediatric sickle cell disease cohort in Malawi. Br J Haematol. 2016;174(2):325–9.
16. Autino B, Noris A, Russo R, Castelli F. Epidemiology of Malaria in Endemic Areas. Mediterr J Hematol Infect Dis [Internet]. 2012 [cited 2016 Aug 20]; 4(1). Available from: http://www.ncbi.nlm.nih.gov/pmc/articles/PMC3499992/.
17. Booth C, Inusa B, Obaro SK. Infection in sickle cell disease: a review. Int J Infect Dis. 2010;14(1):e2–12.
18. Luzzatto L. Sickle Cell Anaemia and Malaria. Mediterr J Hematol Infect Dis [Internet]. 2012 [cited 2016 Aug 20];4(1). Available from: http://www.ncbi.nlm.nih.gov/pmc/articles/PMC3499995/.
19. Leikin SL, Gallagher D, Kinney TR, Sloane D, Klug P, Rida W. Mortality in children and adolescents with sickle cell disease. Cooperative study of sickle cell disease. Pediatrics. 1989 Sep;84(3):500–8.
20. Cox SE, Makani J, Fulford AJ, Komba AN, Soka D, Williams TN, et al. Nutritional status, hospitalization and mortality among patients with sickle cell anemia in Tanzania. Haematologica. 2011;96(7):948–53.
21. Haematology and Blood Transfusion M. Management of Sickle Cell Disease [Internet]. Department of Internal Medicine, Muhimbili National Hospital, Dar es salaam-Tanzania; 2014. Available from: https://www.h3abionet.org/muhas.
22. Vos J, Gumodoka B, van Asten HA, Berege ZA, Dolmans WM, Borgdorff MW. Changes in blood transfusion practices after the introduction of consensus guidelines in Mwanza region, Tanzania. AIDS. 1994;8(8):1135–1140.
23. Gumodoka B, Vos J, Kigadye FC, van Asten H, Dolmans WM, Borgdorff MW. Blood transfusion practices in Mwanza region, Tanzania. Bugando Medical Centre. AIDS. 1993;7(3):387–92.
24. Information NC for B, Pike USNL of M 8600 R, MD B, Usa 20894. TREATMENT OF SEVERE MALARIA [Internet]. World Health Organization; 2015 [cited 2017 Sep 24]. Available from: https://www.ncbi.nlm.nih.gov/books/NBK294445/.

Evaluation and characterization of tumor lysis syndrome before and after chemotherapy among pediatric oncology patients in Tikur Anbessa specialized hospital, Addis Ababa, Ethiopia

Haileleul Micho[1,2], Yasin Mohammed[3], Daniel Hailu[3] and Solomon Genet[2*]

Abstract

Background: Tumor lysis syndrome (TLS) is a life-threatening emergency disorder, caused by an abrupt release of intracellular metabolites after tumor cell death. It is characterized by a series of metabolic manifestations, especially hyperuricemia, hyperkalemia, hyperphosphatemia and hypocalcemia. The aim of this study was to evaluate and characterize the incidence of tumor lysis syndrome among pediatric oncology patients before and after treatment.

Methods: Hospital based prospective cohort study was conducted for 6 months on 61 newly diagnosed pediatric oncology patients. Socio-demographic data was collected by interview administered questionnaire. Patients were followed and the physical diagnosis, imaging and laboratory results were interpreted by senior physicians. Data was entered to and analyzed by SPSS version 23.

Results: Among 61 pediatric oncology patients 39(63.9%) were males. The mean (±SD) age of the pediatric patients was 6.39 (± 3.67) years ranging from 2 months to 14 years. 29.5% of patients were found to have TLS. There were 11.5% and 18.0% of laboratory TLS (LTLS) and clinical TLS (CTLS) cases respectively. There were72.2% spontaneous and 27.8% treatment induced TLS cases with 23% and 21.3% cases of hyperuricemia and 4.9% and 6.6% cases of hyperkalemia incidence before and after treatment respectively. Only two patients died, in the study period, due to TLS.

Conclusion: There was high incidence of TLS irrespective of socio-demographic variation among study participants, suggesting that children with cancer are at risk of developing TLS. As TLS is a life-threatening complication of malignancies, early identification of patients at risk and reducing morbidity and mortality is crucially important.

Keywords: Tumor lysis syndrome, Pediatric oncology, Cell death, Biomarkers

Background

Tumor lysis syndrome (TLS) is one of the most common cancer therapy related complication, first described by Bedrna and Polcák in 1929 [1]. It is a life-threatening condition with high morbidity and mortality, caused by an abrupt release of intracellular metabolites after tumor cell lysis [2]. It usually occurs a few hours to a few days after commencing cytotoxic chemotherapy for tumors with a high percentage of proliferating and drug-sensitive cells. Cell death leads to the release of potassium, phosphate, uric acid, proteins and other purine metabolites into the systemic circulation. These factors will overtax the body's homeostatic mechanisms and overwhelm the capacity of the renal system for normal excretion of these materials. When the renal clearance of these chemical substances is overwhelmed, hyperkalemia, hyperuricemia, hyperphosphatemia and secondary hypocalcemia will result. Serum lactate dehydrogenase (LDH) levels are also often elevated

* Correspondence: solgen73@yahoo.com
[2]Department of Medical Biochemistry, School of Medicine, College of Health sciences, Addis Ababa University, P. O. Box 9086, Addis Ababa, Ethiopia
Full list of author information is available at the end of the article

concurrently [3]. Uncontrolled TLS progresses to lactic acidosis and acute renal failure (ARF). Clinically, this results in multi organ defects such as acute kidney injury (AKI), cardiac arrhythmias, and seizures or sudden death that requires intensive care. TLS is the most common oncologic emergency, and without prompt recognition and early therapeutic intervention, morbidity and mortality is high [4]. Hande and Garrow first initiated a definition of the clinical and pathologic characteristics of patients at risk for developing TLS. They classified TLS as laboratory TLS (LTLS) or clinical TLS (CTLS) [5]. Cairo and Bishop modified these criteria to formulate a commonly used classification system for TLS. This system defines LTLS when two or more of the following abnormalities are met within 3 days before or 7 days after the initiation of che motherapy in the face of adequate hydration and use of uric acid lowering agent: 25% decrease from baseline in serum calcium, and/or 25% increase from baseline in the serum values of uric acid, potassium, or phosphate.

CTLS is defined as LTLS accompanied by one or more clinical manifestations such as cardiac arrhythmia, AKI, seizure, or death with an elevated serum creatinine > 1.5ULN (upper limit of normal) [6]. TLS is the mainstay for the complication and unfavorable outcome of cancer treatments. Specifically cancers with high proliferation and high sensitivity to chemotherapy are highly susceptible to TLS and its complications. In the era of novel agents, there is greater concern that the incidence of TLS in pediatric oncology may occur more frequently. The problem is disturbing and causing a major concern in low income countries like Ethiopia. Unfortunately, due to socio-economic and other factors patients come to health facilities at an advanced stage. To the best of our knowledge, the incidence of TLS has not been specifically addressed in Ethiopia. Therefore, determining the frequency, clinical course and outcome of TLS in pediatric oncology patients in our setup will significantly be important to help shape clinical as well as public health care of the patients and the population. Findings from this work can help TLS diagnosis and improve treatment strategies of malignancies. In addition, the results obtained from this study are expected to pave the way for further broad and extensive related studies. In this study we have tried to give baseline information about TLS incidence and treatment outcome, with special emphasis on measurement of laboratory parameters that predict the onset and progress of TLS in different pediatric oncology, like acute myeloid leukemia (AML), chronic myeloid leukemia (CML), acute lymphoid leukemia (ALL), non-Hodgkin lymphoma (NHL), Burkitt's lymphoma (BL) and some solid tumors.

Methods

A prospective cohort study was conducted from October, 2016 - July, 2017 at the pediatric hematology/oncology unit of Tikur Anbesa Specialized Hospital (TASH), which is the largest referral teaching hospital of the country, located in Addis Ababa, Ethiopia. The hospital has about 800 beds and gives diagnostic and treatment services for about 370,000–400,000 patients per year. The pediatric hematology/oncology unit of TASH is under the department of pediatrics and child health and gives out patient and in patient services. Around 500–600 pediatric oncology patients visit TASH annually. The unit has hemato-oncologists, hemato-patho logysts, residents, and nurses.

Study population and data collection

The study population for this study was all newly admitted pediatric patients with hematologic and solid malignancy during the study period in TASH. The data was collected by using structured questionnaires which has been translated into the local language "Amharic".

Blood sample collection, processing and laboratory analysis

Venous blood sample was collected using two tubes. About 2 ml of blood in EDTA tube was used for total WBC analysis using Sysmex 2000*i* hematology analyzer (Sysmex, Japan). Blood (5 ml) was drawn into serum separator tube (SST) for clinical chemistry tests (uric acid, creatinine, BUN and LDH) using Mindray clinical chemistry analyzer (Shenzhen Mindray Biomedical Electronics, China) and for electrolyte analysis (potassium, sodium, chloride and calcium). This was done before and after chemotherapy; and duration differs based on stage of malignancy. Prophylactic management was done for all admitted patients.

Management of TLS

A prophylactic management with intensive hydration, 3000 ml/m^2/24 h, and a uric acid lowering agent (allopurinol) along with their respective treatments were administered to the patients. Hydration was used to increase urine output via increased kidney clearance.

Statistical analysis

Data was checked, cleaned, coded and entered to SPSS version 23 for analysis. Simple descriptive statistics was used to present the socio-demographic and clinical characteristics of the study subjects. Data distribution was checked by using Kolmogrov-Smirnov and Shapiro Wilk test. Paired sample t test was used for parametric data and wilcoxon signed rank test for the nonparametric data. Data was described by the use of means, standard deviation, median, inter quartile range (IQR) and percentage. While chi-square test was used to compare categorical variables, Pearson and Spearman rho correlation was applied for continuous variables. p-value < 0.05 at

95% confidence interval was considered as statistically significant in all the analysis.

Result

This study enrolled 61 pediatric oncology patients, 39(63.9%) of the study subjects were males. The mean (±SD) age of the pediatric patients was 6.39 (± 3.67) years ranging from 2 months to 14 years. Male to female ratio was 1.77:1. Twenty eight (45.9%) of pediatric patients were found within the age group of 5 to 9 years. Around 95.1% of the study participants were in low income strata. Regarding distribution, 26 (42.6%) of the children were from Oromia region, followed by Southern Nation Nationality Peoples Region 12(19.7%). Forty four (72.1%) of the study participants were from the rural area of the country. Fifty five (90.2%) of the patients, arrived late at the hospital i.e., 7 days from the onset of sign and symptoms of TLS. None of the patients reported history of cancer in their family (Table 1).

Out of 61 pediatric oncology patients 40(65.9%) had hematologic malignancy, while the rest 21(34.4%) had solid malignancy. Majority of the hematologic malignancies in our study were ALL, 34.4% ($n = 21$) followed by NHL, 13.1% ($n = 8$), AML, 11.5% ($n = 7$), BL, 4.9% ($n = 3$) and CML, 1.6% ($n = 1$). Types of malignancies and their corresponding magnitude of TLS are shown in Fig. 1.

A total of 18 (29.5%) patients had TLS. Seven (11.5%) cases had LTLS whereas the rest 11 (18.0%) had CTLS (Fig. 2).

Out of the 18 TLS cases, 13 (72.2%) developed spontaneous TLS while the remaining 5 (27.8%) had treatment induced TLS. Sixteen (88.9%) of the TLS cases in the study resolved while 2 (11.1%) died. Around 44.4% of the patients resolved from TLS within 72 h of management with adequate hydration and uric acid lowering agent (allopurinol). There were two death reports (11.1%) considered to be caused by TLS, during the study period (Table 2).

Acute kidney injury was observed in 9 (14.8%) of patients, while cardiac arrhythmia and seizure were observed in single patient each. Easy fatigability, abdominal pain and prolonged fever were the most prevalent complaints by the study participants. There was also a high prevalence of swelling on different parts of the body (jaw, facial, neck, thigh and lower leg) of the study participants. Some of the patients also complained of having headache, cough and bleeding (nasal and gum).

Out of 44 patients who underwent chest x-ray imaging, 33 were normal, 4 showed pleural effusion, 4 had lung opacity, 2 had cardiomegally and 1 showed solitary calcified nodule. Ultra sound and physical diagnosis results showed that 23 (37.7%) and 20 (32.8%) patients had hepatomegally and splenomegaly respectively, 6 (9.8%) had pleural effusion, 33 (54.1%) had lymph node enlargement at different sites of their body and 9 (14.8%) had edema. In addition palmar and conjuctival pallor were observed in 47 (77%) of the study participants.

The mean ± SD levels of biochemical parameters before and after treatment are shown in Table 3. A Wilcoxon signed rank test showed statistically significant decrease in total WBC count and serum levels of LDH and calcium after treatment ($p < 0.05$). The study also showed that there is a statistically significant increase in the serum levels of uric acid, BUN and creatinine after treatment ($p < 0.05$). There is no statistically significant difference ($p > 0.05$) in serum levels of sodium and chloride before and after treatment in the study participants. A two tailed paired sample t test revealed that there is a difference between potassium level before treatment

Table 1 Socio-demographic characteristics of pediatric oncology patients

Variables	Frequency	Percent (%)
Sex		
Male	39	63.9
Female	22	36.1
Age		
0–4	19	31.1
5–9	28	45.9
10–14	14	23.0
Region		
Addis Ababa	8	13.1
Oromia	26	42.6
Amhara	10	16.4
SNNPR	12	19.7
Others [b]	5	8.2
Residence		
Urban	17	27.9
Rural	44	72.1
Time of arrival in the hospital after the onset of sign and symptom of disease		
Within < 72 h	2	3.3
72 h – 7 days	4	6.6
After 7 days	55	90.2
History of cancer in the family		
Yes	0	0.0
No	61	100.0
Total	100	100.0

[a], the sixth, seventh, ninth and tenth babies of the families are labeled as "others"

[b], Tigray and Somali regions are labeled as "others"

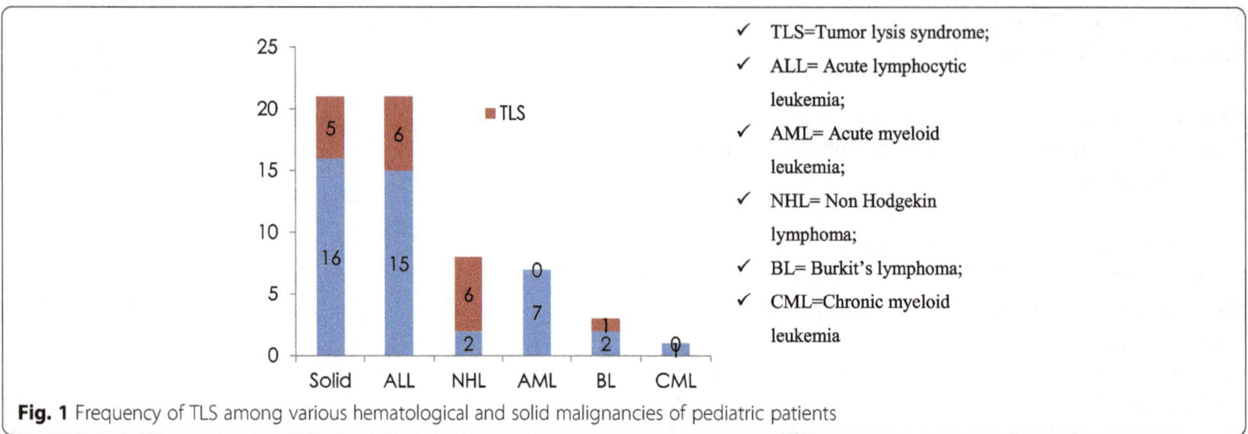

Fig. 1 Frequency of TLS among various hematological and solid malignancies of pediatric patients

(x=4.03, SD = 0.74) and after treatment (x=4.40, SD = 0.50) in the study participants, and this is statistically significant, $t(60) = -4.37$, $p < 0.0001$.

The incidence of hyperuricemia in this study was found to be 23% before treatment and 21.3% after treatment and the incidence of hyperkalemia was 4.9% and 6.6% before and after treatment respectively. The study also revealed two cases of hypocalcemia both before and after treatment.

Bivariate Pearson correlation analysis showed that age was weakly and negatively associated with serum potassium level both before ($r = -0.043$, $p = 0.742$) and after ($r = -0.020$, $p = 0.877$) treatment in the pediatric oncology patients, and this is not statistically significant. Spearman's rho correlation analysis was also used to see correlation between age and some of the dependent variables both before and after treatment in the study participants (Table 4).

Chi-square (x^2) test was implemented to check for the association between the categorical independent variables (gender, residence and family income) and the outcome variable (TLS). The analysis showed that none of the independent variables, gender ($x^2 = 1.378$, $p = 0.240$), residence ($x^2 = 0.105$, $p = 0.746$) and family income ($x^2 = 1.625$, $p = 0.202$) showed significant association with the occurrence of TLS in the study participants (Table 5).

Discussion

The incidence of TLS was 29.5%. Though there is a wide variation in TLS occurrence across the world, this result is comparable with previous researches that reported 26.5% and 30.7% incidence of TLS respectively [7, 8]. The LTLS and CTLS incidences were 11.5% and 18.0%; similar to 11.1% LTLS and 19.6% CTLS reported from a cohort study by Darmon et al. [8] but differs from a report of lower incidence of CTLS (2.9%) in Iran and 6.7% in Saudi Arabia [9, 10]. Out of 18 TLS cases, 13 (72.2%) had spontaneous TLS while the remaining 5 (27.8%) developed treatment induced TLS. This is not in agreement with a previous report of 21.9% spontaneous TLS versus 78.1% therapy induced TLS in Saudi Arabia [10] and 20% spontaneous versus 80% therapy induced TLS elsewhere [11]. The difference in incidence rates reported can be attributed to several factors, such as application of slightly different criteria to recognize TLS, difference in study population, age, underlying malignancy, late presentation of the patients to the health facility, stage of disease at the time of diagnosis and the type of anti-cancer drugs used in our facility. For instance highly myelo-suppressive

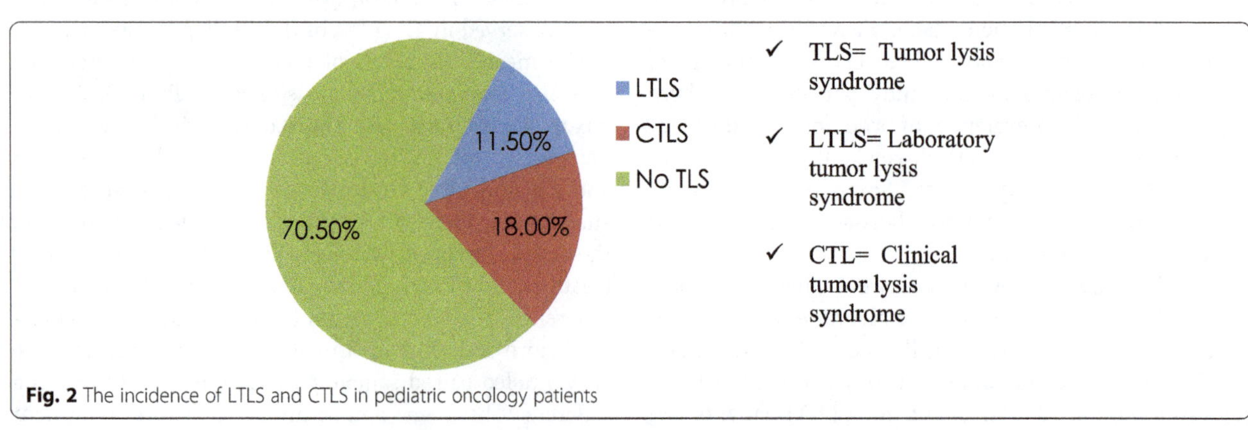

Fig. 2 The incidence of LTLS and CTLS in pediatric oncology patients

Table 2 Management and treatment outcome of TLS in pediatric oncology patients ($n = 18$)

Variables	Frequency	Percent (%)
Resolution		
Yes	16	88.9
No	2	11.1
Total	18	100
Timing of resolution		
Within 72 h	8	44.4
Within 72 - 120 h	5	27.8
Above 120 h	3	16.7
Death	2	11.1

chemotherapies such as high dose methotrexate and cytarabine are used less frequently in our setup. The employment of prophylactic management (i.e., hydration and allopurinol) for all admitted patients may also attribute for a relatively less incidence of chemo induced TLS. But this needs further study to accurately decide on the causes of this discordance.

This study revealed that there were statistically significant decrease in total WBC count and serum levels of LDH after treatment ($p < 0.05$). As the main target of cancer treatment is to eliminate or reduce cancerous cells and a cancer load is mainly manifested by total WBC count (in hematologic malignancies) and serum LDH level, a decrease of these parameters during treatment sounds good outcome of treatment as suggested by Mirrakhimov *et al.* [12]. The decrease in the serum [LDH] after treatment may be due to a decrease in the tumor load. There was statistically significant decrease in the serum level of calcium after treatment ($p < 0.05$). This is because, cytotoxic therapy kills tumor cells leading to rapid release of intracellular phosphate from malignant cells and cancer cells may contain as much as four times the amount of organic and inorganic phosphorous as compared to normal cells [13]. When phosphate concentration is raised, it may lead to precipitation of calcium phosphate crystals, resulting in lowered serum calcium level.

We observed an increase in the serum levels of uric acid, potassium, BUN and creatinine after treatment ($p < 0.05$). As cancer treatment is intended to eliminate or reduce cancerous cells, and when the cells are killed, their intracellular contents will leak out. Thus, there will be an increase in the concentration of these intracellular components and their metabolites in the serum. Uric acid is the end product of purine breakdown. When uric acid is in excess in the serum it results in hyperuricemia. Uric acid may prevent recovery from AKI in TLS, as it has been shown to inhibit proximal tubule cell proliferation [14]. The incidence of hyperuricemia in this study was 23% before treatment and 21.3% after treatment. The result shows that the patients have already developed hyperuricemia before treatment which is in agreement with a result reported from a retrospective study in Turkey which showed a hyperuricemia of 26.5% [6]. But our result is not in agreement with a 40% hyperuricemia, reported from a descriptive study conducted at Liaquat [11]. This variation in the incidence of hyperuricemia may be due to the variation in the types of cancers under study and their response to treatment. It might also be due to late presentation of the patients to the clinics, treatment protocol and difference in study design. Allopurinol was used to reduce or inhibit the formation of uric acid but it has no effect on the already formed uric acid which would have been managed by using a recombinant urate oxidase (rasburicase), but it was not used because it was not available in our set up. The 4.9% and 6.6% incidence of hyperkalemia in the study participants before and after treatment respectively was comparable with a research report from Iran, of 2.9% and 5.8% incidence of hyperkalemia before and after treatment respectively [9]; but discordant with another research which reported a 23% incidence of

Table 3 Laboratory values of biochemical parameters before and after treatment in pediatric oncology patients

Parameters	Before treatment Median(IQR)	After treatment Median(IQR)	*p* value
Potassium(mmol/L)[a]	4.03 ± 0.74	4.40 ± 0.50	**0.0001**
WBC(×10^3/μl)	12.50(8.400–37.700)	10.00(6.250–18.825)	**0.0001**
LDH(IU/L)	749.00(556.95–1274.00)	524.00(371.5–863.5)	**0.0001**
Uric acid(mg/dl)	4.94(3.15–6.90)	6.20(4.69–6.90)	**0.0001**
BUN(mg/dl)	17.00(12.50–25.50)	19.00(13.00–28.25)	**0.006**
Creatinine(mg/dl)	0.70(0.60–0.80)	0.89(0.80–1.00)	**0.0001**
Sodium (mmol/l)	139.0(137.0–140.9)	139.0(138.0–141.0)	0.719
Calcium (mmol/l)	2.01(1.23–2.30)	1.21(1.09–1.90)	**0.0001**
Chloride (mmol/l)	105.0(101.20–109.00)	105.0(100.1–108.0)	0.671

[a]Potassium is normally distributed, expressed as mean ± standard deviation, the rest of the variables are not normally distributed, expressed as median and IQR

Table 4 Spearman's rho correlation between age and some of the dependent variables before and after treatment in pediatric oncology patients

Variable		WBC^a	WBC^b	LDH^a	LDH^b	UA^a	UA^b	BUN^a	BUN^b	Cr^a	Cr^b	Ca^a	Ca^b
AGE	**r**	-.05	-.08	-.07	-.06	-.11	-.04	.14	.20	.27[c]	.15	-.15	-.14
	p	.68	.55	.61	.66	.38	.75	.29	.13	.04	.27	.25	.28

[a] before treatment, [b] after treatment; *UA* uric acid, *Cr* creatinine, *Ca* calcium
[c] Correlation is significant at the 0.05 level (2-tailed)

hyperkalemia and 12% hypokalemia [10]. There was no hypokalemia case in our study.

The majority of the pediatric patients were found within the age group of 5 to 9 years. The result of this study revealed that age is weakly and negatively associated with serum levels of potassium ($r = -0.043$, $p > 0.05$ and $r = -0.020$, $p > 0.05$), calcium ($r = -0.15$, $p > 0.05$ and $r = -0.14$, $p > 0.05$), uric acid ($r = -0.11$, $p > 0.05$ and $r = -0.04$, $p > 0.05$), LDH ($r = -0.07$, $p > 0.05$ and $r = -0.06$, $p > 0.05$), and total WBC count ($r = -0.05$, $p > 0.05$ and $r = -0.08$, $p > 0.05$) respectively before and after treatment, but only serum creatinine level before treatment was statistically significant. At the same time, age was weakly and positively associated with serum BUN ($r = 0.14$, $p > 0.05$ and $r = 0.20$, $p > 0.05$) and creatinine ($r = 0.27$, $p < 0.05$, and $r = 0.15$, $p > 0.05$) respectively before and after treatment. There is a natural tendency that as age increases the muscle mass tends to increase, and also during cancer there is increased muscle wasting leading to a proportioned increase in creatinine level as a catabolic product of amino acids.

Results showed that gender did not have statistically significant association with the occurrence of TLS ($X^2 = 1.378$, $p > 0.240$). This finding does not agree with a previous study which reported that males are more susceptible to TLS [15]. This requires a further elaborated study with a larger sample size and gender balance. Residence ($X^2 = 0.105$, $p > 0.05$) and family income ($X^2 = 1.625$, $p > 0.202$) did not show statistically significant association with the occurrence of TLS in the study participants. But in previous studies, children from low and middle income countries were shown to be at a greater risk of developing TLS [16, 17]. In our case almost all the study participants were in low income stratification hence there was no significant variation within the group with respect to TLS occurrence. Nearly 90% of the patients recovered from TLS during the follow up period. There were 2 (11.1%) death incidences as a consequence of TLS complication. There is a variation in death incidence report due to TLS across different research reports [10, 11]. The variation in the incidence of death report may be due to the difference in the treatment protocols and the management, the variation in the study population and the nature of the underlying malignancies. A recent review can be referred for more information on TLS [18].

Conclusions

In this study TLS occurred irrespective of gender, residence and family income. This suggests that every child with cancer is at risk of developing TLS. Early identification of patients at risk and prevention is of crucial importance. Spontaneous TLS was more prevalent than the drug induced one. This may indicate that patients do not come to health facility early before complication and have advanced malignancy with high tumor burden. The biochemical parameters studied in this research and in other studies have shown strong association with the occurrence of TLS. Thus, these parameters shall be considered in TLS prediction, diagnosis and prognosis. TLS incidence was high irrespective of intensive prophylactic managements (i.e., hydration and allopurinol). A better

Table 5 Chi-square test and cross tabulation between independent variables (gender, residence and family income) and TLS in pediatric oncology patients. (Birr is the Ethiopian currency)

Variables	None TLS, No (%)	TLS, No (%)	X^2	*p*-Value
Gender				
male	30(49.2)	9(14.8)	1.378	0.204
female	13(21.3)	9(14.8)		
Residence				
urban	13(21.3)	4(6.6)	0.105	0.746
rural	30(49.2)	14(22.9)		
Family income				
< 1228 Birr/month/individual)	33(54.1)	17(27.9)	1.625	0.202
> 1228 Birr/month/individual	10(16.4)	1(1.6)		

management strategy shall be adapted in the clinics and valid and efficient diagnostic tests shall be used for better diagnosis and prognosis of cancer and TLS.

Acknowledgements
We would like to thank Addis Ababa University department of Biochemistry and Pediatrics and Child Health for their administrative support, and all study participants and their family for their cooperation.

Funding
This study was funded by Addis Ababa University, School of Graduate Studies.

Authors' contributions
HM conceived the study, participated in data collection and performed data analysis and write up of the paper. YM has done patient identification, diagnosis, follow up and data collection and also assisted in result analysis and interpretation. DH and SG involved in the design, analysis, interpretation of data and the critical review of the manuscript. All authors read and approved the final manuscript. All authors participated in critical appraisal of the manuscript.

Competing interests
The authors declare that they have no competing interests.

Author details
[1]Department of Biomedical Sciences, College of Health Sciences, Dilla University, Dilla, Ethiopia. [2]Department of Medical Biochemistry, School of Medicine, College of Health sciences, Addis Ababa University, P. O. Box 9086, Addis Ababa, Ethiopia. [3]Department of Pediatrics and child Health, School of Medicine, College of Health Sciences, Addis Ababa University, Addis Ababa, Ethiopia.

References
1. Bedrna J, Polc k J. Akuter harnleiterverschluss nach bestrahlung chronischer leuk mien mit r ntgenstrahlen. Med Klin. 1929;25:1700–1.
2. Alakel N, Middeke JM, Schetelig J, Bornhäuser M. Prevention and treatment of tumor lysis syndrome, and the efficacy and role of rasburicase. Onco Targets Ther. 2017;10:597–605.
3. Cairo MS, Bishop M. Tumour lysis syndrome: new therapeutic strategies and classification. Br J Haematol. 2004;127(1):3–11.
4. Gupta S, Howard SC, Hunger SP, et al. Childhood cancers. In: Gelband H, Jha P, Sankaranarayanan R, Horton S, editors. Disease control priorities: volume 3, Cancer. 3rd ed. Washington DC: World Bank; 2015. p. 120.
5. Hande KR, Garrow GC. Acute tumor lysis syndrome in patients with high-grade non-Hodgkin's lymphoma. Am J Med. 1993;94(2):133–9.
6. Sevinir B, Demirkaya M, Baytan B, Güneş AM. Hyperuricemia and tumor lysis syndrome in children with non-Hodgkin's lymphoma and acute lymphoblastic leukemia. Turk J Hernatol. 2011;28:52–9.
7. Wössmann W, Schrappe M, Meyer U, Zimmermann M, Reiter A. Incidence of tumor lysis syndrome in children with advanced stage Burkitt's lymphoma/ leukemia before and after introduction of prophylactic use of urate oxidase. Ann Hematol. 2003;82(3):160–5.
8. Darmon M, Vincent F, Camous L, et al. Tumour lysis syndrome and acute kidney injury in high-risk haematology patients in the rasburicase era. A prospective multicentre study from the Groupe de Recherche en Réanimation Respiratoire et Onco-Hématologique. Br J Haematol. 2013; 162(4):489–97.
9. Esfahani H. The prevalence of tumor lysis syndrome in children and adolescents with Cancer in Hamedan Province, Iran. IJBC. 2015;7(2):97–9.
10. Al Bagshi M, Al Omran S, El Solh H, Al Abaad A. Tumor lysis syndrome in children with acute leukemia: incidence and outcome. J Appl Hematol. 2013;4(3):100–3.
11. Wasim F, Khaskheli AM, Siddiqui AA, Tariq O, Ansari MA. Tumour Lysis Syndrome in Haematological Malignancies. JLUMHS. 2012;11(2):84–9.
12. Mirrakhimov AE, Ali AM, Khan M, Barbaryan A. Tumor lysis syndrome in solid tumors: an up to date review of the literature. Rare Tumors. 2014; 6(2):5389–93.
13. Cairo MS, Gerrard M, Sposto R, et al. Results of a randomized international study of high-risk central nervous system B non-Hodgkin lymphoma and B acute lymphoblastic leukemia in children and adolescents. Blood. 2007; 109(7):2736–43.
14. Han HJ, Lim MJ, Lee YJ, Lee JH, Yang IS, Taub M. Uric acid inhibits renal proximal tubule cell proliferation via at least two signaling pathways involving PKC, MAPK, cPLA 2, and NF-κB. Am J Physiol Renal Physiol. 2007; 292(1):373–81.
15. Mato AR, Riccio BE, Qin L, et al. A predictive model for the detection of tumor lysis syndrome during AML induction therapy. Leuk Lymphoma. 2006;47(5):877–83.
16. Ribeiro RC, Steliarova-Foucher E, Magrath I, et al. Baseline status of paediatric oncology care in ten low-income or mid-income countries receiving my child matters support: a descriptive study. Lancet Oncol. 2008;9(8):721–9.
17. Kellie SJ, Howard SC. Global child health priorities: what role for paediatric oncologists? Eur J Cancer. 2008;44(16):2388–96.
18. La Spina M, Puglisi F, Sullo F, Venti V, et al. Tumor lysis syndrome: an emergency in pediatric oncology. J Ped Biochem. 2015;5(4):161–8.

25

Prevalence, types and determinants of anemia among pregnant women in Sudan: a systematic review and meta-analysis

Ishag Adam[1*], Yassin Ibrahim[2] and Osama Elhardello[3]

Abstract

Background: Anemia during pregnancy is a public health problem especially in developing countries and it is associated with maternal and perinatal adverse outcomes. There is no meta-analysis on anemia during pregnancy in Sudan. The current systemic review and meta-analysis was conducted to assess the prevalence, types and determinant of anemia during pregnancy in Sudan.

Methods: Preferred Reporting Items for Systematic Reviews and Meta-Analyses (PRISMA) guideline was followed. The databases (PubMed, Cochrane Library, Google Scholar, CINAHL, and African Journals Online) were searched using; anemia, pregnancy related anemia and Sudan. Joanna Briggs Institute Meta-Analysis of Statistics Assessment and Review Instrument (JBI-MAStARI) and Modified Newcastle - Ottawa quality assessment scale were used for critical appraisal of studies. The pooled Meta logistic regression was computed using OpenMeta Analyst software.

Results: Sixteen cross-sectional studies included a total of 15, 688 pregnant women were analyzed. The pooled prevalence of anemia among pregnant women in Sudan was 53.0% (95%, CI = 45.9–60.1). The meta-analysis showed no statistical significant between the age (mean difference = 0.143, 95 CI = − 0.033 – 0.319, *P* = 0.112), parity (mean difference = 0.021, 95% CI = − 0.035 – 0.077, *P* = 0.465) between the anemic and no anemic women. Malaria was investigated in six studies. Pregnant women who had malaria infection during pregnancy were 1.94 times more likely to develop anemia than women who had no malaria infection (OR = 1.94, 95% CI =1.33–2.82). Six (37.5%) studies investigated type of anemia. The pooled prevalence of iron deficiency anemia (IDA) among pregnant women in Sudan was 13.6% (95% CI = 8.9–18.2).

Conclusion: There is a high prevalence of anemia among pregnant in the different region of Sudan. While age and parity have no association with anemia, malaria infection was associated with anemia. Interventions to promote the strengthening of antenatal care, and access and adherence to nutrition, and malaria preventive measures are needed to reduce the high level of anemia among pregnant women in Sudan.

Keywords: Prevalence of anemia, Anemia during pregnancy, Age, Parity, Malaria during pregnancy, Sudan, Meta-analysis, systematic review

* Correspondence: ishagadam@hotmail.com
[1]Faculty of Medicine, University of Khartoum, P.O. Box 102, Khartoum, Sudan
Full list of author information is available at the end of the article

Background

Anemia during pregnancy is a public health problem especially in developing countries and it is associated with maternal and perinatal adverse outcomes [1]. World Health Organization (WHO) has defined anemia in pregnancy as the hemoglobin concentration of less than 11 g/dl [2]. According to WHO, anemia is considered of a severe public health significance if its rate of ≥40% [3]. Global data shows that 56% of pregnant women in low and middle income countries have anemia [1]. The prevalence of anemia is highest among pregnant women in sub- Sahara Africa (57%), followed by pregnant women in South-East Asia (48%) and lowest prevalence (24.1%) was reported among pregnant women in South America [3].

The causes of anemia during pregnancy in developing countries are multifactorial; these include micronutrient deficiencies of iron, folate and vitamin A and B12, anemia due to parasitic infections such as malaria and hookworm or chronic infections like tuberculosis and HIV [4, 5]. Contributions of each of the factors that cause anemia during pregnancy vary due to geographical location, dietary practice and season. In Sub Saharan Africa inadequate intake of diets rich in iron is reported as the leading cause of anemia among pregnant women [4–6].

Anemia during pregnancy is reported to have negative maternal and child health effect and increase the risk of maternal and perinatal mortality [7, 8]. The negative health effects for the mother include fatigue, poor work capacity, impaired immune function, increased risk of cardiac diseases and mortality [1, 8]. Some studies have shown that anemia during pregnancy contributes to 23% of indirect causes of maternal deaths in developing countries [1]. Although, there many published studies on anemia during pregnancy in the different setting of Sudan [9–24], there is no systemic review/ meta-analysis on anemia in Sudan. The current systemic review and meta-analysis was conducted to assess prevalence, types and determinant of anemia during pregnancy in Sudan.

Methods

Study design and search strategy

Findings from published studies were used to conduct this systematic review and meta-analysis to determine the prevalence of anemia, types and its determinants (age, parity and malaria) among pregnant women in Sudan. The major databases of PubMed, Cochrane Library, Google Scholar, CINAHL, and African Journals Online were reviewed for all published studies relevant to anemia during pregnancy and its determinant factors.

All studies that were published up to April 03/2018 were retrieved to be assessed for eligibility of inclusion in this review. In addition, the reference list of each included study was also searched, retrieved and assessed for inclusion eligibility.

The terms that used for searching are: "anemia OR anemia during pregnancy OR determinants of anemia AND Sudan". Preferred Reporting Items for Systematic Reviews and Meta-Analyses (PRISMA) guideline was followed for conduction of this systematic review and meta-analysis [25].

Study selection and eligibility criteria

Outcome of interest

The primary outcome of this study was the prevalence of anemia during pregnancy. The WHO defines anemia in pregnancy as low blood hemoglobin concentration, below 11 g/dl or hematocrit level less than 33% dl [2]. The secondary outcomes were; types and determinants (age, parity and malaria) of anemia during pregnancy.

Quality assessment and data collection

The included studies were assessed by using Joanna Briggs Institute Meta-Analysis of Statistics Assessment and Review Instrument (JBI-MAStARI) [26]. Modified Newcastle – Ottawa quality assessment scale for cross sectional studies was used to assess the quality of the study for inclusion [27]. The total score for the modified Newcastle – Ottawa scale for cross sectional studies is nine (9) stars as a maximum for the overall scale with the minimum of zero. A study was considered high quality if it achieved 7 out 9 and medium if it achieved 5out of 9, Table 1, Additional file 1.

Two reviewers (IA & YI) independently assessed the quality of each article for inclusion in the review. The disagreement arise between the reviewers was resolved through discussion and involvement of a third reviewer (OE).

A tool for data extraction was developed to extract the most important relevant information for the review. It consists of tables that include information about the authors' name, year of publication, study location, sample size, age of study participants, and number of pregnancies, malaria with pregnancy, type of anemia and presence and types of complications of anemia.

Data analysis and heterogeneity assessment

OpenMeta Analyst software for Windows [28, 29] was used to perform all the meta-analyses of prevalence and determinants (age, parity and malaria) of anemia. The heterogeneity of the included studies was evaluated using Cochrane Q and the I^2. Cochrane Q with $P < 0.10$ and $I^2 > 50$ was taken as standard to indicate the presence of heterogeneity of the included studies [30]. Based on the results of the analysis of Cochrane Q and I^2 the random effects or fixed model was used to combine the included studies accordingly. A sub-group analysis was

Table 1 Summary and the assessment of the included studies

The study	Year	Location	Sample size	Prevalence of anemia%	Score of the Modified Newcastle Ottawa Scale
Abas et al.,	2017	Khartoum	423	57.68	5
Abdelgadir et al.,	2012	Geizera	292	40.75	6
Abdelrahman	2012	Khartoum	194	24.23	6
Abdelrahim et al.,	2009	Gadarif	300	74.67	7
Abdullahi et al.,	2014	Khartoum	856	47.78	6
Adam a et al.,	2005	New Halfa	744	62.63	7
Adam b et al.,	2005	New Halfa	125	76	7
Adam c et al.,	2007	New Halfa	333	36.94	6
Adam d et al.,	2012	Geizera	324	62.04	7
Ali et al.,	2011	Kassala	9578	41.89	6
Bushra et al.,	2010	Geizera	200	52	7
Elmugabil et al.,	2017	Khartoum	338	49.7	6
Haggaz et al.,	2010	Darfur	403	74.69	6
Mohamed et al.,	2011	Kassala	250	58.4	6
Mubarak et al.,	2014	Khartoum	179	23.46	8

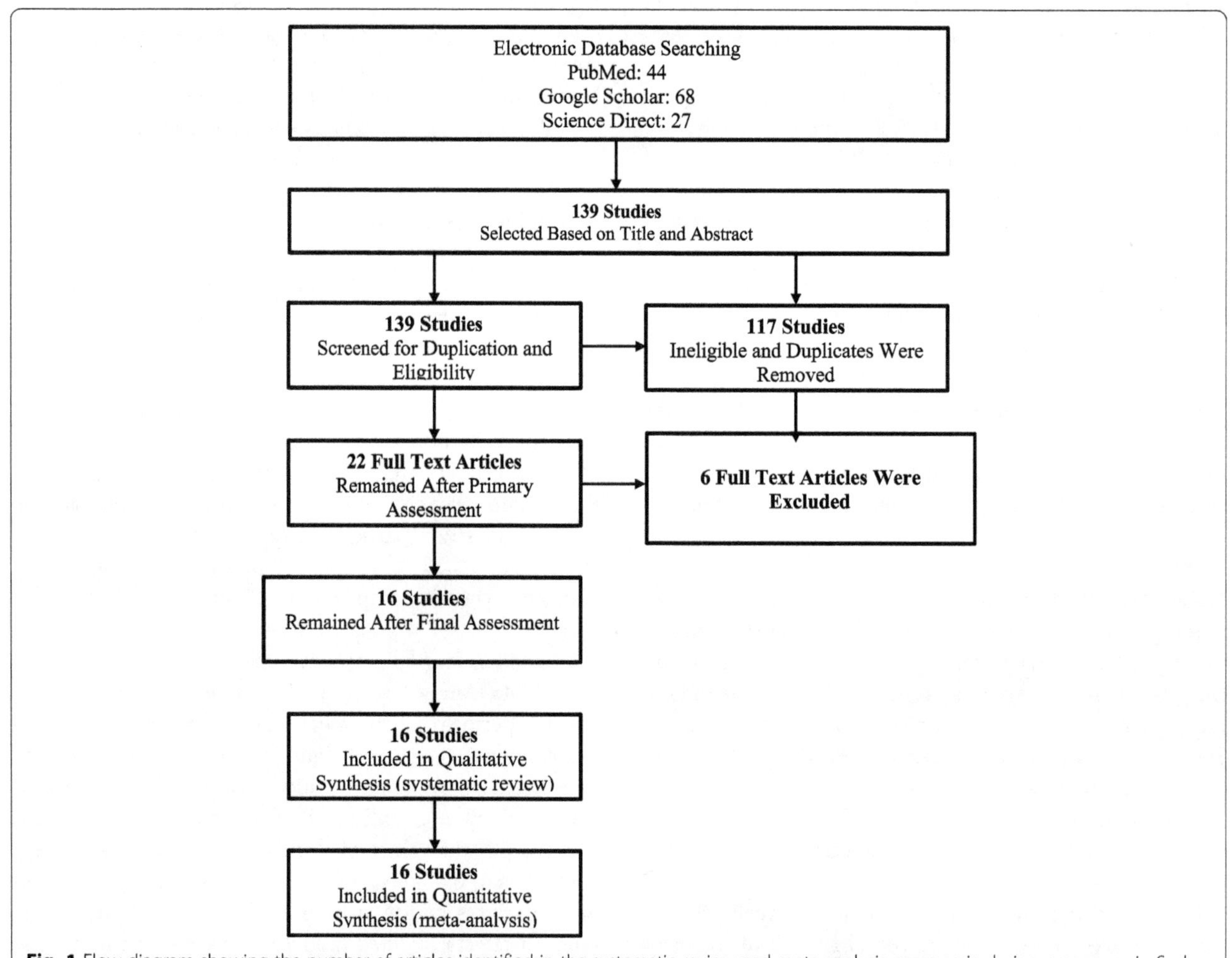

Fig. 1 Flow diagram showing the number of articles identified in the systematic review and meta-analysis on anemia during pregnancy in Sudan

performed to investigate the association between malaria and anemia.

Results

Study selection

The reviewers found a total of 139 published articles initially. Out of these, 117 were removed due to duplicate records and not fulfilling the criteria. A total of 22 full-text articles were screened for eligibility. Out of these 22, 6 articles were excluded (using varied hemoglobin cut- off, case- control studies and included non-pregnant women. Sixteen studies were included in the final analysis, Fig. 1.

Characteristics of included studies

Sixteen cross-sectional studies were included in this meta-analysis [9–24], Fig. 1. All of the included studies were conducted at health institutions, Additional file 2. All the studies used the WHO definition of anemia during pregnancy which is 11 g/dl [2].

Five (31.2%) of the 16 studies in this review were conducted in Khartoum [15, 17–19, 21], six (37.5%) studies were conducted in eastern Sudan (New Half, Kassala and Gadarif) [9, 10, 13, 22–24], three studies were conducted in Geizera [12, 14, 16], one study was conducted in Darfur and one study was conducted in Blue Nile [11, 20], Additional file 2.

The minimum sample size was 125 participants in a study conducted in New Halfa [22]. The higher sample size was 8578 conducted in Kassala in Eastern Sudan [24]. Overall, this meta-analysis included a total of 15, 688 pregnant women. The mean (SD) of the age and parity of pregnant women included in this review was 28.5 years and 2.08, respectively, Additional file 2. Six of 16 studies were conducted during delivery/labour (because investigating other outcome e.g. birth outcome), 2 studies were conducted in early pregnancy and the rest in the early third trimester, Additional file 2.

Prevalence of anemia among pregnant women

The minimum prevalence of anemia was 23.46% observed in a study conducted in Khartoum [15]. The highest, 76.0% was observed in a study conducted in Eastern Sudan [9]. The I^2 test result showed high heterogeneity ($I^2 = 98.2\%$, $p < 0.001$). Using the random effect analysis, the pooled prevalence of anemia among pregnant women in Sudan was 53.0% (95% CI = 45.9–60.1), Fig. 2.

Association between age, parity and anemia

All the included studies (16) reported the age and parity as continuous variables. Therefore the mean (SD) was compared in this review. The meta-analysis showed no statistical significant between the age (mean difference = 0.143, 95% CI = - 0.033 - 0.319, $P = 0.112$), parity (mean difference = 0.021, 95% CI = - 0.035 - 0.077, $P = 0.465$) between the anemic and no anemic women, Figs. 3 and 4. The heterogeneity test showed no statistical evidence of heterogeneity ($p = 0.896$), therefore the fixed model was used.

Association between malaria infection and anemia

Malaria was investigated (peripheral/ placental) in six studies [9, 10, 13, 20, 22, 23], Additional file 3. Pregnant

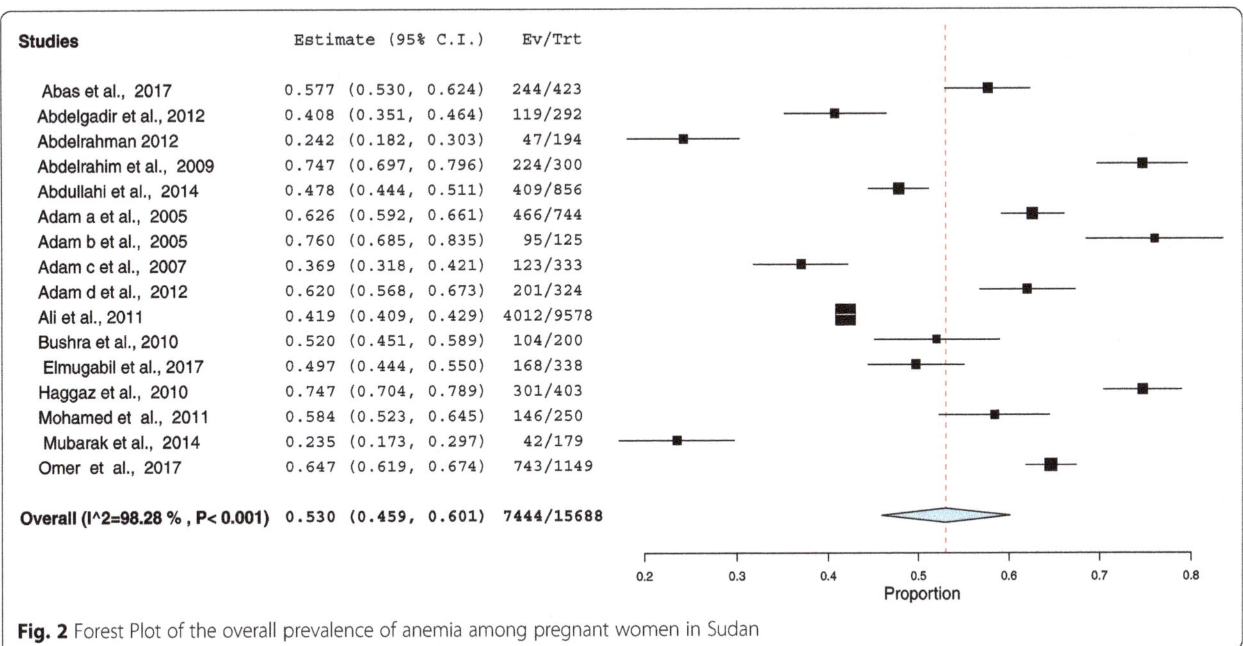

Fig. 2 Forest Plot of the overall prevalence of anemia among pregnant women in Sudan

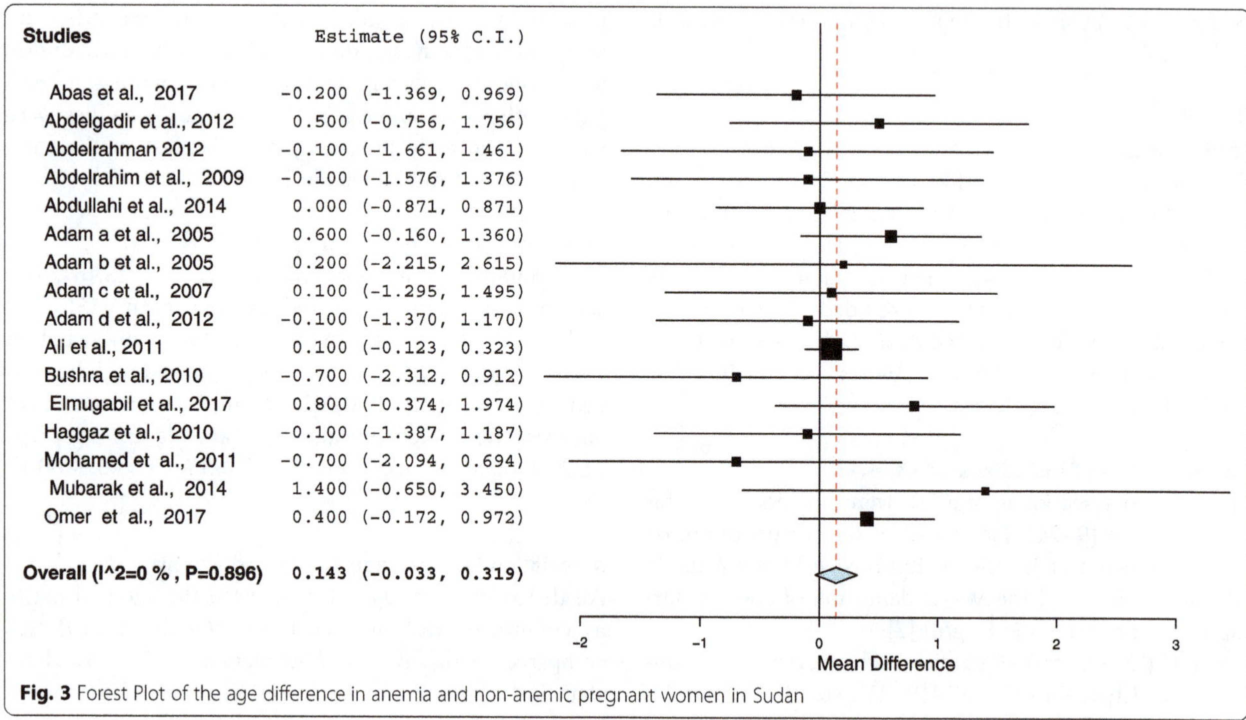

Fig. 3 Forest Plot of the age difference in anemia and non-anemic pregnant women in Sudan

women who had malaria infection during pregnancy were almost two times more likely to develop anemia during pregnancy than women had no such infection (OR = 1.94 (95% CI = 1.33–2.82). The heterogeneity test showed statistical evidence of heterogeneity, $p = < 0.001$. Therefore random-effects analysis was used, Fig. 5.

Type of anemia and micronutrient deficiency

Six (37.5%) out of the 16 included studies investigated type of anemia [10, 12, 13, 15, 17, 19]. The minimum prevalence of iron deficiency anemia (IDA) was 6.5% observed in a study conducted in Geizera [12]. The highest prevalence of IDA was 29.3% which was observed in a study Khartoum [17], Additional file 1. The I^2 test result

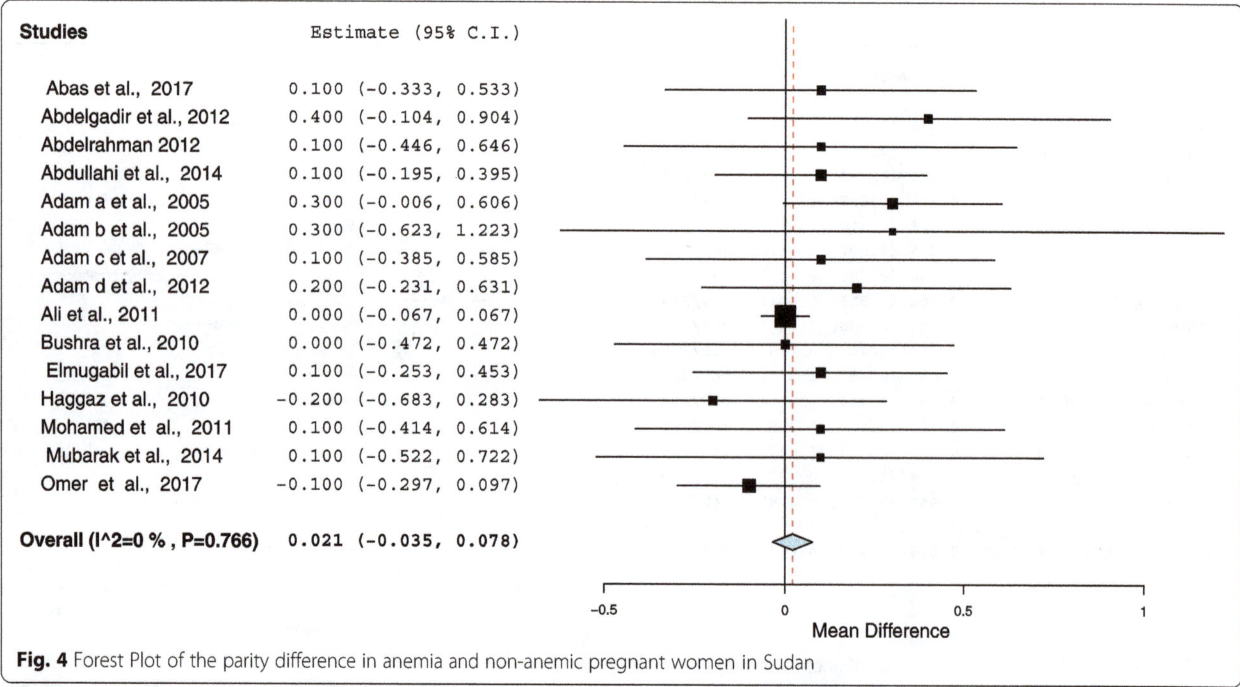

Fig. 4 Forest Plot of the parity difference in anemia and non-anemic pregnant women in Sudan

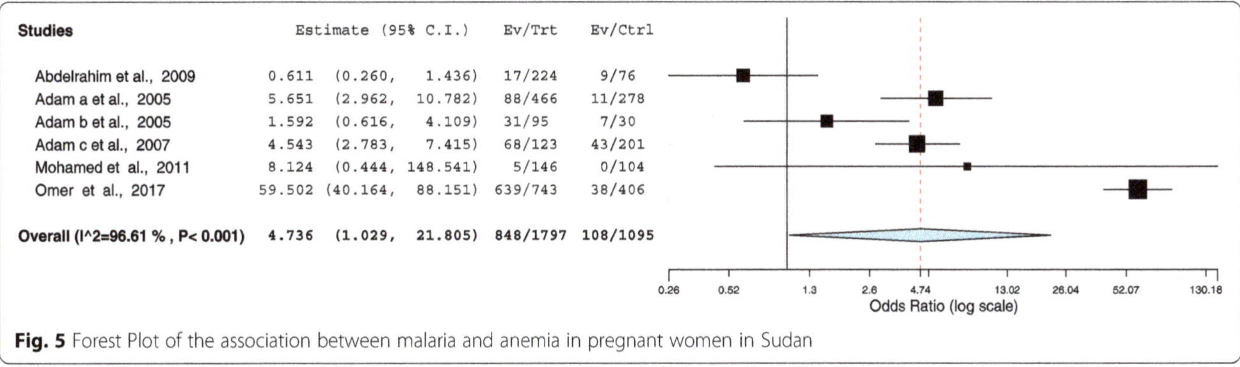

Studies	Estimate (95% C.I.)	Ev/Trt	Ev/Ctrl
Abdelrahim et al., 2009	0.611 (0.260, 1.436)	17/224	9/76
Adam a et al., 2005	5.651 (2.962, 10.782)	88/466	11/278
Adam b et al., 2005	1.592 (0.616, 4.109)	31/95	7/30
Adam c et al., 2007	4.543 (2.783, 7.415)	68/123	43/201
Mohamed et al., 2011	8.124 (0.444, 148.541)	5/146	0/104
Omer et al., 2017	59.502 (40.164, 88.151)	639/743	38/406
Overall (I^2=96.61 %, P< 0.001)	**4.736 (1.029, 21.805)**	**848/1797**	**108/1095**

Fig. 5 Forest Plot of the association between malaria and anemia in pregnant women in Sudan

showed high heterogeneity (I ^{2} 87.6%, $p < 0.001$). Using the random effect analysis, the pooled prevalence of IDA among pregnant women in Sudan was 13.6% (95% CI = 8.9–18.2), Fig. 6.

Two studies; in Geizera [12] and in Kassala [13] reported zinc deficiency rate of 45.0% and 38.0%, respectively. Only one study in Gadarif reported 57.7% and 1% of folate and B12 deficiency, respectively [10]. Only one study reported 4.0% copper deficiency in pregnant women in Geizera [12]. C-reactive protein was investigated in one study [13].

Discussion

The main results of this met- analysis is the high prevalence (53.0%) of anemia among pregnant women in the different regions of Sudan. In neighbouring Ethiopia (meta-analysis of twenty studies and a total of 10, 281 pregnant women) the pooled prevalence of anemia among pregnant women in Ethiopia was 31.66% [31]. The prevalence of anemia in this meta-analyses is higher than the rate of anemia among pregnant women in the other African countries e.g. in Uganda 22.1%; [32]. A recent meta-analysis on global rate of anemia reported a lower rate (38%) of anemia in pregnant women, especially among pregnant women in East Africa where the prevalence of anemia was 36% [33]. This high prevalence of anemia in Sudan, is indicative of a severe public health problem, according to the WHO, anemia is considered a severe health problem if prevalence of anemia of ≥40% in a population [3]. It is worth to be mentioned that all the studies included in this meta-analyses were intuitional studies; therefore their results might not reflect the real situation in the community. Recently Kassa et al., have reported that the rate of anemia in pregnancy was much higher in the pooled meta-analyses (31.66%) that the rate (29.0%) of the anemia reported in the national (Ethiopia) survey [31, 34].

The current pooled meta-analyses showed that the age and parity were not different between anemic and non-anemic women. This reflects that anemia affects pregnant Sudanese women regardless to their age or parity. Recent meta-analyses showed that primigravidae were at lower risk for anemia compared with parous women [31]. Likewise, pregnant women with gravidity three to five and six and above were at 1.78, and 2.59 higher risks for anemia [35]. Wessells and colleauges have recently reported that gravidity and malaria were associated with associated with micronutrient deficiency status in pregnant women in Niger [36]. It is belived that women with high parity have low or no iron staorge as it hass been depleted by the repeated pregnaied hence parous women are more likely to be anemic [8]. Generally various risk factors (residence, parity, nutritional) for anemia during have

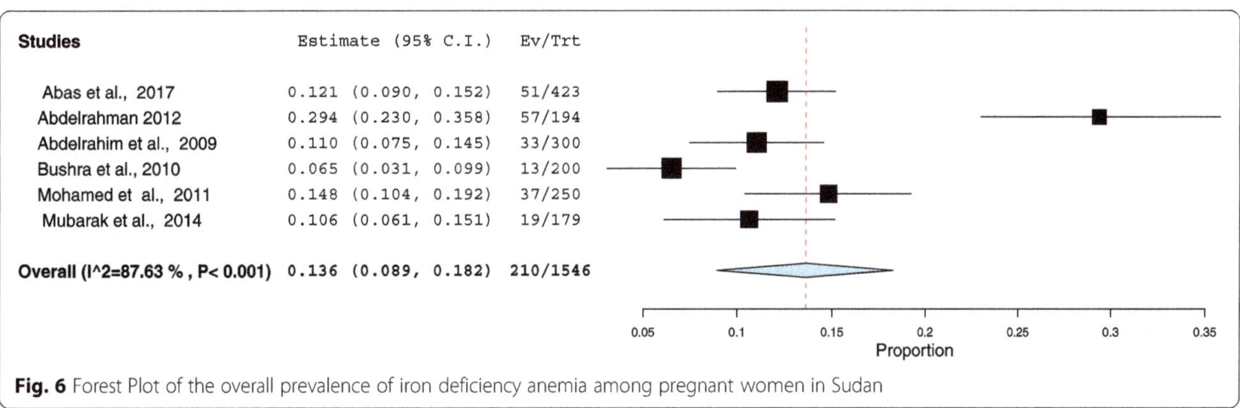

Studies	Estimate (95% C.I.)	Ev/Trt
Abas et al., 2017	0.121 (0.090, 0.152)	51/423
Abdelrahman 2012	0.294 (0.230, 0.358)	57/194
Abdelrahim et al., 2009	0.110 (0.075, 0.145)	33/300
Bushra et al., 2010	0.065 (0.031, 0.099)	13/200
Mohamed et al., 2011	0.148 (0.104, 0.192)	37/250
Mubarak et al., 2014	0.106 (0.061, 0.151)	19/179
Overall (I^2=87.63 %, P< 0.001)	**0.136 (0.089, 0.182)**	**210/1546**

Fig. 6 Forest Plot of the overall prevalence of iron deficiency anemia among pregnant women in Sudan

been reported in Ethiopia [35, 37–41]. In Nigeria pregnant women in the rural communities had high pevalence of anemia and iron deficiency anemia compared to pregnant women in the urban setting [42]. In Ugandan Obai et al., have reported that lower prevalence of anemia (22.1%) among pregnant women and housewife were at 1.7 higher risk of anemia [32].

In the current meta-analysis 13.6% of among pregnant women in Sudan had IDA. This rate (13.6%) of IDA was higher than the rate (5%) of IDA reported among rural women of reproductive age in southern Ethiopia [43]. However, 20.7% of pregnant women in Niger had IDA [36].

The pathophysiological mechanism of anemia and its associations with malaria is not yet fully understood. Howver poor inake of food during illness, hemolysis, anemia of inflammation, bone marrow suppression, and micronutrients deficiency are the plasuible explnations for anemia and malaria [44].

Limitiations

Some points need to be mentioned: fisrtly all of these studies were instituational ones. Thus the the findings of these studies might not indicate what is going at the community level. Secondly anemia during pregnancy in Sudan (included in these studies) has been studied mainly in Khartoum, Eastern Sudan and Geizera. There is a pauxity of reports on anemia during pregnancy in the other regions of Sudan e.g.White Nile, North Sudan and Khordofan. Thirdly, types and predictors for anemia during pregnancy were not deeply investiagted in these studies. Some factors such as antenatal care, food security, dietary diversity, maternal education and income need to be taken in the future research. Other types and causes of anemia e.g. folate and vitamin B12 deficiency need to be addressed in more depth.

Conclusion

There is a high prevalence of anemia among pregnant in the different region of Sudan. While age and parity have no association with anemia, malaria infection was associated with anemia. Interventions to promote the strengthening of antenatal care, and access and adherence to nutrition, and malaria preventive measures are needed to reduce the high level of anemia among pregnant women in Sudan.

Abbreviations

CI: Confidence interval; IDA: Iron deficiency anemia; OR: Odd ratio; WHO: World Health Organization

Acknowledgements

We would like to acknowledge to authors of studies included in this review.

Funding

There are no funding sources for this paper.

Authors' contributions

IA, YI, and OE designed the study and participated in the manuscript drafting. IA, and YI conducted data extraction and statistical analyses. All authors read and approved the final manuscript.

Competing interests

The authors declare that they have no competing interests.

Author details

[1]Faculty of Medicine, University of Khartoum, P.O. Box 102, Khartoum, Sudan. [2]Faculty of Medicine, University of Tabuk, P.O. Box 741, Tabuk, Saudi Arabia. [3]Scarborough General Hospital, Scarborough YO12 6QL, UK.

References

1. Black RE, Victora CG, Walker SP, Bhutta ZA, Christian P, de Onis M, et al. Maternal and child undernutrition and overweight in low-income and middle-income countries. Lancet. 2013;382:427–51. https://doi.org/10.1016/S0140-6736(13)60937-X.
2. World Health Organization. the Global Prevalence of Anaemia in 2011. WHO Rep. 2011;48. doi:https://doi.org/10.1017/S1368980008002401.
3. Worldwide prevalence of anaemia. 1993. http://apps.who.int/iris/bitstream/10665/43894/1/9789241596657_eng.pdf. Accessed 21 Feb 2018.
4. McClure EM, Meshnick SR, Mungai P, Malhotra I, King CL, Goldenberg RL, et al. The association of parasitic infections in pregnancy and maternal and fetal anemia: a cohort study in coastal Kenya. PLoS Negl Trop Dis. 2014;8:e2724. https://doi.org/10.1371/journal.pntd.0002724.
5. Brooker S, Hotez PJ, Bundy DAP. Hookworm-related anaemia among pregnant women: a systematic review. PLoS Negl Trop Dis. 2008;2:e291. https://doi.org/10.1371/journal.pntd.0000291.
6.Ononge S, Campbell O, Mirembe F. Haemoglobin status and predictors of anaemia among pregnant women in Mpigi, Uganda. BMC Res Notes. 2014;7:712. https://doi.org/10.1186/1756-0500-7-712.
7. Levy A, Fraser D, Katz M, Mazor M, Sheiner E. Maternal anemia during pregnancy is an independent risk factor for low birthweight and preterm delivery. Eur J Obstet Gynecol Reprod Biol. 2005;122:182–6. https://doi.org/10.1016/j.ejogrb.2005.02.015.
8. Adam I, AA Ali - Nutritional, 2016 U. Anemia during pregnancy. intechopen.com. https://www.intechopen.com/books/nutritional-deficiency/anemia-during-pregnancy. Accessed 21 Feb 2018.
9. Adam I, Khamis AH, Elbashir MI. Prevalence and risk factors for anaemia in pregnant women of eastern Sudan. Trans R Soc Trop Med Hyg. 2005;99:739–43. https://doi.org/10.1016/j.trstmh.2005.02.008.
10. Abdelrahim II, Adam GK, Mohmmed AA, Salih MM, Ali NI, Elbashier MI, et al. Anaemia, folate and vitamin B12 deficiency among pregnant women in an area of unstable malaria transmission in eastern Sudan. Trans R Soc Trop Med Hyg. 2009;103:493–6. https://doi.org/10.1016/j.trstmh.2008.10.007.
11. Haggaz AD, Radi EA, Adam I. Anaemia and low birthweight in western Sudan. Trans R Soc Trop Med Hyg. 2010;104:234–6. https://doi.org/10.1016/j.trstmh.2009.07.013.
12. Bushra M, Elhassan EM, Ali NI, Osman E, Bakheit KH, Adam II. Anaemia, zinc and copper deficiencies among pregnant women in Central Sudan. Biol Trace Elem Res. 2010;137:255–61. https://doi.org/10.1007/s12011-009-8586-4.
13. Mohamed AA, Ali AAA, Ali NI, Abusalama EH, Elbashir MI, Adam I. Zinc, parity, infection, and severe anemia among pregnant women in Kassla, eastern Sudan. Biol Trace Elem Res. 2011;140:284–90. https://doi.org/10.1007/s12011-010-8704-3.
14. Abdelgadir MA, Khalid AR, Ashmaig AL, Ibrahim ARM, Ahmed A-AM, Adam I. Epidemiology of anaemia among pregnant women in Geizera, Central Sudan. J Obstet Gynaecol. 2012;32:42–4. https://doi.org/10.3109/01443615.2011.617849.
15. Mubarak N, Gasim GI, Khalafalla KE, Ali NI, Adam I. Helicobacter pylori, anemia, iron deficiency and thrombocytopenia among pregnant women at Khartoum, Sudan. Trans R Soc Trop Med Hyg. 2014;108:380–4. https://doi.org/10.1093/trstmh/tru044.
16. Adam I, Ahmed S, Mahmoud MH, Yassin MI. Comparison of HemoCue® hemoglobin-meter and automated hematology analyzer in measurement of hemoglobin levels in pregnant women at Khartoum hospital, Sudan. Diagn Pathol. 2012;7:30. https://doi.org/10.1186/1746-1596-7-30.

17. Abdelrahman EG, Gasim GI, Musa IR, Elbashir LM, Adam I. Red blood cell distribution width and iron deficiency anemia among pregnant Sudanese women. Diagn Pathol. 2012;7:168. https://doi.org/10.1186/1746-1596-7-168
18. Elmugabil A, Rayis DA, Abdelmageed RE, Adam I, Gasim GI. High level of hemoglobin, white blood cells and obesity among Sudanese women in early pregnancy: a cross-sectional study. Futur Sci OA. 2017;3:FSO182. https://doi.org/10.4155/fsoa-2016-0096.
19. Abbas W, Adam I, Rayis DA, Hassan NG, Lutfi MF. Higher rate of iron deficiency in obese pregnant sudanese women. Open access Maced J Med Sci. 2017;5:285–9. https://doi.org/10.3889/oamjms.2017.059.
20. Omer SA, Idress HE, Adam I, Abdelrahim M, Noureldein AN, Abdelrazig AM, et al. Placental malaria and its effect on pregnancy outcomes in Sudanese women from Blue Nile state. Malar J. 2017;16(1):374.
21. Abdullahi H, Gasim GI, Saeed A, Imam AM, Adam I. Antenatal iron and folic acid supplementation use by pregnant women in Khartoum, Sudan. BMC Res Notes. 2014;7:498. https://doi.org/10.1186/1756-0500-7-498.
22. Adam I, A-Elbasit IE, Salih I, Elbashir MI. Submicroscopic *Plasmodium falciparum* infections during pregnancy, in an area of Sudan with a low intensity of malaria transmission. Ann Trop Med Parasitol. 2005;99(4):339-44.
23. Adam I, Babiker S, Mohmmed AA, Salih MM, Prins MH, Zaki ZM. ABO blood group system and placental malaria in an area of unstable malaria transmission in eastern Sudan. Malar J. 2007;6:110.
24. Ali AA, Rayis DA, Abdallah TM, Elbashir MI, Adam I. Severe anaemia is associated with a higher risk for preeclampsia and poor perinatal outcomes in Kassala hospital, eastern Sudan. BMC Res Notes. 2011;4:311. https://doi.org/10.1186/1756-0500-4-311.
25. Moher D, Liberati A, Tetzlaff J, Altman DG, PRISMA Group. Preferred reporting items for systematic reviews and meta-analyses: the PRISMA statement. Ann Intern Med. 2009;151:264–9 W64. http://www.ncbi.nlm.nih.gov/pubmed/19622511. Accessed 15 Apr 2018.
26. Munn Z, Moola S, Lisy K, Rittano D. The systematic review of prevalence and incidence data. Joanna Briggs Inst Rev Man 2014 Ed / Suppl. 2014;1–37. http://joannabriggs.org/assets/docs/sumari/ReviewersManual_2014-The-Systematic-Review-of-Prevalence-and-Incidence-Data_v2.pdf. Accessed 15 Apr 2018.
27. Wells G, Shea B, O'Connell J, Robertson J, Peterson V, Welch V et al. full-text. NewcastleOttawa scale Assess Qual nonrandomised Stud meta-analysis Available http://www.ohrica/programs/clinical_epidemiology/oxfordasp Accessed June 21 2016.
28. Meta-Analyst O. Open Meta-Analyst - The Tool | Evidence Synthesis in Health. https://www.brown.edu/academics/public-health/research/evidence-synthesis-in-health/open-meta-analyst-tool. Accessed 17 Apr 2018.
29. Edwards A, Megens A, Peek M, Wallace EM. Sexual origins of placental dysfunction. Lancet (London, England). 2000;355:203–4. https://doi.org/10.1016/S0140-6736(99)05061-8.
30. Sedgwick P. Meta-analyses: heterogeneity and subgroup analysis. BMJ (Online). 2013;346:f4040. https://doi.org/10.1136/bmj.f4040.
31. Kassa GM, Muche AA, Berhe AK, Fekadu GA. Prevalence and determinants of anemia among pregnant women in Ethiopia; a systematic review and meta-analysis. BMC Hematol. 2017;17:17. https://doi.org/10.1186/s12878-017-0090-z.
32. Obai G, Odongo P, Wanyama R. Prevalence of anaemia and associated risk factors among pregnant women attending antenatal care in Gulu and Hoima regional hospitals in Uganda: a cross sectional study. BMC Pregnancy Childbirth. 2016;16:76. https://doi.org/10.1186/s12884-016-0865-4.
33. Stevens GA, Finucane MM, De-Regil LM, Paciorek CJ, Flaxman SR, Branca F, et al. Global, regional, and national trends in haemoglobin concentration and prevalence of total and severe anaemia in children and pregnant and non-pregnant women for 1995-2011: a systematic analysis of population-representative data. Lancet Glob Heal. 2013;1:e16–25. https://doi.org/10.1016/S2214-109X(13)70001-9.
34. Ethiopia Demographic and Health Survey. 2016. https://dhsprogram.com/pubs/pdf/FR328/FR328.pdf. Accessed 18 Apr 2018.
35. Lebso M, Anato A, Loha E. Prevalence of anemia and associated factors among pregnant women in southern Ethiopia: a community based cross-sectional study. PLoS One. 2017;12:e0188783. https://doi.org/10.1371/journal.pone.0188783.
36. Wessells K, Ouédraogo C, Young R, Faye M, Brito A, Hess S. Micronutrient status among pregnant women in Zinder, Niger and risk factors associated with deficiency. Nutrients. 2017;9:430. https://doi.org/10.3390/nu9050430.
37. Mengist HM, Zewdie O, Belew A. Intestinal helminthic infection and anemia among pregnant women attending ante-natal care (ANC) in east Wollega, Oromia, Ethiopia. BMC Res Notes. 2017;10:440. https://doi.org/10.1186/s13104-017-2770-y.
38. Ebuy Y, Alemayehu M, Mitiku M, Goba GK. Determinants of severe anemia among laboring mothers in Mekelle city public hospitals, Tigray region, Ethiopia. PLoS One. 2017;12:e0186724. https://doi.org/10.1371/journal.pone.0186724.
39. Abay A, Yalew HW, Tariku A, Gebeye E. Determinants of prenatal anemia in Ethiopia. Arch Public Health. 2017;75:51. https://doi.org/10.1186/s13690-017-0215-7.
40. Tadesse SE, Seid O, G/Mariam Y, Fekadu A, Wasihun Y, Endris K, et al. Determinants of anemia among pregnant mothers attending antenatal care in Dessie town health facilities, northern Central Ethiopia, unmatched case -control study. PLoS One. 2017;12:e0173173. https://doi.org/10.1371/journal.pone.0173173.
41. Asrie F. Prevalence of anemia and its associated factors among pregnant women receiving antenatal care at Aymiba Health Center, Northwest Ethiopia. J Blood Med. 2017;8:35–40. https://doi.org/10.2147/JBM.S134932.
42. Okafor IM, Okpokam DC, Antai AB, Usanga EA. Iron status of pregnant women in rural and urban communities of Cross River State, South-South Nigeria. Niger J Physiol Sci. 2017;31:121–5 http://www.ncbi.nlm.nih.gov/pubmed/28262847. Accessed 16 Apr 2018.
43. Gebreegziabher T, Stoecker BJ. Iron deficiency was not the major cause of anemia in rural women of reproductive age in Sidama zone, southern Ethiopia: a cross-sectional study. PLoS One. 2017;12:e0184742. https://doi.org/10.1371/journal.pone.0184742.
44. Gasim G, Deficiency IA-N, 2016 undefined. Malaria, Schistosomiasis, and Related Anemia. intechopen.com. https://www.intechopen.com/books/nutritional-deficiency/malaria-schistosomiasis-and-related-anemia. Accessed 21 Feb 2018.

A pilot study on the usefulness of peripheral blood flow cytometry for the diagnosis of lower risk myelodysplastic syndromes: the "MDS thermometer"

Ana Aires[1,3], Maria dos Anjos Teixeira[1,4,5], Catarina Lau[1,4,5], Cláudia Moreira[1], Ana Spínola[1], Alexandra Mota[1,3], Inês Freitas[2,4], Jorge Coutinho[1] and Margarida Lima[1,3,4,5*]

Abstract

Background: Immunophenotypic analysis of the bone marrow (BM) cells has proven to be helpful in the diagnosis of Myelodysplastic Syndromes (MDS). However, the usefulness of flow cytometry (FCM) for the detection of myelodysplasia in the peripheral blood (PB) still needs to be investigated. The aim of this pilot study was to evaluate the value of FCM-based PB neutrophil and monocyte immunophenotyping for the diagnosis of lower risk MDS (LR-MDS).

Methods: We evaluated by 8-color FCM the expression of multiple cell surface molecules (CD10, CD11b, CD11c, CD13, CD14, CD15, CD16, CD34, CD45, CD56, CD64 and HLA-DR) in PB neutrophils and monocytes from a series of 14 adult LR-MDS patients versus 14 normal individuals.

Results: Peripheral blood neutrophils from patients with LR-MDS frequently had low forward scatter (FSC) and side scatter (SSC) values and low levels of CD11b, CD11c, CD10, CD16, CD13 and CD45 expression, in that order, as compared to normal neutrophils. In addition, patients with LR-MDS commonly display a higher fraction of $CD14^{+}CD56^{+}$ and a lower fraction of $CD14^{+}CD16^{+}$ monocytes in the PB. Based on these results, we proposed an immunophenotyping score based on which PB samples from patients with LR-MDS could be distinguished from normal PB samples with a sensitivity 93% and a specificity of 100%. In addition, we used this score to construct the MDS Thermometer, a screening tool for detection and monitoring of MDS in the PB in clinical practice.

Conclusions: Peripheral blood neutrophil and monocyte immunophenotyping provide useful information for the diagnosis of LR-MDS, as a complement to cytomorphology. If validated by subsequent studies in larger series of MDS patients and extended to non-MDS patients with cytopenias, our findings may improve the diagnostic assessment and avoid invasive procedures in selected groups of MDS patients.

Keywords: Myelodysplastic syndromes, Lower risk MDS, Peripheral blood, Flow cytometry

* Correspondence: mmc.lima@clix.pt
[1]Department of Hematology, Hospital de Santo António (HSA), Centro Hospitalar do Porto (CHP), Porto, Portugal
[3]Instituto de Ciências Biomédicas Abel Salazar, Universidade do Porto (ICBAS/UP), Porto, Portugal
Full list of author information is available at the end of the article

Background

Myelodysplastic Syndromes (MDS) are a group of myeloid neoplasms characterized by inefficient hematopoiesis, peripheral blood (PB) cytopenias and high risk of leukemic progression [1–3]. According to World Health Organization (WHO) classification, lastly updated in 2016, the diagnosis is essentially based on morphological and cytogenetic abnormalities, such as the presence of cytopenias, blasts in the PB and/or bone marrow (BM), and dysplasia in one or more hematopoietic cell lineages [4, 5]. Although PB cytomorphological findings provide information to suspect of MDS, only BM studies are presently accepted to confirm the diagnosis [4, 5].

Five major MDS subtypes are currently recognized (WHO, 2016): MDS with single lineage dysplasia (MDS-SLD), MDS with multilineage dysplasia (MDS-MLD), MDS with ring sideroblasts (MDS-RS), MDS with isolated deletion of chromosome 5q [MDS-del(5q)], MDS with excess of blasts (MDS-EB), and MDS, unclassifiable (MDS-U) [5]. The International Prognostic Scoring System (IPSS), has been used to estimate risk for progression to acute myeloid leukemia (AML) or death from cytopenia-related complications. [6]. Patients categorized as low or intermediate-1 risk using the IPSS are usually referred to as "lower-risk" MDS (LR-MDS), whereas those classified as intermediate-2 or high risk are usually termed "higher-risk" MDS (LR-MDS). In its revised version, the IPSS incorporated new BM blast classes and cytogenetic abnormalities, and included both number and severity of cytopenias, thereby defining five (very low, low, intermediate, high and very high) risk categories, from which the first three correspond to LR-MDS [7]. In general, these include MDS-SLD, MDS-MLD, MDS-RS and MDS-del(5q).

Most of the LR-MDS patients, who account for around 60% of newly diagnosed MDS cases, remain simply on supportive care, being dependent on red blood cell (RBC) and/or platelet transfusions, and/or receiving hematopoietic growth factors; about 1/3 of the patients only require monitoring ("wait and see") [8]. HR-MDS patients may benefit from intensive treatments, although most of them are not eligible due to increased age and/or comorbidities, thereby being selected for low-intensity treatment regimens [8].

Flow cytometry (FCM) is a highly sensitive technique for evaluation of the hematopoietic cells. It has been used with increasing frequency to study the BM from patients with MDS, being considered a promising tool to improve MDS diagnosis, especially in cases of minimal dysplasia, absence of cytogenetic abnormalities, and BM hypocellularity or fibrosis [9–16]. Its value in the diagnosis of Chronic Myelomonocytic Leukemia (CMML) and other Myelodysplastic/myeloproliferative neoplasms (MDS/MPN) has also been documented [17–20].

Flow cytometry has an increasing importance in MDS diagnosis and subtyping, and in predicting the clinical outcome [15, 21]. However, a systematic histological and immuno-histochemical examination of the BM is still required for the final diagnosis and classification of MDS [22].

Several immunophenotypic abnormalities have been reported by FCM in the BM from MDS patients. Some examples are increased numbers of $CD34^+$ precursors, abnormal expression of cell surface molecules on myeloblasts, maturing granulocytic and monocytic cells, or erythroid precursors, and lineage infidelity [13]. For instance, phenotypic abnormalities of $CD34^+$ cells and their compartments have been reported in MDS, with LR-MDS patients typically having an expansion of myeloid $CD34^+$ cells at the expense of lymphoid B-cell precursors, while expansion of immature $CD34^+$ cells occurs in HR-MDS [11, 23]. Aberrant antigen expression (e.g., CD5, CD7 and CD56), and over or under expression of other cell surface markers (e.g. CD13, CD34, CD45, CD117 and HLA-DR) on $CD34^+$ myeloblasts have also been reported [12, 24].

Asynchronous shift to the left in maturing granulocytes is also frequent in the BM from patients with MDS, with neutrophil-precursors and maturing neutrophils having decreased size and granularity, and, consequently, a lower light scatter. Abnormal/Asynchronous expression of CD11b, CD13, CD15 and CD16 molecules has also been described, reflecting an anomalous neutrophil maturation [9, 10, 12]. Likewise, BM monocytes from MDS patients frequently have abnormal maturation patterns, as evaluated by the expression of CD14, CD34, CD36, CD64, and HLA-DR. Erythroid dysplasia has also been documented by FCM, by studying a set of molecules that are expressed differently throughout the maturation of RBC in the BM, such as CD35, CD36, CD44, CD45, CD71, CD105, CD117 and CD235a [9, 12, 25, 26].

Even though the collection of a PB sample is much simpler and much less invasive than a BM aspirate and/or biopsy, nearly all FCM studies in MDS patients have been performed in BM samples; the immunophenotypic alterations in PB cells have been much less explored [27–31].

Taking in consideration the accessibility of PB samples, it would be useful to establish FCM criteria for the diagnosis of myelodysplasia in the PB, especially in patients with LR-MDS. Therefore, the purpose of this study was to search the presence of abnormal and/or aberrant antigen expression in circulating neutrophils and monocytes from these patients. Based on the results obtained, a straightforward FCM-based scoring system is proposed, which allows to distinguish PB samples of patients with LR-MDS from normal PB samples with a high sensitivity and specificity. Using this scoring schema we, conceived the MDS Thermometer, a simple screening tool for detection and monitoring of MDS in the PB in clinical practice.

Methods

Study population and design

This study included 14 patients with LR-MDS, 8 males and 6 females, with a median age of 76 years, ranging from 66 to 88 years, that had been followed in the Hematology Department of Centro Hospitalar do Porto, Porto, Portugal, and that had at least one appointment at the hospital from September 2015 to November 2015.

An equal number of healthy controls (blood donors) were studied in parallel, 8 males and 6 females, with a median age of 55 years, ranging 19 to 63 years. First time donors, and donors with a history of infection in the previous 3 months and/or who have had neoplasms were excluded.

Clinical and laboratory data were retrospectively collected from the hospital records. Patients were considered to have anemia, neutropenia and thrombocytopenia if hemoglobin (Hg) < 12.5 g/dL, neutrophils < 2.000×10^6/L and platelets < 150×10^9/L, respectively.

The diagnosis and classification of MDS were established according to the WHO criteria, revised in 2016 [4, 5], after excluding other conditions that could potentially contribute to BM dysplasia and/or cytopenias. Only the following LR-MDS categories were included: MDS-SLD, MDS-MLD, MDS-RS and MDS-del(5q).

In order to avoid artefactual effects on neutrophil and monocyte immunophenotypes, patients who were being treated with granulocyte (G-CSF) or granulocyte-macrophage (GM-CSF) colony stimulating factors (CSF) at the time of the study or in the preceding 3 months were excluded, as did patients submitted to cytoreductive therapy, lenalidomide, hypomethylating and/or immunosuppressive treatments, and patients with concomitant infections or other neoplastic diseases. Previous or concomitant treatments with erythropoietin (EPO) and thrombopoietin receptor agonists were not exclusion criteria, neither did iron chelating therapies, vitamins or other nutrients.

The IPSS and the revised IPSS (IPSS-R) were calculated for all patients with MDS as previously described [6, 7]. Levels of Hg < 10.0 g/dL, neutrophils < 1800×10^6/L and platelets < 100×10^9/L were considered for risk stratification. The IPSS criteria were used to derive the karyotype-based risk classification [6].

Transfusion-related variables included the cumulative transfusion burden (total number of RBC units) and transfusion intensity (median number of RBC units/month). Transfusion-dependency was defined according to the WHO classification-based Prognostic Scoring System criteria [2].

Given the fact that elevated lactate dehydrogenase (LDH) has been associated with decreased overall survival [32], serum LDH levels were also evaluated. Moreover, as most patients with MDS were RBC transfusion-dependent [14, 33], and iron overload has been associated with worse prognosis in patients with LR-MDS [34], the serum ferritin levels were measured.

Bone marrow aspirate samples were used to prepare BM smears. These were stained with Leishman's stain, and cell morphology was analyzed by conventional light microscopy. In each case, a Perls' Prussian blue stain was performed. Other special stains were used whenever considered helpful. The acceptable quality of samples was defined according to the guidelines of the International Council for Standardization in Hematology [35]. Erythroid and granulocytic dysplasia were defined by the presence of ≥10% BM cells of the respective lineage with morphological alterations; presence of ≥15% ringed sideroblasts was also considered a diagnostic criteria for erythroid dysplasia. Megakaryocytic dysplasia was recognized by the presence of morphological abnormalities. Morphological features used for the definition of myeloblasts were those proposed by the International Working Group on Morphology of MDS [35], and the blast cell percentage was determined using the overall number of BM nucleated cells as denominator.

Bone marrow biopsy specimens were fixed in neutral-buffered formalin or Bouin's fixative solution, decalcified, and embedded in paraffin-wax. Standard routine stains included hematoxylin & eosin and/or Giemsa, and Gömöri's silver stain for the evaluation of BM fibrosis [36]. Immunohistochemistry was done in specific cases. The BM cellularity was estimated based on the age-adapted normal values [36], and dysmyelopoiesis was evaluated as previously described [37, 38].

Cytogenetics studies were performed in BM aspirates, either by conventional cytogenetics and/or fluorescence in situ hybridization (FISH). Conventional cytogenetics was performed on direct and 24- to 48-h unstimulated BM cultures, analyzed following trypsin Giemsa banding; 20 metaphases were evaluated. In FISH studies, VYSIS DNA FISH probes (Abbott Molecular Inc., IL, USA) were used to detect numeric and structural abnormalities on chromosomes 5, 7 and 20, and numeric abnormalities on chromosomes 8 and X. Two hundred interphase nuclei were counted. Cytogenetic classification was performed by grouping patients according to Schanz et al. [39].

Flow cytometry studies

Peripheral blood samples were collected into ethylene-diamine-tetra-acetic acid tripotassium salt containing tubes and processed within 24 h after collection.

Cell immunophenotyping was performed by 8-color FCM using fluorochrome conjugated monoclonal antibodies (mAbs) with different specificities (Table 1). These mAbs were combined in two different tubes, conceived to quantify immature CD34$^+$ cell in the PB and to evaluate cell surface antigen expression in circulating neutrophils (mostly tube 1) and monocytes (mostly tube 2) (Table 2). A normal PB sample was run in parallel with each patient PB sample.

Cell staining was done using a whole blood stain-lyse-and-then-wash method, and the BD FACS™ Lysing Solution, according to the instructions of the manufacturer.

Sample acquisition was performed in a BD FACSCanto II™ flow cytometer. Forward scatter (FSC) and side scatter (SSC) were captured on a linear scale, and SSC was represented with a mathematical transformation (Exp-SSC-Low). For fluorescence parameters, a logarithmic amplification was used, with logical transformation. At least 200,000 cell events per tube were recorded and stored as flow cytometry standard (.fcs) 3.0 files.

Flow cytometer set-up and calibration was performed accordingly to the Euroflow consortium Standard Operating Procedures [40], available in [41]. Daily control was monitored by plotting fluorescence intensity values in Levy Jennings charts. External quality assessment/proficiency testing was performed by participating in the Euroflow Quality Assurance program [42].

Flow cytometry data analysis was done using the Infinicyt™ software (Cytognos, Salamanca, Spain). Neutrophils, monocytes and blast cells were identified and classified according to their SSC and FSC characteristics and antigen expression profiles, as described in Fig. 1.

Table 1 Specificities, clones, isotypes, fluorochromes and manufacturers of the monoclonal antibodies used in this study

Antigen	Clone	Isotype	Fluorochrome	Manufacturer
CD10	ALB1	IgG2a	PE-Cy7	BC-IOT
CD11b	D12	IgG2a	APC	BDB
CD11c	S-HCL-3	IgG2b	APC	BDB
CD13	L138	IgG1	PE	BDB
CD14	HCD14	IgG1	APC-H7	BL
CD15	MMA	IgM	FITC	BDB
CD16	3G8	IgG1	V450	BDH
CD34	8G12	IgG1	PerCP-Cy5.5	BDB
CD45	J.33	IgG1	KO	BC-IOT
CD56	N901-HLDA6	IgG1	PE-Cy7	BC-IOT
CD64	22	IgG1	PE	BC-IOT
HLA-DR	L243	IgG2a	FITC	BDB

Abbreviations: *APC* allophycocyanin, *Cy5.5* Cyanine 5.5, *Cy7* Cyanine 7, *FITC* Fluorescein, isothiocyanate, *KO* Khrome Orange, *PE* Phycoerythrin, *PerCP* Peridinin chlorophyll protein, *V450* Violet 450, *BC* Beckman Coulter, *BDB* Becton Dickinson Bioscience, *BDH* Becton Dickinson Horizon, *BL* Biolegend, *IOT* Immunotech

Monocytes were further subdivided into classical (CD14^{+high}CD16$^-$), intermediate (CD14^{+high}CD16$^+$) and proinflammatory (CD14^{+low}CD16$^+$) monocytes. Non-classical (CD14$^+$CD16$^+$, intermediate + proinflammatory) monocyte subsets were considered together in succeeding analysis. Neutrophils and monocytes were analyzed for the levels of expression of CD10, CD11b, CD11c, CD13, CD15, CD16, CD56, CD64, and HLA-DR, by recording the median fluorescence intensity (MedFI) for each marker. The relative representation of CD14$^+$CD16$^-$ and CD14$^+$CD16$^+$ monocyte subsets and the percentage of CD56$^+$ monocytes were also recorded.

The FSC/SSC values and MedFI values obtained in neutrophils and monocytes from patients with LR-MDS were considered abnormal when they were out of the mean value ±2 standard deviations (SD) of the same parameter obtained in PB neutrophils and monocytes from healthy individuals.

Immunophenotypic scores for myelodysplasia

Neutrophil scores

Two different scoring schemas were used for neutrophils. The scoring schema type 1 was based only on the number of abnormally low parameters found in PB neutrophils (below the mean-2SD of the values found for the same parameter in normal PB neutrophils). The scoring schema type 2 took into account both the number of abnormally low parameters and the severity of each parameter deficiency, as previously described [11, 23].

In both cases, values within the mean ± 2SD or above the mean + 2SD were scored with "0", and in both cases only 8 of the parameters analyzed (FSC, SSC, CD10, CD11b, CD11c, CD13, CD16 and CD45) were considered for scoring. The neutrophil score, ranging from 0 to 8 in both cases, was calculated for each patient by adding up the scores obtained for each of the 8 parameters evaluated. Three groups corresponding to an overall score of "0", 1 and ≥2 were arbitrarily considered equivalent to "no neutrophil dysplasia", "possible neutrophil dysplasia" and "neutrophil dysplasia", respectively. Cases with a neutrophil score ≥ 2 were subsequently arbitrarily classified as having mild (scores 2 and 3), moderate (scores 4, 5 and 6) and severe (scores 7 and 8) neutrophil dysplasia, respectively.

Neutrophil scoring schema 1 Each abnormally low parameter (below the mean-2SD) was scored with 1 point.

Neutrophil scoring schema 2 Values of 0.25, 0.5 or 1.0 were given when the MedFI value obtained for each of the phenotypic variables evaluated were between the mean-2SD and the mean-3SD, between the mean-3SD and the mean-4 SD, or below the mean-4SD of the

Table 2 Eight color-combinations of the fluorochrome-conjugated monoclonal antibodies used in this study

Tubes	FITC	PE	PerCP-Cy5	PE-Cy7	APC	APC-H7	V450	KO
1	CD15	CD13	CD34	CD10	CD11b	CD14	CD16	CD45
2	HLA-DR	CD64	CD34	CD56	CD11c	CD14	CD16	CD45

Abbreviations: *APC* allophycocyanin, *Cy5.5* Cyanine 5.5, *Cy7* Cyanine 7, *FITC* Fluorescein, isothiocyanate, *KO* Khrome Orange, *PE* Phycoerythrin, *PerCP* Peridinin chlorophyll protein, *V450* Violet 450

values found for the same parameter in normal PB neutrophils, respectively.

Monocyte scores

For monocytes, only the percentages of $CD14^+CD56^+$ and $CD14^+CD16^+$ monocytes on total monocytes were used to calculate the FCM monocyte score for myelodysplasia. Aberrant high CD56 expression was defined as a percentage of $CD56^+$ cells exceeding the mean + 2SD of the values found in normal PB monocytes. Abnormal low CD16 expression was defined as a percentage of $CD14^+CD16^+$ monocytes of less than 5% of total monocytes. Depletion of non-classical monocytes was arbitrarily considered mild, moderate or severe when $CD14^+CD16^+$ cells accounted for less than 5%, 2.5% and 1.25% of total monocytes, respectively. The overall monocyte score, ranging from 0 to 2, was calculated for each patient by adding up the scores obtained for each of the 2 parameters evaluated.

As described for neutrophils, two different scoring schemas were used for monocytes: scoring schema type 1, based only on the number abnormal parameters found in PB monocytes, and scoring schema type 2, taking into account both the number of abnormal parameters and the severity of each parameter abnormality. The monocyte score, ranging from 0 to 2, was calculated for each patient by adding up the scores obtained for each of the 2 parameters evaluated. Three groups corresponding to an overall score of 0, 1 and 2, were arbitrarily considered equivalent to "no monocyte dysplasia", "possible monocyte dysplasia" and "monocyte dysplasia", respectively.

Monocyte scoring schema 1 Each abnormal parameter (percentage of $CD56^+$ cells exceeding the mean + 2SD

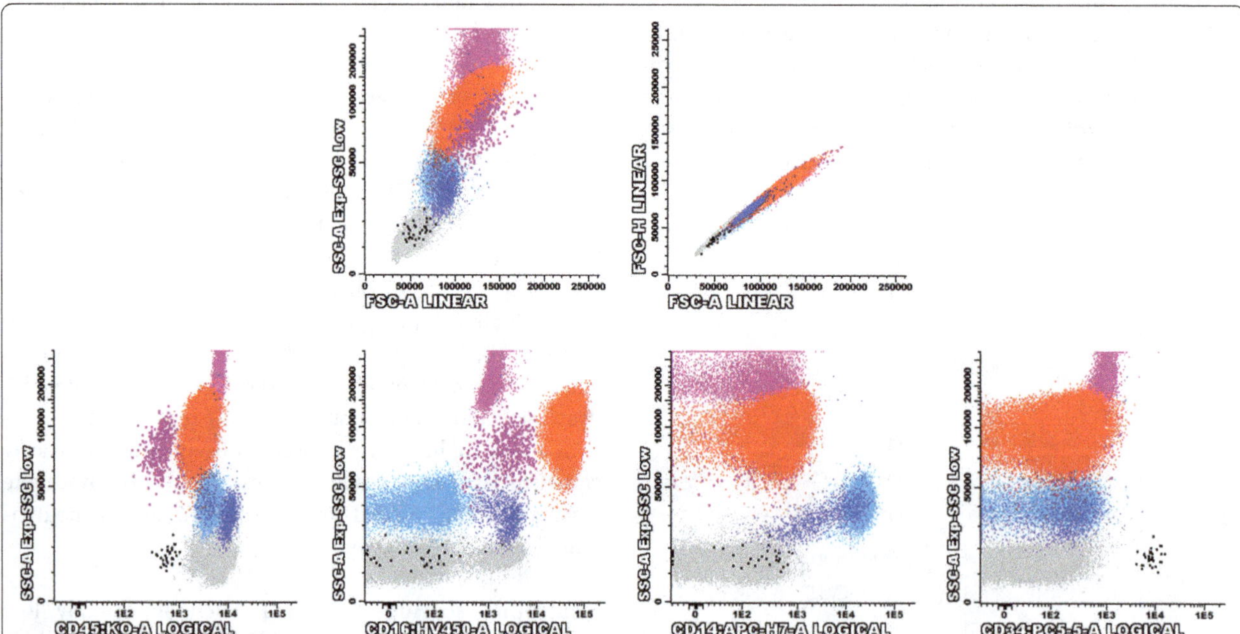

Fig. 1 Bivariate dot-plots obtained from a normal PB sample, illustrating the analysis procedure used for the immunophenotypic identification, quantification and characterization of neutrophils, monocytes, and $CD34^+$ cells, after excluding cell debris and doublets. Neutrophils (red dots; 61.16%) were selected based on their SSC/FSC characteristics and $CD45^{+low}CD16^{+high}$ expression. Monocytes (blue dots; 7.64%) were selected based on SSC/FSC and $CD45^{+int}CD14^+$ expression; subsequently, monocytes were separated into classical (light blue dots; 6.88%) and non-classical (either intermediate $CD14^{+high}CD16^+$ or proinflammatory $CD14^{+low}CD16^+$, dark blue dots; 0.76%) monocyte subsets. Immature CD34+ cells (black dots, 0.02%) were identified based on SSC/FSC and $CD45^{+low}CD34^+$ expression. Other cells: eosinophils (pink dots; 4.93%); immature granulocytes, including promyelocytes, myelocytes and metamyelocytes (purple dots; 0.27%); lymphocytes and basophils (gray dots; 25.97%). Abbreviations: FSC, forward scatter; PB, peripheral blood; SSC, side scatter

and percentage of $CD16^+$ cells < 5%) was scored with 1 point.

Monocyte scoring system 2 Values of 0.25, 0.5 or 1 were given when the % of $CD56^+$ monocytes were between the mean + 2SD and the mean + 3SD, between the mean + 3SD and the mean + 4 SD, or above the mean + 4SD of the values found for the same parameter among normal PB monocytes, respectively. Values of 0.25, 0.5 or 1 were assumed when the percentages of $CD16^+$ monocytes were between the 2.5 and 5.0%, between 1.25% and 2.5% and below 1.25%, respectively.

Myeloid immunophenotypic scores

Two myeloid immunophenotypic MDS scores, type 1 and type 2, both ranging from 0 to 10, were obtained for each patient by adding up the correspondent neutrophil and monocytic MDS scores. Three groups corresponding to overall scores of "0", 1 and ≥2 were arbitrarily considered equivalent to "no myelodysplasia", "possible myelodysplasia" and "myelodysplasia", respectively. Cases with a myeloid score ≥ 2 were subsequently classified as having mild (scores 2 to 4), moderate (scores 5 to 7) and severe (scores 8 to 10) myelodysplasia, respectively.

MDS thermometer

The MDS Thermometer was conceived as a screening tool for detection and monitoring of MDS in clinical practice. It consists in a visual analogue scale rated from 0 to 10 points (myeloid thermometer) with two domains (neutrophil thermometer, rated from 0 to 8, and monocyte thermometer, rated from 0 to 2) based on the immunophenotypic scores defined above. For simplicity, only the neutrophil and monocyte scoring schemas type 1 were used to construct the MDS Thermometer presented in this paper. The concept was based on the Emotion Thermometers Tool, created by Alex J Mitchell [43, 44].

Statistical analysis

Results were expressed as absolute and relative frequencies, or as mean, median, SD, minimum and maximum values. Results obtained in PB samples of MDS patients were compared with those obtained in control PB samples. The non-parametric Mann-Whitney U test was used to compare the MedFI observed for each marker in PB neutrophils and monocytes from MDS patients and controls, as well as to compare blood cell counts at the time of the study with those at diagnosis. P values < 0.05 were considered statistically significant. All statistical analyses were performed using the SOFA Statistics version 1.4.5 (Paton-Simpson & Associates Ltd., Auckland, New Zealand).

Results

Study population

Table 3 summarizes the demographic, clinical and laboratory data of the study population. Detailed data can be found in Supplementary Material (Additional file 1: Table S1).

According to the WHO criteria, 6 patients were classified as MDS-RS, 4 patients had MDS-SLD, 3 patients had MDS-MLD, and 1 patient was classified as MDS-isolated 5q- (Table 3).

Using the IPSS, all patients were categorized as LR-MDS: 8 patients had low IPSS risk and 6 patients had intermediate 1 IPSS risk (Table 3).

Cytogenetic based stratification revealed good or intermediate risk in 9 cases and 1 case, respectively (Table 3).

Table 3 MDS categories and risk stratification of the patients included in this study

Diagnosis (WHO 2016)[a]	
MDS-RS	6/14 (43%)
MDS-SLD	4/14 (29%)
MDS-MLD	3/14 (21%)
MDS-del(5q)	1/14 (7%)
International Prognostic Scoring System (IPSS)	
IPSS score	0.3 ± 0.4; 0 (0–1.0)
Score = 0.0	8/14 (57%)
Score = 0.5	3/14 (21%)
Score = 1.0	3/14 (21%)
Score > 1.0	0/14 (0%)
IPSS risk groups	
Low risk	8/14 (57%)
Intermediate risk 1	6/14 (43%)
Intermediate risk 2	0/14 (0%)
High risk	0/14 (0%)
Cytogenetic based risk classification[b]	
Very good	0/10 (0%)
Good	9/10 (90%)
Intermediate	1/10 (10%)
Poor	0/10 (0%)
Very poor	0/10 (0%)

Abbreviations: *IPSS* International Prognostic Scoring System, *MDS* myelodysplastic syndromes, *MDS-del(5q)* MDS with isolated deletion of chromosome 5q, *MDS-MLD* MDS with multilineage dysplasia, *MDS-RS* MDS with ring sideroblasts, *MDS-SLD* MDS with single lineage dysplasia, *WHO* World Health Organization

Results are expressed as absolute and (relative) frequencies

[a] Patients with MDS unclassifiable or with ≥20% blast in the BM were omitted, as did patients with MDS with excess of blasts, and patients diagnosed with Myelodysplastic/myeloproliferative neoplasms

[b] Cytogenetic scoring: Very good: -Y, del(11q); Good: normal, del(5q), del(12p), del(20q), double including del(5q); Intermediate: del(7q), + 8, + 19, i(17q), any other single or double independent clones; Poor: −7, inv.(3)/t(3q), del3q, double including − 7/del(7q), complex (3 abnormalities); Very poor: complex (> 3 abnormalities)

Overall, metaphase cytogenetics and/or interphase FISH testing for − 5/5q-, − 7/7q-, + 8, and 20q-, identified in cytogenetic aberrancies in only 2 out 10 cases (20%), corresponding to isolated del(5q) (1 patient) and isolated monosomy 8 (1 case); cytogenetic data were unavailable in 4 cases (Additional file 1: Table S1).

The median time from the diagnosis was 7.6 years, ranging from 0.5 to 12.6 years.

At diagnosis, all the MDS patients had anemia, but only 5 (36%) had neutropenia and only 4 (29%) had thrombocytopenia (Additional file 1: Table S1). The median values of the Hg levels, and neutrophil and platelet counts were of 9.1 g/dl, 2567×10^6/L, and 200×10^9/L ranging from 7.2 to 11.9, 575 to 7025 and 61 to 591, respectively. Abnormal RBC morphology in the PB smears were present in all cases, whereas abnormal neutrophil and/or platelet morphological features were observed in 4 patients (29%) each. At the time of the study, the Hg levels were significantly lower than those observed at the diagnosis ($p =$ 0.006), despite of RBC transfusions; no statistically significant differences were found for the neutrophil and platelet counts, neither for the percentage of blasts in the PB ($p >$ 0.05). In addition, although a higher fraction of patients had neutropenia and/or thrombocytopenia, as compared to that observed at diagnosis, differences were also not statistically significant (p > 0.05) (Additional file 1: Table S1 footnote).

Most patients had received RBC transfusions, and most of them had been treated with hematopoietic growth factors at some point during the course of the disease (Additional file 1: Table S1). Concerning blood transfusions, 13 patients (93%) had received at least one RBC unit, and eleven (79%) had been regularly transfused (transfusion-dependent). The median number of RBC units received per transfused patient was of 57, ranging from 15 to 462, and a median number of RBC transfused per patient/month was of 1.4, ranging from 0.3 to 4.0 (Additional file 1: Table S1). The mean ferritin serum levels were of 1854 ± 1126 ng/ml, with 93% of the patients showing increased serum ferritin values, compatible with iron overload. None of the patients was receiving iron-chelating therapies. In addition, none was medicated with myeloid growth factors (exclusion criteria), although 5 patients had been treated with G-CSF in the past. Only 2 patients were being treated with EPO at the time of the study, although most of them had previously received EPO. No patients had ever received GM-CSF or thrombopoietin receptor agonists. Increased serum LDH levels were seen in only 3 cases (23%), at the time of the study (Additional file 1: Table S1).

Flow cytometry studies

Peripheral blood neutrophils

Neutrophils from patients with LR-MDS had lower FSC and SSC values as compared with controls ($p = 0.008$ and $p < 0.001$, respectively) (Figs. 2 and 3, and Additional file 2: Table S2).

In addition, neutrophils from patients with LR-MDS had significantly decreased expression of CD10 ($p <$ 0.001), CD11b ($p < 0.001$), CD11c ($p < 0.001$), CD13 ($p =$ 0.022) and CD16 ($p = 0.002$) when compared to normal individuals. No statistically significant differences were observed for CD15 and CD45 expression ($p > 0.05$), although both markers had a slight reduction in fluorescence intensity in patients, as compared to controls.

When analyzed individually, neutrophils from most LR-MDS patients had abnormally low FSC and/or SSC (71% and 57% of cases, respectively) (Table 4). Among the cell surface molecules evaluated, CD11b, CD11c, CD10, CD16, CD13 and CD45 were the most frequently affected, in that order; the percentage of cases showing reduced levels of expression of these molecules were of 71%, 71%, 64%, 43%, 29% and 14%, respectively (Table 4). Overall, 13 patients (93%) had abnormally low expression of 2 or more (out of 9) molecules on neutrophils, with 7 patients (50%) having abnormally low expression of 5 or more parameters. In addition, 4 cases had abnormally high expression of CD10, CD11b, CD13 or CD45 on circulating neutrophils (1 case each).

In contrast, abnormal levels of cell surface molecules were found in only 4 controls, and the phenotypic abnormalities were restricted to one parameter in all cases (abnormally high CD11b levels: $n = 1$; abnormally high CD15 levels: n = 1; abnormally low CD15 levels: n = 1; abnormally low CD45 levels: n = 1).

The only patient with a normal neutrophil immunophenotype was a 75 year-old female classified as having MDS-SLD, who had mild macrocytic anemia (Hg 9.0 g/dL, MCV 104.1 fL) and mild thrombocytopenia (platelet count of 100×10^6/L). The BM was hypocellular, with 5.3% blast cells, increased myeloid/erythroid ratio (3.9) and mild dyserythropoiesis, with normal myeloid and megakaryocytic lineages. BM cytogenetics have revealed a 46,XX karyotype with 3 metaphases with non-clonal aneuploidies. The time from the diagnosis was of 31 months, the patient had been occasionally transfused (total of 3 RBC units), and the cytopenias have remained stable over time.

When the healthy controls were separated in two groups according to age (< 55 years old, $n = 7$ versus ≥ 55 years old, n = 7), we did not observe statistically significant differences for any of the parameters analyzed on neutrophils; also, no differences were found between males and females ($p > 0.05$ in all cases).

Peripheral blood monocytes

In general, monocytes from patients with LR-MDS had light scatter properties similar to the monocytes from normal individuals (p > 0.05) (Fig. 4 and Additional file 3:

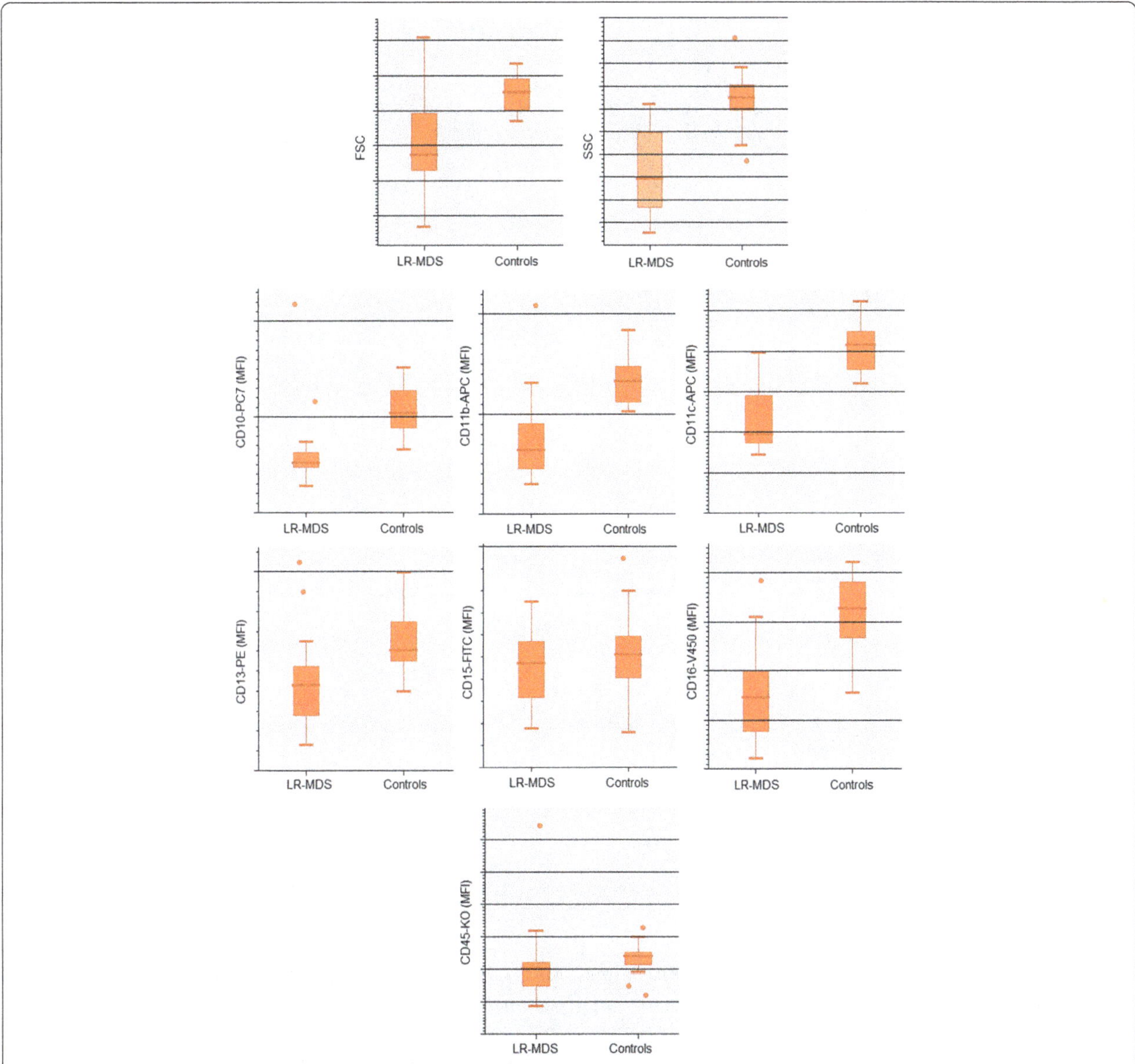

Fig. 2 FSC, SSC and surface antigen expression in PB neutrophils from patients with LR-MDS and healthy individuals (controls). Results as expressed as arbitrary units of fluorescence intensity. Lower whiskers are 1.5 times the Inter-Quartile Range below the lower quartile, or the minimum value, whichever is closest to the middle. Upper whiskers are calculated using the same approach. Outliers are displayed. Abbreviations: FSC, forward scatter; LR-MDS, lower risk myelodysplastic syndromes; MFI, median fluorescence intensity; PB, peripheral blood; SSC, side scatter

Table S3). In the same way, the overall levels of CD13, CD14, CD15, CD45 and CD64 expression on monocytes did not differ significantly from those observed in controls ($p > 0.05$). However, monocytes from patients with LR-MDS had significantly higher levels of CD56 ($p = 0.006$), and lower levels of CD11c ($p = 0.004$), CD16 ($p = 0.005$) and HLA-DR ($p = 0.042$), and showed a tendency for a lower CD11b expression ($p = 0.089$), as compared to controls.

Despite of the above-mentioned differences between monocytes from LR-MDS patients and controls, the individual analysis of the analyzed cell surface markers on monocytes was much less informative than that found in neutrophils, with an abnormal monocyte immunophenotype being found in only a limited number of cases.

One of the most consistent aberrancies found in MDS monocytes consisted in abnormally high levels of CD56 expression, observed in 6 cases (43%), with increased percentages of $CD56^+$ monocytes. In accordance, monocytes from LR-MDS patients had significantly higher percentages of $CD56^+$ cells, as compared to normal individuals (median values of 15% and 7%, ranging from 0 to 99% and from 0 to 15%, respectively; $p = 0.026$) (Fig. 5 and Table 5). Increased percentages of $CD14^+CD56^+$ monocytes (> 18%) were found in 6 (43%) MDS patients but in none of the healthy individuals, and in most of

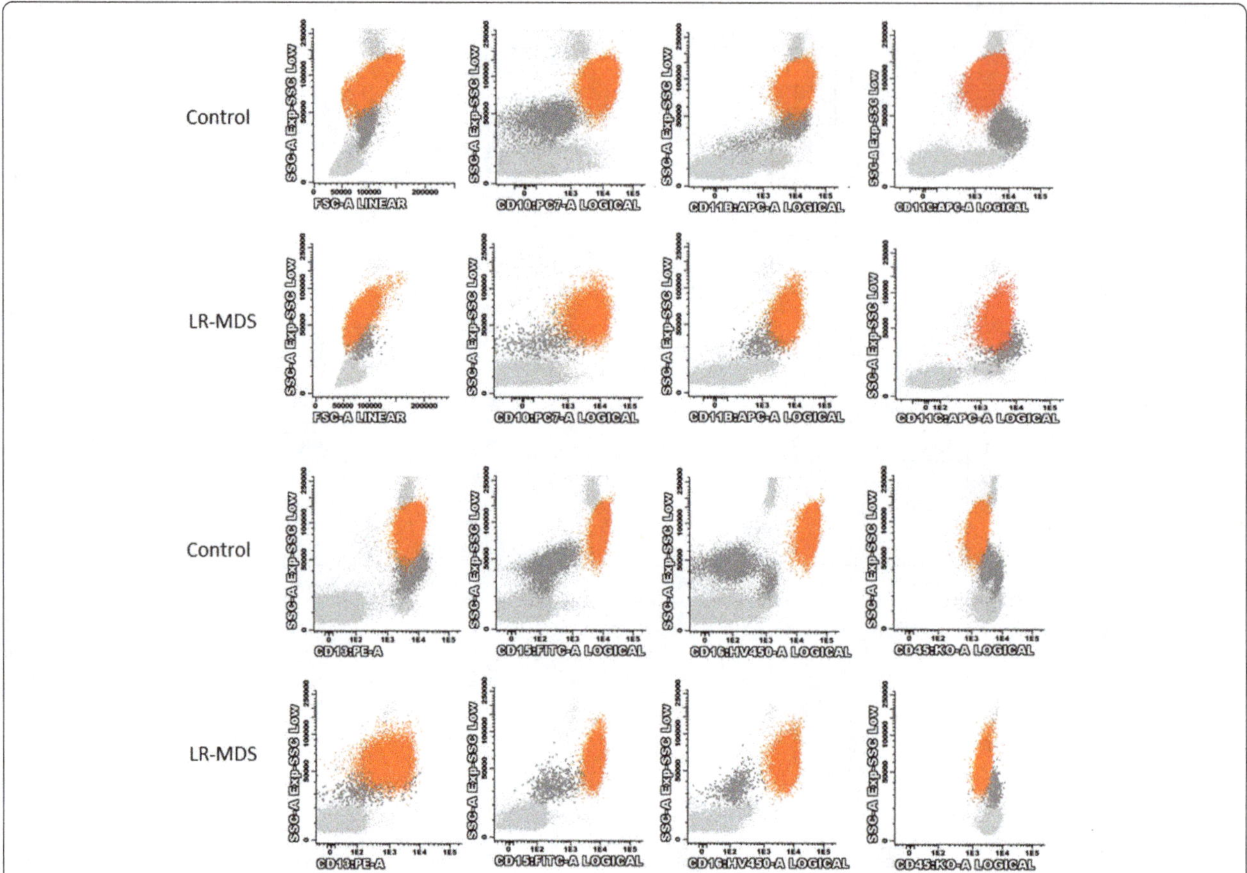

Fig. 3 Bivariate SSC/FSC, SSC/CD10, SSC/CD11b, SSC/CD11c, SSC/CD13, SSC/CD15, SSC/CD16 and SSC/CD45 dot plots illustrating the decreased FSC/SSC and the diminished expression of cell surface molecules (CD10, CD11b, CD13 and CD16) in the PB neutrophils (red dots) from one patient with LR-MDS, as compared to a healthy individual (control). Red dots, neutrophils; light gray dots, lymphocytes and eosinophils; dark gray dots, monocytes. Abbreviations: FSC, forward scatter; LR-MDS, lower risk myelodysplastic syndromes; PB, peripheral blood; SSC, side scatter

the patients (4, 29%), $CD14^+CD56^+$ monocytes were markedly increased (> 28%). CD56 expression was mainly observed on classical $CD14^{+high}CD16^-$ monocytes (Fig. 5, panel B).

Another recurrent aberrancy observed in LR-MDS patients consisted in a marked decrease in the fraction of $CD14^+CD16^+$ monocytes, comparatively to controls (median values of 3% and 12%, ranging from 0 to 8% and from 4 to 28%, in patients and in controls, respectively; $p < 0.001$) (Fig. 5 and Table 5). In overall, 9 patients (64%) had decreased percentages of $CD14^+CD16^+$ monocytes (< 5%), when compared to only 2 (14%) of the controls. Curiously, the severity of the deficiency was higher in patients than in controls, with 50% of the patients, but none of the controls, having a moderate (< 2.5%) or severe (< 1.25%) deficiencies of $CD14^+CD16^+$ monocytes.

Finally, abnormally low CD11b and HLA-DR expression was found in 5 (36%) and 4 (28%) patients, respectively. Less frequent findings included abnormally low levels of CD45 (2 patients, 14%), and decreased CD11c and CD64 expression (1 case each, 7%); moreover, abnormally high levels of CD14 and CD64 were found in 2 cases each, and abnormally high levels of CD11b in only 1 case; cases with abnormal CD13 expression were not found.

When the healthy volunteers aged 55 years or over were compared to those who were younger than 55 years, we observed a tendency for a lower intensity of CD14 expression in monocytes ($p = 0.064$), and a higher percentage of proinflammatory ($CD16^+$) monocytes in the first group (median values of 13.2% and 5.9%, respectively; $p = 0.035$). The other parameters analyzed did not show statistically significant differences between the "youngest" and "oldest" individuals, neither between males and females ($p > 0.05$).

Circulating immature cells

Immature $CD34^+$ cells represented 0.15 ± 0.28% of the WBC in the PB from LR-MDS patients (median value of 0.05%, ranging from 0.01 to 1.05%), as compared to 0.03 ± 0.01% (median value of 0.03%, ranging from 0.01 to

Table 4 Type and frequency of immunophenotypic aberrancies detected in PB neutrophils from LR-MDS patients versus normal individuals (controls)

	LR-MDS (n = 14)		Controls (*n* = 14)	
	Decreased	Increased	Decreased	Increased
Abnormal light scatter characteristics				
FSC	10 (71%)	1 (7%)	0 (0%)	0 (0%)
SSC	8 (57%)	0 (0%)	0 (0%)	1 (7%)
Abnormal expression of cell surface markers				
CD10	9 (64%)	1 (7%)	0 (0%)	0 (0%)
CD11b	10 (71%)	1 (7%)	0 (0%)	1 (7%)
CD11c	10 (71%)	0 (0%)	0 (0%)	0 (0%)
CD13	4 (29%)	1 (7%)	0 (0%)	0 (0%)
CD15	0 (0%)	0 (0%)	1 (7%)	1 (7%)
CD16	6 (43%)	0 (0%)	0 (0%)	0 (0%)
CD45	2 (14%)	1 (7%)	1 (7%)	0 (0%)
Number of individuals with abnormal parameters				
No abnormal parameters	1 (7%)	10 (71%)	12 (86%)	11 (79%)
One abnormal parameter	0 (0%)	3 (21%)	2 (14%)	3 (21%)
Two abnormal parameters	2 (14%)	1 (7%)	0 (0%)	0 (0%)
Three abnormal parameters	1 (7%)	0 (0%)	0 (0%)	0 (0%)
Four abnormal parameters	3 (21%)	0 (0%)	0 (0%)	0 (0%)
Five abnormal parameters	4 (29%)	0 (0%)	0 (0%)	0 (0%)
Six abnormal parameters	2 (14%)	0 (0%)	0 (0%)	0 (0%)
Seven abnormal parameters	0 (0%)	0 (0%)	0 (0%)	0 (0%)
Eight abnormal parameters	1 (7%)	0 (0%)	0 (0%)	0 (0%)
Nine abnormal parameters	0 (0%)	0 (0%)	0 (0%)	0 (0%)

Abbreviations: *LR-MDS* lower risk myelodysplastic syndromes, *PB* peripheral blood
Results are expressed as absolute and (relative) frequencies
Percentages were approximated to the closest full unit

0.04%) in normal individuals. These cells had low SSC and FSC, they were CD45^{+low}, CD34^{+}, CD13^{+}, CD117$^{-/+}$, HLA-DR^{+}, and they virtually fail to express all the other molecules analyzed (CD10, CD11b, CD11c, CD15 and CD16) (data not shown).

Patients with MDS also had increased numbers of circulating immature granulocytes (promyelocytes, myelocytes and metamyelocytes) (1.17 ± 2.03%, with a median value of 0.36%, ranging from 0.06 to 7.72%), as compared to controls (0.11 ± 0.06%; median value of 0.11%, ranging from 0.02 to 0.21%). These cells were SSC^{high}, FSC^{high}, CD45^{+low}, CD15^{+} and CD64^{+}, and they had variable and low CD11b and CD16 expression, being negative for the remaining molecules tested (CD10, CD11c, CD13, CD34, CD56, CD117, HLA-DR) (data not shown).

Differences between patients and controls reached statistical significance for circulating immature granulocytes ($p < 0.001$), but not for immature CD34^{+} cells ($p = 0.056$).

Immunophenotypic scores

As mentioned above, we defined two FCM-based scorings systems (type 1 and 2) to evaluate dysplasia in neutrophils and monocytes, and, for each scoring system, a total myeloid score was calculated. The results obtained are summarized in Tables 6 and 7, respectively.

Immunophenotypic scoring schema 1

Neutrophil score type 1

The mean neutrophil score type 1 obtained in LR-MDS patients was of 4 ± 2, ranging from "0" to 8 (total score rank = 59), while all controls had a score of 1 or lower (total score rank = 1), with only 1 case having a score = 1, corresponding to a normal individual whose neutrophils had dimmer CD45 expression (Table 6). According to this score, four groups of MDS patients were identified: score of "0", no neutrophil dysplasia ($n = 1$, corresponding to the patient with a normal neutrophil immunophenotype mentioned above); score of 1, possible neutrophil dysplasia ($n = 0$); score of between 2 and

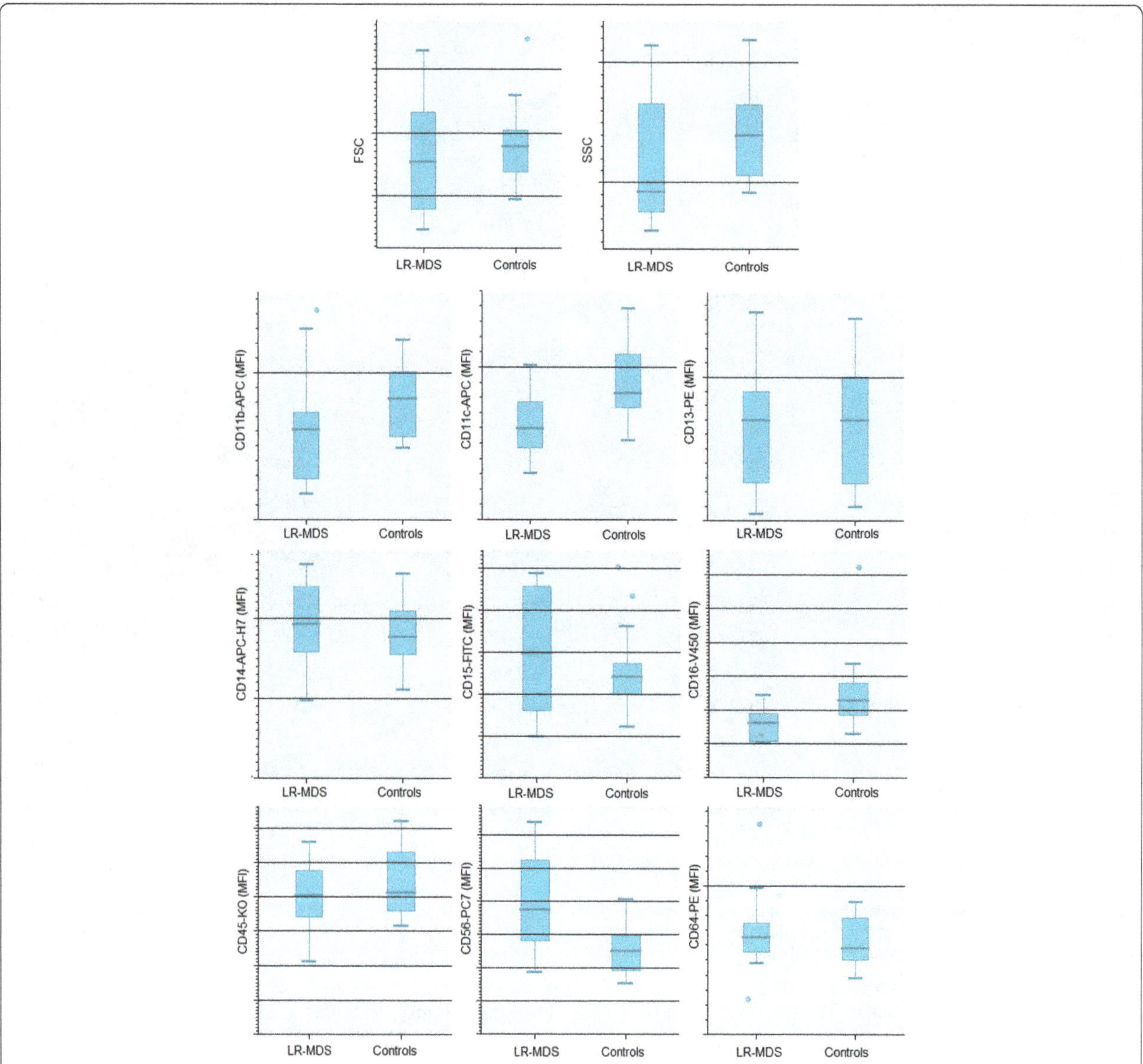

Fig. 4 FSC, SSC and surface antigen expression in PB monocytes from patients with LR-MDS and healthy individuals (controls). Results as expressed as arbitrary units of fluorescence intensity. Lower whiskers are 1.5 times the Inter-Quartile Range below the lower quartile, or the minimum value, whichever is closest to the middle. Upper whiskers are calculated using the same approach. Outliers are displayed. Abbreviations: FSC, forward scatter; LR-MDS, lower risk myelodysplastic syndromes; MFI, median fluorescence intensity; PB, peripheral blood; SSC, side scatter

3, mild neutrophil dysplasia ($n = 3$; 21%); score between 4 and 6, moderate neutrophil dysplasia ($n = 9$; 64%); and score over 6, severe neutrophil dysplasia ($n = 1$; 7%). Thus, assuming a cut-off of >1 points we correctly classified 13 out of 14 LR-MDS patients and 14 out of 14 controls, given a sensitivity of 93% and a specificity of 100% for the diagnosis of MDS.

Monocyte score type 1

The monocytic score type 1 obtained in LR-MDS patients ranged from 0 to 2 (median 1; mean ± SD of 1 ± 1), whereas the score observed in controls ranged from 0 to 1 (Table 6). The total score rank for these groups was of 15 and 2, respectively. Using this score, four groups of MDS patients were identified: score of "0", no monocyte dysplasia ($n = 2$; 14%); score of 1, possible monocyte dysplasia ($n = 8$; 57%); and score of 2, monocyte dysplasia ($n = 4$; 29%). Comparatively, 12 out of 14 controls (86%) had a score of "0", and the remaining 2 cases had a score of 1, due to moderate decrease in the fraction of $CD14^{+}CD16^{+}$ monocytes (4.9% and 4.1% of total monocytes, respectively). Consequently, assuming a cut-off of ≥1 points we correctly categorized 12 out of 14 LR-MDS patients and 12 out of 14 controls, given a sensitivity and a specificity of 86% for the diagnosis of MDS.

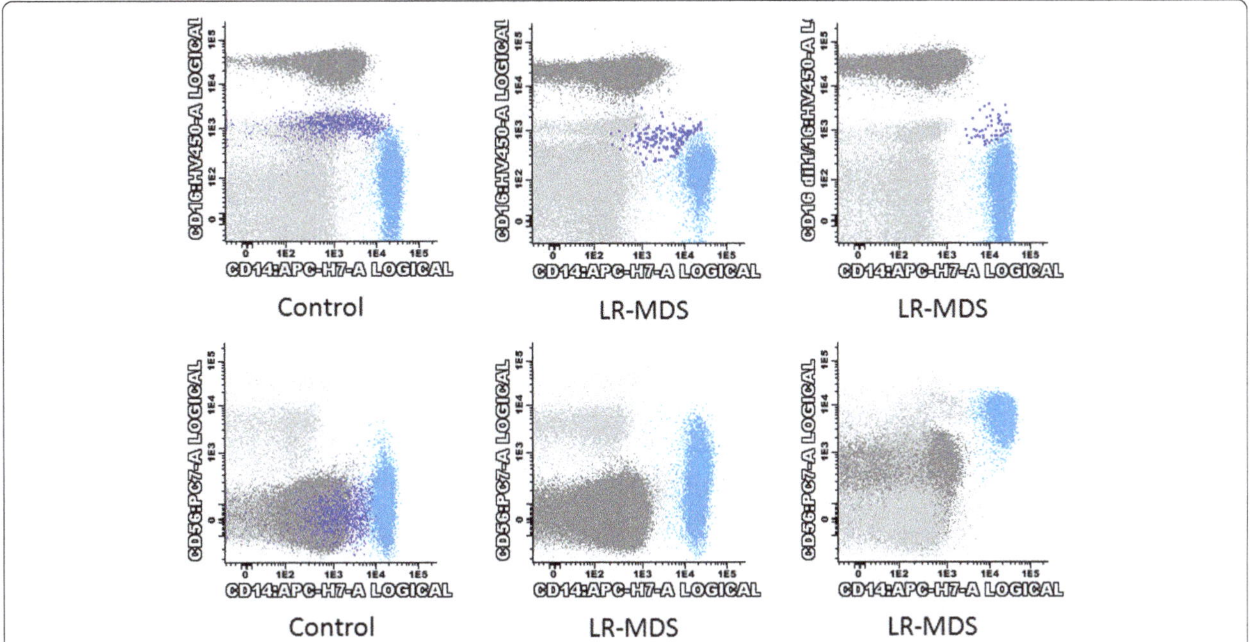

Fig. 5 Bivariate CD16/CD14 and CD56/CD14 dot plots illustrating the depletion of non-classical (intermediate CD14^{+high}CD16^{+} plus proinflammatory CD14^{+low}CD16^{+}) monocytes (upper row) and the aberrant CD56 expression in the PB classical CD14^{+high}CD16^{-} monocytes (lower row) from two patients with LR-MDS, as compared to a normal individual (control). Light blue dots, classical CD14^{+high}CD16^{-} monocytes; dark blue dots, non-classical (intermediate CD14^{+high}CD16^{+} plus proinflammatory CD14^{+low}CD16^{+}) monocytes; light gray dots, lymphocytes and eosinophils; dark gray dots, neutrophils. Abbreviations: FSC, forward scatter; LR-MDS, lower risk myelodysplastic syndromes; PB, peripheral blood; SSC, side scatter

Myeloid score type 1

Considering the total myeloid score type 1, obtained by the sum of the correspondent neutrophil and monocytic scores, we found a score of 5 ± 2 for LR-MDS (median of 6, ranging from 0 to 8), while all controls had a score of 1 or under (Table 6). According to this score, four groups of MDS patients were identified: score of "0" (no myelodysplasia) ($n = 1$; 7%, corresponding to the patient mentioned above); score of 1 (possible myelodysplasia) ($n = 0$); score of between 2 and 4 ($n = 3$; 21%) (mild

Table 5 Immunophenotypic alterations detected in PB monocytes from LR-MDS patients versus normal individuals (controls)

	LR-MDS (n = 14)	Controls (n = 14)
Increased CD56 expression in monocytes		
CD14^{+}CD56^{+} cells (% total CD14^{+} monocytes) (*)	15 (0–99)	7 (0–15)
Increased percentages of CD14^{+} 56^{+} cells (> 18.0% total CD14^{+} monocytes)	6 (43%)	0 (0%)
Severity		
Mild: CD56^{+} cells]18%–23%]	1 (7%)	0 (0%)
Moderate: CD56^{+} cells [23%–28%]	1 (7%)	0 (0%)
Severe: CD56^{+} cells]28%–100%]	4 (29%)	0 (0%)
Decreased CD16 expression in monocytes		
CD14^{+}CD16^{+} cells (% total CD14^{+} monocytes) (**)	3 (0–8)	12 (4–28)
Decreased percentages of CD14^{+}CD16^{+} cells (< 5.0% of total CD14^{+} monocytes)	9 (64%)	2 (14%)
Severity		
Mild: CD16^{+} cells [2.5%–5.0%]	2 (14%)	2 (14%)
Moderate: CD16^{+} cells [1.25–2.5%]	1 (7%)	0 (0%)
Severe: CD16^{+} cells [0.00–1.25%]	6 (43%)	0 (0%)

Abbreviations: *LR-MDS* lower risk myelodysplastic syndromes, *PB* peripheral blood
Results are expressed as absolute and (relative) frequencies or as median (range) values
Percentages were approximated to the closest full unit
Mann-Whitney U test, LR-MDS patients versus controls: (*) $P = 0.026$; (**) $P < 0.001$

Table 6 Neutrophil and monocyte immunophenotypic scores, and total myeloid score for myelodysplasia in the PB from LR-MDS patients versus normal individuals (controls), taking in account the number of phenotypic abnormalities found in each case

	LR-MDS (n = 14)	Controls (*n* = 14)
Neutrophil immunophenotypic score 1 (0–8)		
Score	5 (0–8)	0 (0–1)
Score rank (Σ)	59	1
Score classes		
0 (no dysplasia)	1 (7%)	13 (93%)
1 (possible dysplasia)	0 (0%)	1 (7%)
2–3 (mild dysplasia)	3 (21%)	0 (0%)
4–6 (moderate dysplasia)	9 (64%)	0 (0%)
7–8 (severe dysplasia)	1 (7%)	0 (0%)
Monocyte immunophenotypic score 1 (0–2)		
Score	1 (0–2)	0 (0–1)
Score rank (Σ)	15	2
Score classes		
0 (no dysplasia)	2 (14%)	12 (86%)
1 (possible dysplasia)	8 (57%)	2 (14%)
2 (dysplasia)	4 (29%)	0 (0%)
Myeloid immunophenotypic score 1 (0–10)		
Score	6 (0–8)	0 (0–1)
Score rank (Σ)	74	3
Score classes		
0 (no dysplasia)	1 (7%)	11 (79%)
1 (possible dysplasia)	0 (0%)	3 (21%)
2–4 (mild dysplasia)	3 (21%)	0 (0%)
5–7 (moderate dysplasia)	7 (50%)	0 (0%)
8–10 (severe dysplasia)	3 (21%)	0 (0%)

Abbreviations: *LR-MDS* lower risk myelodysplastic syndromes, *PB* peripheral blood
Results are expressed as absolute and (relative) frequencies or as median (range) values
Percentages were approximated to the closest full unit
Neutrophil score: The following parameters were considered: FSC, SSC, CD10, CD11b, CD11c, CD13, CD16, and CD45. Each abnormally low parameter (< mean - 2D of the values observed in controls) was scored with 1 point. Values within the mean ± SD or above the mean + 2SD were scored with "0"
Monocyte score: The following parameters were considered: % of CD16+ monocytes and % of CD56+ monocytes. These parameters were scored as follows: CD14 + CD56+ monocytes: ≤18% (0 points); > 18% (1 point); CD14 + CD16+ monocytes: ≥5% (0 points); < 5% (1 point)
Myeloid score: obtained by adding up the neutrophil and the monocytic score achieved for each patient
The following score rankings were obtained for each of the parameters analyzed: Patients: FSC = 10; CD11b = 10; CD11c = 10; CD10 = 9; SSC = 8; CD13 = 4; CD15 = 0; CD16 = 6; CD45 = 2. Controls: CD15 = 1; CD45 = 1; other parameters = 0

Table 7 Neutrophil and monocyte immunophenotypic scores, and total myeloid score for myelodysplasia in the PB from LR-MDS patients versus normal individuals (controls), taking in account the number and the severity of the phenotypic abnormalities found in each case

	LR-MDS (n = 14)	Controls (n = 14)
Neutrophil immunophenotypic score 2 (0–8)		
Score	2 (0–3)	0 (0–0)
Score rank (Σ)	28	0
Score classes		
0 (no dysplasia)	1 (7%)	14 (100%)
1 (possible dysplasia)	2 (14%)	0 (0%)
2–3 (mild dysplasia)	11 (79%)	0 (0%)
4–6 (moderate dysplasia)	0 (0%)	0 (0%)
7–8 (severe dysplasia)	0 (0%)	0 (0%)
Monocyte immunophenotypic score 2 (0–2)		
Score	1 (0–2)	0 (0–0)
Score rank (Σ)	12	1
Score classes		
0 (no dysplasia)	5 (36%)	14 (100%)
1 (probable dysplasia)	6 (43%)	0 (0%)
2 (dysplasia)	3 (21%)	0 (0%)
Myeloid immunophenotypic score 2 (0–10)		
Score	3 (0–5)	0 (0–1)
Score rank (Σ)	39	1
Score classes		
0 (no dysplasia)	1 (7%)	14 (0%)
1 (possible dysplasia)	1 (7%)	0 (0%)
2–4 (mild dysplasia)	11 (79%)	0 (0%)
5–7 (moderate dysplasia)	1 (7%)	0 (0%)
8–10 (severe dysplasia)	0 (0%)	0 (0%)

Abbreviations: *LR-MDS* lower risk myelodysplastic syndromes, *PB* peripheral blood
Results are expressed as absolute and (relative) frequencies or as median (range) values
Percentages were approximated to the closest full unit
Neutrophil score: The following parameters were considered: FSC, SSC, CD10, CD11b, CD11c, CD13, CD16, and CD45. Values within the mean ± SD or above the mean + 2SD were scored with "0". Abnormally low parameter (< mean-2D of the values observed in controls) were scored as follows: (< mean-2D: 0.25 points; < mean-3SD: 0.5 points; < mean-3SD: 1 point
Monocyte score: The following parameters were considered: % of CD16+ monocytes and % of CD56+ monocytes. These parameters were scored as follows: CD14 + CD56+ monocytes: ≤18% (0 points); >mean + 2SD (18%): 0.25 points; > mean + 3SD (23%): 0.5 points; > mean + 4SD (28%): 1 point. CD14 + CD16+ monocytes: ≥5%: 0 points; CD14 + CD16+ monocytes < 5%: 0.25 point; CD14 + CD16+ monocytes: < 2.5%: 0.5 points; CD14 + CD16+ monocytes: < 1.25%: 1 point
Myeloid score: obtained by adding up the neutrophil score 1 and the monocytic score achieved for each patient
The following score rankings were obtained for each of the parameters analyzed: Patients: FSC = 6.5; CD11c = 5.5; CD11b = 5.0; SSC = 4.5; CD10 = 2.5; CD16 = 2; CD13 = 1.0; CD15 = 0.0; CD45 = 0.5. Controls: CD15 = 0.25; CD45 = 0.25; other parameters = 0

myelodysplasia); score between 5 and 7 (moderate myelodysplasia) ($n = 7$; 50%); and score over 8 (severe myelodysplasia) (n = 3; 21%). In contrast, in the control group, most of the individuals had a score of "0", with only 3 (21%) having a score of 1. Therefore, assuming a cut-off of ≥2 points we were able to correctly classify 13 out of 14 LR-MDS patients and 14 out of 14 controls, given a sensitivity of 93% and a specificity of 100% for the diagnosis of MDS.

Immunophenotypic scoring schema 2

Neutrophil score type 2

The mean neutrophil score type 2 obtained in LR-MDS patients was of 2 ± 1, ranging from 0 to 3 (total score rank = 28), while all controls had a score of "0" (Table 7). According to this score, four groups of MDS patients were identified: score of "0", no dysplasia (n = 1; 7%); ii) score of 1 ($n = 2$; 14%); score between 2 and 3 (n = 1; 7%); score between 4 and 6 (n = 0); and score over 6 (n = 0). Thus, similarly to that observed with the neutrophil scoring system type 1, assuming a cut-off of > 1 points we were able to correctly classify 13 out of 14 LR-MDS patients and 14 out of 14 controls (sensitivity of 93% and specificity of 100% for the diagnosis of MDS).

Monocyte score type 2

The mean monocyte score type 2 obtained in LR-MDS patients was of 1 ± 1, ranging from 0 to 2 (total score rank = 12), whereas the score observed in controls was of "0" in all cases (Table 7). According this score, four groups of MDS patients were identified: score of "0" ($n = 5$; 36%); score of 1 ($n = 6$; 43%); and score of 2 (n = 3; 21%). Comparatively, all controls had a score of "0". Consequently, assuming a cut off of ≥1 point we were able to correctly classify 9 out of 14 LR-MDS patients and all controls, given a sensitivity and a specificity of 64% for the diagnosis of MDS.

Myeloid score type 2

Considering the total myeloid score type 2, i.e. the sum of the neutrophil and monocytic scores type 2, we obtained a score of 3 ± 1 for LR-MDS (median of 3, ranging from 0 to 8, total score rank = 39), while all controls had a score of 1 or under (Table 7).

As a result, the scoring schemas type 2 apparently do not offer advantages for the diagnosis of myelodysplasia, as compared to the scoring schemas type 1, which are more easily to calculate.

MDS thermometers

The immunophenotypic scoring schemas type 1 were used to conceive the MDS Thermometer tool, aimed for the screening of MDS in PB samples in clinical practice, which can be deployed on two thermometers, for neutrophils and monocytes, respectively (Fig. 6). The neutrophil thermometer is based on the neutrophil score system type 1, i.e., the number of cell surface markers abnormally low expressed in neutrophils, among 8 parameters considered (FSC, SSC, CD10, CD11b, CD11c, CD13, CD16 and CD45). The monocyte thermometer is based on the monocyte scoring system type 1, i.e., increased fraction of $CD56^+$ cells (aberrant CD56 expression) and decreased fraction of $CD16^+$ cells (depletion of proinflammatory monocytes) among total monocytes. The myeloid thermometer was obtained by the sum of the neutrophil and the monocyte type 1 scores.

Discussion

Progresses made in the last years concerning the assessment of MDS by FCM have led to consensus recommendations for the integration of FCM data in the diagnostic work-up of MDS [21]. However, establishing the diagnosis still requires BM aspirate and biopsy, which are invasive procedures and not always conclusive, especially in LR-MDS.

Given the frequency of MDS patients with mild cytopenias that would not demand therapeutic intervention, due the fact that most MDS patients are not eligible for intensive treatment schedules, and taking into account the easy access to PB samples, it would be desirable to have a PB assay to help guide the need for invasive BM evaluation. Nonetheless, immunophenotypic studies in the PB from patients with MDS are surprisingly scarce. Using the PubMed and applying the key words "flow cytometry", "myelodysplastic syndromes", and "peripheral blood", we found only five studies performed in the PB [27–31].

Cherian et al. (2005) observed that neutrophils from MDS patients had lower SSC and higher expression of CD66 and CD11a than did controls; in some cases, PB neutrophils also displayed abnormal CD116 and CD10 expression [27, 28]. Using these markers, they proposed a score that allowed to distinguish MDS patients from normal controls with a sensitivity of 73% and a specificity of 90% [28].

Some years later (2012), using 3-color FCM, Rashidi et al. observed that CD10 expression on PB neutrophils was significantly decreased in patients with HR-MDS and CMML compared to both non-MDS patients with pancytopenia and to LR-MDS patients [30]. In contrast, they found no significant differences in CD11b, CD13, CD14, CD16, CD33, CD56, and CD64 expression in neutrophils and monocytes from the mentioned groups of patients.

More recently (2013), Meyerson et al. realized that low CD177 expression was frequent in PB and BM neutrophils from patients with clonal myeloid disorders; these findings were most pronounced in MDS, with 52% of cases containing less than 40% of $CD177^+$ neutrophils [31].

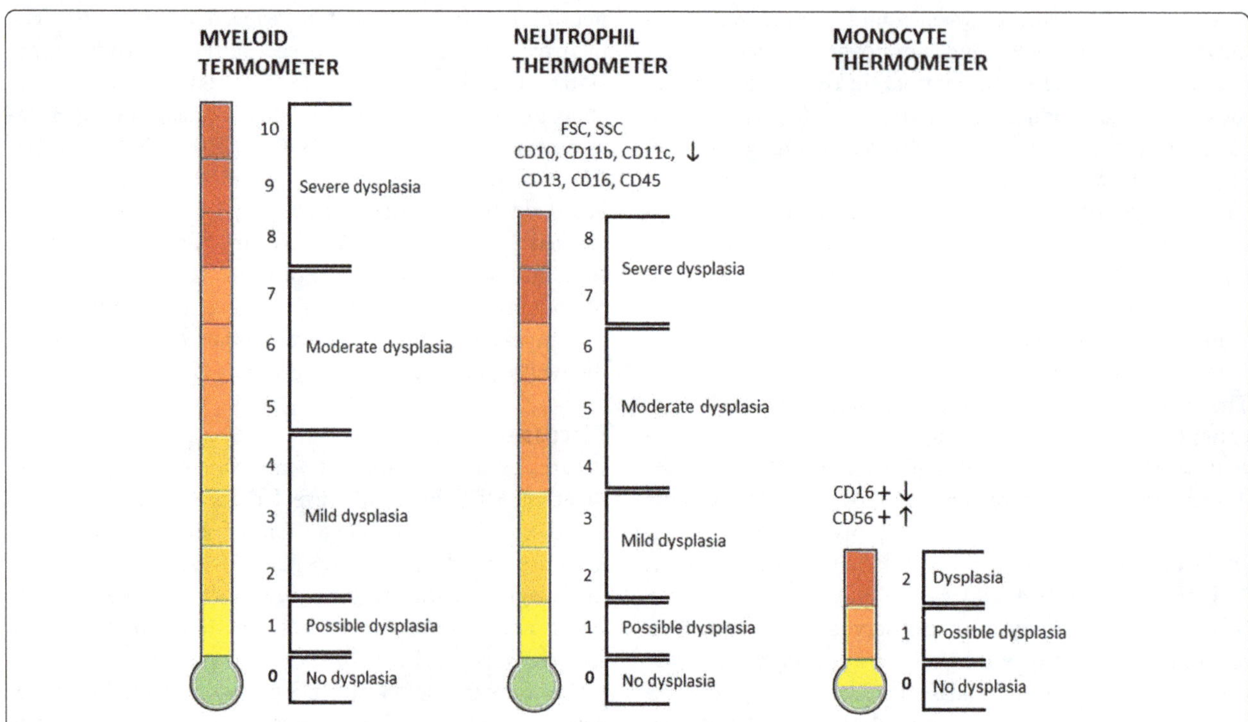

Fig. 6 MDS Thermometers. The neutrophil thermometer is based on the neutrophil score system type 1, i.e., the number of cell surface markers abnormally low expressed in PB neutrophils, among 8 parameters considered (FSC, SSC, CD10, CD11b, CD11c, CD13, CD16 and CD45). The monocyte thermometer is based on the monocyte scoring system type 1, i.e., increased fraction of $CD56^+$ cells (aberrant CD56 expression) and decreased fraction of $CD16^+$ cells (depletion of proinflammatory monocytes) among total PB monocytes. The myeloid thermometer was obtained by the sum of the neutrophil and the monocyte type 1 scores. Abbreviations: FSC, forward scatter; PB, peripheral blood; SSC, side scatter

Altered immunophenotypic features of PB platelets, consisting of abnormal light scatter characteristics, over or under expression of platelet glycoproteins and asynchronous CD34 expression were also described in patients with MDS [29].

Our pilot study revealed, for the first time, that PB neutrophils from LR-MDS not only frequently have decreased FSC and/or SSC, but also commonly display abnormally low levels of CD11b, CD11c, CD10, CD16, CD13 and CD45 expression, as compared to normal neutrophils. The fact that 93% of these patients had abnormally low levels of 2 or more (out of 9) cell surface molecules on neutrophils, as compared to only 29% having abnormal morphology, clearly indicates that FCM is more sensitive for the detection of myelodysplasia in the PB than cytomorphology. In addition, we observed a marked deficiency in proinflammatory $CD16^+$ monocytes and a high frequency of CD56 expression in circulating monocytes from patients with LR-MDS, irrespectively of the monocyte counts.

Human PB monocytes have been divided into distinct subsets, referred to as classical ($CD14^+CD16^-$) and non-classical ($CD14^+CD16^+$) monocytes; in between, there are "intermediate" monocytes, which are transitional cells – for review see [45–48]. $CD14^+CD16^+$ monocytes, which were first described in the late 80 [49], account for about 10% of total PB monocytes in healthy adults and appear to be more mature; they express lower levels of CD14 and higher levels of HLA-DR ($CD14^{+low}CD16^+HLA\text{-}DR^{+high}$) as compared with classical ($CD14^{+high}CD16^-HLA\text{-}DR^{low}$) monocytes [50], and they have distinct patterns of cytokines and chemokine receptors. Specifically, $CD14^+CD16^+$ monocytes have been shown to efficiently produce tumor necrosis factor (TNF), while they produce no or less of the anti-inflammatory cytokine interleukin (IL)-10 [51, 52]. In opposition to classical monocytes, they lack surface expression of CC chemokine receptor type 2 (CCR2), the receptor for monocyte chemotactic protein-1 (MCP-1), and have higher surface expression of CCR5, the receptor for macrophage inflammatory protein 1 alpha (MIP-1alpha) /regulated on activation, normal T cell expressed and secreted (RANTES) chemokine [53]. Their numbers are increased in various pathological conditions, such as HIV infection [54], sepsis [55], inflammatory bowel diseases [56], other inflammatory and autoimmune conditions [57], and tumors [58, 59], and they have been associated with acute or chronic inflammation. In addition, the relative and absolute numbers of the 'non-classical' $CD14^+CD16^+$ monocytes increase with the age [60].

Herein we described, for the first time, a depletion of proinflammatory ($CD14^+CD16^+$) monocytes, with consequent increase in the fraction of classical ($CD14^+CD16^-$)

monocytes, in the PB of LR-MDS patients. This finding may explain the abnormally low levels of CD11c, CD16 and HLA-DR expression we observed in PB monocytes from patients with LR-MDS. The reasons for this abnormal repartition of the PB monocyte subsets observed in patients with MDS are not clear. Patients included were not medicated with corticosteroids, which are known to induce a selective depletion of the $CD14^{+}CD16^{+}$ monocytes [61]. Also, it cannot be explained by aging, as in healthy individuals, proinflammatory $CD14^{+}CD16^{+}$ monocytes significantly increase with age, as we observed in our control group. Maybe this is a consequence of a defective monocyte maturation, as already described for CMML [62]. Curiously, Selimoglu-Buet et al. have recently found an increase in the fraction of classical $CD14^{+}CD16^{-}$ monocytes, in the PB from patients with CMML, as compared to healthy individuals and to patients with reactive monocytosis [18]. Taking in account that, as stated above, an opposite abnormal repartition of the mentioned monocyte subsets, with increased fractions of $CD16^{+}$ monocytes, has been described in inflammatory and autoimmune conditions [56, 57], infections [54, 55, 57, 63], and cancer [58, 59], the selective depletion of $CD14^{+}CD16^{+}$ monocytes in the PB would probably be important for the differential diagnosis between MDS and non-MDS cytopenias.

Abnormal CD56 expression in BM monocytes has already been described in patients with MDS, being observed with higher frequency in HR-MDS, as compared to LR-MDS [64], and is also a frequent in CMML [17, 20, 64], although these findings are not completely understood.

In healthy individuals, around 10% of the monocytes co-express CD56, with the majority of $CD56^{+}$ monocytes being $CD14^{+high}$ [65, 66]. $CD56^{+}$ monocytes are expanded in aging individuals as well as in patients with autoimmune and inflammatory conditions, such as rheumatoid arthritis and inflammatory bowel diseases [66, 67]. Compared to $CD56^{-}$ monocytes, $CD56^{+}$ monocytes spontaneously produce more reactive oxygen intermediates and, upon stimulation, they are stronger producers of cytokines, such as TNF, IL-10 and IL-23 [66]. As so, CD56 expression was recognized as a signal of monocyte activation and/or immunosenescence [66]. Considering the simultaneous decreased fractions of $CD14^{+low}CD16^{+}$ and increased fractions of $CD14^{+high}CD56^{+}$ monocytes observed in MDS patients, we postulate that blockage of differentiation of classical ($CD14^{+high}CD16^{-}$) into proinflammatory ($CD14^{+low}CD16^{+}$) monocytes leads to accumulation of the first monocyte population in the PB, which becomes senescent and then acquire CD56 expression.

The phenotypic aberrancies observed in the PB from patients with LR-MDS are consistent with those that have been previously described in the BM, and the 2-tubes/8-color panel we proposed for the screening of myelodysplasia in the PB would allow to evaluate most of the aberrant immunophenotypic features that have been suggested being included in BM studies for the diagnostic work-up of patients with MDS [13, 21]. The exceptions are lineage infidelity markers and some myeloid-associated markers, which are not evaluated with our protocol. In addition, our FCM panel can also be used to quantify and characterize the immature $CD34^{+}$ cells, both in the PB and BM samples. For the evaluation of the myeloid and lymphoid compartments in $CD34^{+}$ BM cells, CD19 may be used instead of CD15, as this marker did not prove to be useful for the diagnosis of neutrophil dysplasia.

Several FCM scoring schemas have been already proposed for diagnosis and prognosis evaluation in MDS, most of them based on the immunophenotypic features of the BM blast cells and on the abnormal immunophenotypic patterns found in maturing myeloid cells [10, 12, 68]. However, due to the complexity of BM analysis, these schemas are difficult to apply in routine clinical practice. To become clinically applicable, FCM should be not only sensitive and specific, but also reproducible, and the results should be easily understood by clinicians. Therefore, our study fills a gap and refine the accuracy to detect myelodysplasia in the PB.

The visual analogue scale we propose for the screening of myelodysplasia in PB samples – the MDS thermometer, is simple, intuitive and easy to apply. It is based on FCM analysis of 10 parameters, 8 in neutrophils (FSC, SSC, CD10, CD11b, CD11c, CD16, CD45) and 2 in monocytes (CD16, CD56), and it allows to distinguish LR-MDS peripheral blood samples from normal PB samples with a sensitivity of 100% and a specificity of 93%. It could be argued that it does not take into account the severity of the deficiency of each molecule observed in myelodysplastic cells. However, the alternative scoring schema that evaluates this aspect but is more difficult to apply, did not improve the performance of the test; maybe it can be useful in specific cases. With the necessary adaptations, the concept of the MDS Thermometer could probably also be applied to the MDS/MPN, such as CMML, in which monocytic aberrancies are expected to be more pronounced.

There are some limitations to the current study. First, the number of cases studied is small and this study should be considered a pilot study. Secondly, due to the difficulties in finding blood donors older than 60 years, we were not able to pair healthy controls and MDS patients for age, and it could be argued that differences between groups may be age-related; however, the fact that no differences were found in the analyzed parameters when younger and older healthy volunteers were compared, except for a higher fraction of $CD16^{+}$ monocytes in the last group, strongly argue against this possibility.

Thirdly, we did not study non-MDS patients with cytopenias. Finally, attention should be given to the cytometer setup, calibration and stability, and each center should establish its own normal reference values, on the basis of the mAbs and experimental conditions used.

Conclusions

Our pilot study reveals an altered neutrophil immunophenotype, often accompanied by an abnormal monocyte immunophenotype, in the PB from nearly all LR-MDS cases, and suggests that assessment of abnormal antigen expression in PB mature myeloid cells may help to identify patients with LR-MDS. Once translated into a straightforward FCM-based score and converted into a visual analogue scale – MDS thermometer –, these findings can be easily applied in clinical practice. However, due to the low number of cases analyzed, further studies with larger series of patients are needed to confirm our preliminary observations. Furthermore, it would be interesting to evaluate HR-MDS patients, as well as CMML and other MDS/MPN. Additional studies are also required in order to evaluate the specificity of such alterations for the diagnosis MDS, by testing other pathological conditions associated with cytopenias.

Abbreviations

APC: Allophycocyanin; BC: Beckman Coulter; BD: Becton Dickinson; BDB: Becton Dickinson Bioscience; BDH: Becton Dickinson Horizon; BL: Biolegend; BM: Bone marrow; CCR2: C-C chemokine receptor type 2; CCR5: C-C chemokine receptor type 5; CMML: Chronic myelomonocytic leukemia; Cy5.5: Cyanine 5.5; Cy7: Cyanine 7; EPO: Erythropoietin; FAB: French-American-British; FCM: Flow cytometry; FITC: Fluorescein isothiocyanate; FSC: Forward scatter; G-CSF: Granulocyte-colony stimulating factor; GM-CSF: Granulocyte monocyte-colony stimulating factor; Hg: Hemoglobin; HR-MDS: Higher risk myelodysplastic syndrome (IPSS: intermediate-2 + high); IL: Interleukin; IOT: Immunotech; IPSS: International Prognostic Scoring System; IPSS-R: Revised International Prognostic Scoring System; KO: Khrome Orange; LDH: Lactate dehydrogenase; LR-MDS: Lower risk myelodysplastic syndrome (IPSS: low + intermediate-1); mAb: Monoclonal antibody; MCP-1: Monocyte chemotactic protein-1; MCV: Mean corpuscular volume; MDS: Myelodysplastic syndromes; MDS/MPN: Myelodysplastic/myeloproliferative neoplasms; MDS-del(5q): Myelodysplastic syndromes with isolated deletion of chromosome 5q; MDS-EB: Myelodysplastic syndromes with excess of blasts; MDS-MLD: Myelodysplastic syndromes with multilineage dysplasia; MDS-RS: Myelodysplastic syndromes with ring sideroblasts; MDS-RS-MLD: Myelodysplastic syndromes with ring sideroblasts with multilineage dysplasia; MDS-RS-SLD: Myelodysplastic syndromes with ring sideroblasts with single lineage dysplasia; MDS-SLD: Myelodysplastic syndromes with single lineage dysplasia; MDS-U: Myelodysplastic syndromes, unclassifiable; MedFI: Median fluorescence intensity; MIP-1alpha: Macrophage inflammatory protein 1alpha chemokine; NA: Not applicable; PB: Peripheral blood; PBS: Phosphate buffered saline; PE: Phycoerythrin; PerCP: Peridinin chlorophyll protein; PerCP-Cy5.5: Peridinin chlorophyll protein Cy5.5; PMT: Photomultiplier tubes; RANTES: Regulated on activation, normal T cell expressed and secreted chemokine; RBC: Red blood cells; SSC: Side-scatter; TNF: Tumor necrosis factor; V450: Violet 450; WBC: White blood cells; WHO: World Health Organization

Acknowledgements

The authors thank to Marta Gonçalves for cell immunophenotyping, to Ana Sofia Jorge, Cristina Gonçalves, Luciana Pinho, Luciana Xavier, Renata Cabral and Vanessa Mesquita, for patient selection and study implementation, to the other medical doctors and technicians of the Hematology and Pathology Departments for support concerning the routine laboratory tests for MDS diagnosis, and to the nurses for blood collection.

Funding

The Centro Hospitalar do Porto (CHP) made available the necessary infrastructures and equipment, and the Instituto de Ciências Biomédicas Abel Salazar, Universidade do Porto (ICBAS/UP) gave financial support for the purchase of the reagents used in this study. The funders had no role in study design, data collection and analysis, decision to publish, or preparation of the manuscript.

Authors' contributions

AA: study design, data collection, data analysis, and manuscript draft writing. CL and MAT: flow cytometry data analysis. CM: patient selection, study implementation, and clinical data collection, registry and analysis. AS: transfusion data collection and registry, and analysis; AM: cytogenetic data analysis. IF: cytomorphology. JC: contribution to patient selection and study implementation, discussion of the results, and critical revision of the manuscript; ML: study conception and design, flow cytometry data analysis, clinical and laboratory data review, statistical analysis, and manuscript writing and review. All authors read and approved the final version of the manuscript.

Authors' information

AA is a medical doctor undertaking general training for medical specialization; she contributed to this work as a medical student, integrated in the curricular unit of initiation to clinical research. CL and MAT are medical doctors specialized in Immunohemotherapy, with skills in flow cytometry; MAT has expertise in MDS immunophenotyping. AS is a medical doctor specialized in Immunohemoterapy, with skills in transfusion medicine. AM is a medical doctor specialized in Clinical Hematology, with expertise in cytogenetics. IF is a medical doctor specialized in Clinical Pathology, with skills in cytomorphology. JC is a medical doctor specialized in Clinical Hematology, head of the Department of Clinical Hematology, with a large experience in diagnosing and treating patients with MDS. ML is a medical doctor specialized in Immunohemotherapy, head of the flow cytometry laboratory, and an expert in flow cytometry applied to the diagnosis of hemato-oncological disorders.

Competing interests

The authors declare that they have no competing interests.

Author details

[1]Department of Hematology, Hospital de Santo António (HSA), Centro Hospitalar do Porto (CHP), Porto, Portugal. [2]Department of Pathology, Hospital de Santo António (HSA), Centro Hospitalar do Porto (CHP), Porto, Portugal. [3]Instituto de Ciências Biomédicas Abel Salazar, Universidade do Porto (ICBAS/UP), Porto, Portugal. [4]Unidade Multidisciplinar de Investigação Biomédica, Instituto de Ciências Biomédicas Abel Salazar, Universidade do Porto (UMIB/ICBAS/UP), Porto, Portugal. [5]Laboratório de Citometria, Serviço de Hematologia, Hospital de Santo António, Centro Hospitalar do Porto, instalações do Ex-CICAP, Rua D. Manuel II, s/n, 4099-001 Porto, Portugal.

References

1. Adès L, Itzykson R, Fenaux P. Myelodysplastic syndromes. Lancet. 2014;383: 2239–52. https://doi.org/10.1016/S0140-6736(13)61901-7. PMID: 24656536
2. Malcovati L, Hellström-Lindberg E, Bowen D, Adès L, Cermak J, Del Cañizo C, et al. Diagnosis and treatment of primary myelodysplastic syndromes in adults: recommendations from the European LeukemiaNet. Blood. 2013;122: 2943–64. https://doi.org/10.1182/blood-2013-03-492884. PMID: 23980065
3. Meers S. The myelodysplastic syndromes: the era of understanding. Eur J Haematol. 2015;94:379–90. https://doi.org/10.1111/ejh.12443. PMID: 25186093
4. Swerdlow S, Camp E, Harris N, Jaffe E, Pileri S. WHO classification of tumors of haematopoietic and lymphoid tissues. Lyon: IARC; 2008.
5. Arber DA, Orazi A, Hasserjian R, Thiele J, Borowitz MJ, Le Beau MM. The 2016 revision to the World Health Organization classification of myeloid neoplasms and acute leukemia. Blood. 2016;127:2391–405. https://doi.org/10.1182/blood-2016-03-643544. PMID: 27069254
6. Greenberg P, Cox C, LeBeau MM, Fenaux P, Morel P, Sanz G, et al. International scoring system for evaluating prognosis in myelodysplastic syndromes. Blood. 1997;89:2079–88. PMID: 9058730
7. Greenberg PL, Tuechler H, Schanz J, Sanz G, Garcia-Manero G, Solé F, et al. Revised international prognostic scoring system for myelodysplastic syndromes. Blood. 2012;120:2454–65. https://doi.org/10.1182/blood-2012-03-420489. PMID: 22740453
8. Sekeres MA, Schoonen WM, Kantarjian H, List A, Fryzek J, Paquette R, et al. Characteristics of US patients with myelodysplastic syndromes: results of six cross-sectional physician surveys. J Natl Cancer Inst. 2008;100:1542–51. https://doi.org/10.1093/jnci/djn349. PMID: 18957672
9. Stetler-Stevenson M, Arthur DC, Jabbour N, Xie XY, Molldrem J, Barrett AJ, et al. Diagnostic utility of flow cytometric immunophenotyping in myelodysplastic syndrome. Blood. 2001;98:979–87. https://doi.org/10.1182/blood.V98.4.979. PMID: 11493442
10. Wells DA, Benesch M, Loken MR, Vallejo C, Myerson D, Leisenring WM, et al. Myeloid and monocytic dyspoiesis as determined by flow cytometric scoring in myelodysplastic syndrome correlates with the IPSS and with outcome after hematopoietic stem cell transplantation. Blood. 2003;102: 394–403. https://doi.org/10.1182/blood-2002-09-2768. PMID: 12649150
11. Matarraz S, López A, Barrena S, Fernandez C, Jensen E, Flores J, et al. The immunophenotype of different immature, myeloid and B-cell lineage-committed CD34+ hematopoietic cells allows discrimination between normal/reactive and myelodysplastic syndrome precursors. Leukemia. 2008; 22:1175–83. https://doi.org/10.1038/leu.2008.49. PMID: 18337765
12. van de Loosdrecht AA, Westers TM, Westra AH, Drager AM, van der Velden VHJ, Ossenkoppele GJ. Identification of distinct prognostic subgroups in low- and intermediate-1-risk myelodysplastic syndromes by flow cytometry. Blood. 2008;111:1067–77. https://doi.org/10.1182/blood-2007-07-098764. PMID: 17971483
13. Westers TM, Ireland R, Kern W, Alhan C, Balleisen JS, Bettelheim P, et al. Standardization of flow cytometry in myelodysplastic syndromes: a report from an international consortium and the European LeukemiaNet working group. Leukemia. 2012;26:1730–41. https://doi.org/10.1038/leu.2012.30. PMID: 22307178
14. Cazzola M. Flow cytometry immunophenotyping for diagnosis of myelodysplastic syndrome. Haematologica. 2009;94:1041–3. https://doi.org/10.3324/haematol.2009.007682. PMID: 19644135
15. Kern W, Haferlach C, Schnittger S, Haferlach T. Clinical utility of multiparameter flow cytometry in the diagnosis of 1013 patients with suspected myelodysplastic syndrome: correlation to cytomorphology, cytogenetics, and clinical data. Cancer. 2010;116:4549–63. https://doi.org/10.1002/cncr.25353. PMID: 20572043
16. Kern W, Haferlach C, Schnittger S, Alpermann T, Haferlach T. Serial assessment of suspected myelodysplastic syndromes: significance of flow cytometric findings validated by cytomorphology, cytogenetics, and molecular genetics. Haematologica. 2013;98:201–7. https://doi.org/10.3324/haematol.2012.066787. PMID: 22929975
17. Lacronique-Gazaille C, Chaury M-P, Le Guyader A, Faucher J-L, Bordessoule D, Feuillard J. A simple method for detection of major phenotypic abnormalities in myelodysplastic syndromes: expression of CD56 in CMML. Haematologica. 2007;92:859–60. https://doi.org/10.3324/haematol.11118. PMID: 17550865
18. Selimoglu-Buet D, Wagner-Ballon O, Saada V, Bardet V, Itzykson R, Bencheikh L, et al. Characteristic repartition of monocyte subsets as a diagnostic signature of chronic myelomonocytic leukemia. Blood. 2015;125: 3618–26. https://doi.org/10.1182/blood-2015-01-620781. PMID: 25852055
19. Stachurski D, Smith BR, Pozdnyakova O, Andersen M, Xiao Z, Raza A, et al. Flow cytometric analysis of myelomonocytic cells by a pattern recognition approach is sensitive and specific in diagnosing myelodysplastic syndrome and related marrow diseases: emphasis on a global evaluation and recognition of diagnostic pitfalls. Leuk Res. 2008;32:215–24. https://doi.org/10.1016/j.leukres.2007.06.012. PMID: 17675229
20. Xu Y, McKenna RW, Karandikar NJ, Pildain AJ, Kroft SH. Flow cytometric analysis of monocytes as a tool for distinguishing chronic myelomonocytic leukemia from reactive monocytosis. Am J Clin Pathol. 2005;124:799–806. https://doi.org/10.1309/HRJ1-XKTD-77J1-UTFM. PMID: 16203279
21. Porwit A, van de Loosdrecht AA, Bettelheim P, Brodersen LE, Burbury K, Cremers E, et al. Revisiting guidelines for integration of flow cytometry results in the WHO classification of myelodysplastic syndromes-proposal from the international/European LeukemiaNet working Group for Flow Cytometry in MDS. Leukemia. 2014;28:1793–8. https://doi.org/10.1038/leu.2014.191. PMID: 24919805
22. Valent P, Orazi A, Büsche G, Schmitt-Gräff A, George TI, Sotlar K, et al. Standards and impact of hematopathology in myelodysplastic syndromes (MDS). Oncotarget. 2010;1:483–96. https://doi.org/10.18632/oncotarget.101104. PMID: 21317447
23. Sandes AF, Kerbauy DM, Matarraz S, Chauffaille Mde L, López A, Orfao A, et al. Combined flow cytometric assessment of CD45, HLA-DR, CD34, and CD117 expression is a useful approach for reliable quantification of blast cells in myelodysplastic syndromes. Cytometry B Clin Cytom. 2013;84:157–66. https://doi.org/10.1002/cyto.b.21087. PMID: 23475532
24. Alhan C, Westers TM, van der Helm LH, Eeltink C, Huls G, Witte BI, et al. Absence of aberrant myeloid progenitors by flow cytometry is associated with favorable response to azacitidine in higher risk myelodysplastic syndromes. Cytometry B Clin Cytom. 2014;86:207–15. https://doi.org/10.1002/cyto.b.21160. PMID: 24474614
25. Eidenschink Brodersen L, Menssen AJ, Wangen JR, Stephenson CF, de Baca ME, Zehentner BK, et al. Assessment of erythroid dysplasia by "difference from normal" in routine clinical flow cytometry workup. Cytometry B Clin Cytom. 2015;88:125–35. https://doi.org/10.1002/cyto.b.21199. PMID: 25490867
26. Laranjeira P, Rodrigues R, Carvalheiro T, Constanço C, Vitória H, Matarraz S, et al. Expression of CD44 and CD35 during normal and myelodysplastic erythropoiesis. Leuk Res. 2015;39:361–70. https://doi.org/10.1016/j.leukres.2014.12.009. PMID: 25582385
27. Cherian S, Moore J, Bantly A, Vergilio J-A, Klein P, Luger S, et al. Flow-cytometric analysis of peripheral blood neutrophils: a simple, objective, independent and potentially clinically useful assay to facilitate the diagnosis of myelodysplastic syndromes. Am J Hematol. 2005;79:243–5. https://doi.org/10.1002/ajh.20371. PMID: 15981222
28. Cherian S, Moore J, Bantly A, Vergilio J-A, Klein P, Luger S, et al. Peripheral blood MDS score: a new flow cytometric tool for the diagnosis of myelodysplastic syndromes. Cytometry B Clin Cytom. 2005;64B:9–17. https://doi.org/10.1002/cyto.b.20041. PMID: 15668954
29. Sandes AF, Yamamoto M, Matarraz S, Chauffaille M de LLF, Quijano S, López A, et al. Altered immunophenotypic features of peripheral blood platelets in myelodysplastic syndromes. Haematologica. 2012;97:895–902. https://doi.org/10.3324/haematol.2011.057158. PMID: 22271903
30. Rashidi HH, Xu X, Wang H-Y, Shafi NQ, Rameshkumar K, Messer K, et al. Utility of peripheral blood flow cytometry in differentiating low grade versus high grade myelodysplastic syndromes (MDS) and in the evaluation of cytopenias. Int J Clin Exp Pathol. 2012;5:224–30. PMID: 22558477
31. Meyerson HJ, Osei E, Schweitzer K, Blidaru G, Edinger A, Balog A. CD177 expression on neutrophils: in search of a clonal assay for myeloid neoplasia by flow cytometry. Am J Clin Pathol. 2013;140:658–69. https://doi.org/10.1309/AJCPDFBEBQZW1OI7. PMID: 24124144
32. Germing U, Hildebrandt B, Pfeilstöcker M, Nösslinger T, Valent P, Fonatsch C, et al. Refinement of the international prognostic scoring system (IPSS) by including LDH as an additional prognostic variable to improve risk assessment in patients with primary myelodysplastic syndromes (MDS). Leukemia. 2005;19:2223–31. https://doi.org/10.1038/sj.leu.2403963. PMID: 16193087
33. Shenoy N, Vallumsetla N, Rachmilewitz E, Verma A, Ginzburg Y. Impact of iron overload and potential benefit from iron chelation in low-risk myelodysplastic syndrome. Blood. 2014;124:873–81. https://doi.org/10.1182/blood-2014-03-563221. PMID: 24923296

34. Garcia-Manero G, Shan J, Faderl S, Cortes J, Ravandi F, Borthakur G, et al. A prognostic score for patients with lower risk myelodysplastic syndrome. Leukemia. 2008;22:538–43. https://doi.org/10.1038/sj.leu.2405070. PMID: 18079733
35. Mufti GJ, Bennett JM, Goasguen J, Bain BJ, Baumann I, Brunning R, et al. International working group on morphology of myelodysplastic syndrome. Diagnosis and classification of myelodysplastic syndrome: international working group on morphology of myelodysplastic syndrome (IWGM-MDS) consensus proposals for the definition and enumeration of myeloblasts and ring sideroblasts. Haematologica. 2008;93:1712–7. https://doi.org/10.3324/haematol.13405. PMID: 18838480
36. Thiele J, Kvasnicka HM, Facchetti F, Franco V, van der Walt J, Orazi A. European consensus on grading bone marrow fibrosis and assessment of cellularity. Haematologica. 2005;90:1128–32. PMID: 16079113
37. Orazi A. Histopathology in the diagnosis and classification of acute myeloid leukemia, myelodysplastic syndromes, and myelodysplastic/myeloproliferative diseases. Pathobiology. 2007;74:97–114. https://doi.org/10.1159/000101709. PMID: 17587881
38. Horny H-P, Sotlar K, Valent P. Diagnostic value of histology and immunohistochemistry in myelodysplastic syndromes. Leuk Res. 2007; 31:1609–16. https://doi.org/10.1016/j.leukres.2007.05.010. PMID: 17604834
39. Schanz J, Tüchler H, Solé F, Mallo M, Luño E, Cervera J, et al. New comprehensive cytogenetic scoring system for primary myelodysplastic syndromes (MDS) and oligoblastic acute myeloid leukemia after MDS derived from an international database merge. J Clin Oncol. 2012;30:820–9. https://doi.org/10.1200/JCO.2011.35.6394. PMID: 22331955
40. Kalina T, Flores-Montero J, van der Velden VHJ, Martin-Ayuso M, Böttcher S, Ritgen M, et al. EuroFlow standardization of flow cytometer instrument settings and immunophenotyping protocols. Leukemia. 2012;26:1986–2010. https://doi.org/10.1038/leu.2012.122. PMID: 22948490
41. EuroFlow, a division of ESLHO. https://euroflow.org. Accessed 4 Oct 2017.
42. Kalina T, Flores-Montero J, Lecrevisse Q, Pedreira CE, van der Velden VHJ, Novakova M, et al. Quality assessment program for EuroFlow protocols: summary results of four-year (2010-2013) quality assurance rounds. Cytometry A. 2015;87:145–56. https://doi.org/10.1002/cyto.a.22581. PMID: 25345353
43. Mitchell AJ, Baker-Glenn EA, Park B, Granger L, Symonds P. Can the distress thermometer be improved by additional mood domains? Part II. What is the optimal combination of emotion thermometers? Psychooncology. 2010; 19:134–40. https://doi.org/10.1002/pon.1557. PMID: 19296461
44. Mitchell AJ, Baker-Glenn EA, Granger L, Symonds P. Can the distress thermometer be improved by additional mood domains? Part I. Initial validation of the emotion thermometers tool. Psychooncology. 2010;19: 125–33. https://doi.org/10.1002/pon.1523. PMID: 19296462
45. Ziegler-Heitbrock L. The CD14+ CD16+ blood monocytes: their role in infection and inflammation. J Leukoc Biol. 2007;81:584–92. https://doi.org/10.1189/jlb.0806510. PMID: 17135573
46. Ziegler-Heitbrock L, Ancuta P, Crowe S, Dalod M, Grau V, Hart DN, et al. Nomenclature of monocytes and dendritic cells in blood. Blood. 2010;116: e74–80. https://doi.org/10.1182/blood-2010-02-258558. PMID: 20628149
47. Ziegler-Heitbrock L, Hofer TPJ. Toward a refined definition of monocyte subsets. Front Immunol. 2013;4:23. https://doi.org/10.3389/fimmu.2013.00023. PMID: 23382732
48. Ziegler-Heitbrock L. Blood monocytes and their subsets: established features and open questions. Front Immunol. 2015;6:423. https://doi.org/10.3389/fimmu.2015.00423. PMID: 26347746
49. Passlick B, Flieger D, Ziegler-Heitbrock HW. Identification and characterization of a novel monocyte subpopulation in human peripheral blood. Blood. 1989;74:2527–34. PMID: 2478233
50. Ziegler-Heitbrock HW, Fingerle G, Ströbel M, Schraut W, Stelter F, Schütt C, et al. The novel subset of CD14+/CD16+ blood monocytes exhibits features of tissue macrophages. Eur J Immunol. 1993;23:2053–8. https://doi.org/10.1002/eji.1830230902. PMID: 7690321
51. Frankenberger M, Sternsdorf T, Pechumer H, Pforte A, Ziegler-Heitbrock HW. Differential cytokine expression in human blood monocyte subpopulations: a polymerase chain reaction analysis. Blood. 1996;87:373–7. PMID: 8547664
52. Belge K-U, Dayyani F, Horelt A, Siedlar M, Frankenberger M, Frankenberger B, et al. The proinflammatory CD14+CD16+DR++ monocytes are a major source of TNF. J Immunol. 2002;168:3536–42. https://doi.org/10.4049/jimmunol.168.7.3536. PMID: 11907116
53. Weber C, Belge KU, von Hundelshausen P, Draude G, Steppich B, Mack M, et al. Differential chemokine receptor expression and function in human monocyte subpopulations. J Leukoc Biol. 2000;67:699–704. PMID: 10811011
54. Thieblemont N, Weiss L, Sadeghi HM, Estcourt C, Haeffner-Cavaillon N. CD14lowCD16high: a cytokine-producing monocyte subset which expands during human immunodeficiency virus infection. Eur J Immunol. 1995;25: 3418–24. https://doi.org/10.1002/eji.1830251232. PMID: 8566032
55. Blumenstein M, Boekstegers P, Fraunberger P, Andreesen R, Ziegler-Heitbrock HW, Fingerle-Rowson G. Cytokine production precedes the expansion of CD14+CD16+ monocytes in human sepsis: a case report of a patient with self-induced septicemia. Shock. 1997;8:73–5. PMID: 9249916
56. Koch S, Kucharzik T, Heidemann J, Nusrat A, Luegering A. Investigating the role of proinflammatory CD16+ monocytes in the pathogenesis of inflammatory bowel disease. Clin Exp Immunol. 2010;161:332–41. https://doi.org/10.1111/j.1365-2249.2010.04177.x. PMID: 20456413
57. Mukherjee R, Kanti Barman P, Kumar Thatoi P, Tripathy R, Kumar Das B, Ravindran B. Non-classical monocytes display inflammatory features: validation in Sepsis and systemic lupus erythematous. Sci Rep. 2015;5:13886. https://doi.org/10.1038/srep13886. PMID: 26358827
58. Saleh MN, Goldman SJ, LoBuglio AF, Beall AC, Sabio H, McCord MC, et al. CD16+ monocytes in patients with cancer: spontaneous elevation and pharmacologic induction by recombinant human macrophage colony-stimulating factor. Blood. 1995;85:2910–7. PMID: 7742551
59. Feng AL, Zhu JK, Sun JT, Yang MX, Neckenig MR, Wang XW, et al. CD16+ monocytes in breast cancer patients: expanded by monocyte chemoattractant protein-1 and may be useful for early diagnosis. Clin Exp Immunol. 2011;164:57–65. https://doi.org/10.1111/j.1365-2249.2011.04321.x. PMID: 21361908
60. Seidler S, Zimmermann HW, Bartneck M, Trautwein C, Tacke F. Age-dependent alterations of monocyte subsets and monocyte-related chemokine pathways in healthy adults. BMC Immunol. 2010;11:30. https://doi.org/10.1186/1471-2172-11-30. PMID: 20565954
61. Dayyani F, Belge K-U, Frankenberger M, Mack M, Berki T, Ziegler-Heitbrock L. Mechanism of glucocorticoid-induced depletion of human CD14+CD16+ monocytes. J Leukoc Biol. 2003;74:33–9. PMID: 12832440
62. Takuwa N, Kanegasaki S, Asano S, Tomita T, Nakayama E, Sato N, et al. Defective terminal maturation along monocyte-macrophage lineage in chronic myelomonocytic leukemia. Acta Haematol. 1984;72:163–70. PMID: 6438980
63. Soares G, Barral A, Costa JM, Barral-Netto M, Van Weyenbergh J. CD16+ monocytes in human cutaneous leishmaniasis: increased ex vivo levels and correlation with clinical data. J Leukoc Biol. 2006;79:36–9. https://doi.org/10.1189/jlb.0105040. PMID: 16282534
64. Reis-Alves SC, Traina F, Metze K, Lorand-Metze I. Improving the differential diagnosis between myelodysplastic syndromes and reactive peripheral cytopenias by multiparametric flow cytometry: the role of B-cell precursors. Diagn Pathol. 2015;10:44. https://doi.org/10.1186/s13000-015-0259-3. PMID: 25924846
65. Sconocchia G, Keyvanfar K, El Ouriaghli F, Grube M, Rezvani K, Fujiwara H, et al. Phenotype and function of a CD56+ peripheral blood monocyte. Leukemia. 2005;19:69–76. https://doi.org/10.1038/sj.leu.2403550. PMID: 15526027
66. Krasselt M, Baerwald C, Wagner U, Rossol M. CD56+ monocytes have a dysregulated cytokine response to lipopolysaccharide and accumulate in rheumatoid arthritis and immunosenescence. Arthritis Res Ther. 2013;15: R139. https://doi.org/10.1186/ar4321. PMID: 24286519
67. Grip O, Bredberg A, Lindgren S, Henriksson G. Increased subpopulations of CD16(+) and CD56(+) blood monocytes in patients with active Crohn's disease. Inflamm Bowel Dis. 2007;13:566–72. https://doi.org/10.1002/ibd.20025. PMID: 17260384
68. Xu F, Guo J, Wu L-Y, He Q, Zhang Z, Chang C-K, et al. Diagnostic application and clinical significance of FCM progress scoring system based on immunophenotyping in CD34+ blasts in myelodysplastic syndromes. Cytometry B Clin Cytom. 2013;84:267–78. https://doi.org/10.1002/cyto.b.21089. PMID: 23554290

A comparative cross-sectional study of some hematological parameters of hypertensive and normotensive individuals at the university of Gondar hospital, Northwest Ethiopia

Bamlaku Enawgaw*, Nigist Adane, Betelihem Terefe, Fikir Asrie and Mulugeta Melku

Abstract

Background: Hypertension is a major health problem worldwide. It can lead to cardiovascular disease and also leads to functional disturbances including hematological parameters. The abnormalities of haematological parameters may enhance an end-organ damage. Therefore, the aim of this study was to assess some hematological parameters of hypertensive individuals in comparison with normotensive individuals at University of Gondar hospital, northwest Ethiopia.

Methods: A cross sectional comparative study was conducted from October to November 2015 on a total of 126 hypertensive and 126 normotensive individuals at University of Gondar Hospital. All participants after taking informed consent were interviewed for detailed history and 3 ml of blood was collected for hematological test analysis. Independent *t*-test and the Mann Whitney *u*-test were used to find out significant difference and Pearson's and Spearman's correlation were used for correlation test. *P* values less than 0.05 was considered the level of significance.

Result: From a total of 252 study subjects, about 67.5% were females. The mean age of study subjects was 50.3 ± 11 years for hypertensive individuals and 49.8 ± 11.6 years for normotensive individuals with range of 18–65 years. In the present study, the median (IQR) value of WBC, RBC, Hgb, HCT, MCV and the mean value of MCHC, RDW, MPV and PDW were significantly higher in hypertensive group compared to apparently healthy normotensive groups. Additionally, WBC, RBC, Hgb, HCT and PLT showed statistically significant positive correlations with blood pressure indices. Platelet count and MCH did not show statistically significant difference between the two groups.

Conclusion: Hypertension has impact on hematological parameters. In this study, the mean and median values of haematological parameters in hypertensive individuals were significantly different compared to apparently healthy normotensive individuals. Hence, hematological parameters can be used to monitor the prognosis of the disease and manage hypertensive related complications, and it is important to assess hematological parameters for hypertensive individuals which may help to prevent complications associated hematological disorders.

Keywords: Hypertension, Hematological parameters, Blood pressure indices, Gondar, Ethiopia

* Correspondence: bamlak21@gmail.com
Department of Hematology & Immunohematology, School of Biomedical and Laboratory Sciences, College of Medicine and Health Sciences, University of Gondar, Gondar, Ethiopia

Background

Hypertension (HTN) is also called high blood pressure. It is a condition in which systemic arterial pressure is elevated above the threshold value [1]. It is expressed by systolic (maximum) and diastolic (minimum) arterial pressures. Systolic pressure is occurring during contraction of the left ventricle of the heart while diastolic pressure is occurring before the next contraction. Normally at rest the systolic pressure is within 100–140 mm mercury (mmHg) and diastolic pressure is within 60–90 mmHg [2, 3]. Based on the seventh Joint National Committee (7 JNC) report in 2008, normal HTN was defined as systolic blood pressure (SBP) < 120 mmHg and diastolic blood pressure (DBP) < 80 mmHg, pre-HTN with SBP of 120-139 mmHg or DBP 80–89 mmHg, stage I HTN with SBP of 140–159 mmHg or DBP 90–99 mmHg and stage II HTN with SBP ≥ 160 mmHg or DBP ≥ 100 mmHg [1, 4].

HTN can be categorized in to two; primary and secondary hypertensions. Primary HTN, which consists of about 95% cases, can occur without any obvious underlying causes while secondary HTN is developed due to secondary to diseases such as kidney disease, endocrine disorders and narrowing of the aorta or kidney arteries [5, 6].

HTN is a major health problem worldwide that affects 20–30% of the adult population [7]. It is rapidly increased from 3% in rural areas to 30% in urban areas of Sub-Saharan Africa. In 2008, its overall prevalence rate in Sub Saharan Africa was 16.2% ranging from 10.6% (Ethiopia) to 26.9% (Ghana) [8–10].

HTN may lead to severe end-organ damage, coronary heart disease and stroke which constitute the leading cause of mortality [11, 12]. It is strongly associated with functional and structural abnormalities to organs that involve in hematopoiesis [5, 6, 13] and blood viscosity is increased in most hypertensive patient's [14]. Although, the details of this association is unclear, development of HTN is accompanied by reduction in deformability, and an increase in size, number and aggregability of red blood cells. These abnormalities of the red cells may worsen the microcirculation and enhance an end-organ damage [11, 15].

On the other hand, HTN has an impact on hematological parameter such as hematocrit (HCT), hemoglobin (Hgb), red blood cell (RBC) count, white blood cell (WBC) count and platelet (PLT) count. Impaired hematological parameters may strongly indicate hypertensive end-organ damage, specifically kidney failure [7, 16, 17]. Specifically increased Hgb level may cause left ventricular hypertrophy while low Hgb levels causes anemia and heart failure [18].

Generally, there are contradictory results regarding hematological parameters of hypertensive patients in different countries. Moreover, there is lack of information regarding to hematological parameters in hypertensive patients in Ethiopia. Therefore, this study was aimed at assessing hematological parameters in hypertensive patients in comparison with apparently healthy individuals and correlating hematological parameters with blood pressure indices (systolic blood pressure, diastolic blood pressure and mean arterial pressure) at university of Gondar hospital, Northwest Ethiopia.

Methods

Study setting, design and population

A comparative cross-sectional study was conducted from October to November 2015 at university of Gondar hospital chronic illness clinic. The hospital is located in Gondar town which is 740 km from the capital of Ethiopia, Addis Ababa, in the Northwest of Ethiopia. Gondar University Hospital is the only referral hospital in North West Ethiopia serving a population of about 5 million. This hospital gives different types of service for the population including treatment of chronic diseases. A total of 252 (126 hypertensive confirmed and 126 apparently healthy) study subjects were included conveniently in this study. The study subjects with hypertensive and healthy controls were age and sex matched. Study subjects with history of infectious diseases, alcohol consumers, smokers, taking antibiotic, treatment for anemia, patients with systemic diseases and with secondary hypertension were excluded from this study with face to face interview and review of medical records (Additional file 1).

Data collection

Socio-demographic and clinical data collection

After taking a written informed consent data were collected by using structured questionnaire and by reviewing study subjects' medical record (Additional file 1). The questionnaire was validated with pre-test.The data regarding anthropometric variables such as height (to the nearest centimeter without shoes) and weight (to the nearest 0.1 kg) were collected and body mass index (BMI) was calculated as weight in kilograms divided by height in meter squared. Blood pressure (BP) was measured by qualified personnel using an analog sphygmomanometer and stethoscope. All study subjects were recruited during their respective appointment schedule for follow up and newly diagnosed individuals. After interview and detailed review of the medical record, the study subjects were sent to laboratory where blood was collected for determination of complete blood cell count.

Laboratory sample collection and analysis

Laboratory analysis was done at University of Gondar hospital Laboratory. Three milliliters of venous blood were collected by experienced laboratory technologist from each study participants and complete blood cell count (CBC) was analyzed by using Sysmex KX-21 automated hematology analyzer. White blood cells (WBC), red blood cell parameters (RBC, Hgb, HCT, MCV, MCH, MCHC and RDW) and platelet parameters (PLT, MPV and PDW) were analyzed and collected for each study participants by using laboratory result registration form (Additional file 2).

Quality assurance

The anthropometric and blood pressure measurements were taken twice and the average value was used. Protocol for sample collection, processing, and transportation was strictly followed to have safe procedure and reliable specimen. Quality controls and standard operating procedure were strictly followed for hematological parameter analysis. The results were properly documented, transcribed and reviewed.

Statistical analysis

Data were cleaned, edited and checked for completeness and entered in to SPSS version 20 statistical software for analysis. The normality of data distribution was checked by statistical tools of Kolmogorov-Smirnov (K-S). The results were expressed as mean ± standard deviation and median with interquartile range. Comparison of parameters between hypertensive subjects and apparently healthy normotensive controls was done with independent *t*-test for normally distributed data and Mann-Whitney *U* test for non-normally distributed data. The correlation of hematological parameters with blood pressure indices (systolic blood pressure, diastolic blood pressure and mean arterial pressure) was assessed by Pearson's and Spearman's correlation. In any condition, P value < 0.05 was considered as statistically significant.

Results

Characteristics of study subjects

A total of 252 study subjects grouped into two groups (126 Hypertensive and 126 healthy controls) were involved in this study. From them 67.5% (85 hypertensive and 85 healthy) were female study subjects which makes 1:2 ratio of male to female. The mean age of study subjects was 50.3 ± 11 years for hypertensive individuals and 49.8 ± 11.6 years for apparently healthy individuals with range of 18–65 years. About 200 (79.4%) of the total study subjects and 84 (66.7%) of the cases group were urban dwellers. The mean and standard deviation value of the BMI, MAP, SBP and DBP were 24.0 ± 2.3, 109.4 ± 5.4 mmHg, 143.2 ± 8.0 mmHg, and 92.4 ± 4.6 mmHg, respectively. The average duration of illness was 3.47 ± 2.8 years (Table 1).

Table 1 Demographic and anthropometric characteristics of study participants at university of Gondar hospital from October to November 2015

	Variables	Hypertensive (n = 126)	Healthy controls (n = 126)
Age (years)	< 35	15 (51.7%)	14 (48.3%)
	35–55	65 (48.9%)	68 (51.1%)
	> 56	46 (51.1)	44 (48.9%)
Sex	Male	41 (32.5%)	41 (32.5%)
	Female	85 (67.5%)	85 (67.5%)
Residence	Urban	84 (66.7%)	116 (92.1%)
	Rural	42 (33.3%)	10 (7.9%)
BMI	< 18.5	1 (0.8%)	1 (0.8%)
	18.5–24.9	83 (65.9%)	101 (80.2%)
	25–29.9	40 (31.75%)	24 (19.0%)
	> 30	2 (1.6%)	0 (0%)
Duration of illness (years)	< 5	101 (80.2%)	
	5–10	23 (18.3%)	
	> 10	2 (1.6%)	

Comparison of hematological parameters

Hypertensive groups had significantly higher median (IQR) value of WBC, RBC, Hgb, HCT, MCV and mean (SD) value of MCHC, RDW, MPV and PDW were significantly higher in hypertensive patient than apparently healthy normotensive individuals ($P < 0.05$). Although the median (IQR) value of PLT count is relatively higher in hypertensive groups, there is no statistically significant difference between these groups ($P = 0.262$) (Table 2).

Correlation of hematological parameters with blood pressure indices

In the present study correlation of the various haematological parameters and the blood pressure indices among hypertensive individuals was determined. As Table 3 indicates WBC, RBC, Hgb, HCT and PLT showed significant positive correlations with diastolic blood pressure, systolic blood pressure and mean arterial pressure ($r = 0.282–3.96$, $P < 0.01$).

Discussion

A total of 252 study subjects (126 Hypertensive and 126 healthy controls) were involved in this study to compare some hematological parameters among hypertensive and normotensive individuals. The mean age of hypertensive and control individuals were 50.3 ± 11 and 49.8 ± 11.6 years, respectively. Based on the result, hypertensive groups had significantly higher median (IQR) WBC value $6.9 \times 10^3/\mu l$ ($3.7 \times 10^3/\mu l$) when compared to apparently healthy normotensive controls $5.2 \times 10^3/\mu l$ ($2.2 \times 10^3/\mu l$). This finding is in agreement with other similar studies by Babu KR et al. [7] and Al-Muhana et al. [19]. Also, this study showed a significant positive correlation of WBC count with diastolic blood pressure, systolic blood pressure and mean arterial pressure.

Table 2 Comparison of hematological parameters between hypertensive and normotensive groups at university of Gondar hospital from October to November 2015

Variables	Hypertensive ($n = 126$)		Healthy controls ($n = 126$)		P values
	Mean ± SD	Median (IQR)	Mean ± SD	Median (IQR)	
WBC ($10^3/\mu l$)	–	6.90 (3.70)	–	5.20 (2.20)	< 0.001
RBC ($10^6/\mu l$)	–	5.00 (0.88)	–	4.88 (0.58)	0.015
Hgb (g/dl)	–	14.60 (1.85)	–	14.15 (1.00)	0.005
HCT (%)	–	42.70 (5.80)	–	41.3 (3.00)	< 0.001
MCV (fl)	–	86.5 (6.13)	–	86.00 (4.43)	0.011
PLT ($10^3/\mu l$)	–	270.00 (101.00)	–	255.50 (103.25)	0.262
MCH (pg)	29.60 ± 1.75	–	29.61 ± 1.7	–	0.937
MCHC (g/dl)	34.27 ± 1.17	–	34.7 ± 1.13	–	0.003
RDW (SD) (fl)	43.19 ± 2.62	–	42.90 ± 4.42	–	< 0.001
MPV (fl)	10.0 ± 0.95	–	9.8 ± 1.0	–	0.046
PDW (fl)	12.6 ± 1.8	–	12.0 ± 1.7	–	0.007

Note: For hematological parameters expressed by median (IQR), P value is derived from Mann-Whitney U test; while those expressed by mean ± SD, P value is derived from independent T test

There is a causal relationship between vascular function and different hematological disorders [17, 20]. Most hypertensive patient's exhibit increased blood viscosity compared with healthy controls [14]. There is a decreased RBC deformability which could cause an increased microvascular flow resistance, which may result in haemolysis and organ damage [11]. This haemolysis induces release of Hgb in to the plasma which scavenges nitric oxide and causes endothelial dysfunction [21]. There is also functional alterations and abnormalities of platelets in hypertension which is associated with increased risk of clot formation. Activated and large platelets are produced as a result of endothelial dysfunction. These large and activated platelets produce vasoconstrictors. This enhances narrowing of blood vessels; there by high blood pressure and thrombotic disease [22–25].

Table 3 Correlation of haematological parameters with blood pressure indices among hypertensives individuals at university of Gondar hospital from October to November 2015

Variables	DBP (P-value)	SBP (P-value)	MAP (P-value)
WBC ($10^3/\mu l$)	0.362 (0.000) [a]	0.396 (0.000) [a]	0.371 (0.000) [a]
RBC ($10^6/\mu l$)	0.358 (0.001) [a]	0.303 (0.000) [a]	0.301 (0.001) [a]
Hgb (g/dl)	0.341 (0.000) [a]	0.282 (0.001) [a]	0.286 (0.001) [a]
HCT (%)	0.368 (0.000) [a]	0.284 (0.001) [a]	0.300 (0.001) [a]
MCV (fl)	−0.136 (0.130)	−0.147 (0.101)	−0.118 (0.189)
MCH (pg)	−0.088 (0.330)	−0.097 (0.282)	−0.074 (0.410)
MCHC (g/dl)	0.011 (0.904)	0.030 (0.742)	−0.003 (0.904)
RDW (SD) (fl)	−0.031 (0.734)	0.037 (0.685)	0.085 (0.346)
PLT ($10^3/\mu l$)	0.376 (0.000) [a]	0.373 (0.000) [a]	0.362 (0.000) [a]
MPV (fl)	−0.149 (0.97)	−0.062 (0.489)	−0.110 (0.220)

Note: [a]Correlation is significant at the 0.01 level (2-tailed), P value derived from Pearson's and Spearman's correlation coefficient

The relationship between WBC and hypertension may be explained by an increased concentration of stem cell factor (SCF) in serum [26]. During HTN, there is a vascular endothelial dysfunction [27, 28]. Thus, to repair this dysfunction SCF/c-kit increases. The SCF has an important role in differentiation and proliferation of haematopoietic cells [26, 29]. This pathway might increase WBC via its participation in the differentiation and proliferation of haematopoietic cells. Additionally, white blood cells are inflammatory marker and tends to increase during HTN which is supported by Kim D-J et al. [30]. But in contradiction to this study, a study conducted in São Paulo, Brazil showed lower mean value of WBC count in hypertensive individuals when compared to apparently healthy normotensive subjects. But there was no significant association [31]. This difference may be due to differences in the study subjects. The study subjects included in this study were HTN confirmed but the study subjects in São Paulo, Brazil were without a previous diagnosis of high blood pressure.

Similarly, the current study showed significantly higher median (IQR) RBC value $5 \times 10^6/\mu l$ ($0.88 \times 10^6/\mu l$) when compared to apparently healthy controls $4.88 \times 10^6/\mu l$ ($0.58 \times 10^6/\mu l$). This is supported by Babu KR et al. [7], Reis RS et al. [31] and Bruschi G et al. [32]. Also, RBC count showed significantly positive correlation with diastolic blood pressure, systolic blood pressure and mean arterial pressure. The possible mechanisms of the association between RBC and blood pressure are not entirely known but the study showed that it may be associated with stem cell factor. Stem cell factor (SCF)/c-kit signaling proteins are increased in hypertensive individuals [26]. Since it is involved in repairing of damaged blood vessels, the expression of stem cell factor (SCF)/c-kit signaling proteins are relatively high during blood vessel repair. Thus, as a result of SCF, RBC number will be increase via the participation of SCF in the differentiation and proliferation of haematopoietic cells [29].

In the present study, Hgb value was significantly increased in the hypertensive group compared to normotensive groups. This findings is in agreement with supported studies done by Babu KR et al. [7] and Al-Muhana et al. [2, 19] but it contradicts with a study conducted in São Paulo, Brazil [31]. Hgb value has shown a positive correlation with systolic, diastolic and mean arterial pressure in hypertensive groups which is similar to the study conducted by Atsma F et al. in France [33].

The association between HTN and Hgb level may be explained by Hgb and arginase enzyme effects on nitric oxide (NO) bioavailability [21, 34]. During HTN, there is a possibility of hemolysis. But, whether hemolysis is a cause or effect of hypertension remains unclear. Most studies suggest that hypertension is a complication of hemolysis and associated with hemolytic anemia [35]. In addition to this, blood disorders such as polycythemia vera and essential thrombocythemia, causes hypertension [20]. Polycythemia vera will cause an increase in relative red cell mass and whole blood viscosity, and thereby increase peripheral resistance to blood flow. If there is peripheral resistance in the microcirculation, there will be a possibility of hemolysis [21]. During hemolysis, hemoglobin and arginase enzyme are released in to circulation from erythrocytes. This free Hgb is scavenger of nitric oxide which is produced in the endothelial cell that lines the blood vessels and important for relaxation of blood vessels. On the other hand, arginase enzyme depletes the substrate used for NO synthesis by conversion of arginine to ornithine, thus reducing NO production. This conditions leading to endothelial dysfunction and ultimately activation of platelets and clots [21, 36, 37]. Therefore, if free Hgb scavenges nitric oxide and arginase enzyme depletes substrates used for NO production, blood vessel dilation decreases, which in turn causes increased blood pressure.

In our study, the median (IQR) value of HCT significantly increased in hypertensive individuals compare to normotensive individuals. These findings are also familiar to Babu KR et al. [7]. In bivariate correlation analysis, HCT value has shown a positive correlation with systolic, diastolic and MAP blood pressure in hypertensive groups. The reasonable mechanisms underlying the association between HCT and blood pressure is that HCT is a determinant factor for high whole blood viscosity during hypertension. This may lead to a peripheral resistance to blood flow and high blood pressure [7, 11]. The evidence showed that, most hypertensive patients exhibit increased blood viscosity compared with healthy controls [14]. Therefore, high hematocrit in hypertension could reflect a true increase in red blood cell mass as well as hemoconcentration caused by a reduction in plasma volume. In contrary to aforementioned result, contradicted study conducted at University of Port Harcourt teaching hospital, Nigeria [38] and Saudi Arabia [19] reported that HCT was not significantly differ between hypertensive patients and normotensive individuals. This difference may be due to difference in sample size.

In our study, RDW increased significantly in hypertensive groups compared to normotensive individuals. Most studies suggest that higher RDW, which is a measure of the variability in the circulating erythrocytes' size, may be resulted from ineffective erythropoiesis due to chronic inflammation during hypertension [39, 40].

In this study MCV and MCHC were increased significantly in hypertensive groups but there were no significant differences in MCH. But other studies in these parameters showed contradicted ideas. For example a study conducted by Babu KR et al. [7] showed significantly lower MCV, significantly higher MCHC and higher but no difference MCH value. In São Paulo, Brazil, MCV were similar [31], in France MCV is lower by 2% [32] and a study in Saudi Arabia showed no significant differences of MCV, MCH and MCHC [19].

In the present study, the median (IQR) value of PLT count, mean value of MPV and PDW were increased in hypertensive groups than controls. Even though statistically not significant, median value of PLT count was slightly higher in hypertensive groups. The possible explanation for this could be related to consumption of platelets. During hypertension, there is endothelial dysfunction and this leads to platelet activation and clot formation. Then platelets will be consumed and there number does not increase as expected [25, 41, 42]. However, statistically significant increment of MPV and PDW were found in hypertensive groups compared to normotensive groups. This finding is in accordance with the previous findings by Babu et al. [7], Al-Muhana et al. [19], Bruschi et al. [32] and Ates et al. [43].

In our study, PLT count positively correlated with blood pressure indices. The possible mechanisms might be related to vascular complication in hypertensive groups. High blood pressure causes endothelial damage via shear stress, which results in an increase in platelet activation [43]. When platelet production is induced, there could be increment in platelet count, MPV and PDW [44]. Evidence suggests that PLT consumption increase at the site of injured blood vessel. During this condition larger PLTs would be released from the bone marrow because larger PLTs are hemostatically more active than mature PLT. Because larger PLTs are hemostatically more active, the presence of larger PLTs is probably a risk factor for developing coronary thrombosis and myocardial infraction [41, 42].

Since antihypertensive therapy reduces blood pressure and improve endothelial function, their effect didn't assess in this study. Additionally, cell free hemoglobin analysis was not considered. Therefore, further cohort study is required.

Conclusion

In the present study, the median (IQR) value of WBC, RBC, Hgb, HCT, MCV and the mean value of MCHC, RDW, MPV and PDW were significantly higher in the hypertensive group compared to apparently healthy controls. But platelet count and MCH showed no statistically significant difference between hypertensive and normotensive groups. In this study there was statistically significant positive correlations of WBC, RBC, Hgb, HCT and PLT with blood pressure indices (diastolic blood pressure, systolic blood pressure and mean arterial pressure) among hypertensive individuals. Impaired hematological parameters may strongly indicate hypertensive end-organ damage. Hematological complication such as RBCs reduction in deformability and an increase in the size causes hemolysis, high Hgb and low levels are associated with cardiovascular risk and activation of platelets is risk factor for thrombotic diseases observed during hypertension. Therefore, it is important to assess changes in hematological parameters for hypertensive patients which may help to prevent such complications associated hematological disorders.

Abbreviations

BP: Blood pressure; CBC: Complete blood cell count; DBP: Diastolic blood pressure; EDTA: Ethylene diamine tetra-acetate; HCT: Hematocrit; Hgb: Hemoglobin; HTN: Hypertension; MAP: Mean arterial pressure; MCH: Mean cell hemoglobin; MCHC: Mean cell hemoglobin concentration; MCV: Mean cell volume; MI: Myocardial infarction; MmHg: Millimeters mercury; MPV: Mean platelet volume; NO: Nitric oxide; PLT: Platelets; RBC: Red blood cells; RDW: Red blood cell distribution width; SBP: Systolic blood pressure; SCF: Stem cell factor; WBC: White blood cells

Acknowledgements

The authors would like to thank university of Gondar hospital laboratory staff for kind cooperation during data collection and laboratory analysis. We also thank study participants for their willingness to participate in this study and provision of important information.

Funding

Not applicable.

Authors' contributions

BE and NA participated in the design of the study, data collection, performed the statistical analysis and drafted the manuscript. BT, FA and MM involved in analysis, interpretation and drafting of the manuscript along with BE & NA. All authors read and approved the final manuscript.

Competing interests

The authors declare that they have no competing interests.

References

1. Giles TD, Materson BJ, Cohn JN, Kostis JB. Definition and classification of hypertension: an update. The. J Clin Hypertens. 2009;11(11):611–4.
2. Foëx P, Sear J. Hypertension: pathophysiology and treatment. Contin Educ Anaesth Crit Care Pain. 2004;4(3):71–5.
3. Fernández-Arroyo S, Camps J, Menendez JA, Joven J. Managing hypertension by polyphenols. Planta Med. 2015;81:624.
4. Chobanian AVBG, Black HR, Cushman WC, Green LA, Izzo JL, et al. Seventh report of the joint national committee on prevention, detection, evaluation and treatment of high blood pressure. Hypertension. 2003;42(6):1206–52.
5. Kuan Huei Ng AGS, Williams B. Pathogenesis, risk factors and prevention of hypertension. Published by Elsevier ltd. Elsevier Ltd: UK; 2010.
6. Weber MA, Schiffrin EL, White WB, Mann S, Lindholm LH, Kenerson JG, et al. Clinical practice guidelines for the management of hypertension in the community. J Clin Hypertens. 2014;16(1):14–26.
7. Babu KR, Solepure A, Shaikh R. Comparison of hematological parameters in primary hypertensives and normotensives of sangareddy. Int J Biomed Res. 2015;6(5):309–15.
8. Hareri HA, Gedefaw M, Simeng B. Assessment of prevalence and associated factors of adherence to anti-hypertensive agents among adults on follow up in Adama Referal hospital, East Shoa, Ethiopiacross sectional study. Int J Curr Microbiol App Sci. 2014;3(1):760–70.
9. Opie LH, Seedat YK. Hypertension in sub-Saharan African populations. Circulation. 2005;112(23):3562–8.
10. Twagirumukiza M, De Bacquer D, Kips JG, de Backer G, Vander Stichele R, Bortel V, et al. Current and projected prevalence of arterial hypertension in sub-Saharan Africa by sex, age and habitat: an estimate from population studies. J Hypertens. 2011;29(7):1243–52.
11. Karabulut A, Karadag A. Clinical implication of hematological indices in the essential hypertension. World J Hypertens. 2015;5(2):93–7.
12. Bonsa F, Gudina EK, Hajito KW. Prevalence of hypertension and associated factors in Bedele town, Southwest Ethiopia. Ethiop J Health Sci. 2014;24(1):21–6.
13. Yadav R, Bhartiya JP, Verma SK, Nandkeoliar MK. Evaluation of blood urea, creatinine and uric acid as markers of kidney functions in hypertensive patients: a prospective study. Indian J Basic Appl Med Res. 2014;3:682–9.
14. Sandhagen B. Red cell fluidity in hypertension. Clin Hemorheol Microcirc. 1998;21(3–4):179–81.
15. Lominadze D, Schuschke DA, Joshua IG, Dean WL. Increased ability of erythrocytes to aggregate in spontaneously hypertensive rats. Clin Exp Hypertens. 2002;24(5):397–406.
16. AL-Hamdani IH. Estimation of serum uric acid, urea and creatinine in essential hypertensive patients. Tikrit Med J. 2010;16(1):152–8.
17. Jadeja U, Jadeja J, Naik S. Comparative study of haemoglobin concentration in hypertensive and normotensive subjects. Indian J Appl Basic Med Sci. 2011;13(17):7.
18. Smebye ML, Iversen EK, Høieggen A, Flaa A, Os I, Kjeldsen SE, et al. Effect of hemoglobin levels on cardiovascular outcomes in patients with isolated systolic hypertension and left ventricular hypertrophy (from the LIFE study). Am J Cardiol. 2007;100(5):855–9.
19. Al-Muhana F, Larbi E, Al-Ali A, Al-Sultan A, Al-Ateeeq S, Soweilem L, et al. Haematological, lipid profile and other biochemical parameters in normal and hypertensive subjects among the population of the eastern province of Saudi Arabia. East Afr Med J. 2006;83(1):44–8.
20. Mathew R, Huang J, JM W, Fallon JT, Gewitz MH. Hematological disorders and pulmonary hypertension. World J Cardiol. 2016;8(12):703–18.
21. Brittain EL, Janz DR, Austin ED, Bastarache JA, Wheeler LA, Ware LB, et al. Elevation of plasma cell-free hemoglobin in pulmonary arterial hypertension. Chest. 2014;146(6):1478–85.
22. Le Quan Sang KH, Astarie C, Mazeaud M, Structural MAD. Functional alterations of platelet membrane in essential hypertension. In: Bruschi G, Borghetti A, editors. Cellular aspects of hypertension. Berlin: Springer-Verlag; 1991. p. 219–25.

23. Lechi A, Lechi C, Lauciello C, Guzzo P, Arosio E, Minuz P, et al. Platelet abnormalities in human hypertension. In: Bruschi G, Borghetti A, editors. Cellular aspects of hypertension. Berlin: Springer-Verlag; 1991. p. 227–36.
24. Gkaliagkousi E, Passacquale G, Douma S, Zamboulis C, Ferro A. Platelet activation in essential hypertension: implications for antiplatelet treatment. Am J Hypertens. 2010;23(3):229–36.
25. Lande K, Os I, Kjeldsen SE, Westheim A, Hjermann I, Eide I, et al. Increased platelet size and release reaction in essential hypertension. J Hypertens. 1987;5(4):401–6.
26. Zhong H, Lu X, Chen X, Yang X, Zhang H, Zhou L, et al. Relationship between stem cell factor/c-kit expression in peripheral blood and blood pressure. J Hum Hypertens. 2010;24(3):220–5.
27. Higashi Y, Kihara Y, Noma K. Endothelial dysfunction and hypertension in aging. Hypertens Res. 2012;35:1039–47.
28. Dharmashankar K, Widlansky ME. Vascular endothelial function and hypertension: insights and directions. Curr Hypertens Rep. 2010;12(6):448–55.
29. Zeng S, Xu Z, Lipkowitz S, Longley JB. Regulation of stem cell factor receptor signaling by Cbl family proteins (Cbl-b/c-Cbl). Blood. 2005;105(1):226–32.
30. Kim D-J, Noh J-H, Lee B-W, Choi Y-H, Chung J-H, Min Y-K, et al. The associations of total and differential white blood cell counts with obesity, hypertension, dyslipidemia and glucose intolerance in a Korean population. J Korean Med Sci. 2008;23(2):193–8.
31. Reis RS, Benseñor IJ, Lotufo PA. Laboratory assessment of the hypertensive individual. Value of the main guidelines for high blood pressure. Arq Bras Cardiol. 1999;73(2):201–10.
32. Bruschi G, Minari M, Bruschi ME, Tacinelli L, Milani B, Cavatorta A, et al. Similarities of essential and spontaneous hypertension. Volume and number of blood cells. Hypertension. 1986;8(11):983–9.
33. Atsma F, Veldhuizen I, de Kort W, van Kraaij M, Pasker-de Jong P, Deinum J. Hemoglobin level is positively associated with blood pressure in a large cohort of healthy individuals. Hypertension. 2012;60(4):936–41.
34. Hua R, Cao H, Wu Z-Y. Effects of hemoglobin concentration on hyperdynamic circulation associated with portal hypertension. Hepatobiliary Pancreat Dis Int. 2006;5(2):215–8.
35. Wahl S, Vichinsky E. Pulmonary hypertension in hemolytic anemias. F1000 Med Rep. 2010;2:10. http://f1000.com/reports/m/2/10
36. Cabrales P, Friedman JM. HBOC vasoactivity: interplay between nitric oxide scavenging and capacity to generate bioactive nitric oxide species. Antioxid Redox Signal. 2013;18(17):2284–97.
37. Cabrales P, Han G, Nacharaju P, Friedman AJ, Friedman JM. Reversal of hemoglobin-induced vasoconstriction with sustained release of nitric oxide. Am J Phys Heart Circ Phys. 2011;300(1):H49–56.
38. Ighoroje A, Dapper D. Sex variations in the haemorheological parameters of some hypertensive Nigerians as compared to normotensive. Niger J Physiol Sci. 2005;20(1):33–8.
39. Fornal M, Wizner B, Cwynar M, Królczyk J, Kwater A, Korbut RA, et al. Association of red blood cell distribution width, inflammation markers and morphological as well as rheological erythrocyte parameters with target organ damage in hypertension. Clin Hemorheol Microcirc. 2013;56(4):325–35.
40. Inanc T, Kaya MG, Yarlioglues M, Ardic I, Ozdogru I, Dogan A, et al. The mean platelet volume in patients with non-dipper hypertension compared to dippers and normotensives. Blood Press. 2010;19(2):81–5.
41. Sahin I, Karabulut A, Avci II, Okuyan E, Biter HI, Yildiz SS, et al. Contribution of platelets indices in the development of contrast-induced nephropathy. Blood Coagul Fibrinolysis. 2015;26(3):246–9.
42. Yaghoubi A, Golmohamadi Z, Alizadehasl A, Azarfarin R. Role of platelet parameters and haematological indices in myocardial infarction and unstable angina. J Pak Med Assoc. 2013;63:1133–7.
43. Ates I, Bulut M, Ozkayar N, Dede F. Association between high platelet indices and proteinuria in patients with hypertension. Ann Lab Med. 2015;35(6):630–4.
44. Yarlioglues M, Kaya MG, Ardic I, Dogdu O, Kasapkara HA, Gunturk E, et al. Relationship between mean platelet volume levels and subclinical target organ damage in newly diagnosed hypertensive patients. Blood Press. 2011;20(2):92–7.

28

A ten year review of the sickle cell program in Muhimbili National Hospital, Tanzania

Julie Makani[1,2,3*], Furahini Tluway[1], Abel Makubi[1], Deogratius Soka[1], Siana Nkya[1,4], Raphael Sangeda[1], Josephine Mgaya[1], Stella Rwezaula[1,3], Fenella J. Kirkham[5], Christina Kindole[1,3], Elisha Osati[1,3], Elineema Meda[3], Robert W. Snow[2,6], Charles R. Newton[2,6], David Roberts[2], Muhsin Aboud[1], Swee Lay Thein[7], Sharon E. Cox[8], Lucio Luzzatto[1†] and Bruno P. Mmbando[1,9†]

Abstract

Background: Africa has the highest burden of Sickle cell disease (SCD) but there are few large, systematic studies providing reliable descriptions of the disease spectrum. Tanzania, with 11,000 SCD births annually, established the Muhimbili Sickle Cell program aiming to improve understanding of SCD in Africa. We report the profile of SCD seen in the first 10 years at Muhimbili National Hospital (MNH).

Methods: Individuals seen at MNH known or suspected to have SCD were enrolled at clinic and laboratory testing for SCD, haematological and biochemical analyses done. Ethnicity was self-reported. Clinical and laboratory features of SCD were documented. Comparison was made with non-SCD population as well as within 3 different age groups (< 5, 5–17 and ≥ 18 years) within the SCD population.

Results: From 2004 to 2013, 6397 individuals, 3751 (58.6%) SCD patients, were enrolled, the majority (47.4%) in age group 5–17 years. There was variation in the geographical distribution of SCD. Individuals with SCD compared to non-SCD, had significantly lower blood pressure and peripheral oxygen saturation (SpO_2). SCD patients had higher prevalence of severe anemia, jaundice and desaturation ($SpO_2 < 95\%$) as well as higher levels of reticulocytes, white blood cells, platelets and fetal hemoglobin. The main causes of hospitalization for SCD within a 12-month period preceding enrolment were pain (adults), and fever and severe anemia (children). When clinical and laboratory features were compared in SCD within 3 age groups, there was a progressive decrease in the prevalence of splenic enlargement and an increase in prevalence of jaundice. Furthermore, there were significant differences with monotonic trends across age groups in SpO2, hematological and biochemical parameters.

Conclusion: This report confirms that the wide spectrum of clinical expression of SCD observed elsewhere is also present in Tanzania, with non-uniform geographical distribution across the country. Age-specific analysis is consistent with different disease-patterns across the lifespan.

Keywords: Sickle cell anemia, Africa, Tanzania

Background

The highest burden of sickle cell disease (SCD) is in Africa where up to 75% of the 300,000 global births of SCD per year occur [1] and where childhood mortality remains high, ranging between 50 and 90% [2]. Much of what is known about the spectrum of SCD is from cohort studies in USA [3], Europe and Jamaica [4–6], with few studies carried out in Africa [7–10] although it is recognized that there is a need for detailed prospective, epidemiological studies [11]. Tanzania is amongst the 5 countries in the world with the highest estimated number of newborns with SCD a year [12] (Nigeria 85,000, Democratic Republic of Congo 42,000, India 38,000; Tanzania 11,000 and Uganda 10,000 [1, 11]). The World Health Organization (WHO) has formally classified SCD as a major public health problem [13] and Tanzania, like other African countries has included SCD as a priority disease condition

* Correspondence: jmakani@blood.ac.tz
†Lucio Luzzatto and Bruno P. Mmbando contributed equally to this work.
[1]Muhimbili University of Health and Allied Sciences, Dar-es-Salaam, Tanzania
[2]University of Oxford, Oxford, UK
Full list of author information is available at the end of the article

in their strategy for Non-Communicable Diseases (NCD) [13, 14]. In 2004, Tanzania established the Muhimbili Sickle cell (MSC) program [15], integrating research and healthcare in a countrywide referral hospital for all disease conditions, the Muhimbili National Hospital (MNH). The main goal was to conduct research that would delineate the spectrum of disease, identify the main causes of morbidity and mortality and provide evidence-based knowledge that would improve healthcare through the introduction of locally-appropriate interventions and policies. Preliminary information on this population, particularly mortality rates [16], rates and risk factors for malaria [17, 18], bacterial infections [19] and other important clinical features [20–23] has been published. The MSC program has also provided a platform to conduct studies to describe genetic determinants of clinical disease [24], successfully conducting one of the first genome-wide association studies in SCD in Africa [25].

In this paper, we outline the profile of the cohort in the MSC program enrolled over the first 10 years. We then describe the clinical and laboratory features of the SCD population enrolled, as well as the geographical distribution, based on self-reported ethnicity. This program demonstrates the feasibility of conducting longitudinal, cohort studies in Africa and this baseline report is setting the stage for further detailed description of the course and spectrum of disease over time.

Methods

Study site

Tanzania has a population of 45 million and is classified as a low income country. The MSC program was established through collaboration between Muhimbili University of Health and Allied Sciences (MUHAS), the oldest and largest biomedical university in Tanzania and MNH, the national referral hospital which is in Dar-es-Salaam on the Eastern coast.

Study population

Individuals attending MNH who were known or suspected clinically to have SCD or related to SCD individuals were invited to the clinic for enrolment.

Clinic procedures

The hospital had two clinics a week for SCD patients. During the course of the program, a third clinic was started. Patients were encouraged to visit the clinic in the event of an acute illness. All individuals who were enrolled were given a unique identifier number and hospital case number. Case report forms (CRF) were completed including demographic, clinical history and physical examinations. Residence information, including telephone number and consent to contact the family in case the patients did not attend clinic for more than 9 months were obtained. Management of SCD followed hospital guidelines which included prescription of folic acid 5 mg/day, investigations to identify underlying additional causes of anaemia, blood transfusion (BT) for those with haemoglobin< 5 g/dL, or heart failure. Individuals with splenomegaly requiring BT (> 3 times a year) were referred for splenectomy. Oral iron was prescribed to those with iron deficiency, defined by low serum ferritin or empirically to those with low MCV (< 80 fl) and MCHC (< 25 g/dL). Use of insecticide treated nets was emphasized to prevent malaria infections and chloroquine prophylaxis was prescribed until its use was discontinued due to high resistance. From 2010, SCD children under 5 years of age were prescribed daily oral penicillin.

Laboratory procedures

At enrolment visits, peripheral blood samples in EDTA were analyzed for full blood count (haemoglobin (Hb), red blood cell count (RBC), mean corpuscular volume (MCV), mean corpuscular haemoglobin (MCH), mean corpuscular haemoglobin Concentration (MCHC)], white blood cell (WBC) and platelet count (PLT) (Pentra 60, Horiba ABX, Kyoto, Japan; Sysmex XT2000i, Hyogo, Japan). Nucleated RBC could not be differentiated from neutrophils by the haematology analyzer. Reticulocyte count (New methylene blue method; Sysmex XT2000i, Hyogo, Japan) and fetal haemoglobin (HbF) levels by High performance Liquid Chromatography (HPLC) (BioRad, Hercules, CA, USA) were obtained. SCD diagnosis was made by HPLC and Haemoglobin electrophoresis (Helena, Sunderland, Tyne & Wear, UK). Bilirubin total (BIL-T), bilirubin direct (BIL-D)], lactate dehydrogenase (LDH), alkaline phosphatase (ALP) and creatinine were assayed using a chemistry analyzer (Roche Cobas Mira, New York, USA or Abbott Architect, New York, USA). Daytime peripheral oxygen saturation (SpO_2) was determined using a pulse oximeter (pulse oximetry; Nellcor, Pleasanton, CA, USA). Peripheral Oxygen desaturation was defined as < 95%.

Data management and analysis

Data were managed using MySQL database (Sun Microsystems Inc., Santa Clara, California, USA). Analysis was performed using STATA and R statistical software (http://www.R-project.org/). Continuous variables with normal distribution were compared using t-test or ANOVA test and skewed continuous variables were compared using Wilcoxon sign rank or Kruskal Wallis tests, while categorical data were compared using chi-square tests. In order to evaluate the trend of different laboratory parameters, the mean difference between non-SCD and SCD were compared across the age groups. Some mean differences were log transformed to improve visibility of parameters with high and low levels of the difference. Weighted logistic regression was used to determine association between binary response variable and explanatory variables (clinical and haematological factors) accounting for under representation of non-SCD individuals. A p-value < 0.05 was considered to be statistically significant.

Description of the MSC cohort

The description included the age structure and pattern of enrollment. SCD diagnoses were classified into 2 categories: SCD was for SS and non-SCD for those with AS and AA. SCD were almost all β^S/β^S with a small fraction of S/β^0 thalassaemia (estimated at 4% - unpublished data) and very rare β^S/HPFH. SC or CC disease was not encountered. The age of patients was calculated at date of visit from the date of birth and three age group categories were defined: < 5, 5–17 and ≥ 18 (adults) years. Description of clinical and laboratory features between SCD and non-SCD individuals was limited to individuals in age group 5–17 years for the following reasons; 1) < 5 years age group is subject to considerable physiological changes; 2) ≥18 years age group is a heterogeneous group and it is not clear whether it consists of individuals with mild disease who have survived the early mortality of severe disease but who are symptomatic and therefore attend MNH for healthcare. The ethnic group of an individual was from self-reported ethnicity which is patrilineal. If this information was missing, the ethnic group of the mother was used. We plotted the geographical distribution of SCD in Tanzania based on the ethnicity of the SCD cases registered at MNH. The region where a particular ethnic group resides was used as a surrogate for the geographical distribution of SCD. Geographical coordinates of Tanzania and regional administrative boundaries were obtained from Global administrative boundaries website [26].

Results

During the 10-year period (2004–2013), 6397 individuals were enrolled, with 3751 (58.6%) having SCD (> 95% β^S/β^S). 3175 (49.6%) were male and 2393 (37.4%) were children aged < 5 years (Table 1). The median age at testing was higher in non-SCD than in SCD individuals ($p < 0.001$), while the sex ratio was similar between the two groups and there was no difference among those who were coming outside Dar (proxy for distance) compared to those coming from outside Dar es Salaam (Table 1). As the MSC program continued there was a statistically significant ($p < 0.001$) decrease in age of SCD individuals enrolled; the median age decreased from 9.1 years [Interquartile range (IQR): 5.1–14.1] in the first two years (2004–5) to 5.1 years (IQR: 2.3–11.1) during the last two years (2012–3).

The trend of enrolment on annual basis for the SCD patients is shown in Fig. 1a. The largest number of individuals

Table 1 Characteristics of individuals enrolled in the Muhimbili Sickle Cell Programme in Dar-es-Salaam, Tanzania

Variable	Total	Non-SCD	SCD	Test statistic (p-value)
Number screened, n (%)	6397	2646 (41.4)	3751 (58.6)	
Median age (IQR)		9.3 (2.7–24.1)	6.9 (3.3–12.8)	z = 8.7 (< 0.001)
Age group (%)				
0–4	2393 (37.4)	956 (36.1)	1437 (38.3)	$\chi^2 = 346.7$ (< 0.001)
5–17	2592 (40.5)	813 (30.7)	1779 (47.4)	
18+	1360 (21.3)	842 (31.9)	518 (13.8)	
Missing	52 (0.8)	35 (1.3)	17 (0.4)	
Sex (%)				
Male	3175 (49.6)	1294 (48.9)	1881 (50.1)	$\chi^2 = 0.96$ (0.328)
Female	3222 (50.4)	1352 (51.1)	1870 (49.9)	
Place of birth (%)				
Dar es Salaam	3807 (59.5)	1445 (54.6)	2362 (63.0)	$\chi^2 = 41.36$ (< 0.001)
Others	2478 (38.7)	1143 (43.2)	1335 (35.6)	
Missing	112 (1.8)	58 (2.2)	54 (1.4)	
Place living				
Dar es Salaam	4446 (69.5)	1628 (61.5)	2818 (75.13)	$\chi^2 = 1.06$ (0.304)
Others	834 (13.0)	321 (12.1)	513 (13.9)	
Missing	1117 (17.5)	697 (26.2)	420 (11.2)	

Test statistics excluded missing values

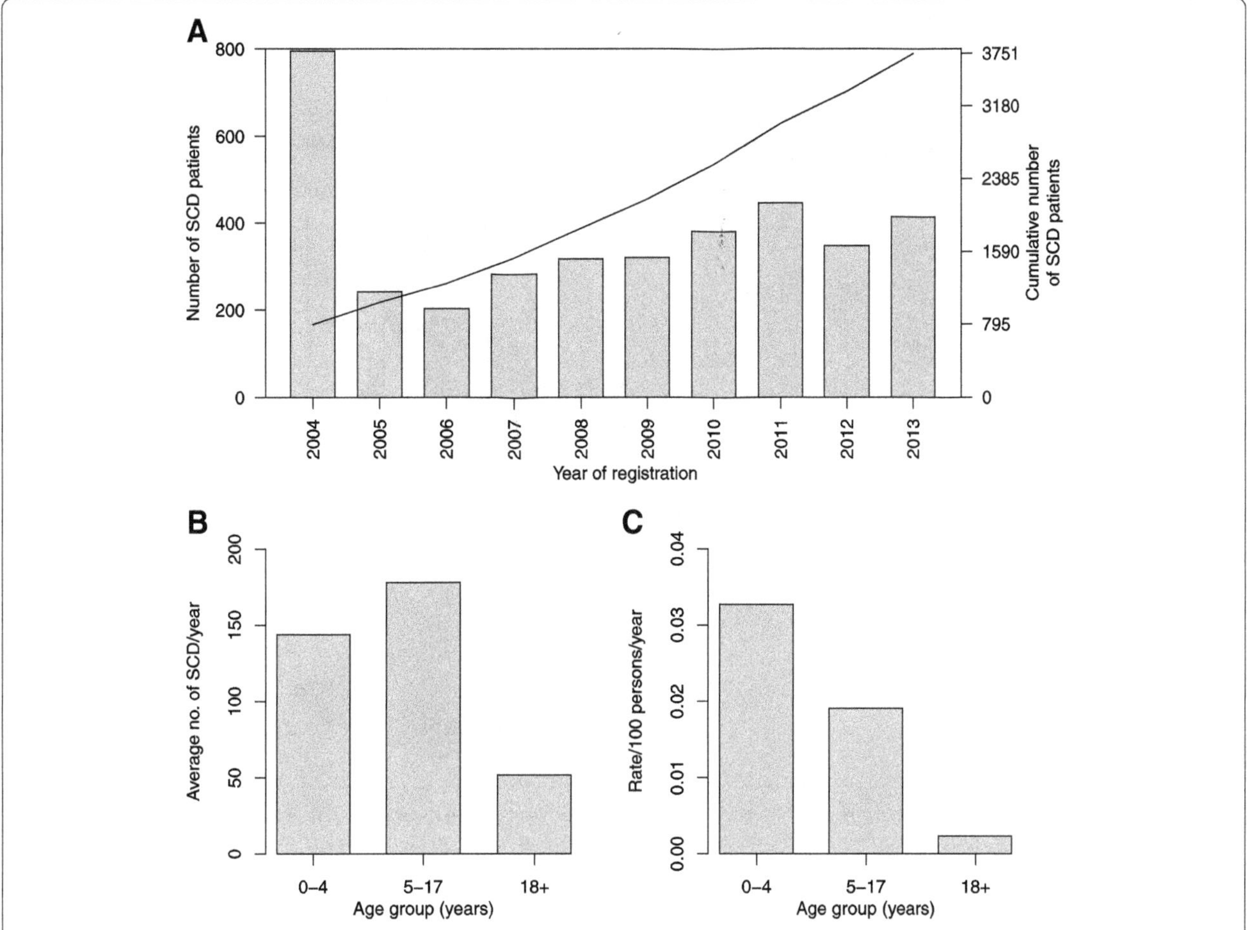

Fig. 1 Pattern of enrollment of individuals with SCD over a 10-year period. Bars and line shows the annual enrolment and cumulative number of enrolment respectively (**a**). Average number of individuals enrolled per year by age group (**b**) and rate of enrolment per 100 persons per year by age group (**c**)

with SCD was enrolled, not surprisingly, during the first year of the program. Subsequently, the annual number enrolled was relatively steady, with the median number enrolled per month being 62 (IQR: 18.5–92). On average, the middle age group (5–17 years) was most abundantly represented (Fig. 1b). However, the rate of enrollment weighted for population size was highest amongst the youngest (< 5 years: Fig. 1c).

Geographical distribution of SCD in Tanzania based on ethnicity of participant

Enrollment is a composite result of the variable prevalence of the Hb S gene, of migration patterns to Dar-es-Salaam and referral practices to MNH. With that proviso, we note that regions with the highest SCD cases were those along the coast (> 10 cases per 100,000 people), the North-Eastern part, which include regions of Coast, Tanga and Zanzibar and along the Lake Victoria zone (Tabora, Shinyanga, Kagera and Mara) with prevalence ranging from 5 to 12 cases per 100,000 people (Fig. 2). In contrast, Arusha, Manyara, Kilimanjaro and Rukwa regions had the lowest representation of SCD (< 2 cases per 100,000).

Comparison of clinical and laboratory features of individuals (5 to 17 years) with and without SCD

Table 2 compares the clinical and laboratory parameters between non-SCD and SCD individuals aged 5–17 years for the reasons outlined under Methods section. Compared to non-SCD, the SCD group had statistically significant higher pulse rate and mean body temperature, but lower levels of blood pressure and peripheral oxygen saturation. The prevalence of low oxygen saturation (< 95%), jaundice and splenomegaly was significantly higher in SCD than in non-SCD group. Regarding laboratory features, SCD is a well-defined disease for which there is no *a priori* appropriate control group. Comparison of SCD and non-SCD individuals enrolled in the MSC programme, we find that all parameters were significantly different. The SCD group had a significantly lower

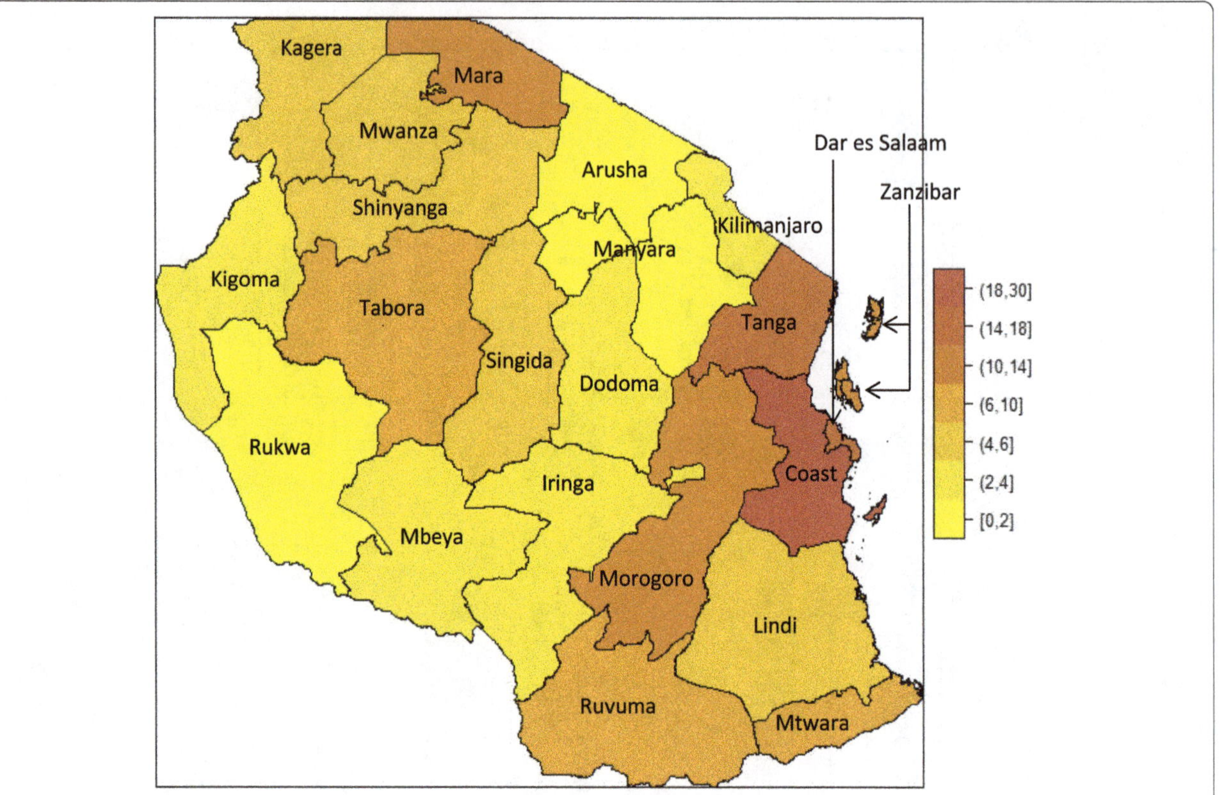

Fig. 2 Geographical distribution of risk of sickle cell disease in Tanzania. Note: Prevalence is expressed (per 100,000) as the ratio of individuals with SCD enrolled in the MSC programme from a particular region to the total population of that region. Ethnicity is self-reported based on patrilineal tribe

Hb (g/dl) (7.4 vs 10.6), alkaline phosphatase and creatinine but higher levels of reticulocyte count, RDW, HbF, MCV, MCH, WBC, platelet count, total, direct and indirect bilirubin, aspartate transaminase, and lactate dehydrogenase. Similar trends for parameter levels were observed even when analysis was extended for all age groups, Fig. 3. The trends of mean difference were similar across the age groups, except for MCHC (non-SCD aged < 5 years had higher levels) and ALP (non-SCD aged > 18 years had lower levels) when compared to other groups. Only mean difference for platelets, ALP and creatinine for children < 5 years were not significantly different between the non-SCD and SCD groups ($p > 0.05$).

Clinical and laboratory features of SCD patients by age group

Evaluation of the clinical and laboratory features in three different age groups within the SCD population is presented in Table 3 and Fig. 4. There were statistically significant differences between the three age groups and interestingly, many of the parameters showed monotonic trends with increasing age. Notably, children aged 0–4 years had a significantly higher pulse rate and prevalence of palpable spleen, whilst peripheral oxygen saturation was lower in older SCD patients and prevalence of jaundice increased with age. The blood pressure (both systolic and diastolic) was significantly higher in the older SCD populations. For 1165 patients (31%), we obtained medical history on the causes of hospitalization in the 12 month period preceding enrollment (Fig. 5). Overall, the three commonest causes of hospitalization were pain, fever (including malaria) and severe anemia. Severe anaemia was the leading cause in children < 18 years (36.9% in 0–4 and 30.7 in 5–17 years), whereas pain was the main cause amongst adults aged ≥18 years (43.2%). Pain (12.9%), fever (12.0%) and malaria (11.2%) contributed equally in children below 5 years, while in children aged 5–17 years pain (27.4%) was the second contributing factor. Out of 469 patients who were admitted with symptoms of severe anaemia as the primary cause, severe anaemia (hb < 5 g.dL) was confirmed in 13.3% of the patients, 36 (7.7%) had pain, while only one patient had jaundice. Contrarily, of patients with Hb results (338) among those admitted with pain as the primary cause, only 11 (3.2%) had confirmed severe anaemia, while only three (out of 388) had jaundice.

The levels of Hb, MCV, MCH and MCHC showed a slight but significant upward trend, whereas RDW

Table 2 Clinical and laboratory features of SCD and non-SCD individuals aged 5–17 years

	Non-SCD (HbAA, AS)		SCD (HbSS)		Test statistic (p-value)
	n	Estimate	n	Estimate	
Clinical features					
Age (years) (Median, IQR]	662	9.91 (7.1–13.1)	1010	9.5 (7.1–12.5)	$\chi^2 = 5.37$ (0.020)
Pulse rate (beats/min) [mean, 95%CI]	680	90.5 (89.2–91.8)	1585	94.0 (93.2–94.7)	$t = -4.79$ (< 0.001)
Temperature(°c) [mean, 95%CI]	694	36.0 (35.8–36.4)	1628	36.5 (36.4–36.5)	$t = -3.63$ (< 0.001)
Systolic Blood pressure (mm/Hg) [mean, 95%CI]	685	107.5 (105.8–109.2)	1462	104.9 (104.1–105.6)	$t = 3.31$ (0.001)
Diastolic blood pressure(mm/Hg) [mean, 95%CI]	684	67.5 (66.3–68.7)	1461	63.9 (63.3–64.5)	$t = 5.96$ (< 0.001)
Peripheral Oxygen saturation,(median, IQR)	662	99 (98,100)	1010	98 (96,100)	$z = 11.78$ ($p < 0.001$)
Peripheral Oxygen desaturation, [n/N (%)]		50/663 (7.5)		162/1009 (16.1)	$\chi^2 = 26.2$ ($p < 0.001$)
Jaundice, [n/N (%)]		45/309 (14.6)		943/1541 (61.2)	$\chi^2 = 224.4$ ($p < 0.001$)
Palpable Spleen, [n/N (%)]		25/451 (5.54)		201/1552 (12.9)	$\chi^2 = 19.16$ (< 0.001)
Laboratory features (95%CI)					
Hemoglobin (Hb) (g/dL)	759	10.6 (10.4–10.8)	1653	7.4 (7.3–7.4)	$t = 32.34$ (< 0.001)
Fetal hemoglobin (HbF)	422	1.7 (0.91–2.5)	803	6.8 (6.4–7.1)	$t = -11.7$ (< 0.001)
Mean Cell Volume (MCV) (fL)	762	75.2 (74.3–76.0)	1653	79.7 (79.1, 80.2)	$t = -8.72$ (< 0.001)
Mean Cell Hb (MCH) (pg)	743	24.5 (24.2–24.7)	1628	26.0 (25.8–26.2)	$t = -9.12$ (< 0.001)
Mean Cell Hb Concentration(MCHC) (g/dL)	760	32.2 (32.1–32.3)	1632	32.5 (32.4–32.6)	$t = -4.00$ (< 0.001)
Red Cell Distribution width (RDW) (%)	761	17.3 (17.0–17.6)	1636	22.6 (22.4–22.8)	$t = -31.49$ (< 0.001)
Reticulocyte (%)	294	7.1 (6.0–8.4)	583	11.2 (10.6–11.8)	$t = -6.15$ (< 0.001)
Absolute reticulocyte (×10^9/L)	274	0.26 (0.21–0.31)	563	0.33 (0.32–0.36)	$t = -2.42$ (0.016)
White Blood Cells (WBC) (× 10^9/L)	868	9.1 (8.6–9.5)	1582	15.6 (15.2–15.9)	$t = -23.5$ (< 0.001)
Platelets (PLT) (× 10^9/L)	763	349.3 (336.5–362.04)	1652	444.4 (434.5–454.3)	$t = -11.55$ (< 0.001)
Bilirubin total (μmol/L)	271	10.3 (9.3–11.4)	930	59.7 (56.7–62.8)	$t = -30.72$ (< 0.001)
Bilirubin direct (μmol/L)	188	3.0 (2.5–3.6)	875	14.4 (13.6–15.2)	$t = -19.08$ (< 0.001)
Bilirubin indirect (μmol/L)	179	8.6 (7.4–9.9)	865	42.1 (39.5–44.8)	$t = -20.52$ (< 0.001)
Aspartate AminoTransferase (AST) (U/L)	295	36.1 (32.6–39.5)	949	52.0 (49.7–54.5)	$t = -7.69$ (< 0.001)
Alkaline phosphatase (ALP) (IU/L)	294	353.6 (329.5–377.7)	953	267.5 (258.8–276.5)	$t = 6.58$ (< 0.001)
Lactate dehydrogenase (LDH) (U/L)	328	593.8 (548.0–639.5)	569	971.6 (932.0–1011.2)	$t = -12.28$ (< 0.001)
Creatinine (μmol/L)	292	46.8 (44.7–48.9)	949	37.6 (36.6–38.5)	$t = 8.36$ (< 0.001)

decreased with age. Reticulocyte counts were elevated in all age groups but they decreased with age. There were significant differences in the WBC counts with counts decreasing with age whereas platelet counts increased with age. Total, direct and indirect bilirubin all increased significantly with age ($p < 0.001$). AST and ALP decreased with age, however the decrease was only significant for ALP ($p < 0.001$).

Discussion

This is the first study that provides a description of the spectrum of SCD in Africa from one of the largest single-centre SCD cohorts in the world. There has been relatively limited information about the spectrum of SCD in Africa when compared to information available from studies outside Africa. Most large series have been from the US, Jamaica and Europe which have involved study populations exceeding 2000 patients with prospective follow up for at least 10 years [4, 27, 28]. In Africa, there has been an increase in the number of similar studies, although the sample size has been smaller (500 to 1000 individuals) and duration has been shorter (up to 5 years) [7–9].

In the first two years of the MSC program, most of the patients enrolled were those already receiving clinical care at MNH, with the majority in the 5–17 year age group (Fig. 1b). This was therefore likely to be a survival cohort and highlighted two unmet needs: the urgency of newborn screening and of strengthening SCD pediatric care. The peak of ongoing enrollment was in 2011 that coincided with optimal number of personnel, weekly clinics and the doctor to patient ratio. This is also the period that the MSC program started working with the Ministry of Health of Tanzania with the aim of strengthening SCD

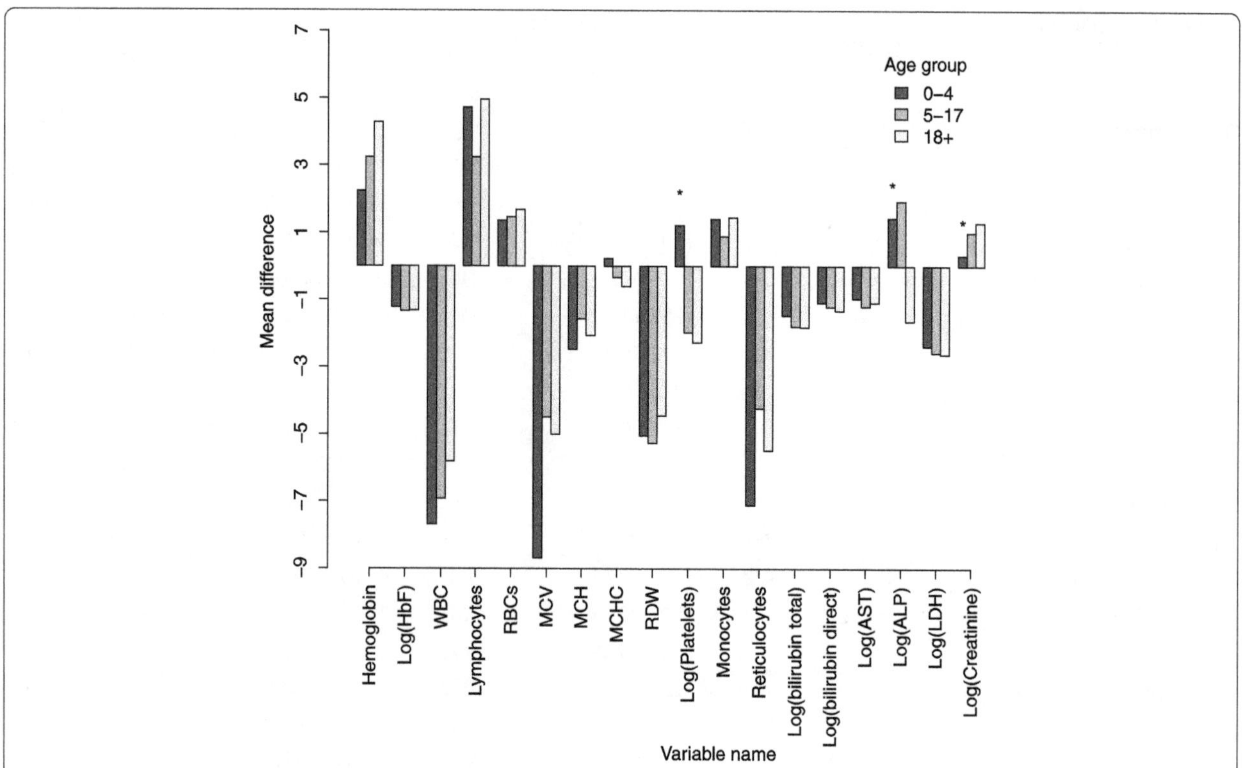

Fig. 3 Distribution of mean difference of hematological parameters between non-SCD and SCD individuals by age-group. Only mean difference for platelets, ALP and creatinine for children < 5 years were not significant difference (*) between the non-SCD and SCD ($p > 0.05$)

services throughout the country, as part of the non-communicable diseases (NCD) program [29]. The age-specific rate of enrollment (Fig. 1c) shows a marked decrease with age: this suggests, unfortunately, a high rate of early mortality in the younger age group, which we have previously reported [16]. At the same time, it is important to note that 518 SCD individuals were aged ≥18 years, providing evidence of survival into adulthood and highlighting the need for adult services. It should be noted that the adult SCD population may comprise two distinct groups: (a) those with severe disease seeking healthcare due to acute and chronic complications, sometimes related to end-organ dysfunction; (b) those with relatively mild disease, who survived childhood.

We report heterogeneity in the geographical prevalence of SCD in Tanzania. The enrollment into the MSC program of patients from different parts of Tanzania will have been influenced by ease of access for residents in regions closer to MNH and/or by socio-economic status, whereby those with higher income are more likely to come to MNH. Nevertheless, it is interesting that the highest numbers were from the coastal regions, including Zanzibar, and from regions around Lake Victoria, despite the long distance between these regions and Dar-es-Salaam. These areas are known to have high malaria transmission˙ On the other hand, there were lower numbers from regions close to Dar-es-Salaam such as Iringa, Manyara, Lindi, Kilimanjaro, where malaria transmission is less. It is noteworthy that, in spite of the ascertainment bias just mentioned, these data agree with previous estimates of β^S gene frequencies in Tanzania [1], although further research is needed to evaluate the genetic and environmental factors, other than malaria, that influence disease prevalence. Detailed micro-mapping of SCD prevalence will also aid planning of optimal health services, targeting areas with high prevalence.

In the initial analysis of features of SCD (Table 2) we compared SCD with non-SCD (HbAA and HbAS) individuals enrolled at the same time. The purpose of this comparison was not to illustrate the differences between SCD and non-SCD, as by definition SCD patients, who have life-long haemolytic anaemia would be discernably different from the non-SCD group. We anticipated that several parameters such as haemoglobin, reticulocytes and bilirubin levels would be higher. What we could not have predicted a priori was that the mean value of all parameters measured would be significantly different - even though, in many cases by a small measure (but, given the large numbers of individuals tested, in nearly all cases the P-value was less than 0.001). The SCD group when compared to non-SCD group had higher prevalence of jaundice and higher pulse rate. The blood pressure was lower in the SCD group, similar to previous reports of a low prevalence of hypertension in this SCD population as

Table 3 Clinical and laboratory features of SCD individuals in 3 age categories (< 5 years; 5–17 years and ≥ 18 years)

Variable	N	Age group (years)			Test statistic	*P*-value
		0–4 years	5–17 years	≥18 years		
Clinical features						
Age (years) (Median,IQR]	3265	2.5 (1·4–3.8)	9.5 (7.1–12.5)	23.7 (20.3–29.5)		
Pulse rate (beats/min) [mean, sd]	3238	110.11 ± 23.1	94.0 ± 15.1	83.5 ± 13.7	446.3↓	< 0.001
Temperature(°c) [mean, sd]	3413	36.5 ± 1.5	36.5 ± 1.0	36.3 ± 1.8	3.16↓	0.042
Systolic Blood pressure (mm/Hg) [mean, sd]	2993	97.9 ± 24.2	104.9 ± 14.4	116.6 ± 16.9	160.8↑	< 0.001
Diastolic blood pressure(mm/Hg) [mean, sd]	2993	58.8 ± 16.4	63.9 ± 11.5	70.7 ± 12.2	127.9↑	< 0.001
Peripheral Oxygen saturation,(median, IQR)	2713	99 (97–100)	98 (96–100)	98 (96–99)	13.7	0.001
Peripheral Oxygen desaturation, [n/N (%)]	2713	170 (15.4)	200 (16.4)	58 (14.9)	0.654	0.721
Jaundice, [n/N (%)]	3171	542 (45.0)	943 (61.2)	292 (68.4)	102.0↑	< 0.001
Pallor, [n/N (%)]	3102	447 (37.8)	573 (38.1)	142 (34.5)	2.06	0.357
Palpable Spleen, [n/N (%)]	3242	192 (15.5)	201 (12.9)	21 (4.7)	35.0↓	< 0.001
Laboratory features						
Hemoglobin (Hb) (g/dL)	3456	7.2 ± 1.4	7.4 ± 1.4	7.6 ± 2.1	10.24↑	< 0.001
Fetal hemoglobin (HbF)	1942	12.2 ± 7.9	6.8 ± 5.63	5.6 ± 4.7	182.9↓	< 0.001
Mean Cell Volume (MCV) (fL)	3454	78.1 ± 11.1	79.7 ± 11.7	82.4 ± 13.8	22.49↑	< 0.001
Mean Cell Hemoglobin (MCH) (pg)	3406	24.6 ± 3.6	26.0 ± 4.1	27.2 ± 5.0	84.11↑	< 0.001
Mean Cell Hemoglobin Concentration(MCHC) (g/dL)	3419	31.4 ± 1.7	32.5 ± 2.1	32.9 ± 2.1	169.58↑	< 0.001
Red Cell Distribution width (RDW) (%)	3440	23.8 ± 4.0	22.6 ± 3.8	21.1 ± 4.4	81.22↓	< 0.001
Reticulocyte (%)	1212	13.3 ± 7.8	11.3 ± 7.5	10.3 ± 7.0	14.45↓	< 0.001
Absolute reticulocyte (×10^9/L)	1153	0.40 ± 0.35	0.33 ± 0.32	0.33 ± 0.62	5.06↓	0.006
White Blood Cells (WBC) (×10^9/L))	3238	19.2 ± 8.3	15.6 ± 6.6	12.4 ± 5.2	170.95↓	< 0.001
Platelets (PLT) (×10^9/L))	3453	377.6 ± 19.8	444.4 ± 205	450.7 ± 213.2	45.92↑	< 0.001
Log(Bilirubin total (μmol/L))	1706	3.62 ± 0.74	4.11 ± -.78	4.16 ± 0.81	76.3↑	< 0.001
Log(Bilirubin direct (μmol/L))	1561	2.45 ± 0.82	2.73 ± 0.80	2.79 ± 0.90	21.3↑	< 0.001
Log(Bilirubin indirect (μmol/L))	1545	3.28 ± 0.83	3.76 ± 0.92	3.80 ± 0.91	47.9↑	< 0.001
Aspartate Aminotransferase (AST) (U/L)	1750	53.2 ± 31.5	52.0 ± 38.3	48.2 ± 39.8	1.64	0.193
Alkaline phosphatase (ALP) (IU/L)	1758	314.2 ± 147.2	267.5 ± 140.5	179.2 ± 156.1	75.69↓	< 0.001
Lactate dehydrogenase (LDH) (U/L)	1196	962.2 ± 428.0	971.6 ± 481.1	918.4 ± 686.9	0.78↑	0.461
Log(Creatinine (μmol/L))	1744	3.49 ± 0.36	3.23 ± 0.39	3.94 ± 0.43	117.0↑	< 0.001

Variables (Hypoxia, Jaundice, Pallor, Palpable Spleen) were compared using χ^2 test, while rest of variables were compared using F-test. ↓ Effect decrease with increase in age while ↑ indicate increase of the effect with age

well as in the USA [23, 30]. The peripheral oxygen saturation was significantly lower in SCD: the difference was small, but in 16.1% of patients it was below 95%. This may be clinically signficant because it is related to the severity of anaemia [31] and to high 2,3-DPG levels, which increases deoxy-Hb S polymerization and sickling [32]. We and others have previously observed that low oxygen saturation is associated with increased cerebral blood flow velocity [33, 34], and higher risk of neurological complications [35, 36]. It was observed that there were low levels of red cell indices (MCV, MCH), which may be attributed in part to the high frequency of α-thalassaemia in this population (about 40% heterozygotes [37]): however, there is no a priori reason why this frequency should be any different in SCD versus non-SCD.

Novel information

Most studies of SCD have focused on children and adults separately, reflecting the fact that most healthcare systems have dedicated but separate paediatric and adult services. The MSC program, instead, aimed to integrate the care of SCD patients across their life span. First, we noted that pain, infection and anaemia were the three most common causes of hospital visits (Fig. 5): but whereas in children the most common cause was anaemia, adults were more affected by painful episodes.

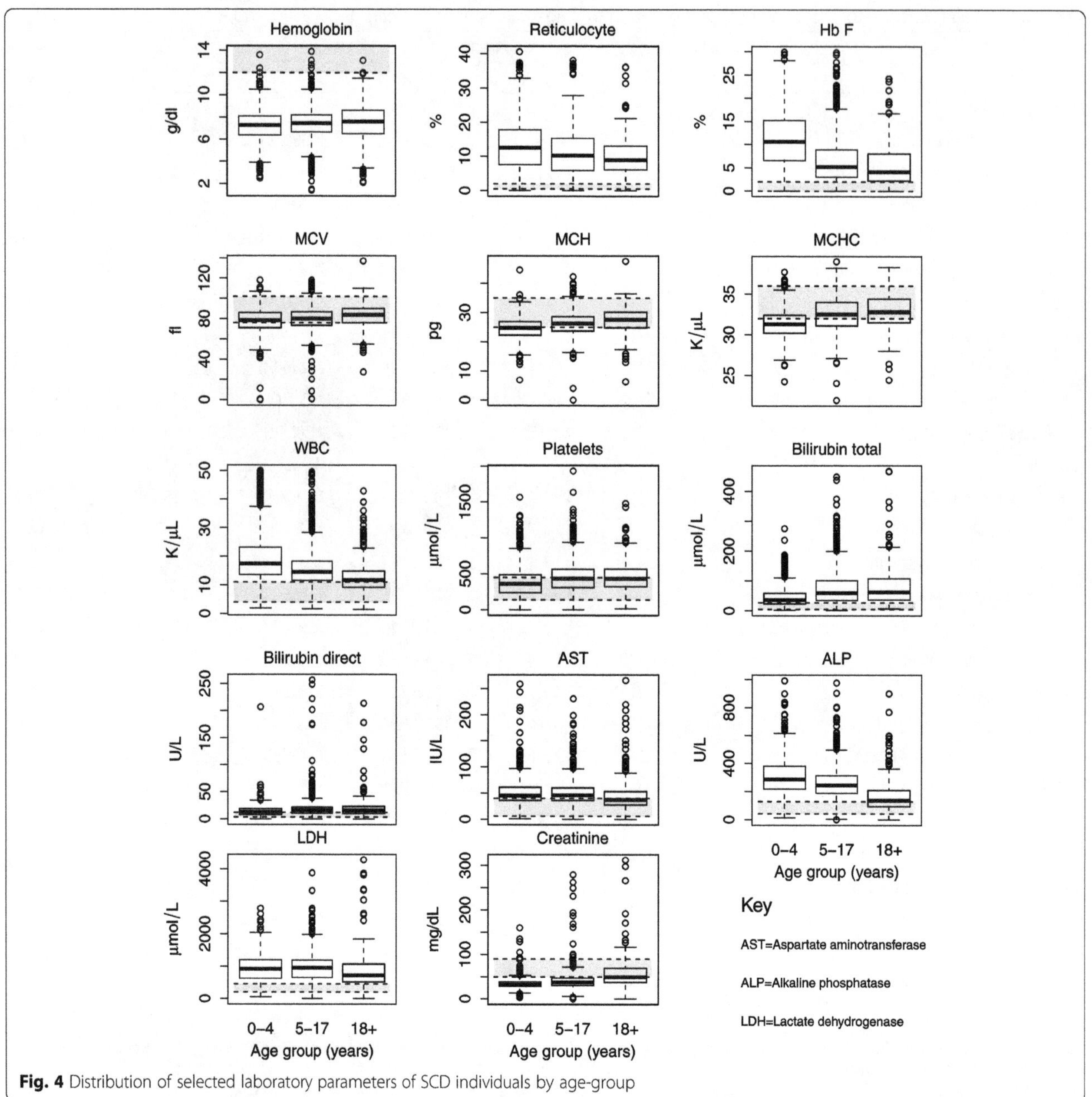

Fig. 4 Distribution of selected laboratory parameters of SCD individuals by age-group

This is similar to findings in other series, where 50% of adults experience painful episodes compared to only 10% in children [38]. Next, we analyzed by age groups all other data over the entire age span from infancy to adulthood. To our knowledge, this is one of the first studies in which such a systematic analysis has been attempted. Here we will focus only on a few observations which we think are important. First, mean level of Hb increased with age, though only slightly, and this was associated with a decrease in the mean reticulocyte count. This correlation is expected, as the increased reticulocyte count reflects a normal compensatory erythropoietic response to anaemia. The decreased reticulocyte count in older patients with SCD may also have reflected reduced erythropoietin levels in the context of the onset of chronic kidney disease, as evidenced by the higher creatinine in the older age group. An alternative explanation may possibly be a direct effect of vaso-occlusive events on the bone marrow resulting in reduced erythropoiesis with impaired reticulocyte production. Second, with respect to HbF, we expected that the mean HbF level would be highest in the youngest age group, since the physiological decrease in HbF from the level of about 80% at birth is much delayed in SS children – compared to controls – in at least the first 30 months of life [39]. However, the further decrease in HbF in the

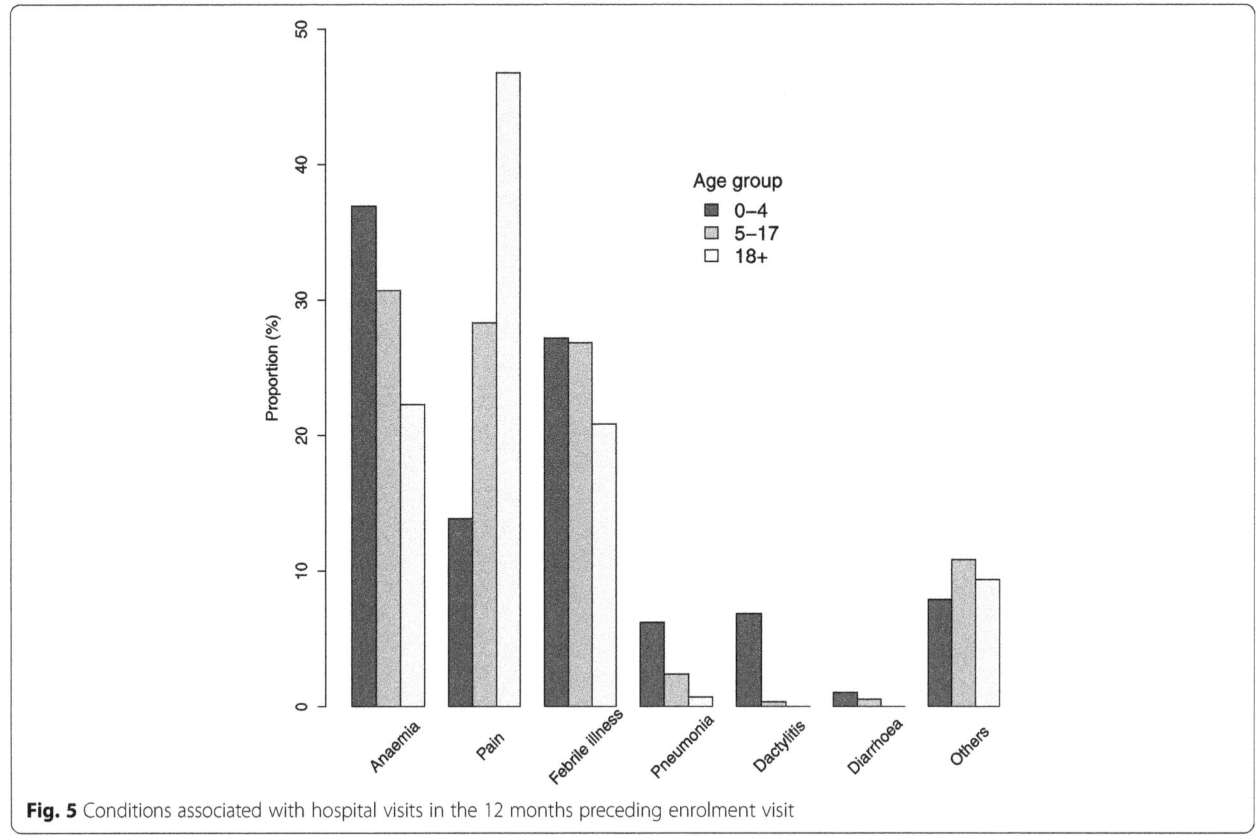

Fig. 5 Conditions associated with hospital visits in the 12 months preceding enrolment visit

transition from the 5–17 age group to adulthood is somewhat paradoxical, because one would have expected that SCD patients with higher HbF would be, if anything, favored in terms of survival: since HbF was seen not to predict mortality in our previous work [33], this finding requires further research. Third, the mean values of red cell indices (MCV, MCH, MCHC) were lower in the younger age group which, in line with the fall in RDW with age, may mean that iron deficiency anemia is more common in the youngest patients (it is indeed common in Tanzania in the < 5 age group). Low MCV and MCH may also result from α-thalassaemia, which is generally regarded as an ameliorating factor in SCD; however, from these data and our previous work [33], low MCV does not seem to confer a survival advantage. Fourth, the mean WBC count decreased with age: which may suggest that the prevalence of infection is higher in children and decreases with age. However, the downward trend in WBC counts may also mean that the older age group is representative of less severe disease. In contrast, the mean platelet count increased with age, probably reflecting a decrease in splenic function: this explanation is supported by a lower prevalence of palpable spleen in the older age groups. The age-specific patterns in the level of WBC counts and platelets warrant further research, as the role of these blood components in the pathophysiology of SCD is being increasingly recognized [40]. Fifth, the mean level of bilirubin increases with age, in keeping with the observation that prevalence of jaundice increased with age. This may be explained by an increase in the rate of extravascular haemolysis; liver dysfunction is less likely since there was a decrease in the mean levels of ALP and AST (albeit not statistically significantly with respect to AST). We must also consider that the higher levels of ALP in the younger age groups could be related to increased bone tissue turnover associated with growth. A striking observation was the high level of LDH (more than 3 times the upper limit of normal) in all age groups, which suggests a significant level of intravascular haemolysis, although cardiac and liver dysfunction may also contribute. Further research is required to quantitate the age-specific rate of haemolysis and whether there is a change with age in the relative rates of intravascular versus extravascular haemolysis. Finally, the mean creatinine level increased with age, although most values remained within the normal range. The creatinine level on its own is not a sensitive index of early renal disease, but one wonders whether in individual cases the trend of creatinine with age may be a prelude to renal insufficiency, a known complication of SCD. It should be noted that the age-related trends in clinical and laboratory parameters in this report were also reported by Aliyu et al. [41] in Nigeria (208 individuals with SCD; Youngest 10 years; 7% > 35 years).

In one of the first systematic studies of SCD patients, Nagel and colleagues [42] noted that the β^S haplotype may account for the great variability in the clinical symptomatology and severity of SCD. In this population in Tanzania, this layer of heterogeneity is largely removed, since nearly all patients are homozygous for the Central African Republic (CAR) haplotype (previously referred to as Bantu haplotype) [43]: However, the spread of values remains just as great (Fig. 4); for example, the mean hematocrit level that Nagel et al. [42] reported for SS patients with CAR haplotype was 23.1, which corresponds almost to the mean Hb of 7.4 in the Tanzania population with the same haplotype, although the range in Tanzania is wider. Although the β-globin haplotype is regarded as a major determinant of HbF production, we found (Fig. 4) a markedly skewed distribution, whereby the top 2.5% of patients had HbF values some 4 times higher than the mean. Genomic studies conducted in SCD in Tanzania have already reported variability in prevalence of and co-existence of genomic loci that influence HbF, α-thalassemia, and G6PD levels [25, 37]. Further research is required, and is ongoing, to increase understanding in the complex interplay of genetic, environmental and socio-economic factors influencing variability of disease spectrum [44].

Limitations

Because enrolment into the SCD cohort was hospital-based, the study may not have captured individuals with mild disease. The non-SCD group was not a population-based age- and sex-matched control group: rather, it was a 'convenient' comparison group consisting of patient family members and of individuals enrolled among those suspected to have SCD: hence they may have other medical conditions. Indeed, the clinical and laboratory features were often not normal. We did not separate controls with HbAA from those with HbAS. This is broadly justified because sickle cell trait subjects have no cells containing exclusively HbS and are haematologically normal. However it is possible that some parameters may differ in AA versus AS subjects: this requires further study. Finally, the work reported here is that from cross-sectional analysis of the enrolment cohort. Although the study was conducted over a 10 year period, we are not yet presenting longitudinal data.

Conclusion

This work demonstrates that in an African country it is feasible to enrol, across all age groups, a large number of SCD patients and to assess in considerable detail their clinical and laboratory manifestations. Not surprisingly, in first approximation the clinical spectrum of SCD is similar to that observed elsewhere. However, the age distribution is different, unfortunately reflecting, at least in part, early mortality and delayed diagnosis due to the absence of newborn screening. The prevalence of severe anaemia is high, probably reflecting less blood transfusion treatment and other environmental factors, including malaria and a higher rate of bacterial infection.

SCD has been recognized as a major public health problem: as such, it was essential for us to establish not just its size, but also its spectrum. While this paper was in its first draft the first SCD patient successfully cured with gene therapy was reported [45] and the American Society of Hematology issued a *Call to Action on Sickle Cell Disease*. We feel strongly that in Africa the transition from taking stock to taking action is overdue: we must implement urgently beneficial measures such as newborn screening, infection prophylaxis, optimization of blood transfusion practice and the use of hydroxyurea; and we must also contribute to research on potentially curative treatments.

Abbreviations

AA: Haemoglobin AA (normal haemoglobin); ALP: Alkaline phosphatase; AS: Haemoglobin AS (sickle cell trait); AST: Aspartate aminotransferase; BIL-D: Bilirubin direct; BIL-T: Bilirubin total; BT: Blood transfusion; CC: Haemoglobin CC; CRF: Case report forms; EDTA: Ethylenediaminetetraacetic acid; Hb: Haemoglobin; HbF: Fetal haemoglobin; HPFH: Hereditary persistence of fetal haemoglobin; HPLC: High performance Liquid Chromatography; IQR: Inter quartile range; LDH: Lactate dehydrogenase; MCH: Mean corpuscular haemoglobin; MCHC: Mean corpuscular haemoglobin Concentration; MCV: Mean corpuscular volume; MNH: Muhimbili National Hospital; MSC: Muhimbili Sickle cell; MUHAS: Muhimbili University of Health and Allied Sciences; NCD: Non-Communicable Diseases; PLT: Platelet count; RBC: Red blood cell count; RDW: Red cell distribution width; SC: Haemoglobin SC; SCD: Sickle cell disease; SS: Haemoglobin SS; UK: United Kingdom; USA: United States of America; WBC: White blood cell; WHO: World Health Organization; β^S: Beta globin

Acknowledgements

We thank the patients and staff of Muhimbili National Hospital and Muhimbili University of Health and Allied Sciences. We thank the following individuals: Data collection: Albert N Komba, Critical comments on statistical analysis: Neal O Jeffries, Nancy L Geller from NHLBI, NIH. Mentorship and support: Thomas Williams, Kevin Marsh, Kisali Pallangyo, Ephata Kaaya.

Funding

This work was supported by the Wellcome Trust, UK (Fellowship Julie Makani 072064, 093727; Project grant 080025; Strategic award 084538; Principal Wellcome Trust Fellowship R W Snow 103602) and Government of United Republic of Tanzania.

Authors' contributions

Contribution: JMa, RWS, CRN, DR, MA, SLT, SEC conceived and designed the study; JMa, FT, AM, DS, SR, CK, EO and EM patients care and clinical data collection; SN and JMg performed sample processing and laboratory analyses; RS and SEC were responsible for data management; BPM analysed the data; JMa, LL and BPM wrote the paper; RWS, CRN, DR, MA, SLT, FJK and SEC critically reviewed the manuscript. All authors read and approved the final manuscript.

Competing interests
The authors declare that they have no competing interests.

Author details
[1]Muhimbili University of Health and Allied Sciences, Dar-es-Salaam, Tanzania. [2]University of Oxford, Oxford, UK. [3]Muhimbili National Hospital, Dar-es-Salaam, Tanzania. [4]Dar-es-Salaam University College of Education, Dar-es-Salaam, Tanzania. [5]University College London, London, UK. [6]Centre for Geographic Medicine Research, Kenya Medical Research Institute, Kilifi, Kenya. [7]National Institutes of Health, Bethesda, USA. [8]London School of Hygiene & Tropical Medicine, London, UK. [9]National Institute for Medical Research Tanga Centre, Tanga, Tanzania.

References

1. Piel FB, Patil AP, Howes RE, Nyangiri OA, Gething PW, Dewi M, et al. Global epidemiology of sickle haemoglobin in neonates: a contemporary geostatistical model-based map and population estimates. Lancet. 2013;281: 142–51.
2. Weatherall D, Akinyanju O, Fucharoen S, Olivieri N, Musgrove P. Inherited disorders of hemoglobin. 2006.
3. Gaston M, Rosse WF. The cooperative study of sickle cell disease: review of study design and objectives. Am J Pediatr Hematol Oncol. 1982;4:197–201.
4. Telfer P, Coen P, Chakravorty S, Wilkey O, Evans J, Newell H, et al. Clinical outcomes in children with sickle cell disease living in England: a neonatal cohort in East London. Haematologica. 2007;92:905–12.
5. Gill FM, Sleeper LA, Weiner SJ, Brown AK, Bellevue R, Grover R, et al. Clinical events in the first decade in a cohort of infants with sickle cell disease. Cooperative Study of Sickle Cell Disease. Blood. 1995;86:776–83.
6. Lee A, Thomas P, Cupidore L, Serjeant B, Serjeant G. Improved survival in homozygous sickle cell disease: lessons from a cohort study. BMJ. 1995;311: 1600–2.
7. Diagne I, Diagne-Gueye ND, Signate-Sy H, Camara B, Lopez-Sall P, Diack-Mbaye A, et al. Management of children with sickle cell disease in Africa: experience in a cohort of children at the Royal Albert Hospital in Dakar. Med Trop (Mars). 2003;63:513–20.
8. Rahimy MC, Gangbo A, Ahouignan G, Adjou R, Deguenon C, Goussanou S, et al. Effect of a comprehensive clinical care program on disease course in severely ill children with sickle cell anemia in a sub-Saharan African setting. Blood. 2003;102:834–8.
9. Tshilolo L, Mukendi R, Girot R. Sickle cell anemia in the south of Zaire. Study of two series of 251 and 340 patients followed-up 1988-1992. Arch Pediatr. 1996; 3:104–11.
10. Dubert M, Elion J, Tolo A, Diallo DA, Diop S, Diagne I, et al. Degree of anemia, indirect markers of hemolysis, and vascular complications of sickle cell disease in Africa. Blood. 2017;130:2215–23.
11. Powars DR, Chan LS, Hiti A, Ramicone E, Johnson C. Outcome of sickle cell anemia: a 4-decade observational study of 1056 patients. Medicine (Baltimore). 2005;84: 363–76.
12. Piel FB, Steinberg MH, Rees DC. Sickle cell disease. N Engl J Med. 2017;377: 305.
13. World Health Organisation. Sickle Cell Anaemia. Agenda item 11.4. 59th World Health Assembly, 27 May 2006. 2006.
14. World Health Organisation. The Brazzaville declaration on non-communicable diseases prevention and control in the WHO African region. 2011.
15. Tluway F, Makani J. Sickle cell disease in Africa: an overview of the integrated approach to health, research, education and advocacy in Tanzania, 2004–2016. Br J Haematol:2017;177:919–29.
16. Makani J, Cox SE, Soka D, Komba AN, Oruo J, Mwamtemi H, et al. Mortality in sickle cell anemia in africa: a prospective cohort study in Tanzania. PLoS One. 2011;6:e14699.
17. Makani J, Komba AN, Cox SE, Oruo J, Mwamtemi K, Kitundu J, et al. Malaria in patients with sickle cell anemia: burden, risk factors, and outcome at the outpatient clinic and during hospitalization. Blood. 2010;115:215–20.
18. Mmbando BP, Mgaya J, Cox SE, Mtatiro SN, Soka D, Rwezaula S, et al. Negative epistasis between sickle and foetal haemoglobin suggests a reduction in protection against malaria. PLoS One. 2015;10:e0125929.
19. Makani J, Mgaya J, Balandya E, Msami K, Soka D, Cox SE, et al. Bacteraemia in sickle cell anaemia is associated with low haemoglobin: a report of 890 admissions to a tertiary hospital in Tanzania. Br J Haematol. 2015;171:273–76.
20. Cox SE, Makani J, Fulford AJ, Komba AN, Soka D, Williams TN, et al. Nutritional status, hospitalization and mortality among patients with sickle cell anemia in Tanzania. Haematologica. 2011;96:948–53.
21. Cox SE, Soka D, Kirkham FJ, Newton CRJ, Prentice AM, Makani J, et al. Tricuspid regurgitant jet velocity and hospitalization in Tanzanian children with sickle cell anemia. Haematologica. 2014;99:e1–4.
22. Cox SE, Makani J, Newton CR, Prentice AM, Kirkham FJ. Hematological and genetic predictors of daytime hemoglobin saturation in Tanzanian children with and without sickle cell anemia. ISRN Hematol. 2013;2013:472909.
23. Makubi A, Mmbando BP, Novelli EM, Lwakatare J, Soka D, Marik H, et al. Rates and risk factors of hypertension in adolescents and adults with sickle cell anaemia in Tanzania: 10 years' experience. Br J Haematol. 2017;177:930–37.
24. Makani J, Menzel S, Nkya S, Cox SE, Drasar E, Soka D, et al. Genetics of fetal hemoglobin in Tanzanian and British patients with sickle cell anemia. Blood. 2011; 117:1390–2.
25. Mtatiro SN, Singh T, Rooks H, Mgaya J, Mariki H, Soka D, et al. Genome wide association study of fetal hemoglobin in sickle cell Anemia in Tanzania. PLoS One. 2014;9:e111464.
26. New. NBS. Geographical Information System (GIS). https://www.nbs.go.tz/nbstz/index.php/english/geographical-information-system-gis. Accessed 30 Oct 2018.
27. Farber MD, Koshy M, Kinney TR, the Cooperative Study of Sickle Cell Disease. Cooperative study of sickle cell disease: Demographic and socioeconomic characteristics of patients and families with sickle cell disease. J Chronic Dis. 1985; 38:495–05.
28. King LGC, Bortolusso-Ali S, Cunningham-Myrie CA, Reid MEG. Impact of a comprehensive sickle cell center on early childhood mortality in a developing country: the Jamaican experience. J Pediatr. 2015;167:702-5.e1.
29. Ministry of Health and Social welfare Tanzania. In: Division of preventative health services, editor. National Strategy for Non-Communicable Diseases 2009–2015: Tanzania Food and Nutrition Centre; 2009.
30. Pegelow CH, Colangelo L, Steinberg M, Wright EC, Smith J, Phillips G, et al. Natural history of blood pressure in sickle cell disease: risks for stroke and death associated with relative hypertension in sickle cell anemia. Am J Med. 1997;102: 171–7.
31. Campbell A, Minniti CP, Nouraie M, Arteta M, Rana S, Onyekwere O, et al. Prospective evaluation of haemoglobin oxygen saturation at rest and after exercise in paediatric sickle cell disease patients. Br J Haematol. 2009;147: 352–9.
32. Poillon WN, Kim BC, Castro O. Intracellular hemoglobin S polymerization and the clinical severity of sickle cell anemia. Blood. 1998;91:1777-83..
33. Makani J, Kirkham FJ, Komba A, Ajala-Agbo T, Otieno G, Fegan G, et al. Risk factors for high cerebral blood flow velocity and death in Kenyan children with sickle cell Anaemia: role of haemoglobin oxygen saturation and febrile illness. Br J Haematol. 2009;145:529–32.
34. Ojewunmi OO, Adeyemo TA, Osuntoki AA, Imaga NA, Oyetunji AI. Haemoglobin oxygen saturation, leucocyte count and lactate dehydrogenase are predictors of elevated cerebral blood flow velocity in Nigerian children with sickle cell anaemia. Paediatr Int Child Health. 2018;38: 34–39.
35. Setty BNY, Stuart MJ, Dampier C, Brodecki D, Allen JL. Hypoxaemia in sickle cell disease: biomarker modulation and relevance to pathophysiology. Lancet. 2003;362:1450–5.
36. Kirkham FJ, Hewes DKM, Prengler M, Wade A, Lane R, JPM E. Nocturnal hypoxaemia and central-nervous-system events in sickle-cell disease. Lancet. 2001;357:1656–9.
37. Cox SE, Makani J, Soka D, L'Esperence VS, Kija E, Dominguez-Salas P, et al. Haptoglobin, alpha-thalassaemia and glucose-6-phosphate dehydrogenase polymorphisms and risk of abnormal transcranial Doppler among patients with sickle cell anaemia in Tanzania. Br J Haematol. 2014;165:699–706.
38. Ballas SK, Gupta K, Adams-Graves P. Sickle cell pain: A critical reappraisal. Blood. 2012;120:3647–56.
39. Maier-Redelsperger M, Noguchi CT, de Montalembert M, Rodgers GP, Schechter AN, Gourbil A, et al. Variation in fetal hemoglobin parameters and predicted hemoglobin S polymerization in sickle cell children in the first two years of life: Parisian Prospective Study on Sickle Cell Disease. Blood. 1994;84: 3182–8.
40. Zhang D, Xu C, Manwani D, Frenette PS. Neutrophils, platelets, and inflammatory pathways at the nexus of sickle cell disease pathophysiology. Blood. 2016;127: 801–9.

41. Aliyu ZY, Gordeuk V, Sachdev V, Babadoko A, Mamman AI, Akpanpe P, et al. Prevalence and risk factors for pulmonary artery systolic hypertension among sickle cell disease patients in Nigeria. Am J Hematol. 2008;83:485–90.
42. Nagel RL, Rao SK, Dunda-Belkhodja O, Connolly MM, Fabry ME, Georges A, et al. The hematologic characteristics of sickle cell anemia bearing the Bantu haplotype: the relationship between G gamma and HbF level. Blood. 1987;69:1026–30.
43. Nagel RL, Ranney HM. Genetic epidemiology of structural mutations of the beta-globin gene. In: Seminars in hematology; 1990;342–59.
44. Makani J, Ofori-Acquah SF, Tluway F, Mulder N, Wonkam A. Sickle cell disease: tipping the balance of genomic research to catalyse discoveries in Africa. Lancet. 2017;389:2355–58.
45. Ribeil J-A, Hacein-Bey-Abina S, Payen E, Magnani A, Semeraro M, Magrin E, et al. Gene therapy in a patient with sickle cell disease. N Engl J Med. 2017; 376:848–55.

Anemia and associated factors among children aged 6–23 months in Damot Sore District, Wolaita Zone, South Ethiopia

Bereket Geze Malako[1], Melese Sinaga Teshome[2*] and Tefera Belachew[2]

Abstract

Background: Anemia affects a significant part of the population in nearly every country in the globe. Iron requirements are greatest at ages 6–23 months when growth is extremely rapid and critically essential in critical times of life. Even though infants and toddlers are highly at risk, they are not considered as separate populations in the estimation of anemia. Despite this, the prevalence of anemia among under 24 months of age is still at its highest point of severity to be a public health problem in Ethiopia. There is no study that documented the magnitude of the problem and associated factors in the study area. The main aim of this study was to assess the prevalence of anemia and to identify associated factors among children 6–23 months of age.

Methods: A community-based cross-sectional study was carried out among 485 children of Damot Sore, South Ethiopia from March to April 2017. Data on socio-demographic, dietary, blood samples for hemoglobin level and malaria infection were collected. Both descriptive and bivariate analyses were done and all variables having a *p*-value of 0.25 were selected for multivariable analyses. A multivariable logistic regression model was used to isolate independent predictors of anemia at a p-value less than 0.05. A principal component analysis was used to generate household wealth score, dietary diversity score.

Results: Out of 522 sampled children, complete data were captured from 485 giving a response rate of 92.91%. For altitude and persons smoking in the house adjusted prevalence of anemia was 255(52.6%). The larger proportion, 128(26.4%) of children had moderate anemia. On multivariable logistic regression analyses, household food insecurity (AOR = 2.74(95% CI: 1.62–4.65)), poor dietary diversity (AOR = 2.86(95% CI: 1.73–4.7)), early or late initiation of complementary feeding (AOR = 2.0(95% CI: 1.23–3.60)), poor breastfeeding practice (AOR = 2.6(95% CI: 1.41–4.62)), and poor utilization of folic acid by mothers (AOR = 2.75(95% CI: 1.42–5.36)) were significantly associated with anemia.

Conclusion: Prevalence of anemia among children (6–23 months) was a severe public health problem in the study area. Most important predictors are suboptimal child feeding practices, household food insecurity, and poor diet. Multi-sectoral efforts are needed to improve health and interventions targeting nutrition security are recommended.

Keywords: Anemia, Children, Damot sore, Wolaita

* Correspondence: Sinmele@gmail.com
[2]Institute of Health, Public Health Faculty, Population and Family Health Department, Nutrition Course Team, Jimma University, Jimma, Ethiopia
Full list of author information is available at the end of the article

Background

Anemia is one of micronutrient deficiency which has serious and common public health significance in the world and it is the second leading nutritional cause of disability. Globally, about 42.6% of children (5–59 months) are suffering from anemia [1, 2]. It affects quarter of world population, primarily pregnant women and young children are at greatest risk [1].

There are many causes of anemia, of the iron deficiency (inadequate iron intake, poor iron absorption or excess iron losses), insufficient hematopoiesis (e.g., from vitamin B-12 deficiency), loss of blood (hemorrhagic anemia), premature red blood cell plasma membrane rapture (hemolytic anemia), deficient or abnormal synthesis of hemoglobin (e.g., thalassemia) or destruction of bone marrow (aplastic anemia were known [3, 4].

Children who live in Asia and Africa are at greatest risk with almost two-thirds of children living in Africa being anemic. Anemia can occur at any time and all stages of life cycle, but young children and pregnant women are the most at risk segment of the community. Iron requirements are greatest at ages 6–11 months when growth is extremely rapid [1, 2, 5].

Even if the prevalence of anemia among under-five children has dropped from 54% in 2005 to 40% in 2011, it increased significantly in Ethiopia according to EDHS 2016 report [6, 7]. Although there have been interventions by the government, prevalence of anemia is still at the highest point of severity to be a public health problem in Ethiopia. According to 2016 EDHS, the prevalence of anemia in this age category is 72.3% [7]. Regardless of efforts done so far, anemia remains to be public health problem especially in this age category [8, 9]. So, identifying factors associated is needed to develop appropriate interventions.

Thus, this study determined the prevalence of anemia among children of age 6–23 months and associated factors in Damot Sore District, Wolaita Zone, South Ethiopia.

Methods

Study area and sample

This study was conducted in Damot Sore District located 326kms south of Addis Ababa. According to the district health office, the total population of the study area for the year 2016/2017 was 128,184 and total numbers of children (6–23 months) were 4499. The altitude of the district is between the ranges of 1500-2500 m. A community-based cross-sectional study was conducted from March 10 to April 10, 2017.

All children aged 6–23 months that were residents of the district for more than 6 months were included, on the other hand, children who had received de-warming, received blood transfusion and diagnosed of anemia and on medication prior (2 months) to data collection and child or mother with health condition that hinders verbal communication were excluded from study. The sample size was estimated using with Epi InfoTM7 by using formula for estimation of a single population proportion for anemia and two population proportion formulas for associated factors with the following assumptions: prevalence of anemia among children 6–23 months of 66.6, 95% confidence level and 5% margin of error from prior study [8] and multiplying 1.5 for the design effect and adding a non-response rate of 10%. Therefore, the subsequent reports were based on the total sample of 522.

Multistage sampling was used to select study participants. For this, first, 6 Kebeles (smallest political administrative unit of government) were selected using lottery method out of 20 "Kebles" in the District. Secondly, within those Kebeles, simple random sampling was used to select the study participants using Kebele health posts family folders of community health information system (CHIS). Households with children 6–23 months were selected using a family folder as a sampling frame.

Measurements

Socio-demographic and economic data were collected by interviewing mothers of the children during house to house data collection by using pretested and interviewer administered a questionnaire that was prepared in the English language, which later was translated into Wolayttattua-local language. The standardized tool for measurement of wealth index was adapted from EDHS 2011 [6]. To determine dietary practices of children food frequency questionnaire [(FFQ) were used. The frequency of consumption of food items by children during the last 1 month prior to data collection was asked. FFQ was developed after pilot study on 5% of a sample size of 24-h recall conducted to list out all foods which were be eaten as a complementary food, and then key informants were asked for additional listing and prioritization, the approach was used in earlier studies [10].

Altitudes of Kebeles were measured by using a hand-held Global Positioning System; Mark: GPS 72H GARMIN. Hemoglobin levels were adjusted for altitude changes. Similarly, hemoglobin levels were adjusted for children who live with smoking individual within the household that smokes indoor [11].

Laboratory investigations were done for hemoglobin measurement and malaria status. Hemoglobin measurement was measured from capillary blood by collecting one drop of blood carefully from the middle finger. The finger of the child pricked after rubbing the fingertip with sterile cotton (immersing in 70% alcohol) with a sterile disposable lancet. Automated HEMOCUE Hb 301, HEMOCUE AB, ANGELHOLM SWEDEN machines were used to determine the hemoglobin concentration, which was recommended elsewhere for the survey in resource-poor settings and the results were expressed in g/dl, then categorized based on criteria of WHO cut off point [11, 12].

Malaria test was also done using rapid diagnostic test (RDT), which was appropriate for community survey to know malaria status [13].

Data analysis

Data were entered into EPI data version 3.1 and then exported to SPSS for data analysis. Statistical analyses were performed using a computer software package SPSS for Windows, version 21.0 (SPSS, Chicago, IL, USA)). Frequency distributions of socio-demographical, environmental health and sanitation related variables, household food insecurity data were first explored using frequencies and cross-tabulations by anemia status and the then binary logistic regression model was fitted with anemia as a dependent variable.

Bivariate analysis was done and All variables which had the association with the outcome variable at $p < 0.25$ on bivariate analyses were selected for entry into multi-variable logistic analyses, which was used to isolate independent predictors of anemia by adjusting for other variables. Adjusted odds ratio (AOR) with 95% Confidence interval (CI) were used to determine the strength of association. Variables with $P < 0.05$ were considered to have statistical significance.

Principal Component Analyses (PCA) were done for household wealth score and dietary diversity score. Then ranked into tertiles (low, middle and high) for wealth and dietary diversity and then dichotomization was done for dietary diversity. The lowest two tertiles were leveled as poor DDS, the highest ranks were categorized as good DDS. Regarding dietary practices, a similar approach was used in a study conducted in Jimma, Ethiopia and elsewhere [14, 15].

An ethical approval was obtained from the Ethical Review Board of Jimma University. Written and informed consents were secured from each mother of children. Children who were found to have malaria were given free treatment from the health posts. Similarly, parents of children diagnosed with severe anemia were given referral papers go to the nearby health center.

Data quality

A two-day training was given for data collectors regarding study objectives, interviewing techniques and ethical issues during data collection. A pretest was done among 5% of the total sample size in Shayamba Kilena Kebele which was not selected into the sample. The questionnaires were checked daily for accuracy, consistency, and completeness.

Proper functionality and technical performance of instruments were cross-checked by using quality control samples, for malaria test result with blood film result by microscope and for Hemocue with CBC machine were checked. Comparisons of Hemocue machines with CBC (Complete blood count) machine, Sysmex analyzer (Sysmex XS-500i, made in China) were done. This was just to be confident on the working instruments by themselves but not on technical issues behind the machines, that how they measure. The results of Pearson correlation coefficients for survey Hemocue machines with Sysmex analyzer were:0.979,0.987, 0.996 and 0.995.

Standard operating procedures and manufacturer's instruction were strictly followed starting from sample collection up to result reporting for laboratory activities. All laboratory procedures were handled by laboratory technologists. Before data analyses cleaning were done and also out layers were identified and managed. Crombach's alpha was checked for household wealth and food frequency.

Results

Out of the total 522 children were included in this study, 485 responded giving a response rate of 92.91%. Twenty-seven 27(7.89%) of sampled children were not included in the analysis due to the incompleteness of their data (Table 1).

Out of 485 children, 247(50.9%) were males and 238(49.1%) were females. The age range of children was 6–23 months and the mean ages were 13.65 ± 5.401 months and while their mother's age range was 15–45 years and their mean age was 30.12 ± 5.807 years. Regarding the severity of anemia, among sampled children, 106(21.9%) were mildly anemic, 128(26.4%) were moderately and 21(4.3%) were severely anemic (Table 1).

In Bivariate analysis a total of 15 variables with a *p*-value < 0.25 were entered into multivariable logistic regression and finally 5 variables (household food insecurity, dietary diversity, introduction time of complementary feeding, iron folate utilization of mothers and quality of breastfeeding) with p-value < 0.05 were isolated to show association with anemia independently. Children with poor dietary diversity score were nearly three times more likely to be anemic than children with good dietary diversity scores (AOR = 2.86 (95% CI: (1.73–4.70)) (Table 2).

Children those introduced complementary feeding earlier than the recommended time, which is at 6 months, or those started late after recommended time were nearly 2 times more likely to be anemic than children which started complementary feeding at 6 months (AOR = 2.0(95% CI: 1.23–3.60) (Table 2).

Children living in food-insecure households were 2.7 times more likely to be anemic than food secure

Table 1 Socio-demographic and economic and care-related characteristics of the family and children 6–23 months aged in Damot Sore District, Wolaita Zone, South Ethiopia, from March to April 2017

Characteristics	Categories	Frequency ($n = 485$)	Percent (%)
Sex of the children	Male	247	50.9
	Female	238	49.1
Age of mothers(years)	15–24	86	17.7
	25–34	267	55.1
	35–49	132	27.2
Age of the children (months)	6–11	193	39.8
	12–17	164	33.8
	18–23	128	26.4
Educational status of mothers	No formal education	312	64.3
	Formal education	173	35.7
Educational status of fathers	No formal education	243	50.1
	Formal education	239	49.3
Mothers occupation	Unemployed	467	96.3
	Government/private employee	18	3.7
Fathers occupation	Unemployed	462	95.3
	Government/private employee	19	3.9
Family size	Less than or equal to 5	221	45.6
	Greater than 5	264	54.4
Under five children within household	More than one child	201	41.4
	One child	284	58.6
Household Wealth	Low	204	42.1
	Middle	74	15.3
	High	207	42.7
Introduction time of complementary feeding	Before or after 6 months	226	46.6
	At 6 months	259	53.4
Breast feeding practice of mothers	Poor	115	23.7
	Good	336	69.3
	Not breast feed	34	7.0
Appropriately utilized iron folate	For less than or equal to 3 months	331	68.2
	For greater than 3 months	62	12.8
	Not utilized at all	92	19
Source of drinking water	Piped inside compound	37	7.6
	Public	357	73.6
	Protected well/spring	91	18.8
Toilet	No facility/bush/field	12	2.5
	Local pit latrine	468	96.5
	VIP latrine	5	1.0
Utilization of ITN	No	46	9.5
	Yes	411	84.7
Diarrhea	No	75	31.2
	Yes	165	68.8
Malaria	No	464	95.7
	P. falciparum	6	1.2

Table 1 Socio-demographic and economic and care-related characteristics of the family and children 6–23 months aged in Damot Sore District, Wolaita Zone, South Ethiopia, from March to April 2017 *(Continued)*

Characteristics	Categories	Frequency ($n = 485$)	Percent (%)
	P.vivax	8	1.6
	P.mixed	7	1.4
Surgery	No	481	99.2
	Yes	4	0.8
DDS	No	319	65.8
	Yes	166	34.2
Fermented foods preparation	No	299	61.6
	Yes	186	38.4
Germinated or soaked foods	No	379	78.1
	Yes	106	21.9

households (AOR = 2.74(95% CI: 1.62–4.65)). Children of mothers those utilized iron folate for less than or equal to 3 months (90 days) during pregnancy were 2.75 times more likely to be anemic than mothers of those utilized more than 3 months children (AOR = 2.75(95%CI:1.42–5.36)). Children from mothers who have had a poor practice of breastfeeding were three times more anemic than children of mothers that have had good breastfeeding practice (AOR = 2.6(95% CI: 1.41–4.62)) (Table 2).

Discussion

This study showed that overall prevalence of anemia among children 6–23 months was 52.6%. After adjusting for various socioeconomic and demographic variables, care related, environmental health and sanitation, dietary and household food modifications, household, and morbidity related variables: having poor dietary diversity, early or late initiation of complementary feeding, poor quality of breastfeeding and children of mothers less utilizes iron folate during pregnancy. The prevalence level of anemia observed in this study among children 6–23 months were classified by WHO as a severe public health problem [16].

Prevalence of anemia in this study was higher than the prevalence of EDHS 2016 regional report for SNNPR which was 49.6% [7]. The possible reasons for the variation may be due to differences in samples size, lifestyles and other reason might be socioeconomic status

Table 2 Independent predictors of anemia among children 6–23 months aged in Damot Sore District, Wolaita Zone, South Ethiopia, from March to April 2017

Predictors	Anemia status		COR (95% C.I.)	AOR (95% C.I.)	p
	Anemic	Not anemic			
DDS			2.89(1.96–4.28)		0.01
Poor	196(40.4%)	123(25.4%)		2.86(1.73–4.70)	
Good	166(34.2%)	107(22.1%)		1.00	
Introduction time of complementary feeding	142(29.4%)	82(17%)	2.3(1.60–3.33)	2.0(1.23–3.60)	0.01[a]
Before or after 6 months of age					
At 6 months of age	111(23%)	148(30.6%)	1.00	1.00	
IFA utilization history	177(45%)	154(39.2%)	2.2(1.27–3.96)	2.75(1.42–5.36)	0.03
≤ 3 months	21(5.3%)	41(10.4%)	1.00	1.00	
> 3 months					
Breast feeding practice	82(18.2%)	33(7.3%)	2.97(1.90–4.70)	2.6(1.41–4.62)	0.02
Poor	153(33.9%)	183(40.6%)	1.00	1.00	
Good					
Household food insecurity	212(43.7%)	119(24.5%)	4.6(3.0–6.90)	2.74(1.62–4.65)	0.04
Food insecure	43(8.9%)	111(22.9%)	1.00	1.00	
Food secure					

[a]Variable with p-value< 0.001

variation. This might be due to fasting time for Orthodox Christianity followers and due to seasonal food scarcity that reduces consumption of diversified foods, as the data were collected in spring "Belg", which were the dry and sunny season and this leads to micronutrient deficiency-related diseases such as anemia.

But it was much lower than EDHS 2016 as a country whole which was 72.7% [7], and also a study conducted in Wag-Himra zone in north Ethiopia which was 66.6% [8]. From abroad still, it was much lower than studies done in Cameroon [17] and Sudan [18] with the prevalence of 66.7 and 86%, respectively. The lower prevalence in this study might be due to the change made by the existing nutritional, public health interventions, easy accessibility of health information through health extension workers and among other factors may be included. But still it lacks adequacy of the sample size to compare with the national data of EDHS with this small cross-sectional study, thus it needs large sample size and also analytic studies to know temporal and seasonal variations.

Regarding food insecurity, children living in food-insecure households were more likely to be anemic than food secure households. This result disagrees with the findings reported from Iran [19] and India [20] that showed, as there were no relations with household food insecurity and anemia status of children. However, this finding was in-line with the study findings from USA [21]. In our study, association with household food insecurity might be due to climate change (El-Niño effect) which shifted seasonal rainfall, reduced yield, and agricultural productivity. So, to cope with food insecurity at the household level, children as other household members reduce consumption of diversified foods (especially, animal source iron-rich and enhancing or vitamin C rich foods) worsen childhood anemia.

Children with poor dietary diversity score were more likely to be anemic than children with good dietary diversity scores. Studies regarding dietary practices of children in some parts of Ethiopia showed that grains, roots, and tubers were eaten by 80.2% of children. And these foods are a source of non-heme iron with low bioavailability and with higher content of phytates, phenols and make children prone to nutritional related deficiencies [22]. This in-line with a study conducted in northern Ethiopia that showed, those children who consumed cereal based monotonous diet were 3.2 times more anemic than those consume diversified diet [8]. In our study, this might be due to tuber, root and cereal-based monotonous diet. In addition, cultural and economic reasons do not allow children to eat iron-rich foods such as meat. In addition to this seasonal unavailability of enhancing citrus fruits such as lemons and oranges might be among reasons. Thus, monotonous diet consumption of cereals and tubers, reduced consumption of iron-rich foods, enhancing [citric fruits] and inhibitors [coffee and tea] were made children be anemic [23].

Children who started complementary feeding earlier than or late to recommended time by WHO, which was at 6 months, were two times more likely to be anemic than children which started complementary feeding just at 6 months. Contrary to this, a study conducted in Nepal on the age of introduction for complementary feeding for infants revealed that early introduction of solid foods at three and 4 months respectively has a significant improvement of iron status among children in developing countries [24]. However, our findings in-line with studies done in Wag-Himra, Ethiopia [8], Brazil [25] and China [26] which revealed that a lower infant Hb was associated with early initiation of complementary feeding and increased EBF duration for more than 6 months. Early exposure of infants (before 6 months of age) to microbial pathogens due to complementary foods increases the risks of infection for diarrheal diseases, thereby leading to mal-absorption (environmental enteropathy). Breast milk has minimal iron to fulfill nutritional requirements of a growing infant, given that providing breast milk alone coupled with rapid iron depletion beyond 6 months also increases the risk of anemia for younger infants [27]. In our study, this might be due to cultural belief of mothers that exclusive breastfeeding is inadequate to infants alone, and they introduce cow milk earlier than 6 months.

Children of mothers those utilized iron folate for less than 3 months during pregnancy were more likely to be anemic than those utilized IFA for more than 3 months. This was similar to a study conducted in India, as children hemoglobin levels were independently associated with maternal hemoglobin level, and antenatal anemia contributes to low birth weight and prematurity, both of which increase the risk of childhood anemia. Severe maternal anemia may also reduce breast milk iron content [20]. In this study, it might due to late initiation of antenatal care, timely shortage of iron folate in health facilities, fear of side effects and lack of awareness among mothers about iron folate had made mothers not to utilize as recommended by the national guideline. These factors might have made a lessened store of iron in mothers to transfer an adequate amount of iron for the fetus. A little store of iron in children during delivery would be a risk factor for anemia in their infancy [5].

Our study showed that children from mothers who had a poor practice of breastfeeding had a statistically significant association with anemia. This study is in-line with other studies conducted in Iran [28], China [26] and Brazil [29] that reported breastfeeding for less than 6 months or exclusive breastfeeding for more than 6 months, early initiation of solid or liquid foods, appropriate position of attachment, switching time from one breast to another and low frequency of breastfeeding per day were associated with childhood anemia. Similarly, in our study, this might be due to lack of awareness among mothers about good breastfeeding practices and lack of advice from health care providers. Mothers were busy with domestic works and greater caring responsibility of the whole family and domestic animals [29].

Although Ethiopia has tried many actions such as NNP, CBN, social protections and others, to reduce nutritional deficiencies, the prevalence of anemia among children remained high over the last few years [6–8]. A landscape analysis and a study conducted in Ghana revealed that there was a significant decline in overall anemia prevalence in children age 6–59 months between 2008 and 2014 (from 78 to 66%). This happened due to multi-sectoral collaboration, daily iron, and folic acid supplementation in pregnant women, intermittent iron and folic acid supplementation in menstruating women and home fortification of foods with multiple micronutrient powders among infants and children 6–23 months, and wheat and maize flour fortification with sodium iron ethylene ediaminetetraacetic acid with malaria prevention [30, 31].

Evidence on the impact of scaled-up iron supplementation across countries in the world on the reduction of anemia prevalence documented that, national programs of Thailand and Nicaragua decreased the prevalence of anemia among children through improving iron folate utilization by pregnant mothers. As they reported in their document, they improved [reduced) the prevalence of anemia by strengthening already existing policy, adopting lessons from successful countries and by strengthening demand and supply system [32].

Food security and diversified diet were important for proper child growth and remains a concern in Ethiopia. There are Programs that would be awaited for changing nutritional problems to scale up, like Seqota declaration [33, 34], and some social protections were implementing. Productive Safety Net Program (PSNP) as one of social protection for food insecure households, were to improve household food security but evaluations of the first three phases of PSNP demonstrated a two-month improvement in food security, but lack of improvement in the quality of children's (6–23 months) diets [33].

Solutions, such as nutrition-sensitive agriculture-specific activities: agriculture based solutions, such as production of nutrient dense crops, livestock/livestock products, agro-processing/storage skills, increasing on-farm or off-farm income for vulnerable households and women need to be further established in order to increase the production and access to diverse, safe, and nutrient-dense foods were considered by government of Ethiopia [33, 34].

It was well documented in a systematic review of thousand day's interventions, interventions in critical times improve irreversible cognitive impairment due to reduced iron. It is a window of opportunity with minimal cost that adds national economy, creative minds and makes healthy old age [5].

Although the micronutrient prevention and control guideline has been developed since 2005 and there have various intervention to prevent anemia at the community level, our results showed the existence high prevalence among children. The practical implication of this updated level of prevalence is, even though it is an area specific, it will use as an input for national nutritional program goal and for Growth and Transformation Plan GTP 2 (2016–2020), which were targeted to reduce micronutrient deficiencies and other nutritional problems. In addition to this, it is an input for declarations that programmed to end up malnutrition problems which were planned by the government such as Seqota declarations. As a country government of Ethiopia planned to be the middle-income country in the year 2030. Sour findings will help FMoH as an input for fortifying its efforts to achieve its plan of enhancing the productivity of individuals who will contribute to the achievement of sustainable development goals.

Limitations of the study

We acknowledge a number of limitations in our study. A cross-sectional design enabled us only to assess hemoglobin levels at one point in time. It is documented in other studies that as intestinal parasites, hereditary diseases, chronic illnesses such as HIV and others could cause anemia, which was not assessed in this study. There were some recall biases among mothers of younger children regarding introduction time of complementary feeding. We minimized this by asking them to remember a time when at least they introduced to water or cow's milk.

Conclusion and recommendations

The prevalence of anemia among children 6–23 months in Damot Sore District, South Ethiopia was 52.6% indicative of the fact that anemia is high public health important problem by WHO classification criteria. Initiation time of complementary feeding, breastfeeding practice, maternal history of iron-folate (IFA) utilization, dietary diversity and household food insecurity were significantly associated with anemia.

Because of this severity of anemia, it requires public health intervention and by taking this into account, the following recommendations are forwarded: Strengthening community-based nutrition activities which were previously integrated into health extension packages. Providing community-based nutrition education on the feeding of diversified diets, increase vitamin C rich foods, reduced consumption of foods that prevent iron absorption (E.g. coffee and tea) and to take an interval to take a milk after consumption of iron-rich foods. Encourage mothers for early follow-up of ANC, IFA utilization, good breastfeeding practices and the right initiation time of complementary feeding. Strengthening integration of services within health facilities. Strengthening activities on identifying households, those in food insecure status and include them in social protection packages. Further analytic studies for temporal relationships of above factors.

Abbreviations

ANC: Antenatal care; AOR: Adjusted odds ratio; CBC: Complete blood count; CBN: Community-based nutrition; CHIS: Community health information system; CI: Confidence Interval; COR: Crude odds ratio; DDS: Dietary diversity score; EBF: Exclusive breast feeding; EDHS: Ethiopian demographic and health survey; FFQ: Food frequency questionnaire; GPS: Global positioning system; Hb: Hemoglobin; HFIAS: Household food insecurity access scale; IFA: Iron folic acid; ITN: Insecticide treated bed net; NNP: National nutrition programme; OR: Odds ratio; PCA: Principal component analysis; RDT: Rapid diagnostic test; SNNPR: South nation's nationalities and peoples regional state; VIP: Ventilation improved pit latrine; WHO: World Health Organization

Acknowledgements

We would also like to pass our deepest gratitude for the research office of Jimma University Institute of Health, Faculty of Public Health for giving us the opportunity to conduct this research and provision of necessary materials for conducting of this study. Damot sore district health office for their whole support. Last but not least, we would really like to thank mothers of children & data collectors.

Funding

This study received financial support from Jimma University and Damot Sore district administrative office. The views expressed in this study are of the authors' and not of funding organizations.

Authors' contributions

BGM; the conception of the research idea, study design and proposal development. BGM; collected and ensured the quality of the data. TBL & MST were supervised overall activities. BGM, TBL& MST analyzed and interpreted the data. All authors critically reviewed the manuscript. After all, authors gave final approval of the paper to be published, MST; the corresponding author had the responsibility to submit the manuscript for publication.

Authors' information

BGM is Nutrition officer in Damot Sore District health office.
MST and TBL(Professor of human nutrition) lecturer in Jimma University Institute of Health, Public Health Faculty, Population and Family Health Department, Nutrition Course Team, PO.Box:1104, Jimma, Ethiopia.

Competing interests

The authors declare that they have no competing interests.

Author details

[1]Damot Sore District Health Office, Wolaita zone, SNNPR, Gununo, Ethiopia. [2]Institute of Health, Public Health Faculty, Population and Family Health Department, Nutrition Course Team, Jimma University, Jimma, Ethiopia.

References

1. McLean E, Cogswell M, Egli I, Wojdyla D, Benoist B. Worldwide prevalence of anaemia, WHO vitamin and mineral nutrition information system: 1993-2005. Public Health Nutrition. 2008;12(4):1–11.
2. WHO. The global prevalence of anaemia in 2011. Geneva, Switzerland 2015 [Accessed: 02 Feb 2017]; Available from: http://apps.who.int/iris/bitstream/10665/177094/1/9789241564960_eng.pdf.
3. Ganong WF. Review of Medical Physiology, Twenty-Second Edition University of California, San Francisco, USA: McGraw-Hill Companies; 2003.
4. Guyton AC, Hall JE. Text Book of Medical Physiology, thirteenth edition. Jackson, Mississippi, USA: Elsevier Inc.; 2006; 11.
5. Burke RM, Leon JS, Suchdev PS. Identification, prevention and treatment of Iron deficiency during the first 1000 days. Nutrients. 2014;6:4093–114.
6. C.S.A. Ethiopia Demographic and Health Survey 2011. Addis Ababa, Ethiopia 2012 [8 Feb 2017]; Available from: https://www.unicef.org/ethiopia/ET_2011_EDHS.pdf.
7. C.S.A. Ethiopia Mini Demographic and Health Survey 2016 Key Indicators Report. Addis Ababa, Ethiopia 2016 [Accessed: 01 Feb 2017]; Available from: https://dhsprogram.com/pubs/pdf/PR81/PR81.pdf.
8. Woldie H, Kebede Y, Tariku A. Factors Associated with Anemia among Children Aged 6–23 Months Attending Growth Monitoring at Tsitsika Health Center, Wag-Himra Zone, Northeast Ethiopia. Journal of Nutrition and Metabolism. 2015;2015(Article ID 928632):9.
9. Roba KT, O'Connor TP, Belachew T, O'Brien NM. Concurrent iron and zinc deficiencies in lactating mothers and their children 6–23 months of age in two agro-ecological zones of rural Ethiopia. Eur J Nutr. 2018; 57(2):655-67. https://doi.org/10.1007/s00394-016-1351-5
10. Fatihah F, Ng BK, Hazwanie H, Norimah K, SiN S, Ruzita AT, et al. Development and validation of a food frequency questionnaire for dietary intake assessment among questionnaire for dietary intake assessment among multi-ethnic primary school-aged children Singapore. Medical Journal. 2015;56(12):687–94.
11. WHO. Haemoglobin concentrations for the diagnosis of anemia and assessment of severity. In: System. VaMNI, editor. Geneva, World Health Organization 2011 (WHO/NMH/NHD/MNM/11.1).
12. Nkrumah B, Nguah SB, Sarpong N, Dekke D, Idriss A, May J, et al. Hemoglobin estimation by the HemoCue® portable hemoglobin photometer in a resource poor setting. BMC Clin Phatol. 2011;11:5.
13. Unicef. Malaria diagnosis: a guide for selecting rapid diagnostic test (RDT) kits - 1st edition Copenhagen 2007 [Accessed 17 Jan 2016]; Available from: https://www.unicef.org/french/supply/files/Guidance_for_malaria_rapid_tests.pdf
14. Belachew T, Lindstrom D, Gebremariam A, Hogan D, Lachat C, Huybregts L, et al. Food Insecurity, Food Based Coping Strategies and Suboptimal Dietary Practices of Adolescents in Jimma Zone Southwest Ethiopia. PLoS One. 2013; 8(3):e57643.
15. Thorpe MG, Milte CM, Crawford D, McNaughton SA. A comparison of the dietary patterns derived by principal component analysis and cluster analysis in older Australians. International Journal of Behavioral Nutrition and Physical Activity 2016(13):30.
16. WHO/UNICEF/UNU. Iron deficiency anaemia: assessment, prevention, and control. Geneva: World Health Organization; 2001. (WHO/NHD/01.3).
17. Sop MMK, Mananga M-J, Tetanye E, Gouado I. Risk factors of anemia among young children in rural Cameroon. Int J Curr Microbiol App Sci. 2015;4(3):925–35.
18. Mahmoud HH, Muddathir AM, Osman SEM, MA AK. K A. Iron Deficiency Anemia among Children under Three years in Kassala, Eastern Sudan. Sudanese J Public Health. 2014;9(1):33–7.
19. Salarkia N, Neyestani TR, Omidvar N, Zayeri F. Household Food Insecurity, Mother's Feeding Practices, and the Early Childhood's Iron Status. Int J Prevent Med. 2015;6:86.
20. Pasricha S-R, Black J, Muthayya S, Shet A, Bhat V, Nagaraj S, et al. Determinants of Anemia among young children in rural India. Pediatrics. 2010;26(1):e140–9.
21. Park K, Kersey M, Geppert J, Story M, Cutts D, Himes JH. Household food insecurity is a risk factor for iron-deficiency anemia in a multi-ethnic, low-income sample of infants and toddlers. Public Health Nutrition. 2009;12(11): 2120–8.
22. Beyene M, Worku AG, Wassie MM. Dietary diversity, meal frequency and associated factors among infant and young children in Northwest Ethiopia: a cross- sectional study. BMC Public Health. 2015;15(1007):1–9.

23. Michaelsen KF, Hoppe C, Roos N, Kaestel P, Stougaard M, Lauritzen L, et al. Choice of foods and ingredients for moderately malnourished children 6 months to 5 years of age. Food Nutrition Bulletin. 2009;30(3):343–404.
24. Chandyo R, Henjum S, Ulak M, Lyman AT, Ulvik R, Shrestha P, et al. The prevalence of anemia and iron deficiency is more common in breastfed infants than their mothers in Bhaktapur, Nepal. Eur J Clin Nutri. 2016;70:456–62.
25. Jordão RE, Bernardi JLD, AdAB F. Feeding pattern and anemia in infants in the city of Campinas, São Paulo, Brazil. Rev Paul Pediatr. 2009;27(7):381–8.
26. Luo R, Shi Y, Zhou H, Yue A, Zhang L, Sylvia S, et al. Anemia and feeding practices among infants in rural Shaanxi Province in China. Nutrients. 2014;6: 5975–91.
27. Iannotti LL, Tielsch JM, Black MM, Black RE. Iron supplementation in early childhood: health benefits and risks. Am J Clin Nutr. 2006;84(6):1261–76.
28. Dalili H, Baghersalimi A, Dalili S, Pakdaman F, Rad F, Kakroodi A, et al. Is there any relation between duration of breastfeeding and anemia? Iranian J Pediatr Hematol Oncol. 2015;15(4):218–26.
29. Castro T, Baraldi L, Muniz P, Cardoso M. Dietary practices and nutritional status of 0–24-month-old children from Brazilian Amazonia. Public Health Nutrition. 2009;12:12.
30. Adu-Afarwuah S, Lartey A, Brown KH, Zlotkin S, Briend A, Dewey KG. Home fortification of complementary foods with micronutrient supplements is well accepted and has positive effects on infant iron status in Ghana. Am J Clin Nutr. 2008;87:929–38.
31. SPRING GHS. Ghana Landscape Analysis of Anemia and Anemia Programming In: Strengthening Partnerships R, and Innovations in Nutrition Globally (SPRING) project., editor. Arlington, VA 2016.
32. Sanghvi TG, Harvey PWJ, Wainwright E. Maternal iron–folic acid supplementation programs: evidence of impact and implementation. Food and Nutrition Bulletin. 2010;31(2):S100–7.
33. FMoH/UNICEF/EU. Situation Analysis of the Nutrition Sector in Ethiopia: 2000-2015. Addis Ababa, Ethiopia 2016; Available from: https://www.unicef.org/ethiopia/ECO_Nutrition_Situation_Analysis_Main_Document.pdf.
34. MoANR. The Federal Democratic Republic of Ethiopia Ministry of Agriculture and Natural resource Nutrition Sensitive agriculture: draft Strategic Plan. Addis Ababa, Ethiopia 2016 [Accessed: February, 2017]; Available from: http://www.moa.gov.et/documents/93665/6308679/Nutrition+Sensitive+agriculture+draft+Strategic+Plan.pdf/2b710b04-2cea-4442-b74c-3ea4033637ef.

Permissions

All chapters in this book were first published in HEMATOLOGY, by BioMed Central; hereby published with permission under the Creative Commons Attribution License or equivalent. Every chapter published in this book has been scrutinized by our experts. Their significance has been extensively debated. The topics covered herein carry significant findings which will fuel the growth of the discipline. They may even be implemented as practical applications or may be referred to as a beginning point for another development.

The contributors of this book come from diverse backgrounds, making this book a truly international effort. This book will bring forth new frontiers with its revolutionizing research information and detailed analysis of the nascent developments around the world.

We would like to thank all the contributing authors for lending their expertise to make the book truly unique. They have played a crucial role in the development of this book. Without their invaluable contributions this book wouldn't have been possible. They have made vital efforts to compile up to date information on the varied aspects of this subject to make this book a valuable addition to the collection of many professionals and students.

This book was conceptualized with the vision of imparting up-to-date information and advanced data in this field. To ensure the same, a matchless editorial board was set up. Every individual on the board went through rigorous rounds of assessment to prove their worth. After which they invested a large part of their time researching and compiling the most relevant data for our readers.

The editorial board has been involved in producing this book since its inception. They have spent rigorous hours researching and exploring the diverse topics which have resulted in the successful publishing of this book. They have passed on their knowledge of decades through this book. To expedite this challenging task, the publisher supported the team at every step. A small team of assistant editors was also appointed to further simplify the editing procedure and attain best results for the readers.

Apart from the editorial board, the designing team has also invested a significant amount of their time in understanding the subject and creating the most relevant covers. They scrutinized every image to scout for the most suitable representation of the subject and create an appropriate cover for the book.

The publishing team has been an ardent support to the editorial, designing and production team. Their endless efforts to recruit the best for this project, has resulted in the accomplishment of this book. They are a veteran in the field of academics and their pool of knowledge is as vast as their experience in printing. Their expertise and guidance has proved useful at every step. Their uncompromising quality standards have made this book an exceptional effort. Their encouragement from time to time has been an inspiration for everyone.

The publisher and the editorial board hope that this book will prove to be a valuable piece of knowledge for researchers, students, practitioners and scholars across the globe.

List of Contributors

Shin-Yeu Ong, Ha-Thi-Thu Truong, Colin Phipps Diong, Yeh-Ching Linn, Aloysius Yew-Leng Ho, Yeow-Tee Goh and William Ying-Khee Hwang
Department of Hematology, Singapore General Hospital, Singapore, Singapore

Patrick Adu, Essel K. M. Bashirudeen, Florence Haruna and Richard K. D. Ephraim
Medical Laboratory Technology Department, School of Allied Health Sciences, University of Cape Coast, Cape Coast, Ghana

Edward Morkporkpor Adela
Haematology unit, Cape Coast Teaching Hospital, Cape Coast, Ghana

Wendy Lim
Departments of Clinical Epidemiology and Biostatistics, McMaster University, Hamilton, Canada

Chatree Chai-Adisaksopha, Alfonso Iorio and Mark Crowther
Departments of Clinical Epidemiology and Biostatistics, McMaster University, Hamilton, Canada
Departments of Medicine, McMaster University, Hamilton, Canada

Christopher Hillis
Departments of Medicine, McMaster University, Hamilton, Canada
Departments of Oncology, McMaster University, Hamilton, Canada

Muriel N. Maeder, Henintsoa M. Rabezanahary, Norosoa J. Zafindraibe and Mala Rakoto Andrianarivelo
Centre d'Infectiologie Charles Mérieux, Université Antananarivo, Antananarivo, Madagascar

Tahinamandranto Rasamoelina
Centre d'Infectiologie Charles Mérieux, Université Antananarivo, Antananarivo, Madagascar
UPFR Biochimie-Centre Hospitalier Universitaire Joseph Ravoahangy Andrianavalona, Antananarivo, Madagascar

Raoelina Randriatiana
Fondation Médicale d'Ampasimanjeva, Manakara, Madagascar

Martin Andry T. Rakotoarivo
UPFR Biochimie-Centre Hospitalier Universitaire Joseph Ravoahangy Andrianavalona, Antananarivo, Madagascar

Jonathan Hoffmann
Laboratoire des Pathogènes Emergents, Fondation Mérieux, Centre International de Recherche en Infectiologie (CIRI), Inserm U1111, CNRS UMR5308, ENS de Lyon, UCBL1 Lyon, France

Philippe Vanhems and Thomas Bénet
Laboratoire des Pathogènes Emergents, Fondation Mérieux, Centre International de Recherche en Infectiologie (CIRI), Inserm U1111, CNRS UMR5308, ENS de Lyon, UCBL1 Lyon, France
Service d'Hygiène, Epidémiologie et Prévention, Hôpital Edouard Herriot, Hospices Civils de Lyon, Lyon, France

Olivat A. Rakoto-Alson
UPFR Hématologie-Centre Hospitalier Universitaire Joseph Ravoahangy Andrianavalona and Département de Microbiologie, Faculté de Médecine, Antananarivo, Madagascar

R. Marchi and M. Linares
Lab. Biología del Desarrollo de la Hemostasia. Instituto Venezolano de Investigaciones Científicas (IVIC), Caracas, Bolivarian Republic of Venezuela

H. Rojas
Instituto de Inmunología, Universidad Central de Venezuela and Lab. Fisiología Celular Centro de Biofisica y Bioquímica (IVIC), Caracas, Bolivarian Republic of Venezuela

A. Ruiz-Sáez
Banco Municipal de Sangre del Distrito Capital, Caracas, Bolivarian Republic of Venezuela

M. Meyer
Medical Engineering and Biotechnology, University of Applied Sciences, Jena, Germany

A. Casini
Division of Angiology and Haemostasis, Faculty of Medicine, University Hospitals of Geneva, Geneva, Switzerland

S.O. Brennan
Molecular Pathology Laboratory, University of Otago, Christchurch, New Zealand

Hirotada Otsuka, Jiro Takito, Nobuaki Yanagisawa, Naoko Nonaka and Masanori Nakamura
Department of Oral Anatomy and Developmental Biology, School of Dentistry, Showa University, 1-5-8 Hatanodai, Shinagawa-ku, Tokyo 142-8555, Japan

Yasuo Endo
Division of Molecular Regulation, Graduate School of Dentistry, Tohoku University, 4-1 Seiryo-machi, Aoba-ku, Sendai 980-8575, Japan

Hideki Yagi
Faculty of Pharmacy, International University of Health and Welfare, 2600-1 Kitakanamaru, Otawara-shi, Tochigi 324-8501, Japan

Satoshi Soeta
Department of Veterinary Anatomy, Nippon Veterinary and Animal Science University, 1 7-1 Kyonan-cho, Musashino-shi, Tokyo 180-8602, Japan

Mustafa I. Elbashir
Department of Medical Biochemistry, Faculty of Medicine, University of Khartoum, Alghasr Street, Khartoum, Sudan

Shiekh Awoda
Department of Medical Biochemistry, Faculty of Medicine, University of Khartoum, Alghasr Street, Khartoum, Sudan
College of Medical Laboratory Sciences, Sudan University of Science& Technology, Khartoum, Sudan

Ahmed A. Daak
Department of Medical Biochemistry, Faculty of Medicine, University of Khartoum, Alghasr Street, Khartoum, Sudan
Center of Molecular Biology and Biotechnology (CMBB), Florida Atlantic University (FAU), Boca Raton, USA
Lipidomics and Nutrition Research Centre, London Metropolitan University, London, UK

Nazik Elmalaika Husain
College of Medical Laboratory Sciences, Sudan University of Science and Technology, Khartoum, Sudan

Kebreab Ghebremeskel
Lipidomics and Nutrition Research Centre, London Metropolitan University, London, UK

Tebit Emmanuel Kwenti
Regional Hospital Buea, Buea, South West Region, Cameroon
Department of Medical laboratory Sciences, Faculty of Health Sciences, University of Buea, Buea, Cameroon
Department of Microbiology and Parasitology, Faculty of Science, University of Buea, Buea, Cameroon

Tayong Dizzle Bita Kwenti
Department of Microbiology and Parasitology, Faculty of Science, University of Buea, Buea, Cameroon

Getachew Mullu Kassa
College of health Sciences, Debre Markos University, Debre Markos, Ethiopia

Achenef Asmamaw Muche
Department of Epidemiology and Biostatistics, Institute of Public Health, University of Gondar, Gondar, Ethiopia.

Abadi Kidanemariam Berhe
Department of Nursing, College of Medicine and Health Science, Adigrat University, Tigray, Ethiopia

Gedefaw Abeje Fekadu
School of Public Health, College of Medicine and Health Sciences, Bahir Dar University, Bahir Dar, Ethiopia

Mikias Negash and Aster Tsegaye
College of Health Science, Department of Medical Laboratory Science, Addis Ababa University, Addis Ababa, Ethiopia

Amha G/Medhin
Department of Internal Medicine, Addis Ababa University, Addis Ababa, Ethiopia

Ted S. Strom
Department of Pathology and Laboratory Medicine, Memphis Veterans Administration Medical Center, 1030 Jefferson Ave, Memphis, TN 38104, USA
Department of Pathology and Laboratory Medicine, University of Tennessee Health Sciences Center, Memphis, TN, USA

Catherine R. Shari, Hendry R. Sawe, Victor G. Mwafongo and Juma A. Mf nanga
Emergency Medicine Department Muhimbili University of Health and Allied Sciences, Dar es Salaam, Tanzania
Emergency Medicine Department, Muhimbili National Hospital, Dar Es Salaam, Tanzania

Michael S. Runyon
Emergency Medicine Department Muhimbili University of Health and Allied Sciences, Dar es Salaam, Tanzania
Department of Emergency Medicine, Carolinas Medical Center, Charlotte, NC, USA

Brittany L. Murray
Emergency Medicine Department Muhimbili University of Health and Allied Sciences, Dar es Salaam, Tanzania
Emergency Medicine Department, Muhimbili National Hospital, Dar Es Salaam, Tanzania
Division of Pediatric Emergency Medicine, Emory University School of Medicine, Emory University, Atlanta, GA, USA

Daniele Kazue Sugioka, Carlos Eduardo Ibaldo Gonçalves and Maria da Graça Bicalho
Departamento de Genética, Laboratório de Imunogenética e Histocompatibilidade (LIGH), Universidade Federal do Paraná, R. Cel. Francisco H. dos Santos S/N, Centro Politécnico - Jardim das Américas, CEP 81.530.990, Curitiba, PR CP 19071, Brazil

Fekede Bekele Daba
Department of Pharmacy, College of Health Sciences, Jimma University, Jimma, Ethiopia

Fisihatsion Tadesse
Department of Internal Medicine, Tikur Anbessa specialized hospital, Addis Ababa University, Addis Ababa, Ethiopia

Ephrem Engidawork
Department of Pharmacology and Clinical Pharmacy, School of Pharmacy, College of Health Sciences, Addis Ababa University, Addis Ababa, Ethiopia

Silvana Sousa da Paz1, and
Laboratório de Hematologia e Genética Computacional, Instituto Gonçalo Moniz - IGM, Fundação Oswaldo Cruz (Fiocruz), Rua Waldemar Falcão, 121, Candeal, Salvador, Bahia CEP 40296-710, Brazil

Milena Magalhães Aleluia, Caroline Conceição da Guarda, Rayra Pereira Santiago, Camylla Villas Boas Figueiredo, Sânzio Silva Santana, Júnia Raquel Dutra Ferreira and Marilda de Souza Gonçalves
Laboratório de Hematologia e Genética Computacional, Instituto Gonçalo Moniz - IGM, Fundação Oswaldo Cruz (Fiocruz), Rua Waldemar Falcão, 121, Candeal, Salvador, Bahia CEP 40296-710, Brazil
Universidade Federal da Bahia (UFBA), Salvador, Bahia, Brazil

Bruna Laís Almeida Cunha
Universidade Federal da Bahia (UFBA), Salvador, Bahia, Brazil

Fábia Idalina Neves
Centro de Referência a Doença Falciforme, Itabuna, Bahia, Brazil

Teresa Cristina Cardoso Fonseca and Regiana Quinto Souza
Centro de Referência a Doença Falciforme, Itabuna, Bahia, Brazil
Universidade Estadual de Santa Cruz (UESC), Ilhéus, Bahia, Brazil

Bruno Antônio Veloso Cerqueira
Universidade Estadual da Bahia (UNEB), Salvador, Bahia, Brazil

Srdjan Denic
Department of Medicine, College of Medicine and Health Sciences, United Arab Emirates University, Al-Ain, United Arab of Emirates

Hassib Narchi, Lolowa A. Al Mekaini, Suleiman Al-Hammadi and Abdul-Kader Souid
Department of Pediatrics, College of Medicine and Health Sciences, United Arab Emirates University, Al-Ain, United Arab of Emirates

Omar N. Al Jabri
Ambulatory Healthcare Services, Abu Dhabi, United Arab of Emirates

Habtom Woldeab Gebresilase
Department of public Health, College of Health Sciences, Adama General
Hospital and Medical College, Adama, Ethiopia

Robera Olana Fite
Department of Nursing, College of Health Sciences and Medicine, Woliata Sodo University, Woliata sodo, Ethiopia

Sileshi Garoma Abeya
Department of Social and Population Health, Adama General Hospital and Medical College, Adama, Ethiopia

Benjamin Ahenkorah
Biochemistry and Hematology Units, Bolgatanga Regional Hospital, Bolgatanga-Upper East Region, Ghana
Department of Biochemistry and Molecular Medicine, School of Medical and Health Science, University for Development Studies, Tamale, Ghana
Department of Molecular Medicine, School of Medical Science, Kwame Nkrumah University of Science and Technology, Kumasi, Ghana

Kwabena Nsiah
Department of Biochemistry and Biotechnology, Kwame Nkrumah University of Science and Technology, Kumasi, Ghana

Peter Baffoe
Obstetrics and Gynecology Unit, Bolgatanga Regional Hospital, Bolgatanga-Upper East Region, Ghana

Enoch Odame Anto
Department of Molecular Medicine, School of Medical Science, Kwame Nkrumah University of Science and Technology, Kumasi, Ghana
Department of Medical Laboratory Technology, Royal Ann College of Health, Atwima-Manhyia, Kumasi, Ghana
School of Medical and Health Science, Edith Cowan University, Perth, WA, Australia

Gashaw Garedew Woldeamanuel and Diresibachew Haile Wondimu
Department of Medicine, College of Medicine and Health Sciences, Wolkite University, Wolkite, Ethiopia
Department of Medical Physiology, School of Medicine, College of Health Sciences, Addis Ababa University, Addis Ababa, Ethiopia

Juthatip Chaloemwong, Adisak Tantiworawit, Thanawat Rattanathammethee, Sasinee Hantrakool, Chatree Chai-Adisaksopha, Ekarat Rattarittamrong and Lalita Norasetthada
Division of Hematology, Department of Internal Medicine, Faculty of Medicine, Chiang Mai University, 110 Intravaroros road, A. Muang, Chiang Mai 50200, Thailand

Olivier Mukuku
Department of Research, High Institute of Techniques Medicales, Lubumbashi, Democratic Republic of Congo

Oscar Numbi Luboya
Department of Research, High Institute of Techniques Medicales, Lubumbashi, Democratic Republic of Congo
Department of Pediatrics, University Hospital of Lubumbashi University of Lubumbashi, Lubumbashi, Democratic Republic of Congo
School of Public Health, University of Lubumbashi, Lubumbashi, Democratic Republic of Congo

Joseph K. Sungu, Augustin Mulangu Mutombo and Stanislas Okitotsho Wembonyama
Department of Pediatrics, University Hospital of Lubumbashi University of Lubumbashi, Lubumbashi, Democratic Republic of Congo

Michel Ntetani Aloni
Division of Hemato-oncology and Nephrology, Department of Paediatrics, University Hospital of Kinshasa, School of Medicine, University of Kinshasa, , Kinshasa, Democratic Republic of Congo

Fekri Samarah
Department of Medical Technology, Faculty of Allied Health Sciences, Arab
American University in Jenin, Jenin, Palestine

Mahmoud A. Srour
Department of Medical Laboratory Sciences, Faculty of Health professions, Al-Quds University, Jerusalem, Palestine
Present address: Department of Biology and Biochemistry, Faculty of Science, Birzeit University, Birzeit, Palestine

Hendry R. Sawe and Juma A. Mfinanga
Emergency Medicine Department, Muhimbili University of Health and Allied Sciences, Dar es salaam, Tanzania
Emergency Medicine Department, Muhimbili National Hospital, Dar es salaam, Tanzania

Teri A. Reynolds
Emergency Medicine Department, Muhimbili University of Health and Allied Sciences, Dar es salaam, Tanzania
Department of Emergency Medicine, University of California San Francisco, San Francisco, CA, USA

Michael S. Runyon
Emergency Medicine Department, Muhimbili University of Health and Allied Sciences, Dar es salaam, Tanzania
Department of Emergency Medicine, Carolinas Medical Center, Charlotte, NC, USA

Brittany L. Murray
Emergency Medicine Department, Muhimbili University of Health and Allied Sciences, Dar es salaam, Tanzania
Division of Pediatric Emergency Medicine, Emory University School of Medicine/Children's Hospital of Atlanta, Atlanta, GA, USA

Lee A. Wallis
Division of Emergency Medicine, University of Cape Town, Cape Town City, South Africa

Julie Makani
Nuffield Department of Medicine, University of Oxford, Oxford, UK
Department of Haematology and blood transfusion, Muhimbili University of Health and Allied Sciences, Dar es Salaam, Tanzania

Haileleul Micho
Department of Biomedical Sciences, College of Health Sciences, Dilla University, Dilla, Ethiopia
Department of Medical Biochemistry, School of Medicine, College of Health sciences, Addis Ababa University, Addis Ababa, Ethiopia

Solomon Genet
Department of Medical Biochemistry, School of Medicine, College of Health sciences, Addis Ababa University, Addis Ababa, Ethiopia

Yasin Mohammed and Daniel Hailu
Department of Pediatrics and child Health, School of Medicine, College of Health Sciences, Addis Ababa University, Addis Ababa, Ethiopia

Ishag Adam
Faculty of Medicine, University of Khartoum, Khartoum, Sudan

Yassin Ibrahim
Faculty of Medicine, University of Tabuk, Tabuk, Saudi Arabia

Osama Elhardello
Scarborough General Hospital, Scarborough YO12 6QL, UK

Cláudia Moreira, Ana Spínola and Jorge Coutinho
Department of Hematology, Hospital de Santo António (HSA), Centro Hospitalar do Porto (CHP), Porto, Portugal

Ana Aires, and Alexandra Mota
Department of Hematology, Hospital de Santo António (HSA), Centro Hospitalar do Porto (CHP), Porto, Portugal
Instituto de Ciências Biomédicas Abel Salazar, Universidade do Porto (ICBAS/UP), Porto, Portugal

Margarida Lima
Department of Hematology, Hospital de Santo António (HSA), Centro Hospitalar do Porto (CHP), Porto, Portugal
Instituto de Ciências Biomédicas Abel Salazar, Universidade do Porto (ICBAS/UP), Porto, Portugal
Unidade Multidisciplinar de Investigação Biomédica, Instituto de Ciências Biomédicas Abel Salazar, Universidade do Porto (UMIB/ICBAS/UP), Porto, Portugal
Laboratório de Citometria, Serviço de Hematologia, Hospital de Santo António, Centro Hospitalar do Porto, instalações do Ex-CICAP, Rua D. Manuel II, s/n, 4099-001 Porto, Portugal

Maria dos Anjos Teixeira and Catarina Lau
Department of Hematology, Hospital de Santo António (HSA), Centro Hospitalar do Porto (CHP), Porto, Portugal
Unidade Multidisciplinar de Investigação Biomédica, Instituto de Ciências Biomédicas Abel Salazar, Universidade do Porto (UMIB/ICBAS/UP), Porto, Portugal
Laboratório de Citometria, Serviço de Hematologia, Hospital de Santo António, Centro Hospitalar do Porto, instalações do Ex-CICAP, Rua D. Manuel II, s/n, 4099-001 Porto, Portugal

Inês Freitas
Department of Pathology, Hospital de Santo António (HSA), Centro Hospitalar do Porto (CHP), Porto, Portugal

Unidade Multidisciplinar de Investigação Biomédica, Instituto de Ciências Biomédicas Abel Salazar, Universidade do Porto (UMIB/ICBAS/UP), Porto, Portugal

Bamlaku Enawgaw, Nigist Adane, Betelihem Terefe, Fikir Asrie and Mulugeta Melku
Department of Hematology and Immunohematology, School of Biomedical and Laboratory Sciences, College of Medicine and Health Sciences, University of Gondar, Gondar, Ethiopia

Furahini Tluway, Abel Makubi, Deogratius Soka, Raphael Sangeda, Josephine Mgaya Muhsin Aboud and Lucio Luzzatto
Muhimbili University of Health and Allied Sciences, Dar-es-Salaam, Tanzania

Julie Makani
Muhimbili University of Health and Allied Sciences, Dar-es-Salaam, Tanzania University of Oxford, Oxford, UK
Muhimbili National Hospital, Dar-es-Salaam, Tanzania

Stella Rwezaula, Christina Kindole and Elisha Osati
Muhimbili University of Health and Allied Sciences, Dar-es-Salaam, Tanzania
Muhimbili National Hospital, Dar-es-Salaam, Tanzania

Siana Nkya
Muhimbili University of Health and Allied Sciences, Dar-es-Salaam, Tanzania
Dar-es-Salaam University College of Education, Dar-es-Salaam, Tanzania

Bruno P. Mmbando
Muhimbili University of Health and Allied Sciences, Dar-es-Salaam, Tanzania
National Institute for Medical Research Tanga Centre, Tanga, Tanzania

David Roberts
University of Oxford, Oxford, UK

Robert W. Snow and Charles R. Newton
University of Oxford, Oxford, UK
Centre for Geographic Medicine Research, Kenya Medical Research Institute, Kilifi, Kenya

Elineema Meda
Muhimbili National Hospital, Dar-es-Salaam, Tanzania

Fenella J. Kirkham
University College London, London, UK

Swee Lay Thein
National Institutes of Health, Bethesda, USA

Sharon E. Cox
London School of Hygiene and Tropical Medicine, London, UK

Bereket Geze Malako
Damot Sore District Health Office, Wolaita zone, SNNPR, Gununo, Ethiopia

Melese Sinaga Teshome and Tefera Belachew
Institute of Health, Public Health Faculty, Population and Family Health
Department, Nutrition Course Team, Jimma University, Jimma, Ethiopia

Index

www.ingramcontent.com/pod-product-compliance
Lightning Source LLC
Chambersburg PA
CBHW061312190326
41458CB00011B/3782
9781632426765